Essentials of
Medical
Biochemistry

Second Edition

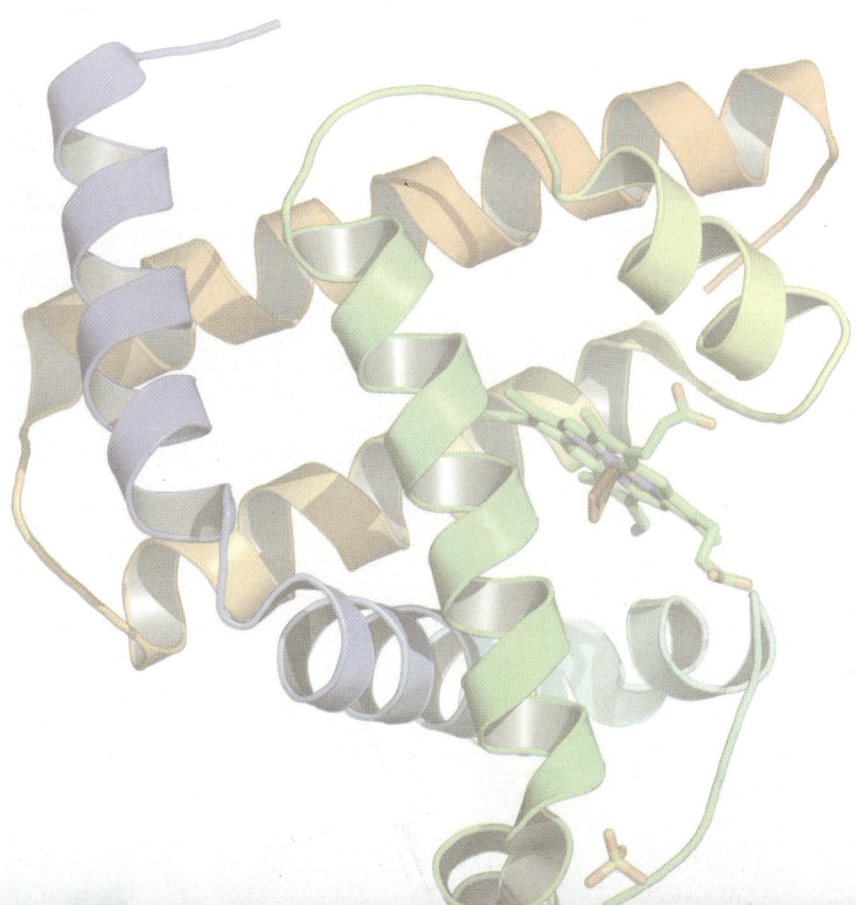

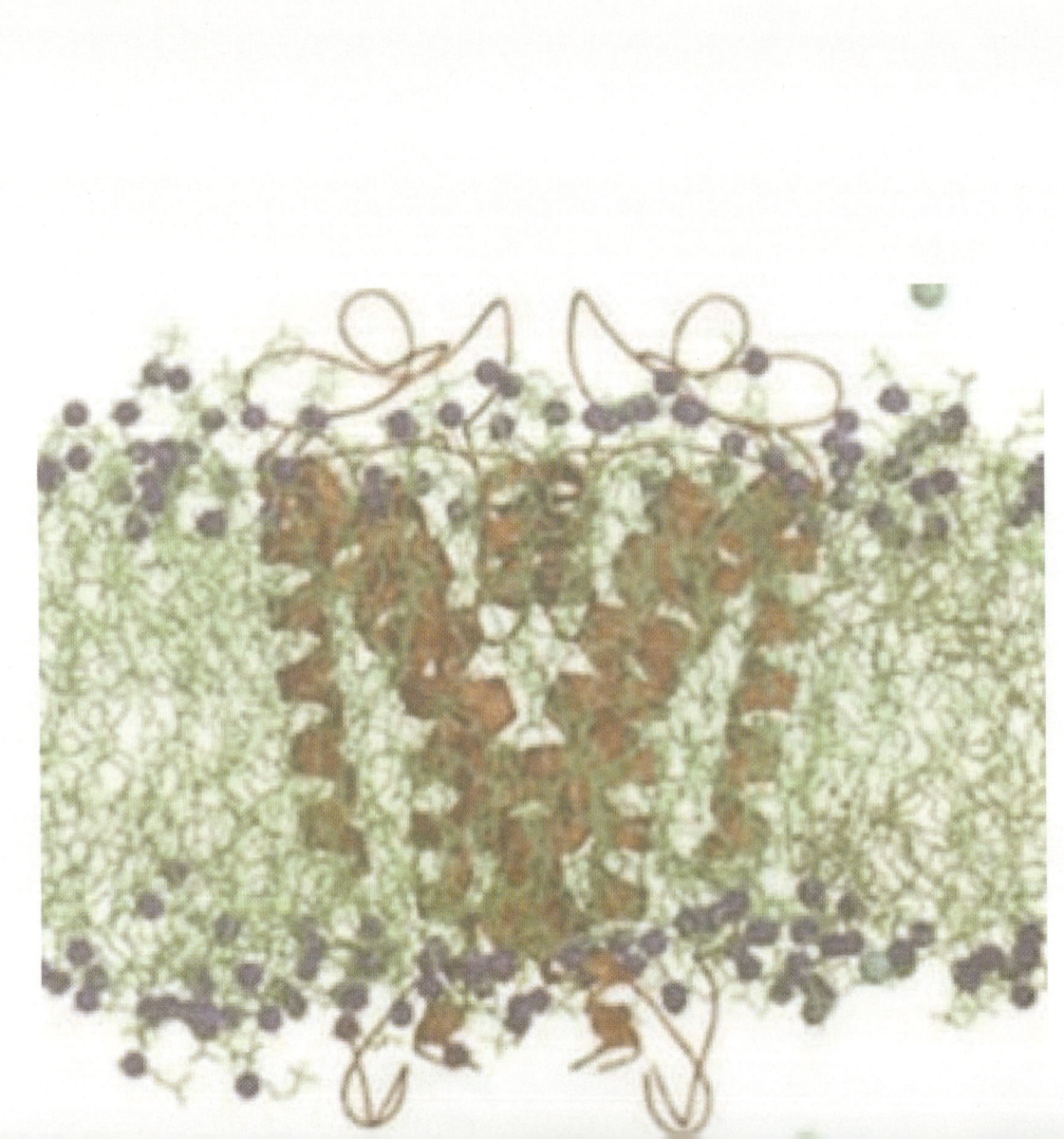

Essentials of
Medical Biochemistry

Second Edition

RC Gupta MD (Biochem)

Professor and Head
Department of Biochemistry
NIMS Medical College
Jaipur, Rajasthan

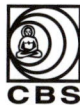

CBS Publishers & Distributors Pvt Ltd

New Delhi • Bengaluru • Pune • Kochi • Chennai
Mumbai • Kolkata • Hyderabad • Patna • Manipal

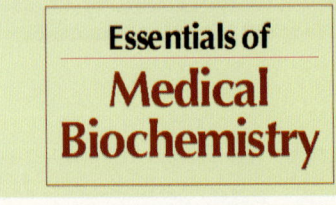

Essentials of
Medical
Biochemistry

Second Edition

ISBN: 978-81-239-2199-0

Second Edition 2013

Reprint 2014

Published by Satish Kumar Jain for

CBS Publishers & Distributors Pvt Ltd

4819/XI Prahlad Street, 24 Ansari Road, Daryaganj, New Delhi 110 002, India.
Ph: 23289259, 23266861, 23266867   Fax: 011-23243014

Website: www.cbspd.com
e-mail: delhi@cbspd.com; cbspubs@airtelmail.in

Corporate Office: 204 FIE, Industrial Area, Patparganj, Delhi 110 092
Ph: 4934 4934   Fax: 4934 4935

e-mail: publishing@cbspd.com; publicity@cbspd.com

Branches

* **Bengaluru:** Seema House 2975, 17th Cross, K.R. Road,
  Banasankari 2nd Stage, Bengaluru 560 070, Karnataka
  Ph: +91-80-26771678/79   Fax: +91-80-26771680   e-mail: bangalore@cbspd.com
* **Pune:** Bhuruk Prestige, Sr. No. 52/12/2+1+3/2 Narhe, Haveli
  (Near Katraj-Dehu Road Bypass), Pune 411 041, Maharashtra
  Ph: +91-20-64704058, 64704059, 32342277   Fax: +91-20-24300160   e-mail: pune@cbspd.com
* **Kochi:** 36/14 Kalluvilakam, Lissie Hospital Road, Kochi 682 018, Kerala
  Ph: +91-484-4059061-65   Fax: +91-484-4059065   e-mail: cochin@cbspd.com
* **Chennai:** 20, West Park Road, Shenoy Nagar, Chennai 600 030, Tamil Nadu
  Ph: +91-44-26260666, 26208620   Fax: +91-44-42032115   e-mail: chennai@cbspd.com

Representatives

* **Mumbai** 0-9833017933   * **Kolkata** 0-9831437309   * **Hyderabad** 0-9885175004
* **Patna** 0-9334159340   * **Manipal** 0-9742022075

Printed at Magic International, Greater Noida, UP

Preface to Second Edition

I am glad to place the second edition of Essentials of Medical Biochemistry in the hands of the readers. Much against my wishes, the second edition was inordinately delayed due to personal reasons.

Many of the chapters have been rewritten to bring them up-to-date. The chapters on molecular biology, immunochemistry and cancer have undergone thorough revision. New material has been added to several other chapters.

Many diagrams have been redrawn, and several new ones added. The diagrams are now in colour.

I am thankful to Mr YN Arjuna and his team at CBS Publishers and Distributors Pvt Ltd, New Delhi, for bringing the book to its present shape. I am also thankful to my colleagues who have given valuable suggestions for improving the book. I will welcome comments, criticism and suggestions from the readers.

RC Gupta

Preface to First Edition

Wide acceptance of my two earlier books and prodding from some of my colleagues prompted me to write a textbook on biochemistry. The writing began with a clear idea that the book was meant specifically for 1st MBBS students. After completing the manuscript, I felt that it was oversized for the 1st MBBS course in view of the limited time available now for learning biochemistry. Considerable pruning had to be done to bring the book to its present size. I have tried to condense and optimise the contents so that the undergraduate medical student finds very little in the book that can be skipped. At the same time, I hope that reference to other sources for additional information will be needed sparingly. I am aware that this is a vain hope as new information is coming in at an explosive rate.

A common accusation against teachers in biochemistry is that they overemphasise chemical fromulae and structures which are rarely required by the student in his future clinical practice. My answer is that chemical formulae and structures have been included in the book as an aid to understanding, and not for retention and reproduction.

Illustrations are another aid to understanding. However, intricate illustrations can frustrate rather than facilitate comprehension. I have tried to illustrate the text with diagrams wherever required but have kept the diagrams very simple for easy comprehension and reproduction.

After graduation, the average student will be dealing more with disease than with health. For understanding disease, diagnosis and treatment, a sound foundation in biochemistry is invaluable. With this objective, I have tried to provide the biochemical basis of aetiology, pathogenesis, symptomatology, diagnosis and at places, treatment of common inherited and acquired diseases.

I am grateful to my friends and colleagues, Dr VS Chowdhary (Jodhpur), Dr KL Mali (Udaipur), Dr VD Bohra (Jaipur), Dr AS Rathore (Jaipur) and Dr GG Kaushik (Ajmer) for reading various chapters and favouring me with their candid comments and useful suggestions. I am thankful to Dr Usha Gupta (Kota) for preparing the preliminary sketches of diagrams and for reading the proofs. I acknowledge the contribution of the team of Academa Publishers for giving a practical shape to my conceptualisation. But above all, I am thankful to the thousands of my students with whom I have interacted during the last three decades, and who have been my raison d'etre for learning Biochemistry. This humble offering is dedicated to them. If it helps the present and the future students, I will feel amply rewarded.

RC Gupta

Contents

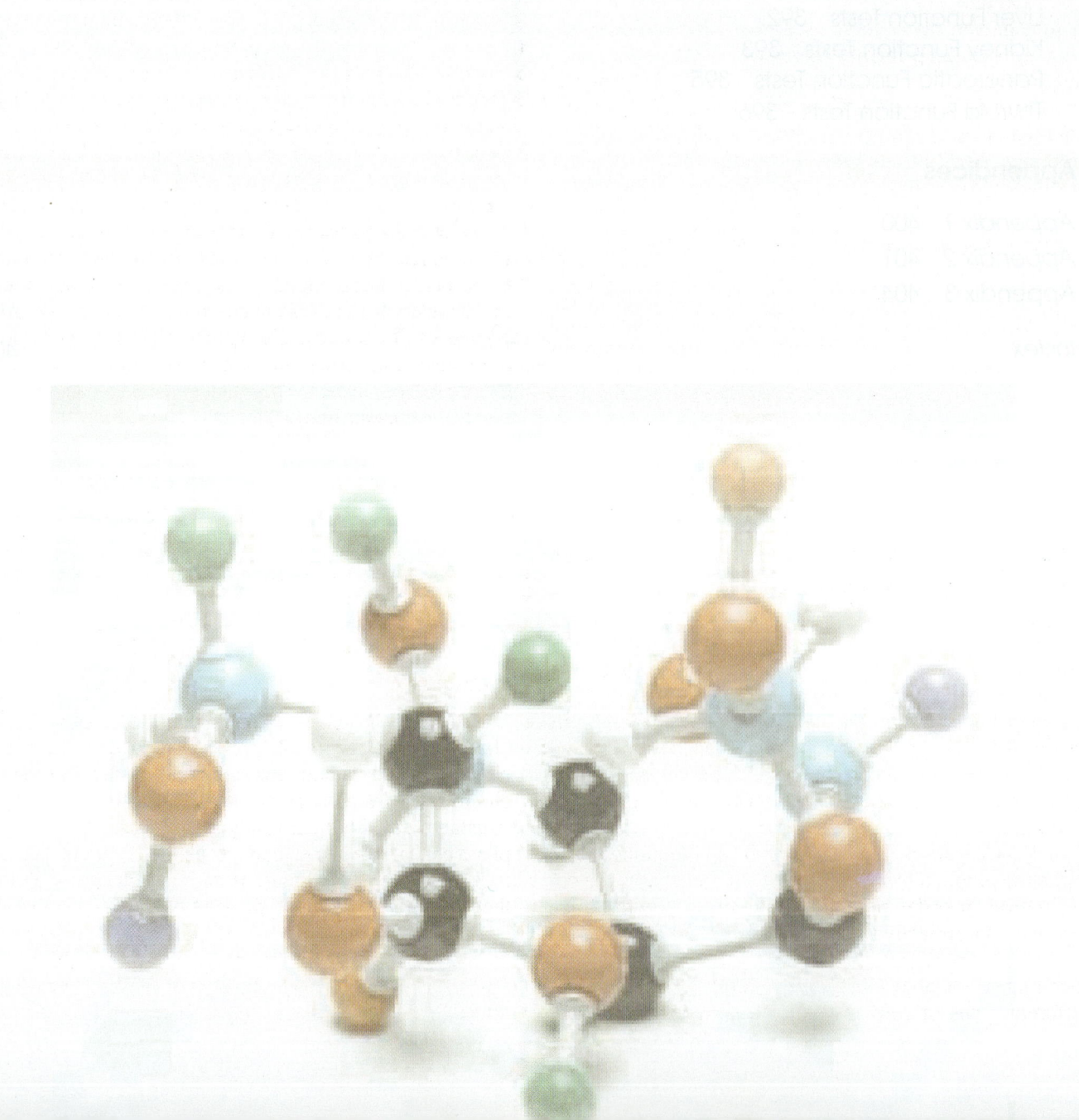

1

Biochemistry: An Overview

INTRODUCTION

Living organisms are made up of chemical elements organised into biomolecules. The important biomolecules include nucleic acids, proteins, carbohydrates, lipids, etc. They are made up mainly of carbon, hydrogen, oxygen and nitrogen with small amounts of some other elements. Several inorganic elements are also present in living organisms. By themselves, the biomolecules and the inorganic elements are non-living but when they come together in a cell, they confer the property of "life" to the cell.

Cell is the structural and functional unit of all living organisms. It obtains raw materials required for sustaining itself from its environment. From raw materials, it produces the biological catalysts (enzymes) that catalyse biochemical reactions in the cell. With the help of enzymes, it oxidises the biomolecules to extract energy. It can convert the raw materials into complex biomolecules and supramolecular assemblies. Chemical events occurring in the cell maintain it in a dynamic steady state in a continually changing, and even inhospitable, environment. And finally, it has the remarkable ability to reproduce itself. Biochemistry encompasses the study of biomolecules and elements essential for life and the chemical reactions they undergo in the living organism to subserve the various functions of the organism.

Unicellular organisms, e.g. bacteria, are made up of a single cell having a simple architecture. Multicellular organisms have a highly organised cellular architecture. An adult human being has nearly 10^{14} cells. These cells are of different types having different shapes, sizes and functions. The cells are organised into tissues and tissues into organs. While this differentiation gives us the advantage of division of labour with different cell types, tissues and organs performing specialised functions, it also poses the problem of intercellular communication and co-ordination in order that the organism as a whole can respond appropriately to changes in internal and external environment. A simple event like removing our hand on touching a hot object involves a series of reactions in different types of cells involving a number of ions and

molecules. Biochemistry seeks to explain the complex biological phenomena at the molecular level.

Though the structural organisation of cells differs from organism to organism and within a multicellular organism, there is a remarkable degree of unity in this diversity. The biomolecules present in different types of cells are similar. The information molecules, deoxyribonucleic acid (DNA) and ribonucleic acid (RNA), are similar and made up of the same nucleotides. The genetic code is the same. The proteins are made up of the same twenty amino acids. The biological catalysts are similar. The currency of energy is the same. The metabolic pathways are similar. Due to this similarity, information obtained in one organism can be extrapolated to others. A large amount of information about human biochemistry has been obtained from experiments in simple organisms like bacteria. Though the scope of biochemistry is very wide covering plants, animals, microbes, industry, etc. we will be concerned here mainly with human (medical) biochemistry. Our study of human biochemistry will cover:

Chemistry of Amino Acids and Proteins

Amino acids are the building blocks for the synthesis of proteins which form the structural framework of tissues besides performing a variety of other important functions in the form of enzymes, hormones, receptors, antibodies, etc.

Enzymes

Enzymes are the universal catalysts of the living world. No chemical reaction in living organisms can occur at a significant rate without enzymes. With a few exceptions, all enzymes are proteins having unique three-dimensional structures suited to their catalytic functions. Enzymes also play a crucial role in metabolic regulation. Rates of reactions in a metabolic pathway are usually regulated by altering the concentration or catalytic activity of one or a few key enzyme(s) in the pathway. Many diseases can be diagnosed by measuring the levels of some enzymes in biological fluids, e.g. plasma. Many inhibitors of enzymes are used as drugs. Some enzymes are used as therapeutic agents also.

Chemistry of Carbohydrates and Lipids

These are biomolecules used mainly as sources of energy. Carbohydrates constitute the largest component of our daily diet. Lipids constitute the major storage form of energy. Some carbohydrates and lipids perform structural roles as well.

Metabolism of Carbohydrates, Lipids, Amino Acids and Proteins

The chemical reactions undergone by these compounds in the body constitute metabolism. The process begins with the digestion of dietary carbohydrates, lipids and proteins followed by absorption of the products of digestion, and includes anabolism, i.e. synthesis of large molecules from small precursors and catabolism, i.e. breakdown of large molecules. Anabolism and catabolism occur by a series of reactions which constitute a metabolic pathway. While studying metabolic pathways, we will be interested in their tissue distribution, intracellular location, reactions, energetics, regulation and importance. We will also be interested in disorders which occur due to a block in some reaction of the pathway owing to a mutated, dysfunctional enzyme.

Bio-energetics and Oxidative Phosphorylation

Energy is released during catabolism of carbohydrates, lipids and amino acids. This energy is utilised in anabolic pathways and for muscle contraction, active transport, etc. Adenosine triphosphate (ATP) is the universal carrier of energy. It is formed during exergonic (energy-yielding) reactions, and is utilised in endergonic (energy-consuming) activities. Oxidative phosphorylation is the process by which the energy released during catabolism of carbohydrates, lipids and amino acids is captured in the form of ATP.

Molecular Biology

Molecular biology comprises the chemistry and metabolism of nucleic acids, i.e. DNA and RNA, and their building blocks, the nucleotides. DNA and RNA are information molecules. Genetic information is present in DNA in the form of genes. A gene possesses coded information about the amino acid sequence of a protein. An RNA transcript of the gene carries the information from the DNA to the ribosomes on which the protein is synthesised. During cell division, DNA of the cell is exactly replicated so that the daughter cells acquire the genetic information present in the parent cell. Our study of molecular biology will cover processes like replication (synthesis of DNA), transcription (synthesis of RNA) and translation (synthesis of proteins).

A recent and revolutionary development in molecular biology is the advent of recombinant DNA technology. This technology is finding wide-ranging applications in medicine, agriculture, animal husbandry, industry, etc. We will study the tools and techniques of this technology and its applications in medical science.

Vitamins

Vitamins are a group of chemically diverse organic compounds required in minute quantities but essential for life. Many of these act as coenzymes, and are essential for the catalytic activity of a number of enzymes. Others are required for growth, differentiation, vision, etc. Deficient intake of most, and excessive intake of some, vitamins produces specific diseases. Our study of vitamins will cover their chemistry, functions, requirements, dietary sources and the diseases resulting from their deficient or excessive intake.

Minerals

Several minerals are essential for human beings, and these perform a variety of functions, e.g. formation of bones (calcium and phosphorus), nerve conduction (sodium and potassium), formation of haemoglobin (iron), as cofactors for enzymes (iron, copper, zinc, etc.), and so on. Their deficiency or excess can cause disease.

Hormones

Hormones are mobile molecules that carry signals from one organ, tissue or cell to another, and help the organism to respond in an appropriate and coordinated manner to any change in internal or external environment. Small changes in the concentrations of hormones produce profound biochemical and physiological effects. Under- or over-production of hormones produces serious disorders. Diagnosis of these disorders usually requires measurement of hormone concentrations in blood.

Maintenance of pH, Water and Electrolyte Balance

Water, in intra- and extra-cellular compartment, constitutes nearly two-thirds of the body weight in an adult man. Water is the universal solvent of the living world, and is the medium in which all biochemical reactions occur. Small changes in the water content of a compartment, distribution of electrolytes and pH of body fluids can disturb the normal biochemical and physiological activities. Such changes can occur in a variety of diseases, and correction of the imbalance requires a sound understanding of the normal regulatory mechanisms.

Nutrition and Dietetics

We obtain all the nutrients we require, viz. carbohydrates, lipids, proteins, vitamins and minerals, from food. Malnutrition (under- and over-nutrition) is common all over the world. Diseases resulting from undernutrition afflict large sections of population in poor societies while overnutrition is the bane of the rich. Ignorance contributes significantly to both. A sound knowledge of the principles of nutrition and dietetics is essential to prevent and to treat the nutritional disorders.

Cancer

Cancer (malignancy) has emerged as a leading cause of death worldwide. Though a number of physical, chemical and biological agents are known to play a role in the development of cancer, the molecular mechanisms that transform a healthy cell into a cancer cell have eluded scientists for a long time. Advances in molecular biology are now revealing the complex interplay of anti-oncogenes, proto-oncogenes and oncogenes resulting in transformation of a normal cell into a cancer cell. We will look at the role of these genes in malignant transformation.

Immunochemistry

We are exposed to a bewildering range of foreign antigens that can cause disease. We also have a highly competent immune system to protect us against these antigens. The immune system comprises innate immunity and adaptive immunity. A number of molecules are involved in the recognition and inactivation of foreign antigens. We will study the molecules of immune recognition and the mechanisms by which the foreign antigens are dealt with.

Xenobiotics

Apart from the antigens, we are also exposed to a vast variety of foreign chemicals (xenobiotics) that can cause toxicity. We will look at the mechanisms by which the xenobiotics are detoxified and excreted.

Our study of human biochemistry, thus, will provide us insights into the molecular basis of complex biological phenomena. Biochemistry is described as the chemical language of life. It helps us not only in understanding the normal functioning of the body at the molecular level but also unravels the molecular basis of diseases, provides laboratory tools for diagnosis and is now providing even treatment in the form of gene therapy.

Cell Structure

Cells are the structural and functional units of all living organisms. In unicellular organisms, a single cell constitutes the entire organism. Multicellular organisms have a large and varying number of cells. Living organisms can be broadly divided into prokaryotes and eukaryotes. Prokaryotes, e.g. bacteria, do not have a well-delineated nucleus. Nuclear DNA is not bounded by a membrane, and is known as nucleoid. The cell does not have subcellular organelles and intracellular compartments. All biochemical events occur in cytoplasm which is surrounded by a plasma (cell) membrane.

In eukaryotes, e.g. yeast, plants and animals, the cells have a well-defined nucleus surrounded by a nuclear membrane or envelope. The cytoplasm has a number of subcellular organelles. Specific biochemical events occur in different intracellular compartments. Though eukaryotic cells differ greatly in size, shape and cellular architecture, certain features are common to all eukaryotic cells. For instance, most of the animal cells possess subcellular organelles like endoplasmic reticulum, Golgi apparatus, mitochondria, lysosomes, peroxisomes, etc. In addition to the subcellular organelles, which are membrane-bound compartments, some other subcellular structures, e.g. ribosomes and cytoskeleton, are also present in most cells (Fig. 2.1).

Subcellular organelles and structures create different intracellular compartments having different environments in which specific biochemical events can occur. Functions of different organelles can be studied in vitro by isolating them after disrupting the cell and subjecting it to differential centrifugation.

Plasma Membrane

Plasma membrane or cell membrane surrounds the intracellular contents, and separates them from the external environment. It is made up mainly of lipids and proteins with some carbohydrates occurring as prosthetic groups of both.

Glycerophospholipids are the predominant lipids in the plasma membrane. Small amounts of sphingolipids and cholesterol are also present. Phospholipid molecules are amphipathic. One region of the molecule made up of

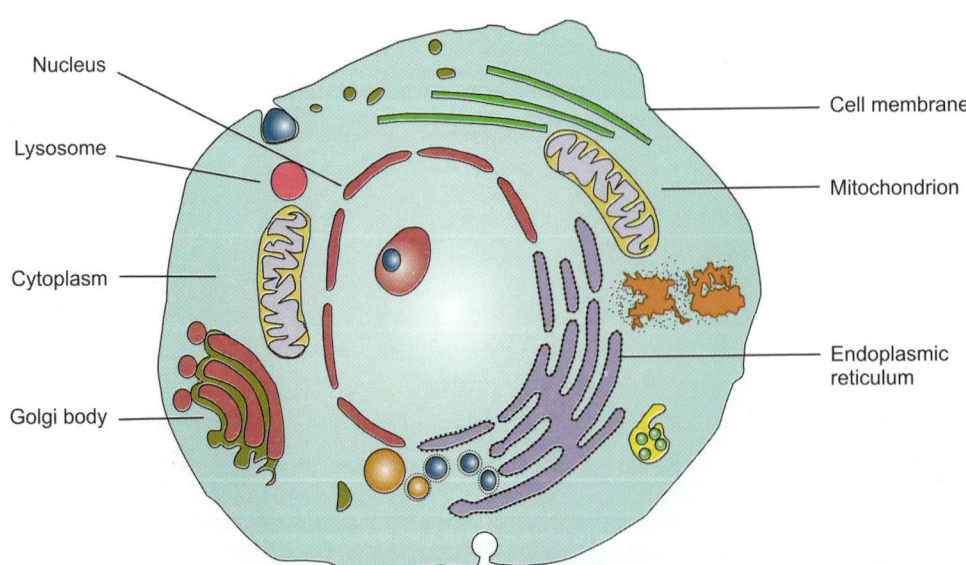

Fig. 2.1: Diagrammatic depiction of a typical animal cell with its common subcellular structures and organelles

Nucleus
Lysosome
Cytoplasm
Golgi body
Cell membrane
Mitochondrion
Endoplasmic reticulum

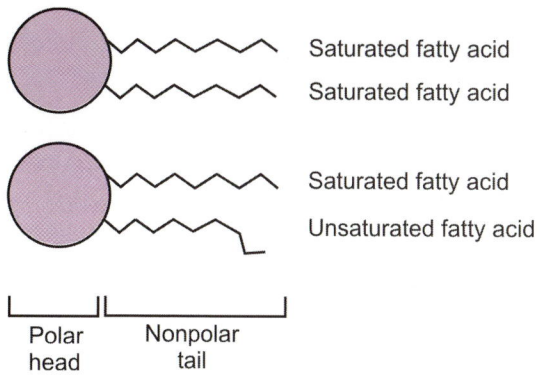

Saturated fatty acid
Saturated fatty acid

Saturated fatty acid
Unsaturated fatty acid

Polar head   Nonpolar tail

Fig. 2.2: Glycerophopholipids having a polar head and a nonpolar tail. Unsaturated fatty acids are kinked at the double bonds

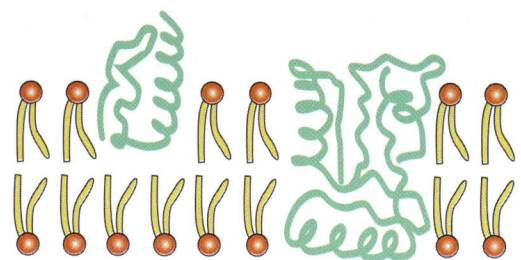

Fig. 2.3: Plasma membrane made up of lipid bilayer, integral proteins and peripheral proteins

phosphate and nitrogenous base is hydrophilic (polar head). The other region made up of fatty acyl chains is hydrophobic (nonpolar tail) (Fig. 2.2).

The lipids are arranged in a bilayer in the membrane with the polar heads on the two surfaces and the nonpolar tails in between. Cholesterol molecules are present in the nonpolar interior. Fluidity of the membrane is important for its functioning, and depends upon the nature of fatty acids and the amount of cholesterol in the membrane. The temperature at which the membrane changes from a relatively rigid *gel* form into a more fluid *sol* form is known as the transition temperature of the membrane. The transition temperature is increased by long chain fatty acids, saturated fatty acids and cholesterol. The *cis* double bonds present in the naturally occurring unsaturated fatty acids produce kinks in the fatty acyl chains and make the membrane less compact and more fluid. The proteins present in the membrane may be divided into peripheral (extrinsic) proteins and integral (intrinsic) proteins. Peripheral proteins are present on the external and internal surfaces, and may be removed without disrupting the membrane. Integral proteins span the membrane, and can be removed only by disrupting the membrane (Fig. 2.3).

The amino acid residues of integral proteins embedded in the lipid bilayer are usually nonpolar. The membrane proteins are not only structural constituents of the membrane but also perform other important functions as enzymes, receptors, signal transducers and transporters.

Plasma membrane is dynamic and selectively permeable. Lipophilic substances can easily diffuse through the lipid bilayer but hydrophilic substances require special transport mechanisms, e.g. facilitated diffusion and active transport, to move in and out of cells. Selective permeability is important in maintaining a constant environment in the cell. Plasma membrane has a role in cell-cell communication also which is essential for coordinated functioning of the organism.

In bacteria, the plasma membrane is usually surrounded by a relatively rigid cell wall that protects the cell from osmotic rupture. Peptidoglycan confers rigidity and osmotic resistance to the cell wall. Many antibiotics, e.g. penicillins, cephalosporins, vancomycin, bacitracin, etc. kill bacteria by inhibiting the synthesis, assembly or cross-linking of peptidoglycan.

Nucleus

Nucleus is the largest intracellular organelle visible under the microscope. It is the site of DNA and RNA synthesis. DNA encodes the proteins synthesised by the cell. Various types of RNA assist in protein synthesis. DNA is associated with some specific proteins to form chromosomes and chromatin. Nucleolus is another structure present within the nucleus. It is the site for RNA processing and ribosome synthesis. Nucleus is enveloped by a double membrane having a number of pores through which most molecules except the very large macromolecules can enter and exit. The outer nuclear membrane is continuous with endoplasmic reticulum.

Ribosomes

Ribosomes are synthesised in the nucleus, and move out into cytosol where many are present as free particles while others are attached to endoplasmic reticulum. They are made up of two subunits. Based on their sedimentation constant, the subunits are called 40S and 60S subunits. Each is made up of some specific proteins and ribosomal RNA (rRNA). The subunits associate to form the 80S ribosome. The eukaryotic ribosome is larger than the 70S prokaryotic ribosome. Ribosome is the structure on which proteins are synthesised.

Endoplasmic Reticulum

This is a network of extensively folded membranes enclosing narrow channels (cisternae). It can be divided into rough endoplasmic reticulum and smooth endoplasmic reticulum. A number of ribosomes are attached to the cytosolic surface of rough endoplasmic reticulum giving it a rough appearance. The bound ribosomes synthesise proteins destined for export from the cells and proteins meant for incorporation in the membranes. These proteins enter the cisternae and, after some modifications, are transferred to the Golgi apparatus for onward transport.

Smooth endoplasmic reticulum appears smooth because of the absence of ribosomes on its cytosolic surface. It synthesises membrane lipids and hydroxylates a variety of endogenous and exogenous substrates.

When the cell is disrupted for fractionation of organelles, the membranes of endoplasmic reticulum are broken and spontaneously resealed to form vesicles known as microsomes.

Golgi Apparatus

This is another network of folded sheet-like membranes and vesicles. The proteins coming to the Golgi apparatus from endoplasmic reticulum are further modified here, usually by addition of carbohydrate and lipid prosthetic groups. The modified proteins enter the vesicles, and are secreted. Endoplasmic reticulum and Golgi apparatus also form some other subcellular organelles, e.g. lysosomes and peroxisomes.

Mitochondria

Mitochondria are described as the powerhouse of the cells as they are the site of ATP synthesis. The inner space (matrix) of the mitochondria is surrounded by two membranes. The inner membrane is heavily folded to form cristae which project into the mitochondrial matrix (Fig. 2.4). Many oxidative pathways which generate energy, e.g. β-oxidation of fatty acids and citric acid cycle, are located in the mitochondrial matrix. The components of the respiratory chain, together with vectorial ATP synthetase which synthesises ATP, are located in the inner mitochondrial membrane.

Some DNA is also present in mitochondria (mitochondrial DNA) along with the replication, transcription and translation machinery. Mitochondrial DNA is maternally inherited, and encodes some proteins used within the mitochondria for oxidative phosphorylation.

Lysosomes

Lysosomes are membrane-bound sacs containing hydrolytic enzymes that can digest nucleic acids, proteins, lipids and carbohydrates. They can digest extracellular as well as intracellular substrates. The extracellular substrates to be digested, e.g. components of micro-organisms, enter the

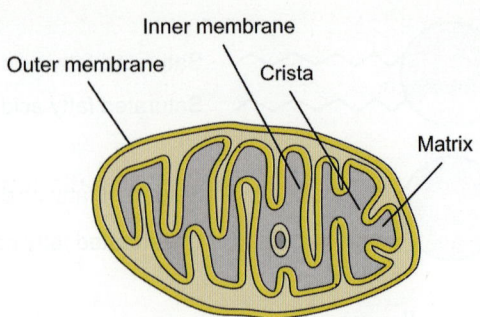

Fig. 2.4: Sub-compartments of a mitochondrion

cell by endocytosis. A portion of the plasma membrane invaginates and surrounds the extracellular material. This membrane fuses with the lysosomal membrane, and the lysosomal hydrolases digest the foreign material. Intracellular material to be digested, e.g. portions of endoplasmic reticulum, Golgi apparatus, mitochondria, etc. also fuse with the lysosomal membrane followed by hydrolysis of their contents.

Peroxisomes

Peroxisomes are granular, membrane-bound subcellular structures that contain enzymes involved in the metabolism of hydrogen peroxide. These include flavoprotein enzymes that produce hydrogen peroxide, e.g. L-amino acid oxidase, xanthine oxidase, etc. and catalase that degrades hydrogen peroxide. By segregating enzymes that produce and degrade hydrogen peroxide in one compartment, the cell is protected from the harmful effects of toxic hydrogen peroxide.

Enzymes involved in the synthesis of plasmalogens and conversion of very long chain fatty acids into long chain fatty acids are also present in peroxisomes. Congenital absence of functional peroxisomes results in Zellweger syndrome (cerebro-hepato-renal syndrome) which is fatal in early infancy.

Cytoskeleton

Cells also contain networks of proteins that constitute the cytoskeleton (skeleton of the cell). The cytoskeletal proteins maintain the morphology of the cell, and assist in cell motility and cell division. Cytoskeleton consists of microfilaments, intermediate filaments and microtubules.

Table 2.1: Markers* for subcellular organelles			
Organelle	*Marker*	*Organelle*	*Marker*
Nucleus	DNA	Mitochondria	Glutamate dehydrogenase
Endoplasmic reticulum	Glucose-6-phosphatase	Golgi apparatus	Galactosyl transferase
Lysosomes	Acid phosphatase	Peroxisomes	Catalase

* Markers are compounds restricted to an organelle and, hence, useful in detection of organelles in fractions obtained by differential centrifugation.

Microfilaments are polymers of actin. Intermediate filaments are polymers of several proteins, e.g. keratin. Microtubules are polymers of α-tubulin and β-tubulin.

Cytosol

The fluid left after removal of all subcellular organelles and structures by centrifugation is known as cytosol. Several metabolic pathways are located either completely or partially in cytosol. The pathways which are located completely in cytosol include glycolysis, hexose monophosphate shunt, glycogenesis, glycogenolysis, lipogenesis, lipolysis, de novo synthesis of fatty acids, de novo synthesis of purine nucleotides, etc. The pathways which are located partially in cytosol include gluconeogenesis, cholesterol synthesis, urea synthesis, porphyrin synthesis, de novo synthesis of pyrimidine nucleotides, etc.

3

Chemistry of Carbohydrates

Carbohydrates are synthesised in plants by the process of photosynthesis, and are used by animals as food. They constitute the largest source of energy in our daily diet. Besides providing energy, some carbohydrates perform other important functions. Ribose and deoxyribose are constituents of nucleotides and nucleic acids. Glycolipids are a component of nervous tissue. Glycoproteins form the blood group substances and some hormones. Mucin, a mucoprotein, is a component of mucous secretions. As mucopolysaccharides, carbohydrates serve as structural constituents of tissues.

DEFINITION

Carbohydrates can be defined as polyhydroxyaldehydes and polyhydroxyketones or compounds that give polyhydroxyaldehydes and/or polyhydroxyketones on hydrolysis. Or the carbohydrates can be defined as the aldehyde or ketone derivatives of polyhydric alcohols.

CLASSIFICATION

Carbohydrates can be divided into three classes:
  i. Monosaccharides,
  ii. Disaccharides, and
  iii. Polysaccharides.

1. Monosaccharides

These are the simplest carbohydrates that cannot be hydrolysed into smaller carbohydrates. They are made up of carbon, hydrogen and oxygen. Their general formula is $C_nH_{2n}O_n$. The monosaccharides having an aldehyde group as carbonyl functional group are known as aldoses, and those having a ketone group are known as ketoses. Each of these may be sub-divided, on the basis of the number of carbon atoms present in them, into trioses (three carbon atoms), tetroses (four carbon atoms), pentoses (five carbon atoms), hexoses (six carbon atoms) and heptoses (seven carbon atoms). Some common examples of monosaccharides are given in Table 3.1.

2. Disaccharides

These are made up of two molecules of monosaccharides which may be similar or dissimilar. One molecule of water is lost during their union. Therefore, their general formula is $C_n(H_2O)_{n-1}$. Some common examples of disaccharides, and their constituent monosaccharides, are given in Table 3.2.

Monosaccharides and disaccharides are commonly known as **sugars** because of their sweet taste.

3. Polysaccharides

These are made up of a large number of monosaccharide molecules. Sometimes, polysaccharides made up of three to six molecules of monosaccharides are termed as **oligosaccharides**, and those made up of seven or more molecules of monosaccharides are termed as polysaccharides. In general, polysaccharides are very large molecules (macromolecules) made up of a very large number of monosaccharide molecules.

Carbohydrates are generally found in nature in the form of polysaccharides. These are of two types: homopolysaccharides and heteropolysaccharides. The homopolysaccharides yield only one type of monosaccharide on

Table 3.1: Some common monosaccharide

	Number of carbon atoms	Aldoses	Ketoses
Trioses	3	Glyceraldehyde	Dihydroxyacetone
Tetroses	4	Erythrose	Erythrulose
Pentoses	5	Ribose	Ribulose
Hexoses	6	Glucose	Fructose

Table 3.2: Some disaccharides and their constituents

Disaccharide	*Constituent monosaccharides*
Sucrose	Glucose + Fructose
Maltose	Glucose + Glucose
Lactose	Glucose + Galactose

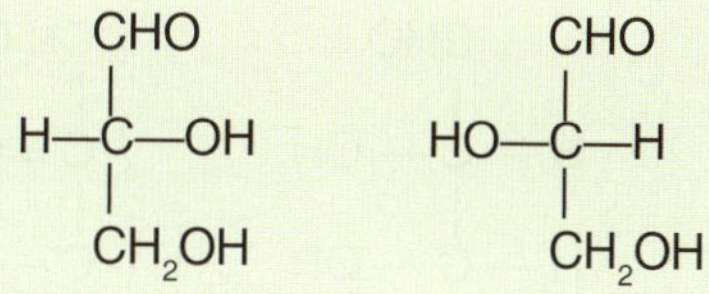

D-Glyceraldehyde L-Glyceraldehyde

Fig. 3.2: D- and L-isomers of glyceraldehyde

hydrolysis. The common homopolysaccharides are starch, dextrin, cellulose, inulin, glycogen, etc. The heteropolysaccharides yield more than one type of monosaccharides on hydrolysis. Mucopolysaccharides are the most important heteropolysaccharides in human beings. Important examples of mucopolysaccharides include hyaluronic acid, heparin and chondroitin sulphate.

Majority of the polysaccharides are made up of hexoses, and are collectively known as hexosans. Those which are made up of pentoses are known as pentosans.

MONOSACCHARIDES

Trioses

The smallest monosaccharides are the two trioses—glyceraldehyde (glycerose) and dihydroxyacetone. These may be considered to be the aldehyde and ketone derivatives, respectively of the trihydric alcohol, glycerol. Thus, glyceraldehyde is an aldotriose and dihydroxyacetone a ketotriose (Fig. 3.1). The trioses are formed in the body during the metabolism of hexoses.

Glyceraldehyde and dihydroxyacetone may be considered to be isomers of each other as they share the same molecular formula ($C_3H_6O_3$) but differ in their structural formulae. This is a simple aldose-ketose isomerism. In addition, glyceraldehyde shows another type of isomerism. It contains an **asymmetric carbon atom**. All the four groups attached to the second carbon atom (C_2) are different from each other. This asymmetry produces two **stereoisomers** of glyceraldehyde. The isomer having the –OH group on the right hand side of C_2 is termed as D-glyceraldehyde and the one having the –OH group on the left hand side of C_2 is termed as L-glyceraldehyde.The presence of asymmetric carbon atom also makes the compound optically active. When polarised light is passed through the solution of such a compound, its plane is rotated to the left (laevorotation) or the right (dextrorotation). Of the two stereoisomers, one causes laevorotation and the other causes dextrorotation. However, the prefixes L- and D- refer to the orientation of the –OH group relative to the asymmetric carbon atom and not to optical rotation. The latter is shown by a (+) or a (–) sign, denoting dextro- and laevo-rotation respectively, preceding the name of the compound. Thus, glyceraldehyde could be denoted as D(+)-glyceraldehyde or L(–)-glyceraldehyde. But it is not necessary that the D-isomer of every compound will be dextrorotatory and the L-isomer will be laevorotatory. The reverse is also seen.

Stereoisomerism and optical activity are also present in higher monosaccharides. In fact, the higher monosaccharides possess more than one asymmetric carbon atoms. The total number of stereoisomers in a compound having n asymmetric carbon atoms is 2^n. But whether the compound belongs to the D-series or L-series is determined by the orientation of the –OH group relative to the asymmetric carbon atom most remote from the aldehyde or the ketone group. This will be carbon atom 3 in tetroses, carbon atom 4 in pentoses and carbon atom 5 in hexoses. If the –OH group is on the right of these carbon atoms, the carbohydrate will belong to the D-series and if it is on the left, the carbohydrate will belong to the L-series.The D- and L-isomers are mirror images of each other, and are known as **enantiomers**. Most of the carbohydrates important in human biochemistry belong to the D-series.

Tetroses

The only tetrose of some importance in human beings is D-erythrose (Fig. 3.3). This is formed as an intermediate (as erythrose-4-phosphate) during the metabolism of glucose via the hexose monophosphate shunt pathway. The corresponding ketotetrose is D-erythrulose.

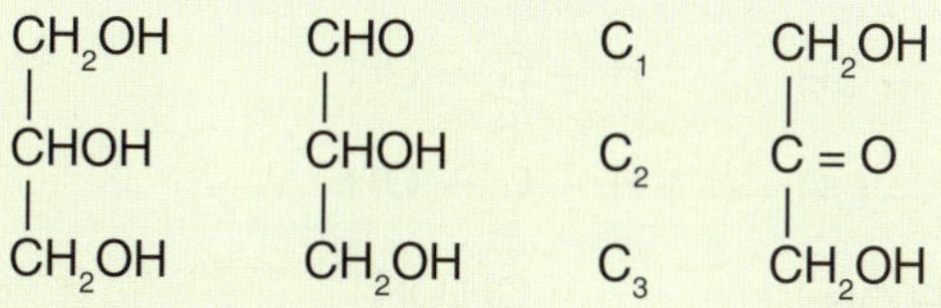

Glycerol Glyceraldehyde Dihydroxyacetone

Fig. 3.1: Trioses and their relationship with glycerol

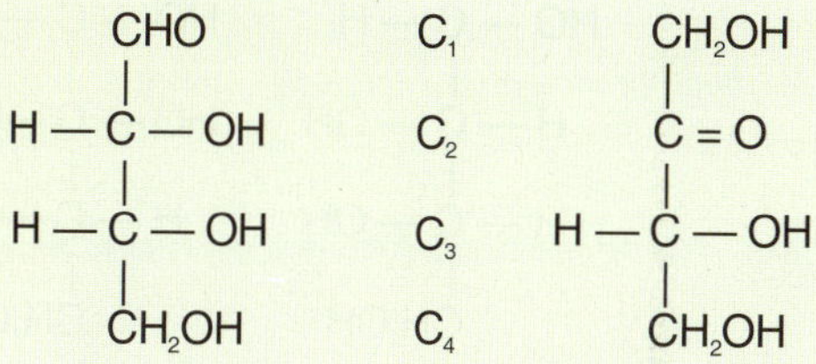

D-Erythrose D-Erythrulose

Fig. 3.3: An aldotetrose and a ketotetrose

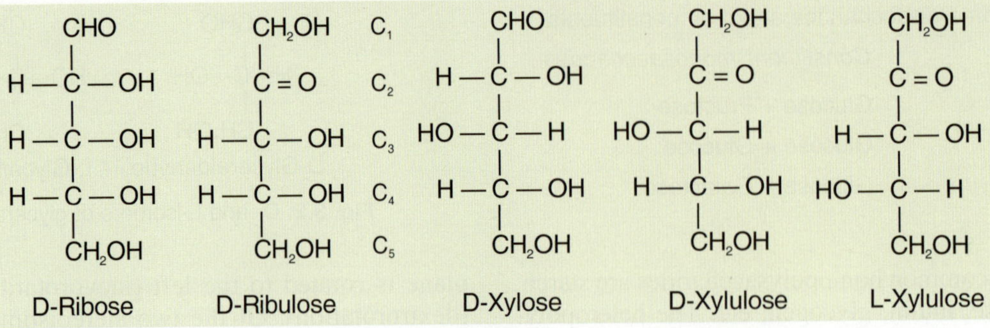

Fig. 3.4: Some important aldo- and keto-pentoses

Pentoses

D-Ribose and its deoxy derivative (2-deoxy-D-ribose) are the most important pentoses. These are constituents of nucleic acids and nucleotides. D-Ribose is present in ribonucleic acid (RNA). 2-Deoxy-D-ribose (deoxyribose) is present in deoxyribonucleic acid (DNA). D-Ribose is a constituent of several nucleotides, e.g. adenosine triphosphate (ATP), cyclic adenosine monophosphate (cAMP), cyclic guanosine monophosphate (cGMP), etc. It is also present in some coenzymes, e.g. flavin mononucleotide (FMN), flavin adenine dinucleotide (FAD), nicotinamide adenine dinucleotide (NAD), coenzyme A (CoA), etc. D-Ribose and its corresponding ketopentose, D-ribulose are formed as intermediates in the hexose monophosphate shunt. Another pentose formed in this pathway is D-xylulose. Its corresponding aldopentose is D-xylose (Fig. 3.4). D-xylose is used as a diagnostic agent to study intestinal absorption.

An L-pentose occurring in human beings is L-xylulose. This is formed as an intermediate in the uronic acid pathway of carbohydrate metabolism. It is excreted in urine in detectable amounts in a hereditary disease known as **essential pentosuria**.

Hexoses

The important aldohexoses in human biochemistry are D-glucose, D-galactose and D-mannose. The important

ketohexose is D-fructose which is the ketoisomer of D-glucose (Fig. 3.5).

D-Glucose is the most important carbohydrate in human beings. The carbohydrates are transported in blood in the form of D-glucose. It is also the form in which carbohydrates are used by the tissues to obtain energy. Most other carbohydrates are converted into D-glucose in the body. The important polysaccharides, starch, dextrin and glycogen are made up of D-glucose. Concentration of glucose in blood is delicately regulated. A disturbance in regulation can cause diabetes mellitus in which the concentration of glucose in blood is elevated. This can lead to a variety of clinical abnormalities.

D-Galactose is present in glycolipids which are an important constituent of nervous tissue. The dietary source of galactose is milk in which galactose is present in the form of the disaccharide, lactose. Amino derivatives of D-galactose and D-mannose are present in mucopolysaccharides and glycoproteins.

D-Fructose is the predominant carbohydrate in honey. It is present in many fruits. Is a constituent of the disaccharide, sucrose. It is formed in human beings in some pathways of carbohydrate metabolism. It is present in a high concentration in seminal fluid where it provides nourishment to the sperms.

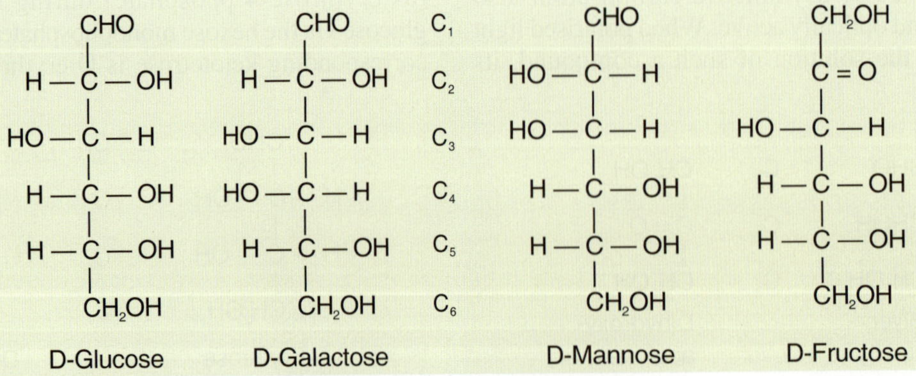

Fig. 3.5: Some important hexoses

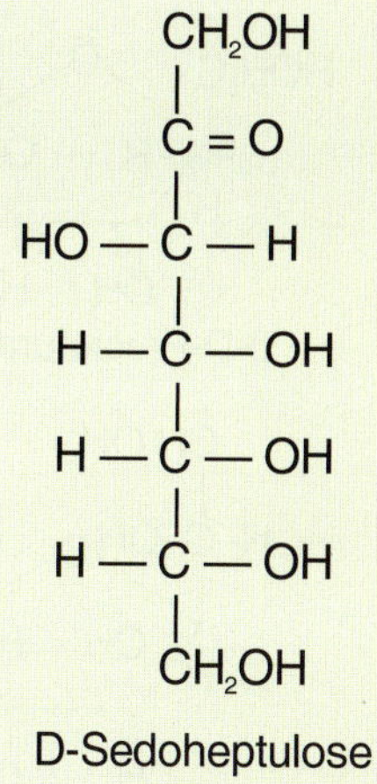

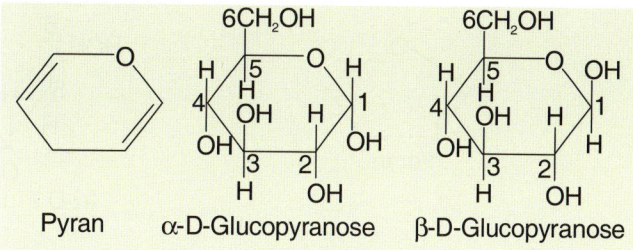

Fig. 3.8: Anomers of glucose having pyranose ring structure

Fischer did not extend the concept of the cyclic structure of methyl glucosides to the structure of glucose itself. This was later done by Haworth and his associates. They proposed a cyclic 1,5-oxide structure for glucose in which the C_1 aldehyde group forms a hemiacetal linkage with C_5 alcohol group. Since this structure resembled the pyran ring, they named glucose as glucopyranose. Not only glucose but other aldohexoses also exist in solution mainly in the pyran ring form because this form has the lowest energy and is thermodynamically favoured. The three-dimensional representation of the ring structure is known as Haworth projection formula.

In this representation, the plane of the ring is perpendicular to the plane of the paper. The substituent groups project upwards or downwards from the ring. Carbon atom 1 is known as the **anomeric carbon atom** as it constitutes an additional centre of asymmetry in the molecule. It can have either α- or β-configuration. In α-**D-glucopyranose**, the hydroxyl group attached to carbon atom 1 projects below the plane of the ring. In β-**D-glucopyranose**, it projects above the plane of the ring (Fig. 3.8). The α- and β- forms of glucopyranose are said to be anomers of each other, and this phenomenon is termed as **anomerism**.

Ketohexoses, aldopentoses and sometimes even the aldohexoses exist in the form of a five-membered ring resembling furan. Carbohydrates having this type of structure are known as furanoses. In case of ketohexoses, the additional centre of asymmetry is at carbon atom 2. If the hydroxyl group attached to this carbon atom projects below the plane of the ring, it is known as the α-anomer. In the β-anomer, it projects above the plane of the ring (Fig. 3.9).

Heptoses

The only heptose of interest in human biochemistry is D-sedoheptulose which is a ketoheptose (Fig. 3.6). It is formed as an intermediate in the hexose monophosphate shunt pathway of carbohydrate metabolism.

In the following description, the prefixes L- and D- will not be used. It should be assumed that the carbohydrates are the D-isomers unless mentioned otherwise.

ISOMERISM

Mention has been made of the simple aldose-ketose isomerism, stereoisomerism and optical isomerism earlier. The higher monosaccharides, viz. pentoses, hexoses and heptoses, exhibit another type of isomerism. It was shown by Fischer that when glucose is treated with methanol in the presence of a mineral acid, two distinct methyl glucosides are formed. One can be hydrolysed by maltase but not by emulsin. The other is hydrolysed by emulsin but not by maltase. The two glucosides were named **methyl-α-D-glucoside** and **methyl-β-D-glucoside**, both having cyclic structures (Fig. 3.7).

Mutarotation

It has been mentioned earlier that carbohydrates possessing an asymmetric carbon atom are optically active. The specific rotation caused by each carbohydrate is quite characteristic. Before the ring structures of carbohydrates were established, it had been shown that glucose existed in two optically distinct forms. When glucose, crystallised from alcohol-water, is dissolved in water, its specific rotation is +112°. When glucose, crystallised from boiling pyridine or a concentrated aqueous solution at 110°C, is

CH₂OH
|
C = O
|
HO — C — H
|
H — C — OH
|
H — C — OH
|
H — C — OH
|
CH₂OH

D-Sedoheptulose

Fig. 3.6: A ketoheptose

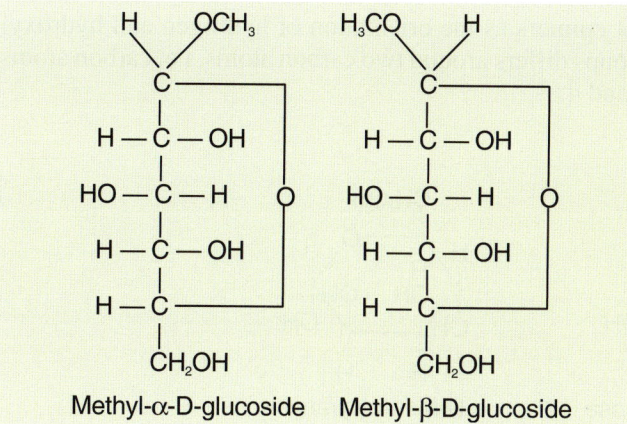

Methyl-α-D-glucoside   Methyl-β-D-glucoside

Fig. 3.7: Cyclic methyl glucosides

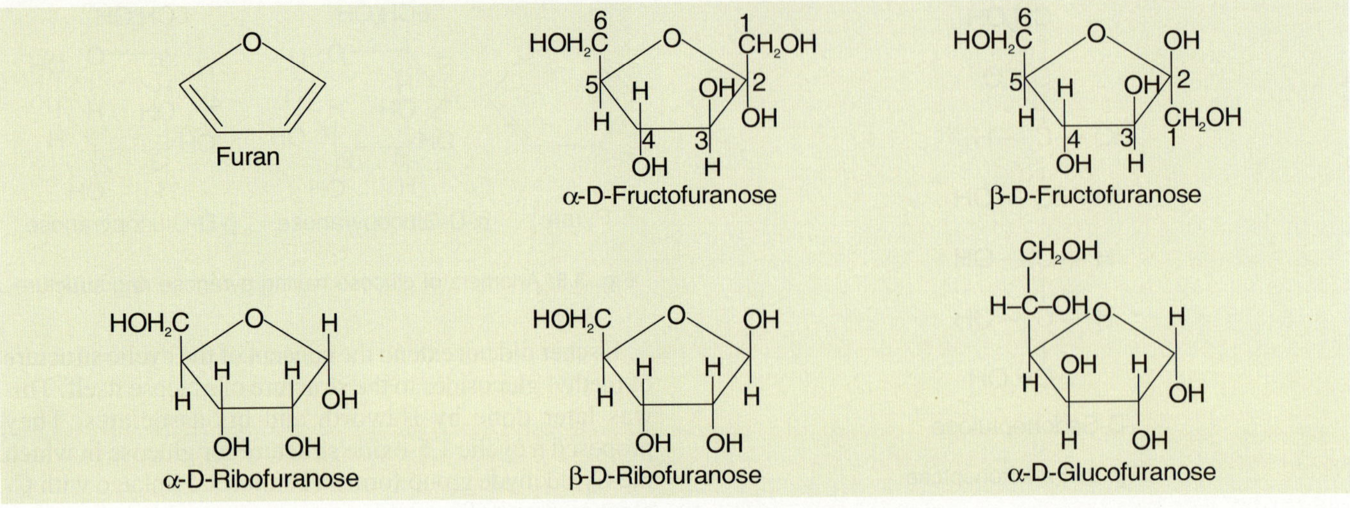

Fig. 3.9: Furanose forms of ribose, glucose and fructose

dissolved in water, it has a specific rotation of +19°. When either form is allowed to stand, the specific rotation gradually changes to +52.5°, and then becomes constant. This change in specific rotation is known as mutarotation.

When ring structures of carbohydrates were discovered, it was shown that the glucose crystallised from alcohol-water is α-D-glucose which has a specifc rotation of +112°. On the other hand, the glucose crystallised from boiling pyridine or a concentrated aqueous solution at 110°C, is β-D-glucose which has a specific rotation of +19°. On standing, α-D-glucose changes into β-D-glucose and vice versa until an equilibrium mixture having 36% α-D-glucose and 64% β-D-glucose is formed. This equilibrium mixture has a specific rotation of +52.5°. The interconversion of the α- and β-forms occurs via the formation of straight-chain glucose monohydrate which does not exceed 0.0025% in concentration.

It was later shown that the property of mutarotation is not confined to glucose alone but is present in all carbohydrates that possess a cyclic structure and have an anomeric carbon atom. In aldoses, e.g. D-ribose and D-glucose, the additional centre of asymmetry is present at carbon atom 1 (Fig. 3.9).

A practical importance of mutarotation in biochemistry laboratories is in the measurement of blood glucose

concentration by glucose oxidase method. Glucoseoxidase acts only on β-glucose. As β-glucose gets depleted, α-glucose is converted into β-glucose, and the reaction continues. A freshly prepared standard solution of glucose contains only α-glucose. Before use, it should be allowed to stand for 12–18 hours so that an equilibrium mixture of α-glucose and β-glucose is formed.

Epimerism

Glucose, galactose and mannose show another type of isomerism. Glucose and galactose differ from each other with respect to the orientation of the hydrogen and hydroxyl groups around carbon atom 4 only. They are said to be epimers of each other. Similarly, glucose and mannose are also epimers of each other as they differ from each other only with respect to the orientation of hydrogen and hydroxyl groups around carbon atom 2 (Fig. 3.10). Thus, those carbohydrates which differ from each other with respect to the orientation of substituent groups around a single carbon atom are known as epimers of each other, and this phenomenon is known as epimerism. In the above example, it can be seen that galactose and mannose are not epimers as the orientation of hydrogen and hydroxyl groups differs around two carbon atoms, i.e. carbon atoms 2 and 4.

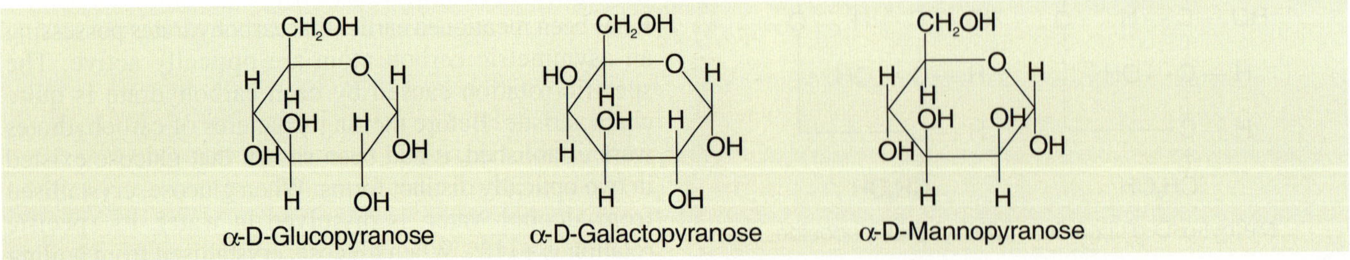

Fig. 3.10: Epimers of glucose

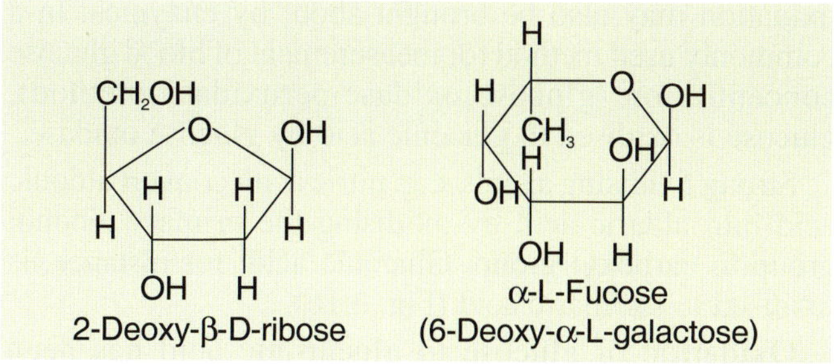

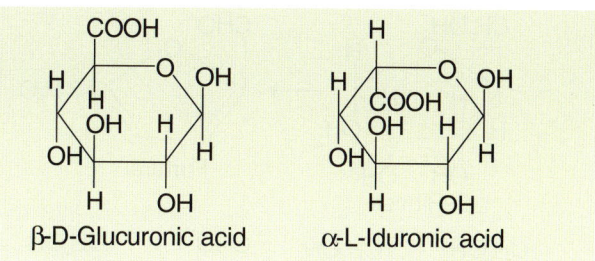

2-Deoxy-β-D-ribose

α-L-Fucose
(6-Deoxy-α-L-galactose)

Fig. 3.11: Deoxysugars

β-D-Glucuronic acid

α-L-Iduronic acid

Fig. 3.13: Uronic acid derivatives of hexoses

DERIVATIVES OF MONOSACCHARIDES

Some important derivatives of monosaccharides are formed by substitution of certain atoms or groups in the monosaccharide molecules. Three important groups of carbohydrates formed in this way are deoxysugars, amino sugars and uronic acids.

1. Deoxysugars

There are two important carbohydrates in this group. The most important deoxysugar is the pentose, 2-deoxy-D-ribose (deoxyribose) which is formed by substitution of the hydroxyl group attached to carbon atom 2 of ribose with hydrogen. It is generally present in the form of its β-anomer in deoxyribonucleic acid (DNA). Another imporant deoxysugar is L-fucose which may be considered as the 6-deoxy derivative of L-galactose (Fig. 3.11). It is commonly found in glycoproteins.

2. Amino Sugars

Amino sugars are formed by substitution of a hydroxyl group of the sugar with an amino group. Since most amino sugars are derived from hexoses, they are also known as hexosamines. Some important amino sugars are glucosamine, galactosamine and mannosamine (Fig. 3.12). These are found in hyaluronic acid, chondroitin sulphate and glycoproteins respectively. The amino sugars are generally present in mucopolysaccharides in the form of their N-acetyl derivatives in which an acetyl group is attached to the amino group.

The amino sugars may also be sulphated. The sulphate group may be attached to the amino group (as in heparin) or to one of the carbon atoms (as in chondroitin sulphate, dermatan sulphate and keratan sulphate).

3. Uronic acids

Uronic acids are formed by substitution of the terminal hydroxymethyl (–CH$_2$OH) group of monosaccharides with a carboxyl group. Thus, hexuronic acids have a carboxyl group at carbon atom 6. The most important uronic acid in human beings is glucuronic acid. Glucuronic acid is formed in the body enzymatically from glucose in the uronic acid pathway. It is used to detoxify a number of harmful endogenous and exogenous compounds. Conjugation of these substances with glucuronic acid makes them water soluble and, hence, easily excretable. Glucuronic acid is also a constituent of several mucopolysaccharides either as such or in the form of its sulphate. L-Iduronic acid is another uronic acid found in some mucopolysaccharides (Fig. 3.13).

Reactions of Monosaccharides

1. Dehydration

Monosaccharides are dehydrated by strong mineral acids, e.g. hydrochloric acid and sulphuric acid, to furfural or furfural derivatives (Fig. 3.14).

Furfural or its derivatives condense with various phenols to form characteristically coloured complexes. This reaction forms the basis of a number of tests for identification of carbohydrates. Furfural derivatives of carbohydrates condense with **α-naphthol** to form a violet coloured complex. This reaction is the basis of **Molisch's test.** Molisch's test is a class test for carbohydrates, and is

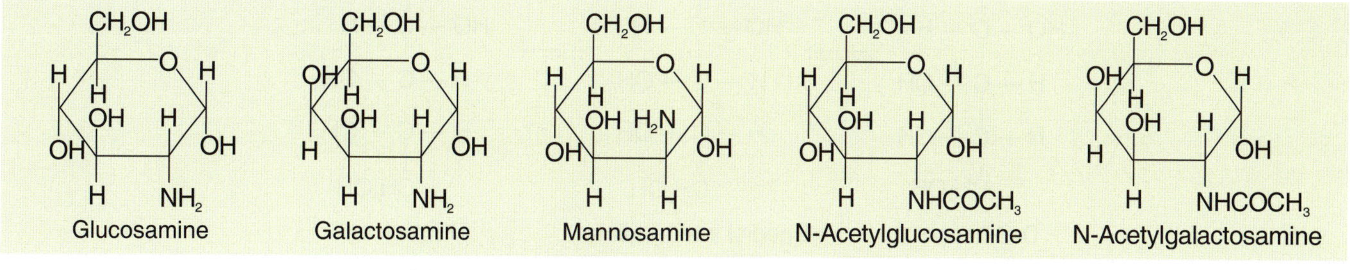

Glucosamine

Galactosamine

Mannosamine

N-Acetylglucosamine

N-Acetylgalactosamine

Fig. 3.12: Hexosamines and N-acetyl hexosamines

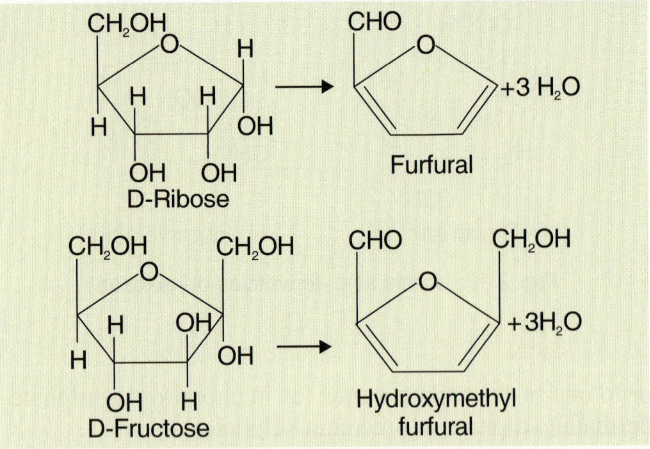

Fig. 3.14: Dehydration of sugars by strong mineral acids

given by all the carbohydrates. Furfural derivatives of ketoses condense with **resorcinol** to form a red coloured complex. This reaction is the basis of **Selivanoff's test.** Selivanoff's test is given by ketoses, e.g. fructose. This reaction can also be used for quantitative measurement of fructose concentration.

2. Interconversion

If glucose or fructose is disolved in a dilute alkali and allowed to stand for a few hours, each of them forms a mixture containing both the monosaccharides. This is due to very poor stability of the monosaccharides in alkaline solutions. The interconversion occurs via the formation of a common enediol intermediate (Fig. 3.15). This reaction shows that the structures of glucose and fructose are identical as far as carbon atoms 3, 4, 5 and 6 are concerned. Mannose also undergoes a similar type of interconversion with glucose or fructose.

3. Oxidation

The aldehyde group of aldoses is readily oxidised to a carboxyl group by mild oxidising agents in acidic medium. The general name of the resulting product is aldonic acid. Glucose, for example, is oxidised to gluconic acid. Such oxidation may also be brought about by enzymes. In a commonly used method for measurement of blood glucose concentration (glucose oxidase-peroxidase method), glucose is oxidised to gluconic acid by glucose oxidase.

Strong oxidising agents, e.g. nitric acid, convert aldonic acid into aldaric acid by oxidising the primary alcohol group to carboxyl group. Gluconic acid, for instance, is oxidised to saccharic acid (Fig. 3.16).

Oxidation of glucose to glucuronic acid has been described earlier which occurs enzymatically and in which the primary alcohol group at carbon atom 6 of glucose is oxidised to a carboxyl group while carbon atom 1 remains unaffected.

4. Reduction

Monosaccharides can be reduced in the presence of sodium amalgam to their parent sugar alcohols. Glucose, mannose and galactose are reduced to sorbitol, mannitol and galactitol respectively. Reduction of glucose occurs enzymatically in the body. Excessive reduction of glucose to sorbitol in lens cells in diabetes mellitus is believed to be the cause of premature cataract in this disease. Premature cataract is common in diabetics. Similarly, reduction of excess galactose to galactitol in lens cells is believed to be the cause of premature cataract in congenital galactosaemia.

Mannitol is not metabolised in the body, is fully filtered in the glomeruli and is not reabsorbed by the renal tubular cells. It is used pharmacologically as a diuretic to increase the output of urine in some pathological conditions.

Fructose gives both sorbitol and mannitol on reduction. Ribose and ribulose are reduced to ribitol. Erythrose is reduced to erythritol. Glyceraldehyde and dihydroxyacetone are reduced to glycerol. The general reaction involving the reduction of sugars is shown in Fig. 3.17. The aldehyde group is reduced in aldoses and the keto group is reduced in ketoses.

5. Reduction of Metal Ions

The aldehyde and ketone groups of monosaccharides possess reducing property. Many qualitative tests and

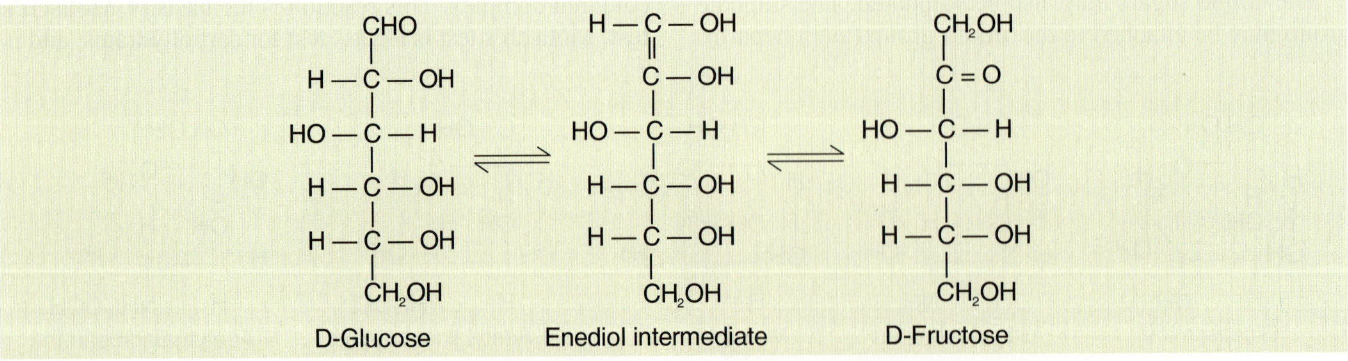

Fig. 3.15: Interconversion of glucose and fructose

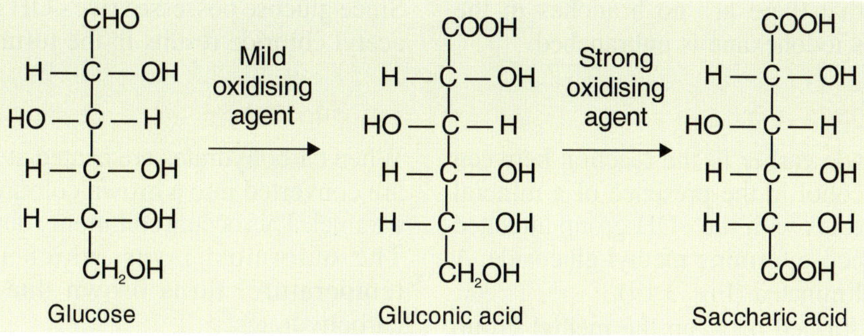

Fig. 3.16: Oxidation of glucose

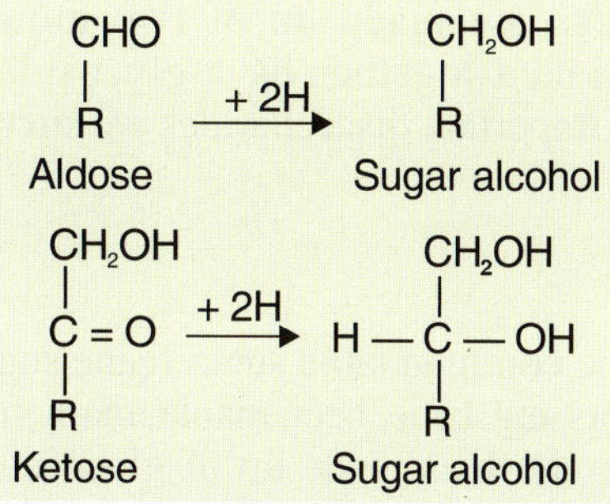

Fig. 3.17: Reduction of aldoses and ketoses

quantitative analytical methods for sugars are based on the reduction of certain metal ions, e.g. copper, iron, bismuth, silver, etc. caused by the sugars. The best known example is **Benedict's test** in which the sugar is boiled with a solution of copper sulphate, sodium carbonate and sodium citrate. Copper sulphate is hydrolysed to cupric hydroxide. Cupric hydroxide is reduced by the sugar to cuprous oxide which separates out of the solution as a red precipitate. If the sugar solution is dilute, the precipitate may be orange, yellow or green in colour depending upon the concentration of the sugar. This is a valuable means of differentiating carbohydrates that possess a free aldehyde or ketone group from those that do not.

6. *Formation of Osazones*

This is another reaction given by carbohydrates that possess a free aldehyde or ketone group. The reaction involves carbon atoms 1 and 2 of the aldoses and ketoses. When the carbohydrate is heated with phenylhydrazine in a boiling water-bath in the presence of acetate buffer (pH 4.3), a series of reactions occur leading to the formation of osazone of the given carbohydrate (Fig. 3.18).

Since the differences between carbon atoms 1 and 2 are obliterated in these reactions, those carbohydrates that differ only with respect to these two carbon atoms, e.g. glucose, mannose and fructose, will form identical osazones. The other carbohydrates will form distinctive osazones which differ in their time of formation, solubility, melting point and crystalline structure. These diferences may be used to identify the carbohydrates.

7. *Reaction with Hydroiodic Acid*

If an aldohexose, e.g glucose, is heated with hydroiodic acid, it results in the formation of iodohexane ($C_6H_{13}I$).

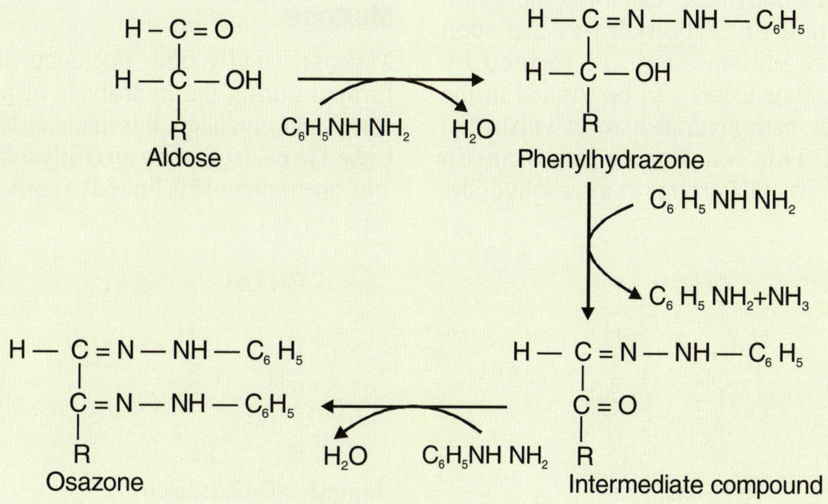

Fig. 3.18: Formation of osazone

This reaction shows that there are no branches in the structures of aldoses as iodohexane is unbranched.

8. *Reaction with Alcohols*

Reference has been made earlier to the reaction between glucose and methyl alcohol in the presence of a mineral acid. Methyl alcohol reacts with the –OH group attached to carbon atom 1 of glucose forming methyl glucoside. A molecule of water is eliminated (Fig. 3.19).

The bond which is formed between the methyl group of alcohol and the carbon atom of glucose is known as a **glycosidic bond**. If the carbon atom of glucose has an α-configuration, the bond is known as α-glycosidic bond. A similar reaction occurs between other carbohydrates and alcohols as well leading to the formation of various glycosides. The alcohol group reacting with the mono-saccharide may be provided by another monosaccharide or by an organic alcohol. In the former case, the product will be a disaccharide. In all disaccharides and poly-saccharides, the constituent monosaccharides are linked with each other through glycosidic bonds. The glycosidic bond is formed in living cells under the influence of specific enzymes rather than inorganic catalysts.

If the alcohol group is provided by a non-carbohydrate, it is known as the aglycone portion of the glycoside. In methyl glucoside, for example, the methyl group consititutes the aglycone portion. **Cardiac glycosides**, such as digoxin and ouabain, are an important group of drugs which increase the force of contraction of heart. The aglycone portion of these glycosides is made up of sterols.

If methyl glucoside is treated with dimethyl sulphate in the presence of an alkali, the other –OH groups of glucose are also methylated forming pentamethyl glucose. This reaction also proves that glucose contains five –OH groups.

9. *Esterification*

The hydroxyl groups of carbohydrates can form esters with acids. Phosphoric esters of carbohydrates are seen commonly in living organisms and are formed by enzymatic reactions. Acetate esters can be formed in the laboratory by allowing the carbohydrate to react with acetyl chloride (CH_3COCl). This reaction is important in determining the number of –OH groups in a carbohydrate.

Since glucose possesses five –OH groups, its reaction with acetyl chloride results in the formation of a pentaacetate.

10. *Caramelisation*

When carbohydrates are heated at high temperatures, they are converted into a brown coloured degradation product, caramel. This occurs commonly during the baking of bread. The outermost layer, which is exposed to a high temperature, turns brown due to caramelisation of carbohydrates.

DISACCHARIDES

Disaccharides are made up of two monosaccharide molecules linked together by a glycosidic bond. The biologically important disaccharides are **sucrose**, **maltose** and **lactose**.

Sucrose

Sucrose is the common table sugar (cane sugar). It occurs in many plants, e.g. cane, beet, maple, many fruits, flowers, roots, seeds, etc. It is made up of glucose and fructose. Carbon atom 1 of glucose is linked to carbon atom 2 of fructose by a glycosidic bond. Since the anomeric carbon of fructose (carbon atom 2) has got a β-configuration, the glycosidic bond is said to be a β-glycosidic bond. Therefore, sucrose may be described as **α-D-gluco-pyranosyl-β-D-fructofuranoside** (Fig. 3.20).

Sucrose is dextrorotatory (+66.5°). When it is hydrolysed, an equimolar mixture of glucose and fructose is formed. Of these, glucose is dextrorotatory (+52.5°) and fructose is laevorotatory (–92.3°). As fructose causes greater laevorotation as compared to the dextrorotation caused by glucose, the hydrolysate is laevorotatory. As the optical rotation is inverted on hydrolysis, sucrose is described as invert sugar.

Maltose

Maltose usually does not occur as such in nature. It is formed during the hydrolysis of polysaccharides such as starch and glycogen. It is made up to two glucose molecules linked to each other by an α-glycosidic bond. Carbon atom 1 of one molecule is linked to carbon atom 4 of the second.

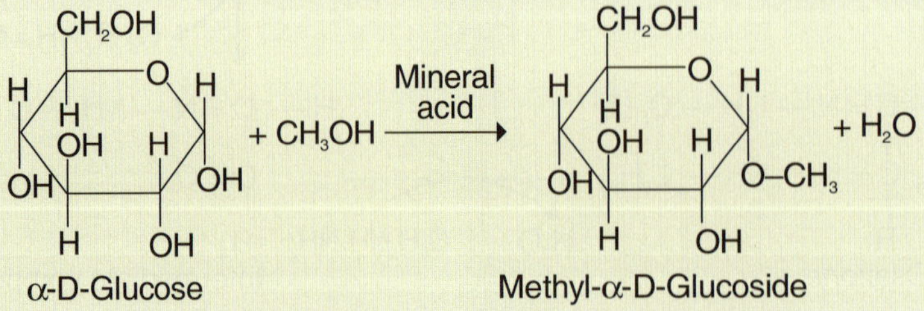

Fig. 3.19: Reaction of glucose with methyl alcohol

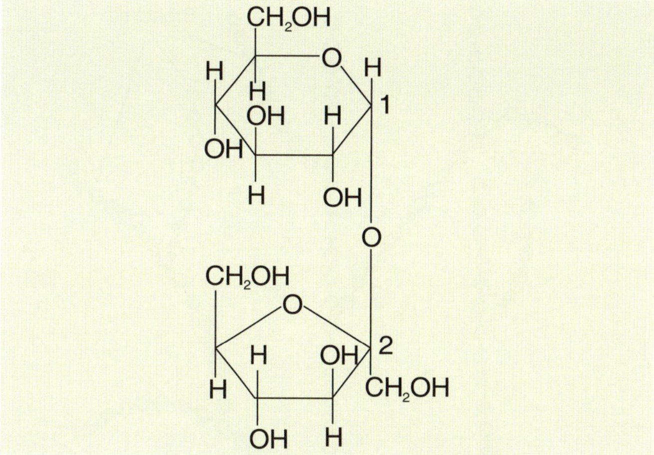

Fig. 3.20: Sucrose (invert sugar)

The carbon atom 1 (anomeric carbon) of the second glucose molecule is free, and may possess an α- or a β-configuration. Therefore, maltose may exist as α-maltose or β-maltose. However, the anomeric carbon of the first glucose molecule, involved in the bonding, always possesses an α-configuration. Therefore, the bond is an α-glycosidic bond. The α form of maltose may be described as **α-D-glucopyranosyl-α-D-glucopyranoside** (Fig. 3.21).

Lactose

Lactose is found only in mammals. Since it is present in milk, and is the principal sugar of milk, it is commonly described as **milk sugar**. It is made up of galactose and glucose. Since galactose is required for the formation of glycolipids of the nervous tissue, its importance in the diet of the young ones of mammals is obvious.

In lactose, carbon atom 1 of galactose is linked with carbon atom 4 of glucose by a β-glycosidic bond. Lactose may exist in α- and β-forms depending upon the orientation

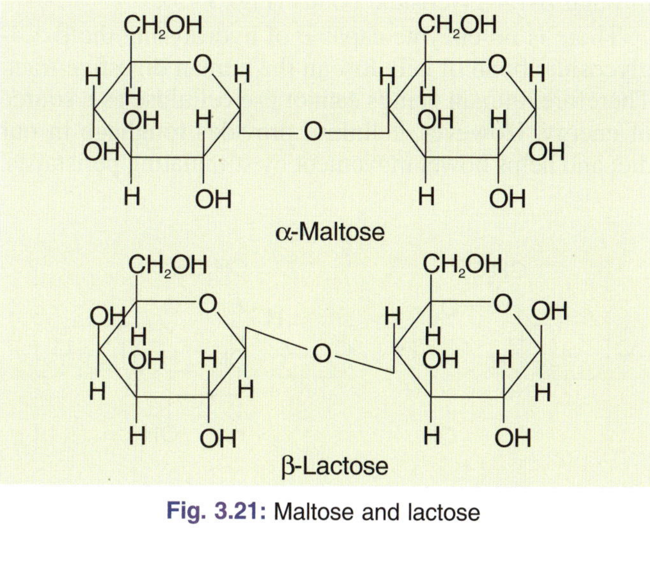

Fig. 3.21: Maltose and lactose

of –H and –OH groups around carbon atom 1 of the glucose residue which is free. The β-form would be described as **β-D-galactopyranosyl-β-D-glucopyranoside** (Fig. 3.21).

Reactions of Disaccharides

The glycosidic bond of disaccharides can be hydrolysed by specific enzymes, e.g. sucrase, maltase and lactase. As mentioned earlier, hydrolysis of sucrose leads to a change in the direction of optical rotation. Therefore, sucrase, which hydrolyses sucrose, is also known as invertase. The disaccharides can also be hydrolysed by heating them in the presence of mineral acids.

Mineral acids first hydrolyse the disaccharides into monosaccharides, and then dehydrate the monosaccharides to form furfural derivatives. The furfural derivatives would condense with phenols, e.g. α-naphthol (Molisch's test), to form coloured complexes. Therefore, Molisch's test is also given by disaccharides.

Disaccharides also give reactions characteristic of hydroxyl, aldehyde and ketone groups. Sucrose, however, has no free aldehyde or ketone group, and does not give any of the reactions characteristic of these groups. On the other hand, maltose and lactose form distinctive osazones and reduce metal ions, e.g. cupric ions, in hot alkaline solutions.

POLYSACCHARIDES

Polysaccharides, as mentioned earlier, are made up of a large number of monosaccharide molecules, and include homopolysaccharides and heteropolysaccharides.

Homopolysaccharides

The most important homopolysaccharide in human body is **glycogen**. The plant homopolysaccharides include **starch**, **cellulose**, **inulin,** etc.

Glycogen

Glycogen (animal starch) is the form in which carbohydrates are stored in our body. Glycogen is made up of a large number of glucose molecules.

The glucose molecules are linked with each other through **α-1,4-glycosidic bonds**. A long chain of glucose molecules is formed in this way (Fig. 3.22). However, after every 8–12 glucose units, there is a branch point. At branch points, a glucose molecule is attached to one of the glucose units in the linear chain by an **α-1, 6-glycosidic bond**. Thus, the glucose molecule at a branch point is involved in two glycosidic linkages. An α-1,4-glycosidic bond links it with the main linear chain, and an α-1,6-glycosidic bond links it with a branch (Fig. 3.23). The branch also continues linearly until a secondary branch arises from it after 8 to 12 glucose units. In this way, a very big and highly branched molecule of glycogen is formed (Fig. 3.24).

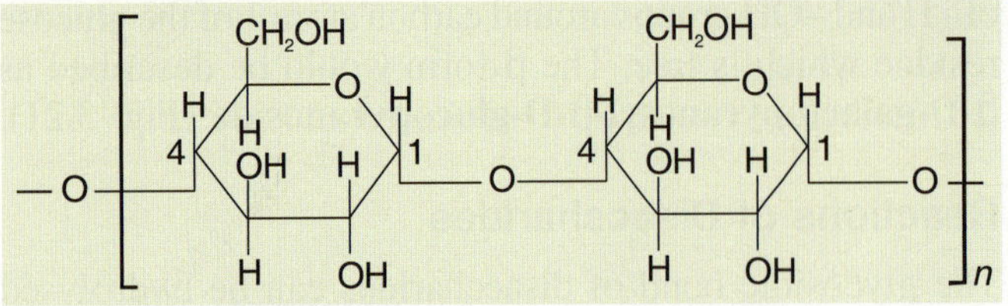

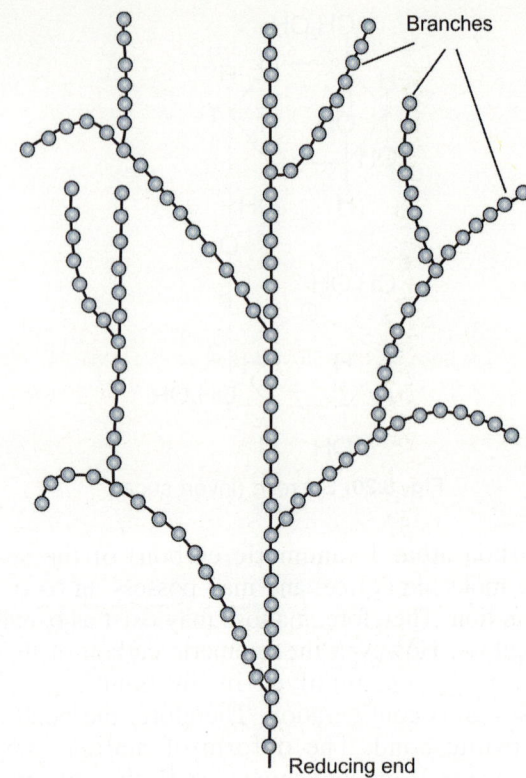

Fig. 3.22: Repeating unit of glycogen

Starch

Starch is the most abundant source of energy in our daily diet. It is a polymer of glucose. It is synthesised in plants by the process of photosynthesis. Potatoes, other tubers, cereals and legumes are rich in starch. It is made up of a large number of glucose units. Starch, in fact, is made up of two different types of molecules – **amylose** and **amylopectin**.

Amylose is a straight-chain molecule made up of glucose units linked with each other by means of α-1, 4-glycosidic bonds. The chain is coiled to form a helical structure. The structure of amylose is similar to that of glycogen with the difference that it has no branches. It constitutes about 15–20 percent of starch.

Amylopectin constitutes the remaining 80–85 percent of starch. It has greater structural similarity with glycogen. It contains linear portions made up of glucose units linked by α-1,4-glycosidic bonds, and branches arising from the straight chains by means of α-1,6-glycosidic bonds. It differs from glycogen in that the branch points are 24–30 glucose units apart. Therefore, amylopectin has fewer branches than glycogen.

Dextrin

Dextrin is not a naturally occurring polysaccharide. It is a hydrolytic product of starch. When starch is hydrolysed, its molecular size decreases progressively until it is converted into maltose or glucose. The intermediate products, between starch and maltose, are known as dextrins. Thus, dextrin is not a single molecular species

Fig. 3.24: A portion of the glycogen molecule

but is a mixture of several products with progressively decreasing molecular size. They are generally divided, on the basis of the colours that they give with iodine, into amylodextrin (violet), erythrodextrin (red) and achrodextrin (no colour).

Cellulose

Cellulose is also a polymer of glucose. It forms the structural framework of plants. It is a straight-chain molecule made up of glucose units linked with each other through β-1,4-glycosidic bonds (Fig. 3.25).

There is no enzyme capable of hydrolysing the β-1,4-glycosidic bond of cellulose in the human digestive tract. Therefore, human beings cannot use cellulose as a source of energy. However, cellulose provides roughage in our diet and helps bowel movement by stimulating peristalsis.

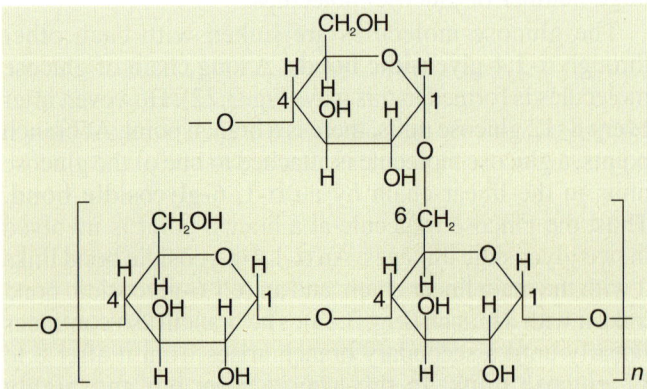

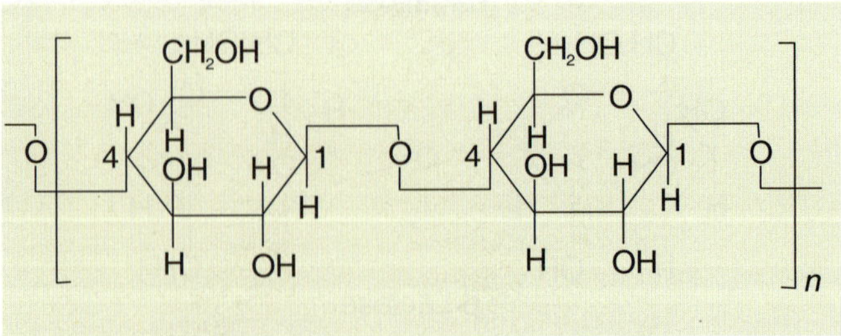

Fig. 3.23: A branch point in glycogen

Fig. 3.25: Repeating unit of cellulose

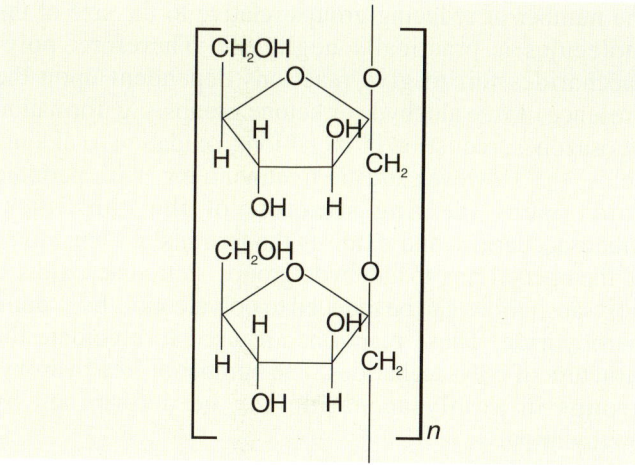

Fig. 3.26: Repeating unit of inulin

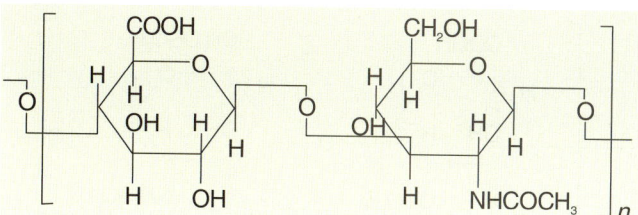

Fig. 3.27: Repeating unit of hyaluronic acid

Inulin

Inulin is present in Jerusalem artichoke and some other plants. It is a straight-chain molecule made up of fructose units joined to each other by β-1, 2-glycosidic bonds (Fig. 3.26). The fructose molecules possess furanose ring structure. There are 33 to 35 fructose residues in each molecule of inulin. The molecular weight is about 5,000.

Like cellulose, inulin cannot be metabolised by human beings. If it is injected intravenously, it is completely filtered by the glomeruli, and is neither secreted nor reabsorbed by the renal tubules. For these reasons, inulin is used as a diagnostic agent to measure the glomerular filtration rate.

Heteropolysaccharides

The heteropolysaccharides are made up of more than one kind of monosaccharides and/or monosaccharide derivatives. The most important heteropolysaccharides in human beings are the **mucopolysaccharides** (glycosaminoglycans). These are present in connective tissues and mucous secretions. They are often combined with proteins. Hexosamines and uronic acids are the prominent constituents of mucopolysaccharides. These are usually present in the form of repeating disaccharide units. The important mucopolysaccharides are the following:

Hyaluronic Acid

Hyaluronic acid has a very wide tissue distribution. It forms the ground substance of the mesenchymal tissue. It is made up of glucuronic acid and N-acetyl glucosamine. Anomeric carbon atoms of both of these possess the β-configuration. Carbon atom 1 of glucuronic acid forms a glycosidic bond with carbon atom 3 of N-acetylglucosamine. Carbon atom 1 of the latter forms a similar bond with carbon atom 4 of the next glucuronic acid residue in the chain (Fig. 3.27). This basic structure is repeated over and over again to form a very large molecule having a molecular weight of 150,000–1,500,000.

Hyaluronic acid acts as a cementing substance. It helps in retaining water in the interstitial spaces. It is a very efficient lubricant. The last function is particularly important in joints where hyaluronic acid is present in the synovial fluid.

Chondroitin Sulphate

Chondroitin sulphate has a restricted tissue distribution. It is mainly found in cartilages and bones. It is present in some other tissues also but in very small amounts. It is made up of glucuronic acid and N-acetylgalactosamine sulphate. The glycosidic bonds are similar to those in hyaluronic acid. There are two types of chondroitin sulphate. In chondroitin-4-sulphate, the sulphate group is esterified with carbon atom 4 of galactosamine. In chondroitin-6-sulphate, it is esterified with carbon atom 6 of galactosamine (Fig. 3.28).

Heparin

Heparin is secreted by mast cells which are present in many tissues including the walls of large arteries, lungs, liver, etc. It is an anticoagulant and prevents intravascular clotting. It also releases lipoprotein lipase from the walls of capillaries and, thus, helps in the catabolism of chylomicrons and very low density lipoproteins.

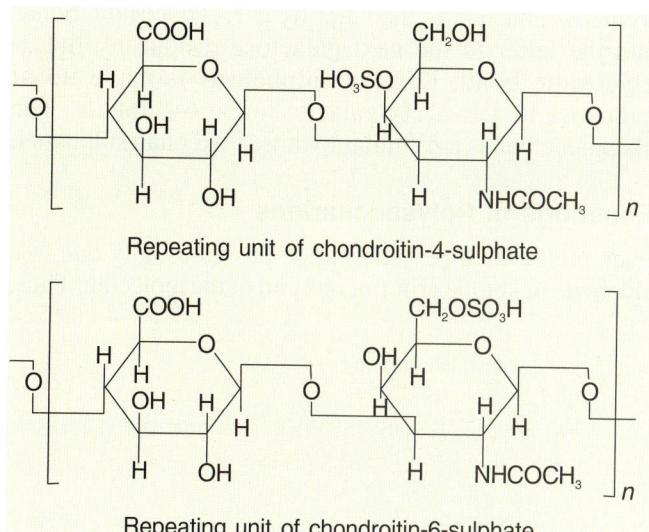

Repeating unit of chondroitin-4-sulphate

Repeating unit of chondroitin-6-sulphate

Fig. 3.28: Repeating units of chondroitin sulphate

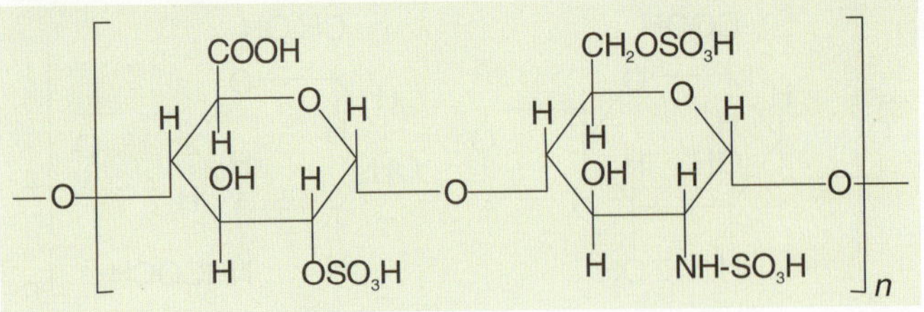

Fig. 3.29: Repeating unit of heparin

Heparin is made up of glucuronic acid and glucosamine, both of which are sulphated. These two are linked to each other by α-1,4-glycosidic bonds (Fig. 3.29). Some L-iduronic acid residues also occur in heparin. Naturally occurring heparin comprises molecules of varying length ranging in molecular weight from 3,000 to 30,000. A low molecular weight heparin (MW 5,000) is used clinically as an anticoagulant drug.

Heparan Sulphate

Heparan sulphate has a much wider tissue distribution than heparin. It is a less powerful anticoagulant. It differs from heparin in that some of the glucosamine residues carry an N-acetyl group instead of a sulphate group on carbon atom 2.

Dermatan Sulphate

Dermatan sulphate is found in skin, tendons and valves of the heart. It differs from chondroitin sulphate in that it has L-iduronic acid as the uronic acid component instead of D-glucuronic acid.

Keratan Sulphate

Keratan sulphate is widely distributed in tissues. It is found in cornea, costal cartilages, intervertebral discs and walls of aorta. It is of two types. Keratan sulphate I is made up of galactose and N-acetylglucosamine-6-sulphate. The former is attached to the latter by β-1,4-glycosidic bonds and the latter to the next galactose residue by β-1,3-glycosidic bond. Keratan sulphate II is made up of galactose and N-acetylgalactosamine-6-sulphate. The glycosidic bonds are similar to those in keratan sulphate I.

Reactions of Polysaccharides

Each molecule of polysaccharide possesses only one free aldehyde or ketone group at one end of the molecule. Thus, the number of reducing groups relative to the size of the molecules is practically negligible. Therefore, polysaccharides fail to give reactions dependent upon the presence of free aldehyde or ketone groups, e.g. formation of osazones, reduction of metal ions, oxidation to aldonic acids, etc. However, drastic treatment, e.g. with periodic acid, opens the ring structure of the constituent monosaccharides and oxidises the terminal carbon atoms of the opened ring to aldehyde groups. Periodate-oxidised polysaccharides can be reduced to polyalcohols by sodium borohydride. These reactions are used to elucidate the structure of polysaccharides. The number of free hydroxyl groups in a polysaccharide can be determined by methylation.

Some important reactions of polysaccharides depend upon their large size. As polysaccharides are macromolecules, they form colloidal solutions. When a solution of iodine in potassium iodide is added to the polysaccharide solution, iodine is adsorbed on the surface of the polysaccharide forming a complex having a characteristic colour. Thus, starch gives a blue colour with iodine, glycogen gives a red colour, and dextrin gives a violet colour.

Polysaccharides can be precipitated from their colloidal solutions by adding neutral salts, e.g. ammonium sulphate. Each polysaccharide molecule possesses a number of electric charges on its surface and is surrounded by a film of water (shell of hydration). These two factors prevent the coalescence of the molecules and keep them in solution. When ammonium sulphate is added, it neutralises the electric charges and removes the shell of hydration. The molecules come together and are precipitated. The amount of the salt required to precipitate the polysaccharides is inversely proportional to their molecular weights. Starch is precipitated when its solution is half-saturated with ammonium sulphate. Glycogen and dextrin are precipitated when their solutions are fully saturated with ammonium sulphate.

Polysaccharides are hydrolysed into monosaccharides, and monosaccharides are dehydrated to furfural derivatives by mineral acids, e.g. sulphuric acid. The furfural derivatives give characteristic colours when condensed with phenolic compounds, e.g. violet colour with α-naphthol (Molisch's reaction). Molisch's test is, thus, given by all the carbohydrates.

EXERCISE

1. Define carbohydrates. Classify them giving one example from each class/subclass.
2. Describe the structures and functions of glycosaminoglycans.
3. Write short notes on:
   a. Anomerism,
   b. Mutarotation,
   c. Epimerism,
   d. Inversion,
   e. Glycogen,
   f. Mucopolysaccharides,
   g. Glycosidic bonds, and
   h. Cardiac glycosides
4. Write 'true' or 'false':
   a. Dihydroxyacetone has no stereoisomers.
   b. Galactose and mannose are epimers of each other.
   c. Glucose and galactose form identical osazones.
   d. D-Fructose is dextrorotatory.
   e. Lactose is also known as invert sugar.
   f. Sucrose is a non-reducing carbohydrate.
   g. Both α-1,4- and α-1,6-glycosidic bonds are present in amylose.
   h. Inulin is a homopolysaccharide made up of fructose.
   i. Heparin is made up of glucuronic acid and N-acetylgalactosamine sulphate.
   j. Heparin prevents intravascular coagulation of blood.
5. Fill in the blanks:
   a. A carbohydrate not having D- and L-isomers is …….….…..….….. .
   b. A carbohydrate present in DNA is …….….…..….….. .
   c. Monosaccharides differing in the orientation of –H and –OH on a single carbon atom are known as …….….…..….….. of each other.
   d. Hydrolysis of invert sugar yields …….….…..... and …….….…..... .
   e. Galactose and glucose are linked by …….….…..….….. bond in lactose.
   f. A monosaccharide present in sucrose as well as inulin is …….….…..….….. .
   g. A monosaccharide present in maltose as well as lactose is …….….…..….….. .
   h. Hyaluronic acid is made up of …….….…..... and …….….…..... .
   i. …….….…..….….. is present in hyaluronic acid as well as chondroitin sulphate.
   j. Heparin is secreted by …….….…..….….. cells.

ANSWERS TO SHORT QUESTIONS

4. a. True
   b. False
   c. False
   d. False
   e. False
   f. True
   g. False
   h. True
   i. False
   j. True

5. a. Dihydroxyacetone
   b. Deoxyribose
   c. Epimers
   d. Glucose, fructose
   e. β-1, 4-glycosidic
   f. Fructose
   g. Glucose
   h. Glucuronic acid, N-acetylglucosamine
   i. Glucuronic acid
   j. Mast

Chemistry of Lipids

Lipids are not a chemically homogeneous group of compounds. They include different compounds which share the following properties:

1. They are insoluble in water and soluble in organic solvents.
2. They are related to fatty acids either actually or potentially.
3. They can be used as a source of energy by animals.

Lipids are widely distributed in nature. Their tissue distribution in human beings is also widespread. They perform a number of important functions in human beings. These include:

1. They are a rich source of energy. Their calorific value is much higher than that of carbohydrates and proteins.
2. They provide polyunsaturated fatty acids which are an essential component of human diet.
3. They carry fat-soluble vitamins viz. vitamins A, D, E and K.
4. They provide insulation in the form of subcutaneous fat.
5. A layer of fat is present around several delicate organs which acts as a mechanical shock absorber.
6. They are the structural constituents of tissues in the form of glycolipids, phospholipids and cholesterol.

CLASSIFICATION

Lipids can be broadly divided into three classes:

1. Simple lipids,
2. Compound lipids, and
3. Derived lipids.

Simple Lipids

These are the esters of fatty acids with alcohols. These can be further divided into two groups.

(i) Fats

Fats are the esters of fatty acids with glycerol. Fats are solid at room temperature. Some of them are liquid at room temperature, and are known as oils. The physical state depends upon the nature of fatty acids. Fats have a preponderance of saturated fatty acids while oils are rich in unsaturated fatty acids.

(ii) Waxes

These are the esters of fatty acids with higher alcohols. Cetyl alcohol is a common constituent of waxes. Other higher alcohols are also found.

Compound Lipids

Compound lipids contain some substances in addition to fatty acids and alcohols. They can be further divided into the following subclasses:

(i) Phospholipids

These are made up of fatty acids, an alcohol which may or may not be glycerol, phosphoric acid and a nitrogenous base. Some examples of phospholipids are lecithin, cephalin and sphingomyelin.

(ii) Glycolipids

Glycolipids contain a fatty acid, an alcohol and some carbohydrates. They can be subdivided into cerebrosides and gangliosides. Cerebrosides contain a fatty acid, sphingosine (an amino alcohol) and a carbohydrate (galactose). Gangliosides contain a fatty acid, sphingosine, N-acetylneuraminic acid and some hexoses.

(iii) Sulpholipids

These are also known as sulphatides. They are similar to cerebrosides with the difference that galactose is sulphated.

(iv) Lipoproteins

Lipoproteins may be considered to be conjugated proteins or compound lipids. They are made up of various lipids which are combined with some specific proteins. The lipid fraction includes triglycerides, phospholipids, cholesterol and fatty acids which are present in varying proportions.

The lipoproteins are soluble in water because of their protein content. Therefore, this is the form in which lipids are transported in circulation.

Derived Lipids

These are the compounds obtained on hydrolysis of simple and compound lipids but still possessing the properties of lipids, e.g. fatty acids, higher alcohols, sterols, steroids, hydrocarbons, etc. Glycerol is generally studied with lipids because of its widespread occurrence in lipids but is not strictly a lipid as it is soluble in water.

Some important lipids from each of the above classes will now be considered in detail.

FATTY ACIDS

These are aliphatic acids having a carboxyl group. Most of them are straight chain compounds. They generally contain an even number of carbon atoms because two carbon atoms are added at a time during their synthesis. Each fatty acid possesses a carboxy terminal and a methyl terminal. The carbon atoms are numbered from the carboxy terminal, the carboxyl atom being numbered 1. The second, third and fourth carbon atoms are also known as α, β and γ carbon atoms respectively. The methyl carbon is known as ω (omega) carbon.

The fatty acids may be saturated or unsaturated. The saturated fatty acids have no carbon-carbon double bonds. Their general formula is $C_nH_{2n+1}COOH$. Some important saturated fatty acids are shown in Table 4.1.

Monounsaturated Fatty Acids

The unsaturated fatty acids contain one or more double bonds in their structure. The fatty acids having only one double bond are known as monounsaturated fatty acids (MUFA). The principal example of this class is oleic acid. It is an 18-carbon fatty acid having a double bond between carbon atoms 9 and 10. Its formula is $CH_3-(CH_2)_7-CH=CH-(CH_2)_7-COOH$. It is formed in the body from stearic acid. Palmitoleic acid is similarly formed from palmitic acid. Its formula is $CH_3-(CH_2)_5-CH=CH-(CH_2)_7-COOH$.

Polyunsaturated Fatty Acids

Fatty acids having more than one double bonds are known as polyunsaturated fatty acids (PUFA). Examples include linoleic acid, linolenic acid and arachidonic acid. Linoleic acid is an 18-carbon fatty acid having two double bonds. The double bonds are present between carbon atoms 9 and 10, and between carbon atoms 12 and 13. A simpler representation of linoleic acid is 18:2; 9,12. The first number (18) shows the number of carbon atoms, the second digit (2) shows the number of double bonds, and the succeeding digits (9 and 12) show the positions of double bonds. Similarly, α-linolenic acid, which has got 18 carbon atoms and three double bonds, is represented as 18:3;9,12,15 (γ-linolenic acid is 18:3;6,9,12). Arachidonic acid has got 20 carbon atoms and four double bonds, and is represented as 20:4;5,8,11,14.

Essential Fatty Acids

Human beings require PUFA but cannot synthesise them. Therefore, these must be provided in the diet. For this reason, PUFA are known as essential fatty acids. Most of the vegetable oils, e.g. groundnut oil, sesame oil, mustard oil, cottonseed oil, soyabean oil, safflower oil, etc. are good sources of essential fatty acids.

Essential fatty acids (EFA) are constituents of several lipids. Their deficiency can impair the synthesis of these lipids. EFA deficiency causes dermatitis and hair loss. It can also raise the plasma cholesterol concentration, which predisposes the individual to atherosclerotic diseases. Essential fatty acids also act as the precursors of a class of hormone-like compounds known as eicosanoids, e.g. prostaglandins, thromboxanes and leukotrienes.

Some fatty acids have hydroxyl groups in their acyl chains, e.g. cerebronic acid and oxynervonic acid which are present in cerebrosides. The active principle of the laxative castor oil is ricinoleic acid which has a hydroxyl group in its acyl chain. Some fatty acids have a ring in their acyl chain, e.g. chaulmoogric acid which was used in the treatment of leprosy in the past but is of only historic interest now. Some eicosanoids also have cyclic rings in their acyl chains.

Table 4.1: Some saturated fatty acids			
Fatty acid	*Formula*	*Fatty acid*	*Formula*
Acetic acid	CH_3COOH	Propionic acid	C_2H_5COOH
Butyric acid	C_3H_7COOH	Caproic acid	$C_5H_{11}COOH$
Caprylic acid	$C_7H_{15}COOH$	Capric acid	$C_9H_{19}COOH$
Lauric acid	$C_{11}H_{23}COOH$	Myristic acid	$C_{13}H_{27}COOH$
Palmitic acid	$C_{15}H_{31}COOH$	Stearic acid	$C_{17}H_{35}COOH$
Arachidic acid	$C_{19}H_{39}COOH$	Behenic acid	$C_{21}H_{43}COOH$
Lignoceric acid	$C_{23}H_{47}COOH$	Cerotic acid	$C_{25}H_{51}COOH$

Eicosanoids

Prostaglandins were the first eicosanoids to be discovered. They were first found in seminal fluid and were believed to be synthesised in prostate gland alone. Hence, they were named prostaglandins. But it was later discovered that their tissue distribution is very wide. They produce profound physiological and biochemical effects on various organs and systems, e.g. reproductive system, cardiovascular system, gastrointestinal tract, central nervous system, etc.

There are six primary prostaglandins, viz. PGE_1, PGE_2, PGE_3, $PGF_{1\alpha}$, $PGF_{2\alpha}$, and $PGF_{3\alpha}$. There are several secondary prostaglandins.

The other eicosanoids, thromboxanes and leukotrienes also produce profound physiological effects. The important thromboxanes are thromboxane A_1 (TXA_1), thromboxane A_2 (TXA_2) and thromboxane A_3 (TXA_3).

Leukotriene C_4 (LTC_4), leukotriene D_4 (LTD_4) and leukotriene E_4 (LTE_4) are important leukotrienes (Fig. 4.1).

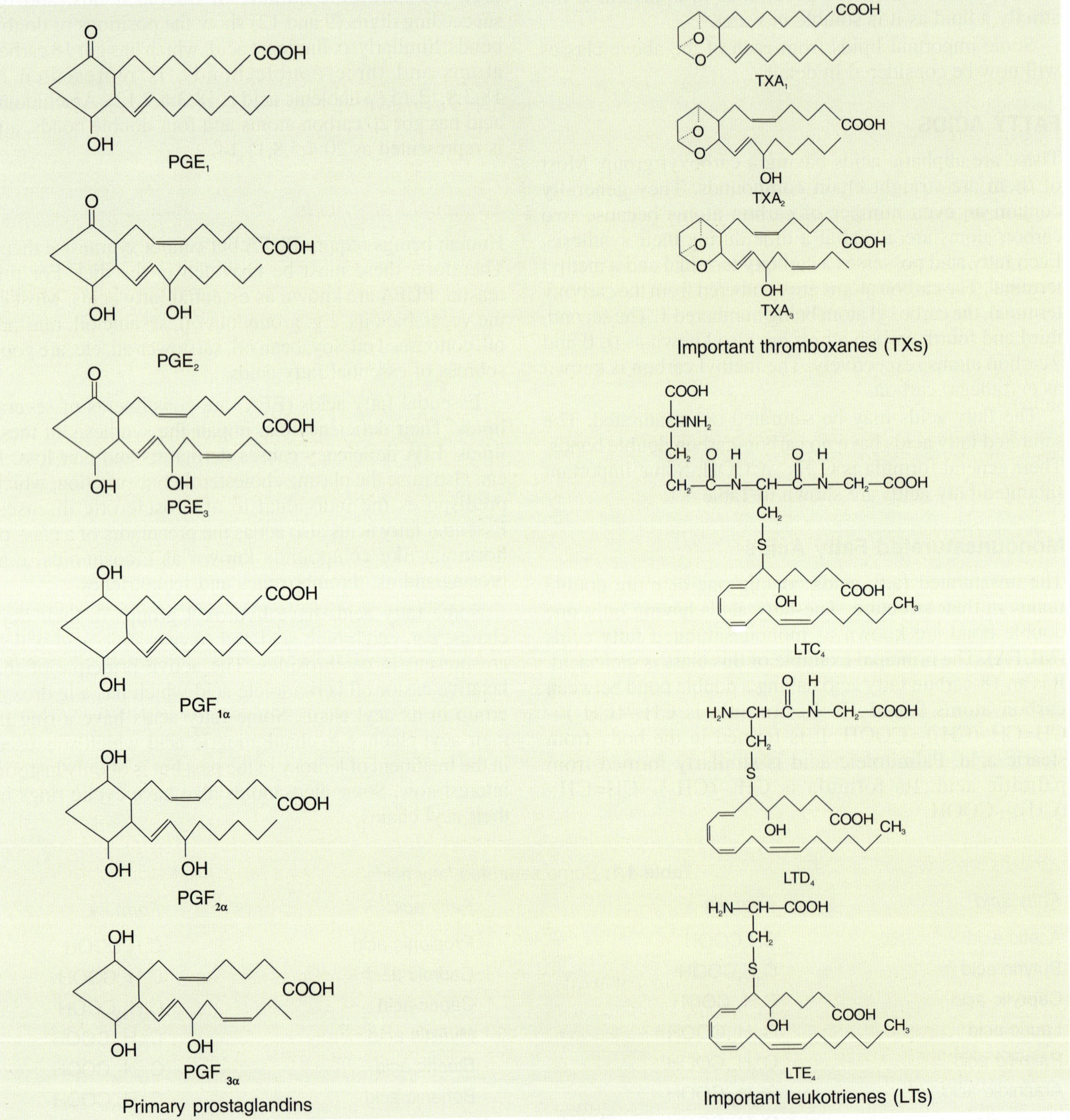

Primary prostaglandins

Important thromboxanes (TXs)

Important leukotrienes (LTs)

Fig. 4.1: Eicosanoids

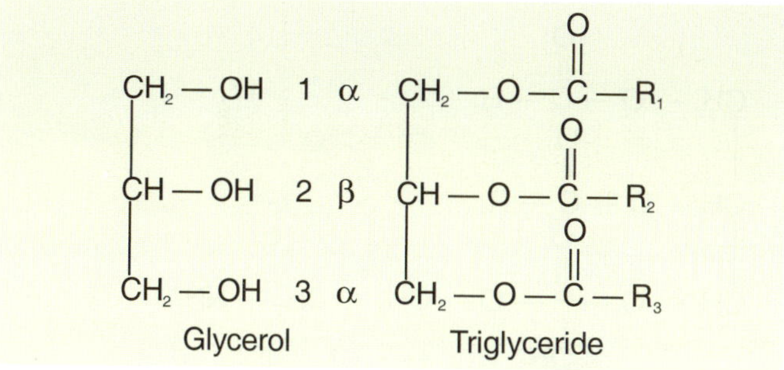

Fig. 4.2: Glycerol and triglyceride (triacylglycerol)

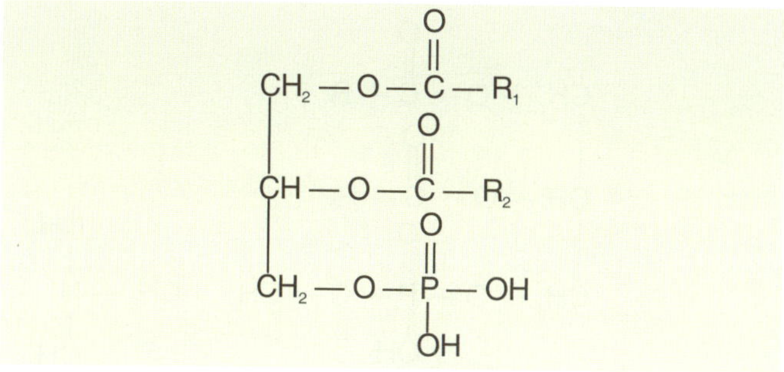

Fig. 4.3: Phosphatidic acid

GLYCEROL

Glycerol, though not a lipid itself, is found in many lipids, e.g. triglycerides and phospholipids. It is a trihydric alcohol.

In the past, the top and the bottom carbon atoms were termed as α-carbon atoms and the middle carbon atom was termed as the β-carbon atom. According to modern stereochemical numbering, the carbon atoms are numbered 1, 2 and 3 starting from top. The three–OH groups of glycerol can be esterified with acids, including fatty acids.

TRIGLYCERIDES

Triglycerides (TG) are formed by esterification of one molecule of glycerol with three molecules of fatty acids. They are also known as **triacylglycerols (TAG)** or neutral fats. They are the major storage form of energy. A large number of triglyceride molecules can coalesce with each other because of their hydrophobic nature to form fat globules. Triglycerides are stored mainly in cells known as adipocytes. A tissue rich in adipocytes is known as adipose tissue. Carbohydrates require an appreciable quantity of water for their storage in the body. Since lipids do not require water for their storage, a large amount of triglycerides can be stored in the body without too much increase in body weight. However, excessive accumulation of triglycerides in the body leads to obesity with its attendant health risks.

The fatty acids present in a triglyceride are generally different from each other. In Fig. 4.2, R_1, R_2 and R_3 represent the acyl groups of fatty acids. The first fatty acid is generally saturated, and the second and the third are generally unsaturated.

PHOSPHOLIPIDS

Phospholipids are widely distributed in the body. Some of them contain glycerol as the alcohol component while others contain sphingosine (sphingol). The former are known as **glycerophospholipids**, and the latter are known as **sphingophospholipids**.

Glycerophospholipids may be considered to be the derivatives of phosphatidic acid in which the –OH groups at positions 1 and 2 of glycerol are esterified with fatty

acids, and the –OH group at position 3 is esterified with phosphoric acid (Fig. 4.3).

The phosphate group of phosphatidic acid is linked with choline in phosphatidyl choline (lecithin), with ethanolamine in phosphatidyl ethanolamine (cephalin), with serine in phosphatidyl serine and with inositol in phosphatidyl inositol. Choline, ethanolamine and serine are nitrogenous compounds while inositol is a cyclic polyhydric alcohol. Two molecules of phosphatidic acid are linked, through their phosphate groups, with a molecule of glycerol in diphosphatidyl glycerol (cardiolipin). In plasmalogens, an unsaturated alcohol is linked with carbon 1 of glycerol by an ether bond.

Though lipids are nonpolar in general, some of them possess some polar groups. For example, glycero-phospholipids contain phosphoric acid and a nitrogenous base or inositol which are polar. Such lipids are said to be **amphipathic,** i.e. a part of the molecule is polar and a part nonpolar. Many functions of glycerophospholipids depend upon their amphipathic nature. Such functions include:

1. They are the predominant constituent of cell membrane and intacellular membranes. Due to their amphipathic nature, they form lipid bilayers with the hydrophobic tails oriented inwards when exposed to water.

2. Lecithin is a constituent of bile. Along with bile salts, it helps in the digestion of dietary lipids by emulsifying them.

3. Cardiolipin, which was first discovered in animal heart, is a major constituent of mitochondrial membrane.

4. Phosphatidyl inositol, present in cell membrane, is a precursor of inositol triphosphate and diacyl glycerol which are important in intracellular signalling.

5. Dipalmitoylphosphatidylcholine (DPPC), also known as disaturated phosphatidyl choline or dipalmitoyl lecithin, is a major constituent of lung surfactant.

Lung surfactant is a complex of some phospholipids and proteins. It is formed by type II alveolar cells in the lungs. Lipids constitute 90% of the complex and proteins form the rest. DPPC forms half of the lipid component.

The sphingophospholipids contain sphingosine as the alcohol portion. Sphingosine is a long chain amino alcohol

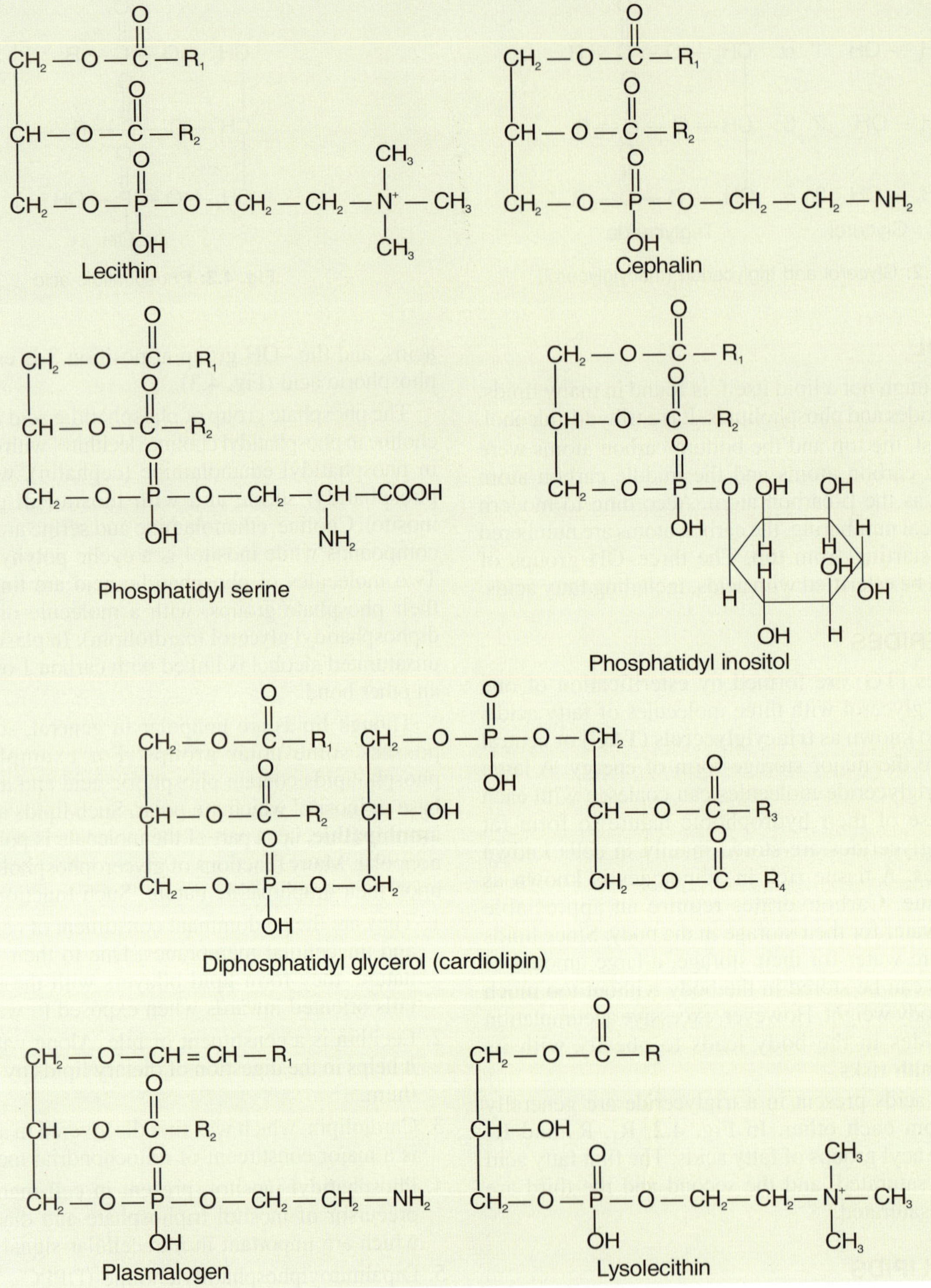

Fig. 4.4: Glycerophospholipids

which is synthesised from palmitic acid and serine. The most important sphingophospholipid in our body is sphingomyelin which is a constituent of nervous tissue and membranes. It is also present in lungs. Lecithin: sphingomyelin ratio in amniotic fluid is an indicator of foetal lung maturity. A ratio of less than 2 shows immaturity, and increases the risk of respiratory distress syndrome. Sphingomyelin is made up of sphingosine, a fatty acid, phosphoric acid and choline (Fig. 4.5).

CEREBROSIDES

Cerebrosides are glycolipids containing sphingosine, a fatty acid and galactose (Fig. 4.6). They are found in brain

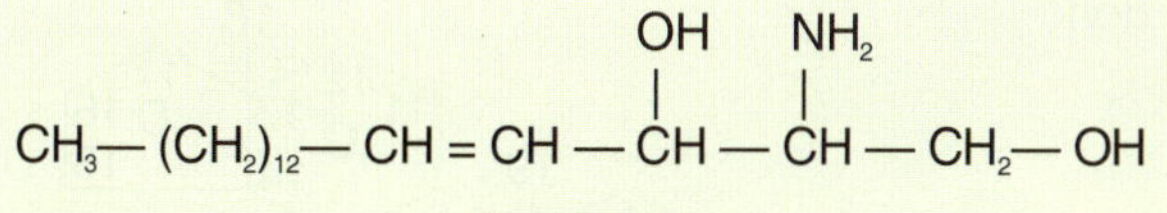

Fig. 4.5: Sphingosine and sphingomyelin

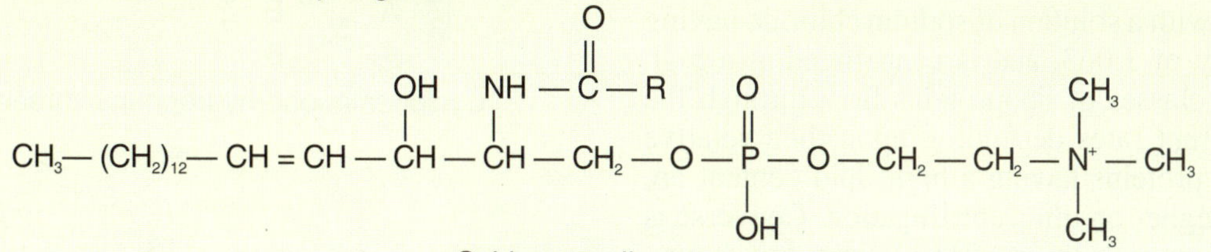

and some other tissues. Important cerebrosides are kerasin, cerebron, nervon and oxynervon which contain lignoceric acid, cerebronic acid, nervonic acid and oxynervonic acid respectively as the fatty acid component. These are very long chain (24-carbon) fatty acids.

SULPHATIDES

Sulphatides are also known as cerebroside sulphates. They differ from cerebrosides in that they contain galactose-3-sulphate instead of galactose (Fig. 4.6).

GANGLIOSIDES

Gangliosides are also glycolipids occurring in nervous tissue. They are made up of sphingosine, a fatty acid, N-acetylneuraminic acid (NANA), a number of hexoses and hexosamines (Fig. 4.6). Sphingosine linked with a fatty acid is known as acyl sphingosine or ceramide.

LIPOPROTEINS

Lipids constitute an important source of energy in our body. As they are insoluble in water, their transport in the aqueous environment of plasma poses a problem. This difficulty is overcome by combining the more insoluble lipids, e.g. triglycerides and cholesterol, with more polar ones, e.g. phospholipids, and then combining them with some proteins. The complex, so formed, is known as a lipoprotein. The lipoproteins contain some specific proteins, known as **apolipoproteins** or **apoproteins**, and variable amounts of lipids, e.g. triglycerides, cholesterol, phospholipids and free fatty acids.

Different types of lipoproteins are present in plasma. Increase in the concentration of certain lipoproteins is associated with an increased risk of developing athero-sclerosis. Therefore, separation and measurement of different plasma lipoproteins is often needed to identify the individuals who are prone to this disease. Separation

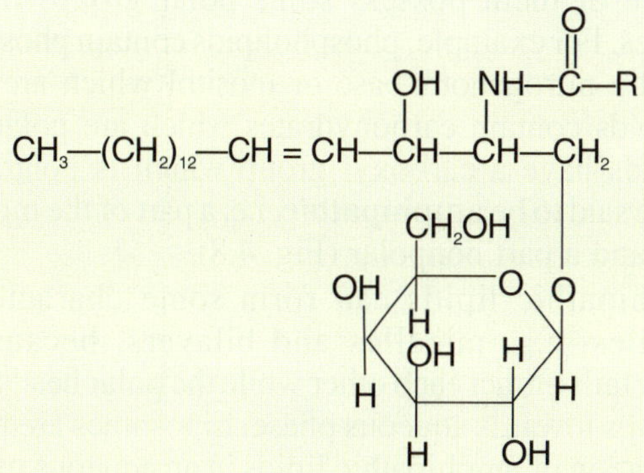

Cerebroside 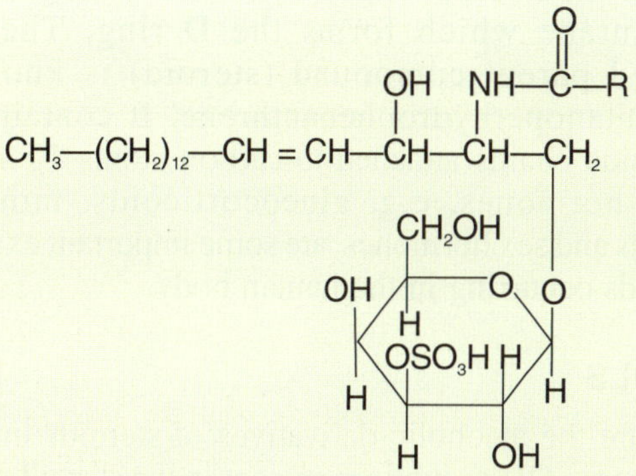   Sulphatide (cerebroside sulphate)

Ceramide – Glucose – Galactose – N-Acetyl galactosamine– Galactose
|
NANA

G_{M1} ganglioside

Fig. 4.6: Cerebroside, sulphatide and G_{M1} ganglioside

and quantitation of plasma lipoproteins is generally done by the following techniques:

1. Ultracentrifugation

Plasma is mixed with a solution of sodium chloride having a specific gravity of 1.063, and is centrifuged at a high speed. Different classes of lipoproteins float through the medium at different rates depending upon their relative density. The lipoproteins having a high lipid content are lighter and rise higher on ultracentrifugation. Converse is true of lipoproteins rich in proteins. After a few hours, four different layers are formed. From above downwards, these are:

   i. Chylomicrons (CM),
   ii. Very low density lipoproteins (VLDL),
   iii. Low density lipoproteins (LDL), and
   iv. High density lipoproteins (HDL).

2. Electrophoresis

Plasma is placed in an electric field in the presence of an appropriate buffer. Different classes of lipoproteins migrate at different speeds depending upon the electric charges present on them. After a few hours, four bands are formed:

   i. Chylomicrons (CM),
   ii. β-Lipoproteins,
   iii. Pre-β-lipoproteins, and
   iv. α-Lipoproteins.

The β-lipoproteins are chemically identical with LDL, the pre-β-lipoproteins with VLDL and the α-lipoproteins with HDL.

STEROIDS

Steroids are found in the unsaponifiable residue of lipids. They contain phenanthrene nucleus, made up of three six-membered rings (A, B and C rings) and a cyclopentane which forms the D ring. The fully saturated parent compound (steroid) is known as cyclopentanoperhydrophenanthrene. It contains two methyl side chains attached to carbon atoms 10 and 13. Steroid hormones, e.g. glucocorticoids, mineralocorticoids and sex hormones, are some important examples of steroids occurring in the human body.

STEROLS

Sterols are the alcoholic derivatives of steroids in which one or more –OH groups are present in the steroid nucleus but there are no carboxyl or carbonyl groups. Cholesterol, ergosterol, coprosterol and sitosterol are some important sterols. Cholesterol is the most important of these. It possesses an –OH group at carbon atom 3, a double bond between carbon atoms 5 and 6, and a side chain of eight carbon atoms at carbon atom 17. Cholesterol is the precursor of many important compounds in our body, e.g.

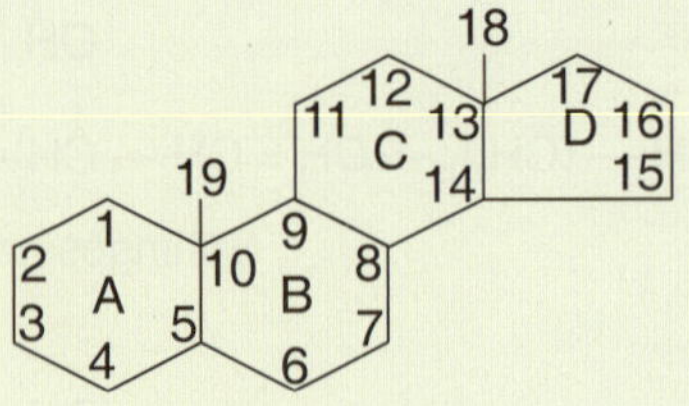

Cyclopentanoperhydrophenanthrene

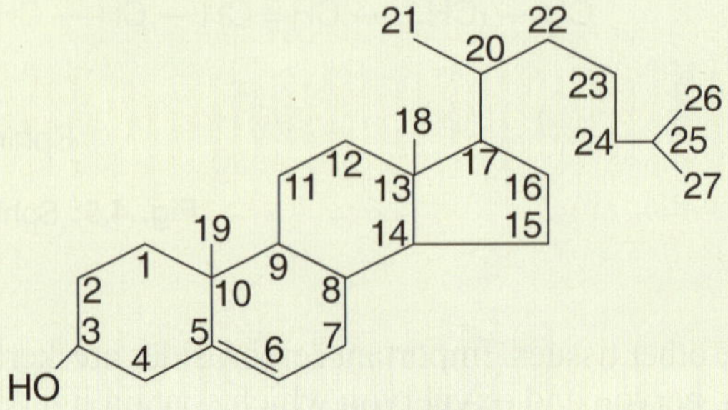

Cholesterol

Fig. 4.7: Steroid nucleus and cholesterol

vitamin D_3, steroid hormones, bile acids and bile salts. If an excess of cholesterol is present in plasma, it tends to get deposited in the walls of arterioles causing atherosclerosis.

Unsaturated sterols are dehydrated by strong dehydrating agents to form coloured products. Cholesterol is often detected by Salkowski's and Liebermann-Burchard reactions. In the former, cholesterol is treated with concentrated sulphuric acid, and is dehydrated to cholestadiene and its polymers which are red in colour. In the latter, cholesterol is treated with concentrated sulphuric acid and acetic anhydride. Cholesterol is dehydrated to cholestadiene and its polymers which are sulphonated to form a green or blue complex.

As mentioned earlier, the lipids are nonpolar in general but some of them possess some polar groups in their molecules. For example, phospholipids contain phosphoric acid and a nitrogenous base or inositol which are polar. Glycolipids contain carbohydrates which are polar. Free fatty acids have a carboxyl group which is polar. Such lipids are said to be **amphipathic,** i.e. a part of the molecule is polar and a part nonpolar (Fig. 4.8).

Amphipathic lipids can form some characteristic assemblies, e.g. micelles and bilayers, because the nonpolar tails attract each other while the polar heads orient themselves towards aqueous phase. Liposomes are formed by sonication of amphipathic lipids in an aqueous medium (Fig. 4.9). They can be used for drug delivery. The drug present in the hydrophilic core of the liposome is delivered inside a cell when the lipid bilayer of the cell fuses with the lipid bilayer of the liposome.

Lipid bilayers constitute the basic structure of membranes (Fig. 4.10). In addition to lipids such as phospholipids and cholesterol, membranes also contain

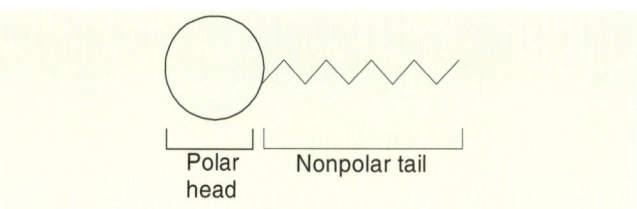

Fig. 4.8: Amphipathic lipid

simple proteins and glycoproteins which may be present on the inner and outer surface (peripheral proteins) or across the membrane (integral proteins).

One of the important attributes of membranes is their fluidity which is important to permit passage of various molecules and ions through the membrane. A membrane changes from the rigid, *gel* form into a fluid, *sol* form at a particular temperature which is known as the **transition temperature** of the membrane. If the transition temperature is high, the membrane tends to be rigid. The transition temperature depends upon:

a. The length of fatty acids,

b. The degree of saturation of fatty acids, and

c. The cholesterol content of the membrane.

Long chain fatty acids and saturated fatty acids increase the transition temperature. In the naturally occurring unsaturated fatty acids, the double bonds are in *cis* configuration which introduce kinks in the hydrocarbon chain (Fig. 4.11). Kinked or bent hydrocarbon chains make the membrane less compact and more fluid. Cholesterol

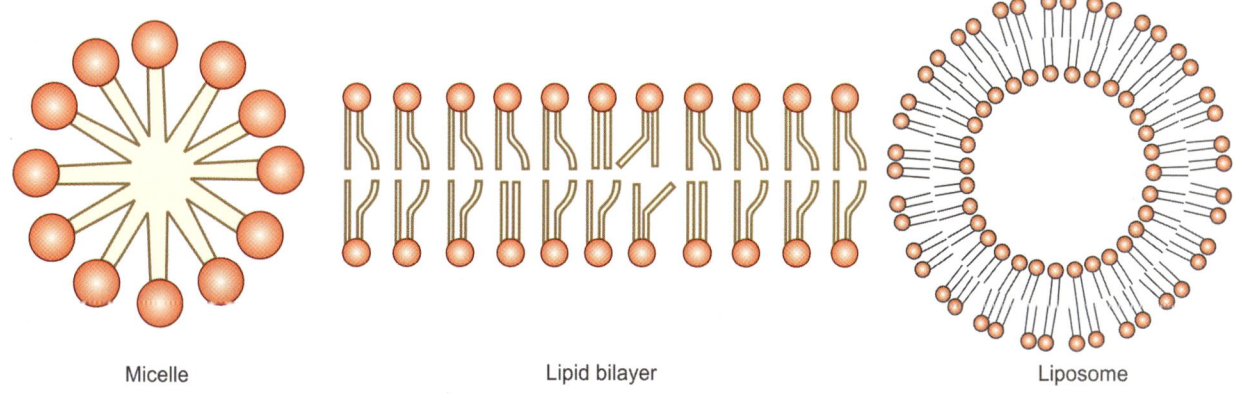

Micelle   Lipid bilayer   Liposome

Fig. 4.9: Different lipid assemblies

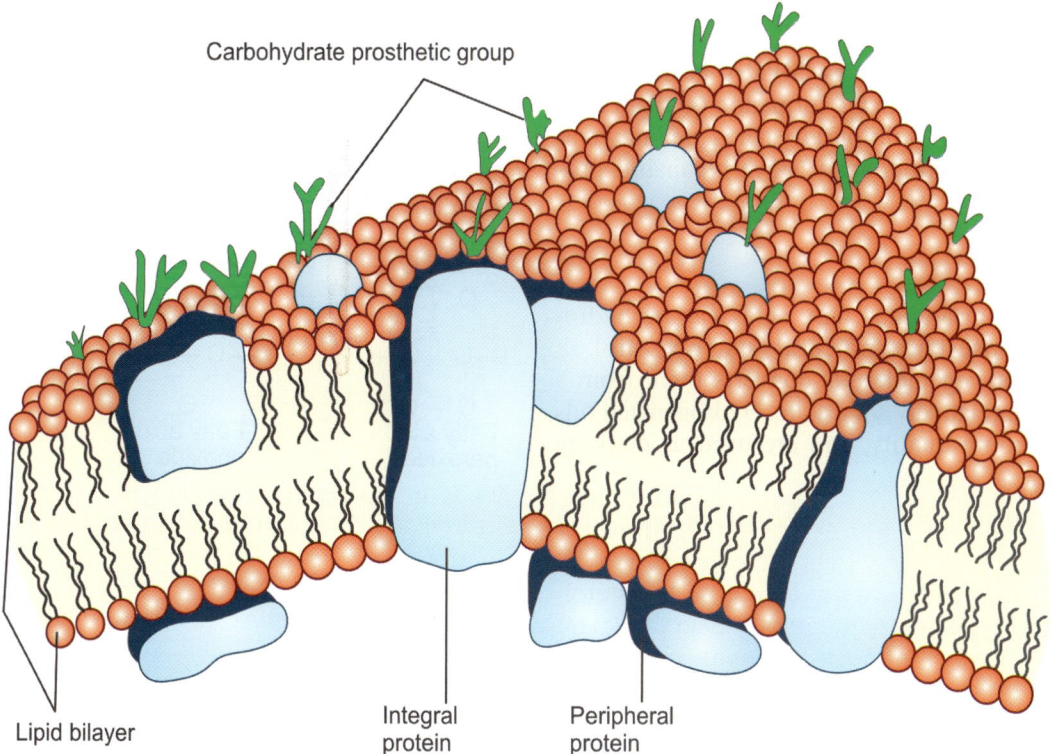

Carbohydrate prosthetic group

Lipid bilayer   Integral protein   Peripheral protein

Fig. 4.10: Fluid mosaic model of a membrane

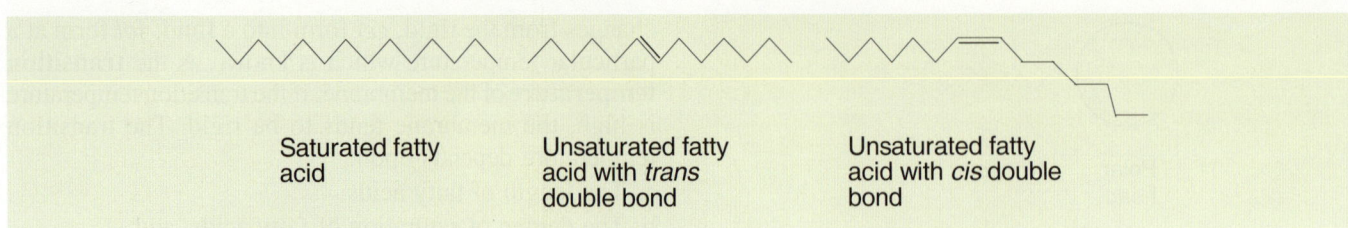

Saturated fatty acid   **Unsaturated fatty acid with *trans* double bond**   **Unsaturated fatty acid with *cis* double bond**

Fig. 4.11: Bends or kinks are produced in the hydrocarbon chain by *cis* double bonds

increases the transition temperature and makes the membrane rigid.

Physical Properties of Lipids

As mentioned earlier, lipids are insoluble in water and soluble in organic solvents. They are greasy in nature. If a small amount of a lipid dissolved in an organic solvent is put on a filter paper, the solvent evaporates leaving a transluscent greasy spot on the filter paper. Triglycerides having a preponderance of unsaturated fatty acids (oils) are liquid at room temperature. Others are solid at room temperature. Oils have a high boiling point (food gets cooked quickly in oils due to their high boiling point).

Chemical Reactions of Lipids

1. Hydrolysis

The ester bonds of lipids can be hydrolysed by specific enzymes.

2. Saponification

Hydrolysis of triglycerides by alkalis is known as saponification, and results in the formation of alkali salts of fatty acids. The alkali salts of fatty acids are known as soaps. Being amphipathic, soaps have cleansing pro-perties.

3. Hydrogenation

Double bonds of unsaturated fatty acids can be hydro-genated in the presence of catalysts, e.g. nickel. Hydrogenation of vegetable oils converts them from a liquid state into a relatively solid state. Hydrogenated oils have better keeping quality, and are used as cooking mediums.

$$-C=C- \xrightarrow[H_2]{Ni} -\overset{\overset{\displaystyle H}{|}}{C}-\overset{\overset{\displaystyle H}{|}}{C}-$$

4. Iodination

Iodine can also reduce the double bonds of unsaturated fatty acids.

$$-C=C- \xrightarrow{I_2} -\overset{|}{C}-\overset{|}{C}-$$

The degree of unsaturation is an important property of a lipid which can be ascertained by measuring its iodine number. Iodine number is the number of gm of iodine required to saturate all the double bonds in 100 gm of the lipid. A higher iodine number means a greater degree of unsaturation.

5. Oxidation

Unsaturated fatty acids can spontaneously react with atmospheric oxygen to form fatty acid peroxides, fatty acids epoxides and fatty acid aldehydes. Fat which undergoes this type of oxidation becomes rancid. Rancid fat is unpleasant in taste and smell, and can be toxic. Rancidity is prevented by anti-oxidants, e.g. vitamin E.

$$-C=C- \xrightarrow{O_2} -C=C-$$
Fatty acid peroxide

$$-C=C- \xrightarrow{[O]} -C-C-$$
Fatty acid epoxide

$$-C=C- \xrightarrow{O_2} -CH + HC-$$
Fatty acid aldehyde

EXERCISE

1. Classify lipids giving examples. Describe the structure and functions of cholesterol.

2. What are lipoproteins? Describe the composition and methods of separation of plasma lipoproteins.

3. Write short note on:
   a. Essential fatty acids
   b. Eicosanoids
   c. Sphingolipids
   d. Transition temperature

4. Write 'true' or 'false':
   a. Oleic acid is a polyunsaturated fatty acid.
   b. Arachidonic acid is a 20-carbon polyunsaturated fatty acid.
   c. Vegetable oils are poor in essential fatty acids.
   d. Prostaglandins, thromboxanes and leukotrienes are collectively known as eicosanoids.
   e. Sphingosine is present in sulphatides and gangliosides.
   f. Cerebrosides are made up of glycerol, a fatty acid and galactose.
   g. Cerebrosides contain very long chain fatty acids.
   h. Cholesterol increases the fluidity of membranes.
   i. Unsaturated fatty acids increase the transition temperature of membranes.
   j. Naturally occurring unsaturated fatty acids have *cis* double bonds.

5. Fill in the blanks:
   a. Fatty acids having more than one double bonds are known as .... fatty acids.
   b. Linoleic acid, linolenic acid and arachidonic acid are .... fatty acids for human beings.
   c. .... oils are good sources of essential fatty acids.
   d. Eicosanoids are synthesised from .... fatty acids.
   e. The nitrogenous base in lecithin is ....
   f. Sphingosine can be synthesised from palmitic acid and ....
   g. Ceramide is made up of .... and a ....
   h. Vitamin D_3 can be synthesised from ....

ANSWERS TO SHORT QUESTIONS

4. a. False
   b. True
   c. False
   d. True
   e. True
   f. False
   g. True
   h. False
   i. False
   j. True

5. a. Polyunsaturated
   b. Essential
   c. Vegetable
   d. Polyunsaturated
   e. Choline
   f. Serine
   g. Sphingosine, fatty acid
   h. Cholesterol

Chemistry of Amino Acids and Proteins

Proteins are among the most important biomolecules. Living cells produce a vast array of proteins which perform a variety of biological functions. Proteins are polymers of amino acids. Structures and functions of proteins depend upon the nature of amino acids present in them, the sequence in which the amino acids are present and the spatial relationship of the amino acids with one another.

AMINO ACIDS

Amino acids are carboxylic acids having one or more amino groups. The carbon atoms of the amino acids are numbered 1, 2, 3, etc. starting from the carboxyl group. They are also named α, β, γ, etc. starting from the carbon atom next to the carboxyl group (Fig. 5.1).

The amino group may be attached to any of the carbon atoms next to the carboxyl group. The amino acid is accordingly known as α-amino acid (2-amino acid), β-amino acid (3-amino acid), γ-amino acid (4-amino acid), etc (Fig. 5.2).

Proteins are made up of only α-amino acids. The α-amino acids contain at least one **asymmetric carbon atom**. Therefore, they exhibit **stereoisomerism** and **optical isomerism**. The amino acid can exist as a D-isomer and an L-isomer. The amino group is present on the right hand side of the asymmetric α-carbon in D-amino acids, and on the left hand side in L-amino acids (Fig. 5.3).

Glycine is the only amino acid that has no asymmetric carbon atom and, hence, no stereoisomers. Threonine, isoleucine, hydroxylysine and hydroxyproline have two asymmetric carbon atoms, and have four stereoisomers each. The asymmetric carbon atom also confers optical activity on the amino acid. One of the stereoisomers is dextrorotatotry (+), and the other laevorotatory (–).

$$R - CH_2 - CH_2 - \underset{\underset{NH_2}{|}}{CH} - COOH$$

α-Amino acid (2-amino acid)

$$R - CH_2 - \underset{\underset{NH_2}{|}}{CH} - CH_2 - COOH$$

β-Amino acid (3-amino acid)

$$R - \underset{\underset{NH_2}{|}}{CH} - CH_2 - CH_2 - COOH$$

γ-Amino acid (4-amino acid)

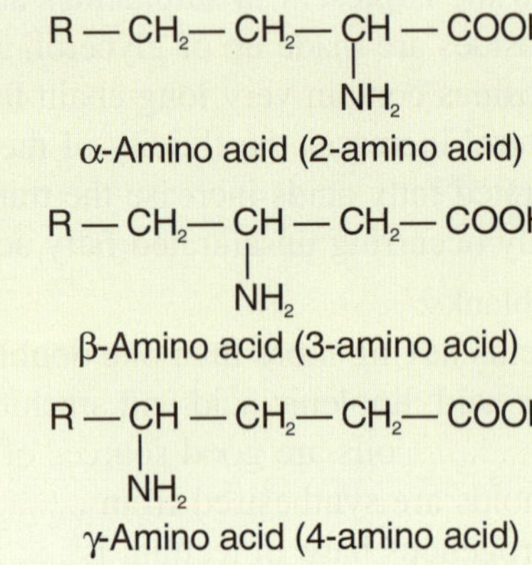

Fig. 5.2: α-, β- and γ-amino acids

About 300 amino acids have been found in nature but only 20 of these are used to synthesise proteins in all life forms whether animal, plant or microbial. These 20 amino acids are frequently described as **standard amino acids**. All the amino acids used to synthesise proteins are L-amino acids. If the prefix L- or D- is not shown, it is presumed that the given amino acid is an L-amino acid.

Each amino acid is also described by a one-letter abbreviation and a three-letter abbreviation. The sequence of amino acids in proteins is generally shown by these abbreviations. The standard amino acids, with their three-letter abbreviations in parentheses, are glycine (gly), alanine (ala), valine (val), leucine (leu), isoleucine (ile), serine (ser), threonine (thr), cysteine (cys), methionine (met), aspartate (asp), asparagine (asn), glutamate (glu), glutamine (gln), arginine (arg), histidine (his), lysine (lys), phenylalanine (phe), tyrosine (tyr), tryptophan (trp) and proline (pro). After the synthesis of a protein, lysine and

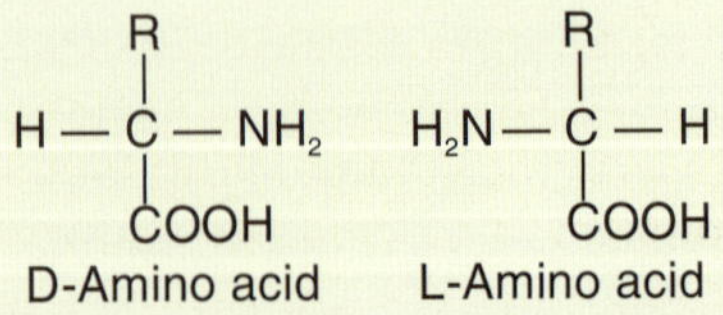

$$\underset{4}{R} - \underset{3}{CH_2} - \underset{2}{CH_2} - \underset{\alpha}{CH_2} - COOH$$
$$ \quad \gamma \qquad \beta \qquad \alpha$$

Fig. 5.1: A carboxylic acid

$$H - \underset{\underset{COOH}{|}}{\overset{\overset{R}{|}}{C}} - NH_2 \qquad H_2N - \underset{\underset{COOH}{|}}{\overset{\overset{R}{|}}{C}} - H$$

D-Amino acid   L-Amino acid

Fig. 5.3: Stereoisomers of an α-amino acid

proline residues of the protein may be hydroxylated to hydroxylysine and hydroxyproline respectively.

CLASSIFICATION

The standard amino acids can be classified in several ways. Three commonly used systems of classification are:

According to Nutritional Importance

The amino acids are classified, according to their nutritional importance, into three groups:

1. *Essential Amino Acids*

These include valine, leucine, isoleucine, threonine, methionine, lysine, phenylalanine and tryptophan. These amino acids can not be synthesised in human beings, and must be provided in diet. Their deficiency or absence from the diet can seriously impair the normal functioning of the body.

2. *Semi-essential Amino Acids*

Arginine and histidine are included in this group. These can be synthesised in the human body to some extent. However, their synthesis is not sufficient to meet the requirements of growing children. Therefore, these must be provided in the diet of children.

3. *Non-essential Amino Acids*

The remaining amino acids which are not included in the above two groups, i.e. glycine, alanine, serine, cysteine, glutamate, glutamine, aspartate, asparagine, tyrosine and proline are considered to be non-essential for human beings because these can be synthesised in the human body. However, this does not mean that these amino acids are not required by human beings. All the 20 amino acids occurring in proteins are required by human beings. The non-essential amino acids are only nutritionally non-essential because of their endogenous synthesis in the human body.

According to Polarity

The carboxyl and amino groups attached to the α-carbon atom are electrically charged, and are, therefore, polar in all the α-amino acids. However, the side chain (–R) attached to the α-carbon atom may be polar or nonpolar. Those amino acids that contain some dissociable groups in the side chain are known as polar amino acids, and are highly soluble in polar solvents such as water. These include glycine, serine, threonine, cysteine, aspartate, asparagine, glutamate, glutamine, arginine, lysine, histidine and tyrosine. The amino acids that have no ionisable groups in the side chain are known as non-polar amino acids, and include alanine, valine, leucine,

isoleucine, methionine, phenylalanine, tryptophan and proline. However, these amino acids are not absolutely nonpolar. These are less polar and less soluble in polar solvents than the polar amino acids. In transmembrane proteins, nonpolar amino acids are generally embedded in the lipid bilayer while the polar amino acids are present outside or inside the membrane.

According to Chemical Nature of Side Chain

The amino acids can be divided into seven groups according to the chemical nature of their side chains (Fig. 5.4).

1. *Amino Acids with Aliphatic Side Chains*

This group includes glycine, alanine, valine, leucine and isoleucine. Glycine is the smallest amino acid, having no asymmetric carbon, stereoisomers and optical isomers. Its side chain is made up of a single hydrogen atom. Because of its small side chain, it can easily fit into crowded regions of protein molecules. It is the most abundant amino acid in collagen. Beside proteins, many other specialised products are formed from glycine (*see* Chapter 12). It also acts as a neurotransmitter.

The side chain in alanine is a methyl group. Valine, leucine and isoleucine have bulky aliphatic side chains which are branched. Isoleucine has got an additional asymmetric carbon atom (β-carbon), and has four stereoisomers. The aliphatic side chains of these amino acids attract each other because of their hydrophobic nature. These amino acids tend to occupy the core of globular proteins. In transmembrane proteins, they are usually embedded in the lipid bilayer of the membrane.

2. *Amino Acids with Side Chains having Hydroxyl Group*

This group includes serine and threonine. The –OH group in the side chain of these amino acids can form an ester bond with phosphoric acid and a glycosidic bond with carbohydrates. Many regulatory proteins undergo reversible phosphorylation-dephosphorylation. In such proteins, the phosphate group is generally bonded to the –OH group of serine residues. In O-linked glycoproteins, the oligosaccharide prosthetic group is bonded to the –OH group of a serine residue in many cases, and to that of a threonine residue in some cases. Serine residues are present at the catalytic site of many enzymes, and play a role in catalysis. Threonine has an additional asymmetric carbon atom (β-carbon) in its side chain, and has four stereoisomers.

3. *Amino Acids with Side Chains containing Sulphur*

Cysteine and methionine belong to this group. The sulphur atom is present in the form of a sulphydryl (–SH) group in cysteine while it is bonded to a methyl group in methionine.

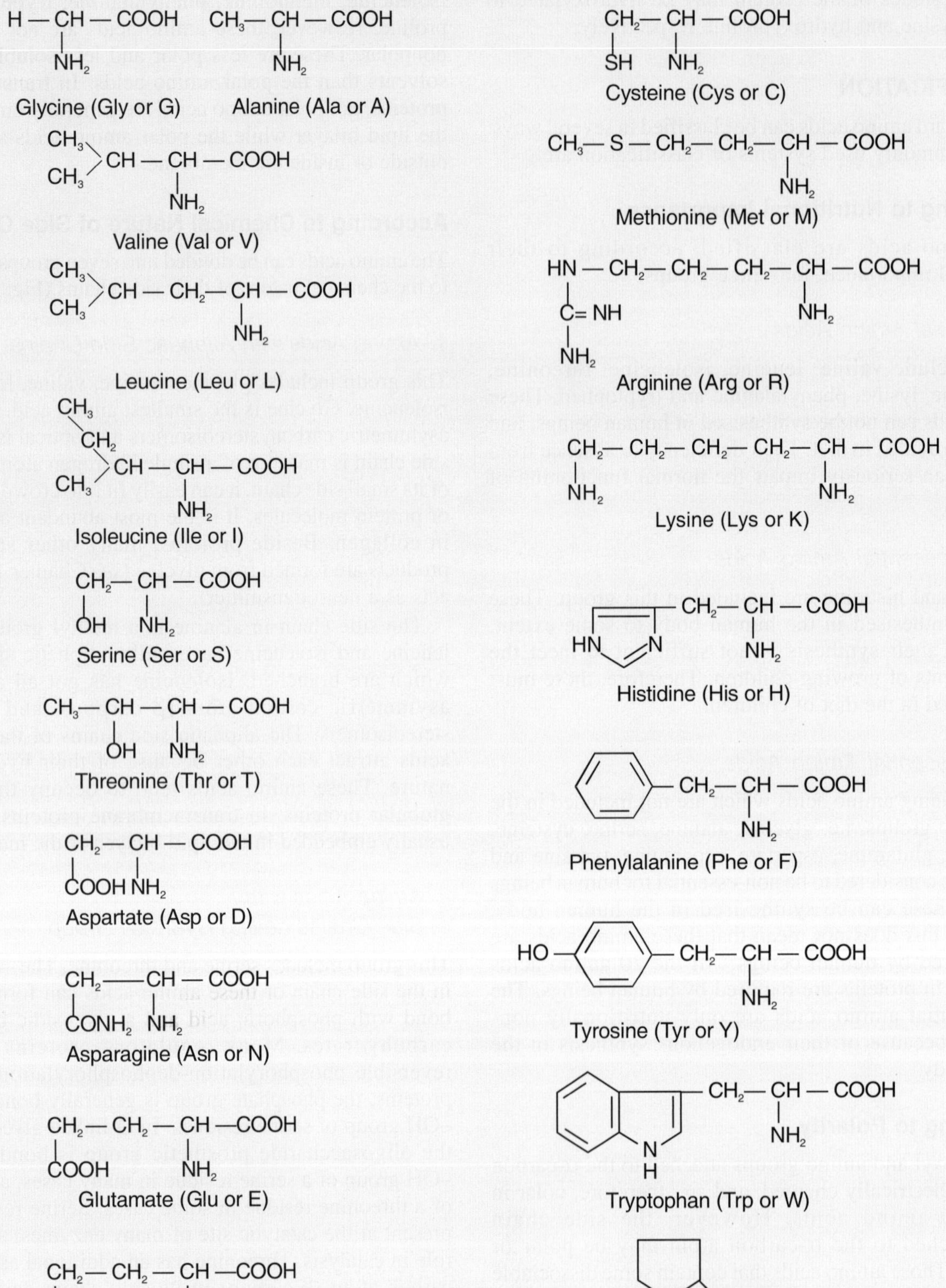

H — CH — COOH
    |
    NH$_2$

Glycine (Gly or G)

CH$_3$— CH — COOH
    |
    NH$_2$

Alanine (Ala or A)

CH$_3$
    \
     CH — CH — COOH
    / |
CH$_3$ NH$_2$

Valine (Val or V)

CH$_3$
    \
     CH — CH$_2$— CH — COOH
    / |
CH$_3$ NH$_2$

Leucine (Leu or L)

CH$_3$
 |
CH$_2$
  \
   CH — CH — COOH
  / |
CH$_3$ NH$_2$

Isoleucine (Ile or I)

CH$_2$— CH — COOH
 | |
OH   NH$_2$

Serine (Ser or S)

CH$_3$— CH — CH — COOH
     | |
     OH NH$_2$

Threonine (Thr or T)

CH$_2$— CH — COOH
 | |
COOH NH$_2$

Aspartate (Asp or D)

CH$_2$——CH — COOH
 | |
CONH$_2$ NH$_2$

Asparagine (Asn or N)

CH$_2$— CH$_2$— CH —COOH
 | |
COOH   NH$_2$

Glutamate (Glu or E)

CH$_2$— CH$_2$— CH —COOH
 | |
CONH$_2$ NH$_2$

Glutamine (Gln or Q)

CH$_2$— CH — COOH
 | |
SH   NH$_2$

Cysteine (Cys or C)

CH$_3$— S — CH$_2$— CH$_2$— CH — COOH
                        |
                        NH$_2$

Methionine (Met or M)

HN — CH$_2$— CH$_2$— CH$_2$— CH — COOH
 | |
C= NH   NH$_2$
 |
NH$_2$

Arginine (Arg or R)

CH$_2$— CH$_2$— CH$_2$— CH$_2$— CH — COOH
 | |
NH$_2$ NH$_2$

Lysine (Lys or K)

CH$_2$— CH — COOH
         |
         NH$_2$

Histidine (His or H)

(benzene ring)— CH$_2$— CH — COOH
                   |
                   NH$_2$

Phenylalanine (Phe or F)

HO —(benzene ring)— CH$_2$— CH — COOH
                           |
                          NH$_2$

Tyrosine (Tyr or Y)

(indole ring)— CH$_2$— CH — COOH
                    |
                    NH$_2$

Tryptophan (Trp or W)

(pyrrolidine ring)
  N   COOH
  |
  H

Proline (Pro or P)

Fig. 5.4: Structural formulae of standard amino acids with their three-letter and one-letter abbreviations in parentheses

The –SH groups of cysteine residues play a vital role in the functioning of several enzymes, and other peptides and proteins, e.g. glutathione, thioredoxin, etc. Mercury, lead and iodoacetamide can combine with the free –SH groups and inactivate these proteins. The –SH groups of cysteine residues also play a role in structural organisation of proteins by forming disulphide bonds (explained later).

The methyl group in the side chain of methionine is used in many methylation reactions. Methionine is converted into S-adenosyl methionine (active methionine) which is a donor of labile methyl groups.

4. Amino Acids with Side Chains having Acidic Groups or their Amides

This group includes aspartate, glutamate, asparagine and glutamine. Aspartate and glutamate have a second carboxylic group in their side chains, and are known as dicarboxylic amino acids. Asparagine and glutamine are the amide derivatives of aspartate and glutamine respectively. Aspartate is present at the catalytic site of some proteolytic enzymes (aspartyl proteases). Glutamate plays an important role in the disposal of amino nitrogen of proteins. It also acts as an excitatory neurotransmitter in brain. The amide group in the side chain of asparagine takes part in the formation of hydrogen bonds. In N-linked glycoproteins, the carbohydrate prosthetic group is bonded to the amide group of asparagine residues.

Glutamine is the most abundant amino acid in our body. Conversion of glutamate into glutamine is an important mechanism for detoxification of ammonia in brain. Converion of glutamine into glutamate and ammonia in renal tubular cells is important in renal regulation of blood pH.

5. Amino Acids with Side Chains having Basic Groups

The amino acids in this group are arginine, lysine and histidine. Lysine and arginine possess an additional amino group in their side chains, and are known as diamino acids. In arginine, the additional –NH$_2$ group is present as part of a guanidino group. An imidazole group is present in the side chain of histidine. Lysine and hydroxylysine residues play a role in stabilising the structure of collagen (explained later). Some prosthetic groups, e.g. biotin and retinal, are bonded to the epsilon-amino groups of lysine residues in the proteins. Arginine is the precursor of urea and nitric oxide. Histidine residues are present at the catalytic site of some proteases. Histidine residues of heamoglobin bind iron. Histidine residues of proteins play an important role in pH regulation.

6. Amino Acids with Side Chains containing Aromatic Rings

This group includes phenylalanine, tyrosine and tryptophan. These are also known as aromatic amino acids.

The side chain of phenylalanine contains a phenyl group while that of tyrosine has a hydroxyphenyl group. Tyrosine can be synthesised in the body by hydroxylation of phenylalanine. A number of specialised products are synthesised from phenylalanine and tyrosine.

An indole group is present in the side chain of tryptophan. Tryptophan is the bulkiest amino acid amongst the twenty standard amino acids. A number of specialised products are synthesised from tryptophan.

7. Imino Acids

Instead of an amino group, an imino group is present which is a part of a heterocyclic ring. Proline is the only member of this group. α-Amino group of proline is bonded with C$_5$ of the side chain, and is converted into an imino group. C$_2$,C$_3$, C$_4$, C$_5$ and L-imino group form a rigid heterocyclic ring. The imino group can from a peptide bond with the carboxyl group of another amino acid, which may have a *cis* or a *trans* configuration.

Lysine and proline can be hydroxylated to hydroxylysine and hydroxyproline respectively after their incorporation into proteins. Therefore, hydrolysis of proteins may yield hydroxylysine and hydroxyproline also. Two cysteine residues in a protein may be linked through their –SH groups to form a cystine residue (Fig. 5.5). Some enzymes contain an unusual amino acid, selenocysteine, at their catalytic site. Selenocysteine is formed from serine by replacement of the oxygen atom in the side chain of serine by selenium. This transformation occurs before the incorporation of serine into the protein. Glutathione peroxidase is an example of a selenocysteine-containing enzyme.

$$CH_2 - CH - COOH$$
$$| \qquad |$$
$$SeH \quad NH_2$$

Selenocysteine

Besides the standard amino acids, some other L-α-amino acids are also found in human beings either as intermediates or as products of various metabolic pathways. These are shown in Fig. 5.6.

Some non-α-amino acids are also present in human beings, e.g. β-alanine, taurine, β-aminoisobutyric acid, γ-aminobutyric acid, etc (Fig. 5.7). β-Alanine is a constituent of the vitamin, pantothenic acid and of acyl carrier protein and coenzyme A. The amino group is attached to the β-carbon in this amino acid. Taurine is a neurotransmitter, and is a constituent of bile acids and bile salts. Taurine has a sulphonic acid group instead of a carboxylic group attached to the α-carbon atom. Its amino group is attached to the β-carbon atom. β-Amino-isobutyric acid is a metabolite of some pyrimidines. γ-Aminobutyric acid is formed by decarboxylation of glutamic acid. The amino group is attached to the γ-carbon atom. It acts as a neurotransmitter in brain.

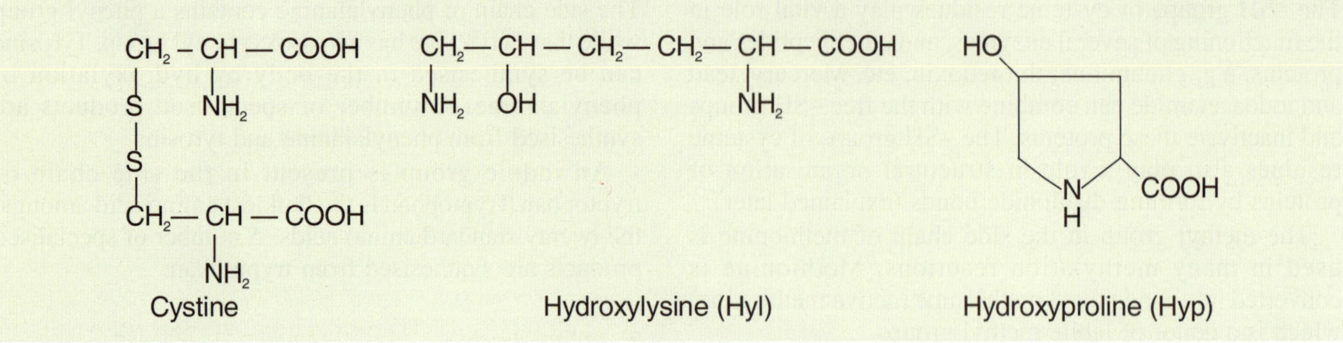

CH₂ – CH — COOH
| |
S   NH₂
|
S
|
CH₂— CH — COOH
|
NH₂

Cystine

CH₂— CH — CH₂— CH₂— CH — COOH
| | |
NH₂   OH   NH₂

Hydroxylysine (Hyl)

Hydroxyproline (Hyp)

Fig. 5.5: Cystine, hydroxylysine and hydroxyproline are formed from standard amino acids after the synthesis of proteins

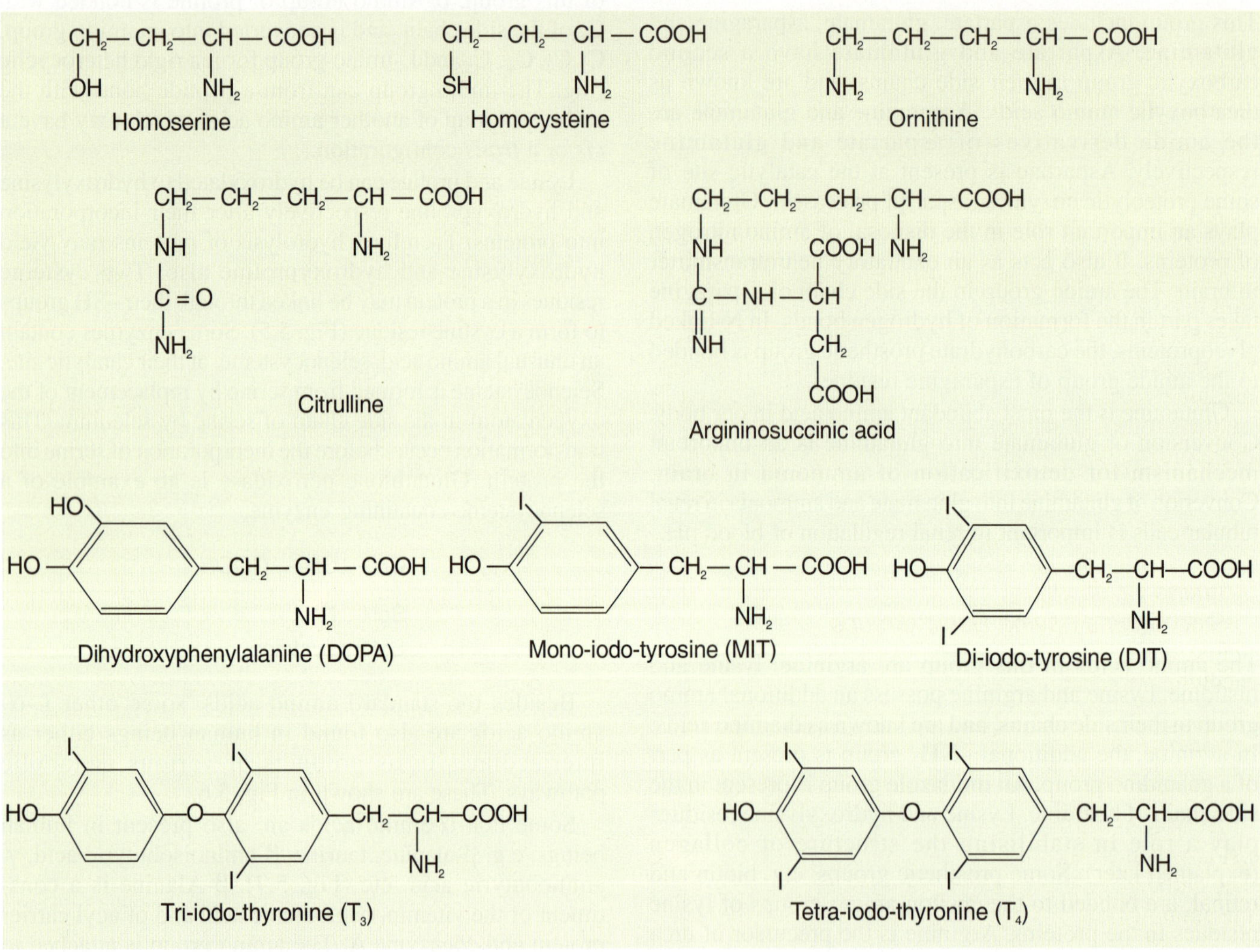

CH₂— CH₂— CH — COOH
| |
OH   NH₂

Homoserine

CH₂— CH₂— CH — COOH
| |
SH   NH₂

Homocysteine

CH₂— CH₂— CH₂— CH — COOH
| |
NH₂   NH₂

Ornithine

CH₂— CH₂— CH₂— CH — COOH
| |
NH   NH₂
|
C = O
|
NH₂

Citrulline

CH₂— CH₂— CH₂— CH — COOH
| |
NH   COOH NH₂
| |
C — NH — CH
‖ |
NH   CH₂
                    |
                   COOH

Argininosuccinic acid

CH₂— CH — COOH
|
NH₂

Dihydroxyphenylalanine (DOPA)

CH₂— CH — COOH
|
NH₂

Mono-iodo-tyrosine (MIT)

CH₂—CH—COOH
|
NH₂

Di-iodo-tyrosine (DIT)

CH₂—CH—COOH
|
NH₂

Tri-iodo-thyronine (T₃)

CH₂—CH—COOH
|
NH₂

Tetra-iodo-thyronine (T₄)

Fig. 5.6: Some non-standard α-amino acids

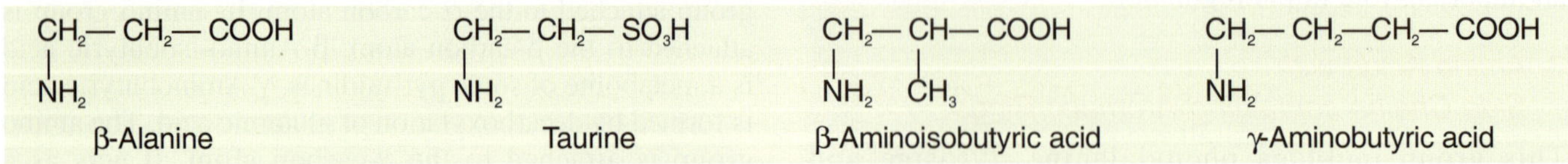

CH₂— CH₂— COOH
|
NH₂

β-Alanine

CH₂— CH₂— SO₃H
|
NH₂

Taurine

CH₂— CH— COOH
| |
NH₂   CH₃

β-Aminoisobutyric acid

CH₂— CH₂—CH₂— COOH
|
NH₂

γ-Aminobutyric acid

Fig. 5.7: Some β- and γ-amino acids

Physical Properties

Amino acids are crystalline solids. They are soluble in polar solvents, e.g. water and ethanol, and insoluble in nonpolar solvents, e.g. ether, chloroform, etc. The aromatic amino acids absorb ultraviolet light. All amino acids have high melting points.

Chemical Properties

1. Amphoteric Nature

All amino acids have at least one carboxyl and one amino group. Both of these are ionisable. Carboxyl group can donate a proton. Amino group can accept a proton.

$$R - COOH \underset{+ H^+}{\overset{- H^+}{\rightleftharpoons}} R - COO^-$$

$$R - NH_2 \underset{- H^+}{\overset{+ H^+}{\rightleftharpoons}} R - NH_3^+$$

R–COOH and R–NH$_3$$^+$ are the acidic forms as they can donate hydrogen ions (protons). R–COO$^-$ and R–NH$_2$ are conjugate bases as they can accept hydrogen ions. Thus, amino acids can act as acids (proton donors) as well as bases (proton acceptors). Therefore, they are said to be amphoteric in nature. Whether they will behave as acids or bases at a given time depends upon the pH of the medium in which they are present. In an alkaline medium, the carboxyl group is dissociated while ionisation of the amino group is suppressed. The amino acid, therefore, behaves as an acid in an alkaline medium.

$$\underset{NH_2}{R-CH-COOH} \rightleftharpoons \underset{NH_2}{R-CH-COO^-} + H^+$$

In an acidic medium, the amino group is ionised while ionisation of the carboxyl group is suppressed. Thus, the amino acid acts as a proton acceptor (base) in an acidic medium.

$$\underset{NH_2}{R-CH-COOH} + H^+ \rightleftharpoons \underset{NH_3^+}{R-CH-COOH}$$

Between these two extremes, there is a certain pH at which both carboxyl and amino groups are ionised. The carboxyl group exists in the unprotonated form and the amino group in the protonated form.

$$\underset{NH_3^+}{R-CH-COO^-}$$

This form of amino acid is known as a **zwitterion** as it has both an anionic and a cationic group. Though both carboxyl and amino groups are ionised, the molecule as a whole is electrically neutral, and does not move when placed in an electric field. The pH at which an amino acid exists in the zwitterion form is known as its isoelectric pH or isoelectric point (i.e.p.). This is constant for every amino acid. The solubility of the amino acid is the least at its **isoelectric pH**. It should be remembered that the completely undissociated form of amino acids, shown frequently for the sake of simplicity, does not exist in solution at any pH.

The strength of an acid depends upon the degree to which it dissociates and liberates hydrogen ions or protons. Strength of acids is generally expressed in terms of their dissociation constants. Since amino acids are very weak acids, their strength is expressed in terms of pK which is the negative log of the dissociation constant. The pK of the α-carboxyl groups of amino acids is around 2.1, and that of the α-amino groups is around 9.8. This means that the protonated α-amino groups (R–NH$_3$$^+$) are less stronger than the α-carboxyl groups (R–COOH) as acids.

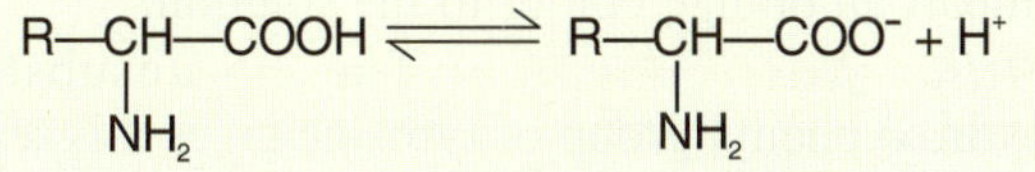

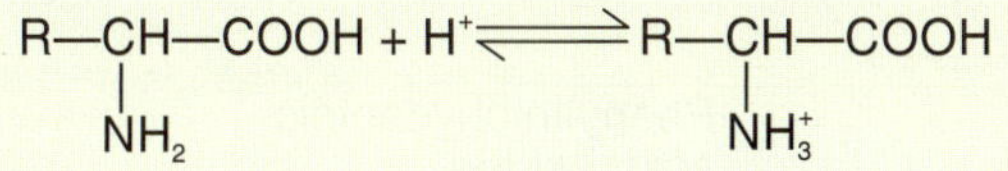

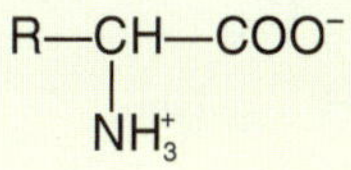

2. Formation of Peptide Bonds

One of the most important reactions of amino acids is formation of peptide bonds. This is the bond by which amino acids are linked with each other in peptides and proteins. The peptide bond is formed between the carboxyl group of one amino acid and the amino group of another amino acid with elimination of one molecule of water.

The actual formation of peptide bonds in living cells is complex. The reaction occurs in stages, and requires enzymes, coenzymes, different types of RNA and other factors. The dipeptide shown in Fig. 5.8 has a free amino group at one end and a free carboxyl group at the other. The former is known as the amino end (N-terminus) and the latter as the carboxy end (C-terminus). All peptides and proteins possess an N-terminus and a C-terminus.

3. Reactions of Carboxyl and Amino Groups

The carboxyl and amino groups of amino acids can undergo their usual reactions, e.g. acylation, esterification, formation of salts, etc.

4. Reactions of Sulphydryl Groups

The sulphydryl group of cysteine can undergo reversible oxidation and reduction. Formation of disulphide bonds

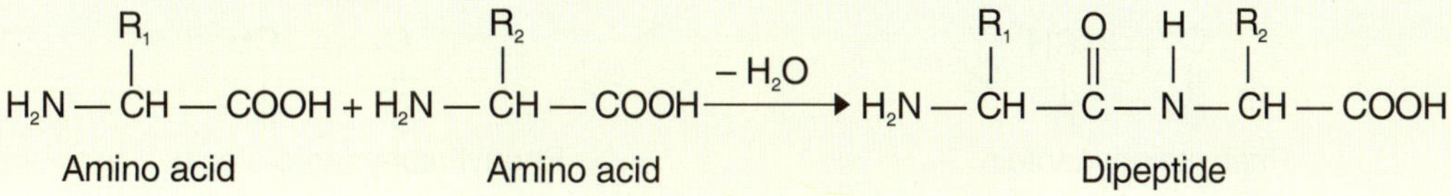

$$\underset{Amino\ acid}{\underset{NH_2}{H_2N-CH-COOH}} + \underset{Amino\ acid}{\underset{NH_2}{H_2N-CH-COOH}} \xrightarrow{-H_2O} \underset{Dipeptide}{\underset{}{H_2N-\underset{R_1}{CH}-\underset{O}{C}-\underset{H}{N}-\underset{R_2}{CH}-COOH}}$$

Fig. 5.8: Formation of peptide bond

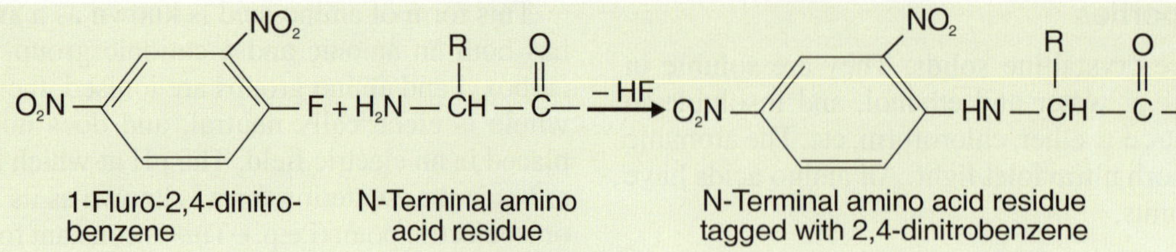

Fig. 5.9: Sanger's reaction

between the sulphydryl groups of two cysteine molecules has been mentioned earlier. The sulphydryl groups of cysteine residues are essential for the biological activity of many proteins.

5. Reactions used for Determination of the Amino Acid Sequence of Peptides and Proteins

Determination of the sequence of amino acids is important in elucidating the structures of peptides and proteins. Generally, the N-terminal amino acid is tagged with some reagent. It is split off by hydrolysis, and the tagged amino acid is identified. The reaction is, then, repeated with the new N-terminal amino acid and so on. Complete sequence of amino acids can, thus, be determined. The most frequently used reactions for this purpose are Sanger's reaction and Edman's reaction.

   i. *Sanger's reaction:* The amino group of the N-terminal amino acid residue is tagged with 1-fluoro-2,4-dinitrobenzene or Sanger's reagent (Fig. 5.9).
   ii. *Edman's reaction:* The amino group of the N-terminal amino acid residue is tagged with phenylisothiocynate (Edman's reagent) to form phenylthiohydantoic acid. The latter is converted into

phenylthiohydantoin in the presence of an acid and nitromethane (Fig. 5.10).

6. Reactions used for Identification and Quantitation of Individual or Groups of Amino Acids

These reactions are frequently used for qualitative detection and/or quantitative measurement of various amino acids. The reactions are given both by free amino acids and by amino acids present in peptides and proteins. Some of the important reactions are:

   i. *Ninhydrin reaction:* This reaction is given by all amino acids and small peptides. The α-amino acids react with two molecules of ninhydrin to form a blue-purple coloured complex (proline gives a yellow colour). The reaction occurs in stages (Fig. 5.11).
   ii. *Xanthoproteic reaction:* This reaction is given by the aromatic amino acids, phenylalanine, tyrosine and tryptophan. On boiling with concentrated nitric acid, their phenyl groups are converted into nitrophenyl groups. These ionise on addition of an alkali, and impart an orange colour to the solution.
   iii. *Millon-Nasse reaction:* The 3,5-unsubstituted hydroxyphenyl group of tyrosine gives this reaction.

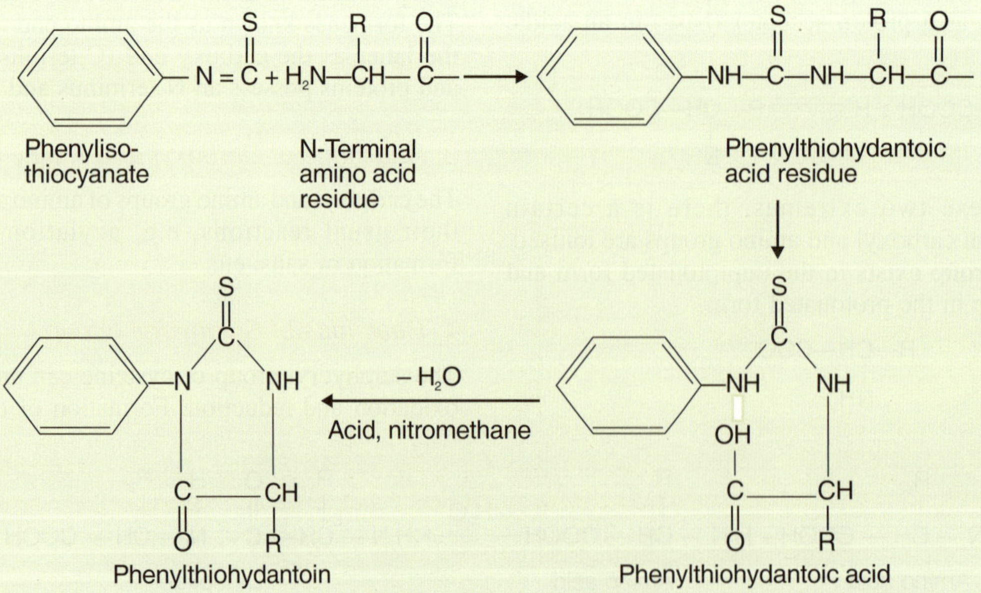

Fig. 5.10: Edman's reaction

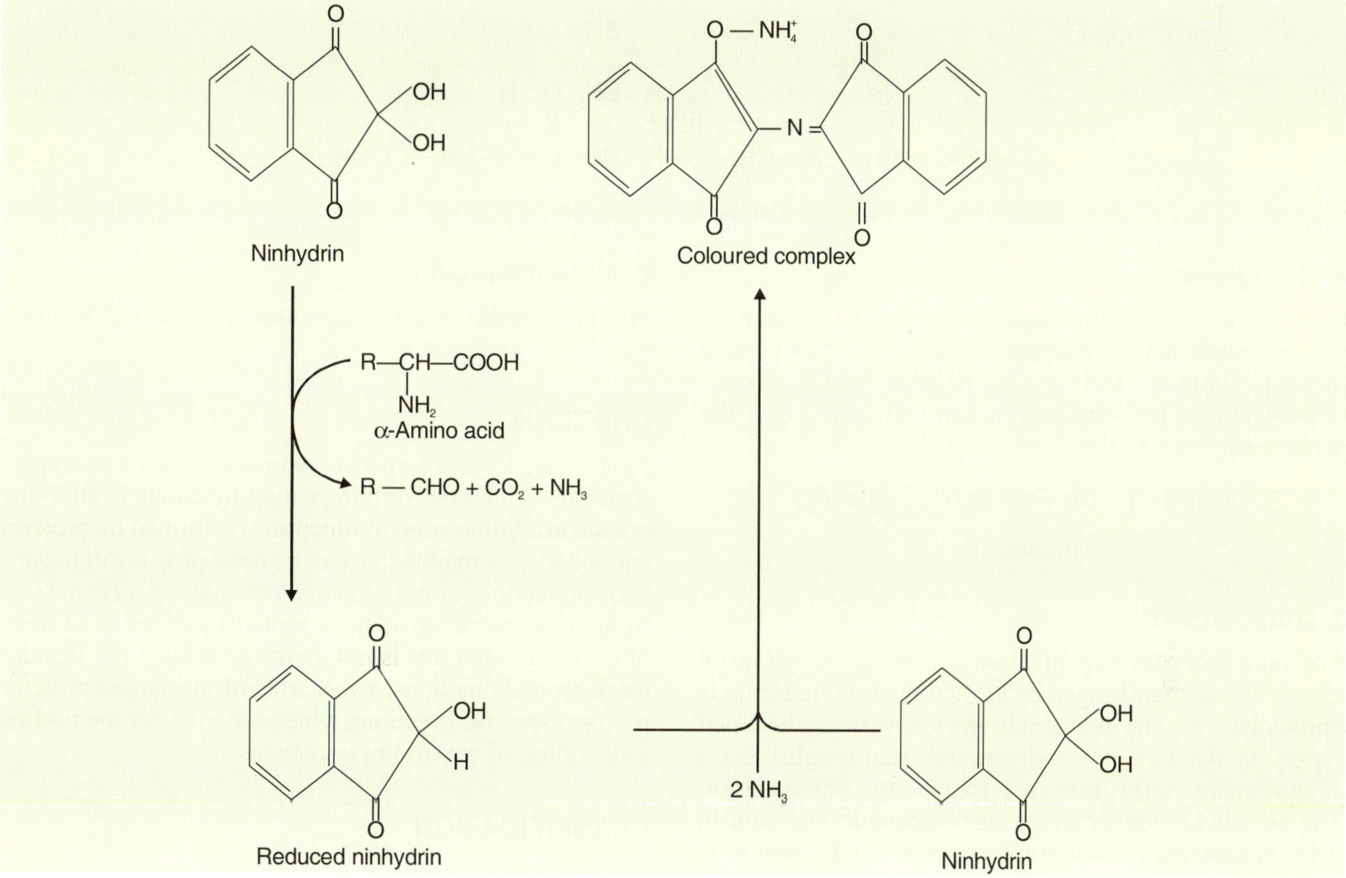

Fig. 5.11: Ninhydrin reaction

Treatment with mercuric sulphate and nitrous acid causes mercuration and nitration or nitrosation of the hydroxyphenyl group of tyrosine giving a red colour.

iv. *Aldehyde reaction:* This reaction is given by the indole ring of tryptophan. The indole ring reacts with aldehydes, e.g. formaldehyde, in the presence of sulphuric acid to form a violet coloured complex.

v. *Hopkins-Cole reaction:* This is similar to the Millon-Nasse reaction. Glyoxylic acid (HOOC–CHO) reacts with the indole ring of tryptophan in the presence of sulphuric acid to form a violet coloured complex.

vi. *Sakaguchi's reaction:* This reaction is given by the guanidino group of arginine. In an alkaline medium, α-naphthol combines with the guanidino group to form a complex which is oxidised by sodium hypobromite or sodium hypochlorite to produce a red colour.

vii. *Lead sulphide reaction:* This reaction is given by sulphur-containing amino acids, cysteine and cystine. On boiling with sodium hydroxide, the sulphur present in these amino acids is released in the form of sodium sulphide. This reacts with lead acetate to form a brown or black precipitate of lead sulphide. Though methionine contains sulphur, it does not give this reaction as the sulphur present in it is not released on boiling with sodium hydroxide.

PEPTIDES

Peptides are formed by the union of several amino acids through peptide bonds. They are synthesised in the body by a complex process. Generally, the molecules made up of 100 amino acids or less are known as peptides or polypeptides, and molecules made up of more than 100 amino acids are known as proteins.

But this distinction is not hard and fast. A number of small peptides found in the human body are just catabolic products of proteins, and have no definite function. But some of the small peptides are formed purposely to perform specific physiological functions. Some physiologically active peptides are:

1. Glutathione

Glutathione is a tripeptide made up of glutamate, cysteine and glycine (γ-glutamyl-cysteinyl-glycine). The sulphydryl (–SH) group of cysteine residue is the reactive portion of glutathione which can undergo oxidation and reduction (Fig. 5.12). Reduced form of glutathione is generally shown as G–SH, and the oxidised form as G–S–S–G. Glutathione is required for the catalytic activity of many enzymes and for detoxification of hydrogen peroxide, fatty acid peroxides and some xenobiotics.

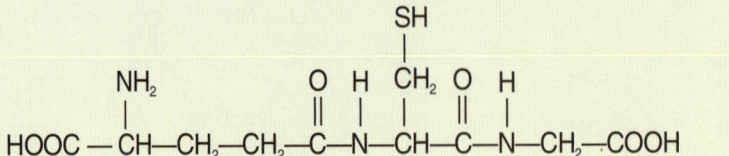

Fig. 5.12: Glutathione

2. Bradykinin

Bradykinin is formed in plasma from an α_2-globulin by the proteolytic action of trypsin or some enzymes present in snake venom. It is a nonapeptide which causes vasodilatation, bronchoconstriction and increase in the permeability of capillaries.

Arg–Pro–Pro–Gly–Phe–Ser–Pro–Phe–Arg

Bradykinin

3. Angiotensin

Angiotensin is formed in plasma from an α_2-globulin known as angiotensinogen by the action of renin. Renin is a proteolytic enzyme released from kidneys when the blood supply to the kidneys is decreased. Renin splits off a decapeptide, angiotensin I from angiotensinogen. Angiotensin I is converted into an octapeptide, angiotensin II by angiotensin converting enzyme (ACE) which is present in plasma, endothelial cells and lungs.

Angiotensinogen $\xrightarrow{\text{Renin}}$ Angiotensin I

Angiotensin I $\xrightarrow{\text{ACE}}$ Angiotensin II

Angiotensin II causes vasoconstriction, increases the force of contraction of heart and raises blood pressure. Renin-angiotensin system plays an important role in the regulation of blood pressure. Some inhibitors of ACE are used as antihypertensive drugs.

4. Vasopressin

Vasopressin or antidiuretic hormone (ADH) is a cyclic nonapeptide hormone released from the posterior pituitary gland.

5. Oxytocin

Oxytocin is another cyclic nonapeptide hormone released from the posterior pituitary gland.

6. Thyrotropin-releasing Hormone (TRH)

TRH is a tripeptide hormone released from the hypothalamus which acts on the anterior pituitary gland, and increases the secretion of thyrotropin (thyroid–stimulating hormone).

7. Met-enkephalin

Met-enkephalin is a pentapeptide synthesised in brain which acts as a pain reliever.

PROTEINS

Proteins are large polymers of amino acids having complex structures which perform important functions in all living organisms. Some general functions performed by proteins in our body are maintenance of osmotic pressure of plasma and intracellular fluid, and maintenance of pH of body fluids. In some circumstances, proteins are used as a source of energy though this is not their major function. Besides these general functions, a vast array of specialised proteins perform specific functions which are vital for the normal functioning of any living organism.

CLASSIFICATION

There is no universally accepted classification of proteins as the complete structure of proteins is not known in majority of cases. A satisfactory and comprehensive classification will be possible only when the structures of all the proteins have been defined. The following classification is based on the composition and solubility of proteins:

Simple Proteins

These are the proteins made up of amino acids only. Simple proteins can be sub-divided into the following groups:

1. Albumins

These are soluble in water and dilute salt solutions. They are heat-coagulable. They are precipitated when their solutions are saturated with ammonium sulphate. Some common albumins are ovalbumin (present in eggs), lactalbumin (present in milk) and serum albumin (present in blood).

2. Globulins

These are soluble in dilute salt solutions but are insoluble in water. They are heat-coagulable. They are precipitated when their solutions are half-saturated with ammonium sulphate. Examples are ovoglobulin (present in eggs), lactoglobulin (present in milk) and serum globulin (present in blood).

3. Glutelins

These are soluble in dilute acids and alkalis but are insoluble in water. Examples are glutenin and oryzenin. Glutenin is found in wheat and oryzenin in rice. Glutelins are found in plants only.

4. Prolamins

These are soluble in 70% ethanol but insoluble in water and absolute ethanol. These are rich in proline. Examples are gliadin and zein which are found in wheat and corn respectively.

5. Protamines

These are soluble in water and ammonium hydroxide. They have relatively low molecular weights. Examples of protamines include salmine and sturine which are found in the sperms of the fishes, salmon and sturgeon respectively.

6. Histones

Histones are soluble in water but are insoluble in ammonium hydroxide. They are rich in arginine. They have relatively high molecular weights. Histones (H1, H2A, H2B, H3 and H4) are present in nucleus in association with DNA.

7. Albuminoids

They are also known as scleroproteins. They are insoluble in most of the solvents. Examples are collagen, keratin, elastin, etc. These are structural constituents of tissues, and provide strength to the tissues. Collagen, made up of three intertwined polypeptide chains, is the most abundant protein in mammals.

Conjugated Proteins

These are made up of amino acids and a non-protein part which may be organic or inorganic. The non-protein component is known as the prosthetic group. Depending upon the nature of the prosthetic group, the conjugated proteins may be sub-divided into:

1. Glycoproteins

The prosthetic group is made up of carbohydrates. In the past, proteins having up to 4% carbohydrates were known as glycoproteins and those having more than 4% carbohydrates were known as mucoproteins. Examples of glycoproteins are mucin, leutinising hormone, human chorionic gonadotropin, etc. All the plasma proteins except albumin are glycoproteins.

2. Lipoproteins

The prosthetic group is made up of lipids. Lipoproteins are found in eggs, nervous tissue, plasma, etc. The lipoproteins in plasma include chylomicrons (CM), very low density lipoproteins (VLDL), low density lipoproteins (LDL) and high density lipoproteins (HDL).

3. Nucleoproteins

The prosthetic group is made up of nucleic acids. An example is nucleohistone. Since histones are usually found as components of nucleoproteins, some authorities do not consider them as simple proteins.

4. Phosphoproteins

The protein is combined with phosphate group (but not in the form of phospholipids or nucleic acids). Examples are casein and vitelline which are found in milk and eggs respectively.

5. Chromoproteins

The prosthetic group is a pigment. Examples include haemoglobin, myoglobin, rhodopsin, etc.

6. Metalloproteins

Prosthetic group is a metal. However, chromoproteins, e.g. haemoglobin, which contain metals are not included in this group. Some important metalloproteins are ferritin, haemosiderin, ceruloplasmin, carbonic anhydrase, glutathione peroxidase, carboxypeptidase, etc.

Derived Proteins

These proteins do not occur in nature. They are formed from naturally occurring proteins by the action of physical agents, e.g. heat, ultrasonic waves, etc. or chemical agents, e.g. acids, alkalis, enzymes, etc. They can be sub-divided into:

1. Primary Derived Proteins

These are formed by some intramolecular changes in the native proteins not involving hydrolysis of the proteins. These are insoluble and biologically inactive. Examples are metaproteins, denatured proteins and coagulated proteins.

2. Secondary Derived Proteins

These are formed by hydrolysis of native proteins. These include primary proteoses, secondary proteoses and peptones in the decreasing order of size.

STRUCTURAL ORGANISATION OF PROTEINS

Proteins perform a variety of functions. These functions are closely related to the structures of proteins. Fundamentally, all proteins are made of amino acids linked to one another by peptide bonds. However, coiling and

```
— HN — CH — CO —                      — HN — CH — CO —
        |                                     |
       CH₂                                   CH₂          Disulphide
        |        A cysteine                   |           bond
       SH        residue                      S           between
    _____                  |           two
                                              S            cysteine
       SH                                      |           residues
        |        Another                      CH₂
       CH₂       cysteine                      |
        |        residue                — HN — CH — CO —
— HN — CH — CO —
```

Fig. 5.13: Disulphide bond

folding of peptide chains and union of several peptide chains with one another produce a very complex three-dimensional structure. The three-dimensional structure, which is also known as the conformation of the protein, is unique to each protein. The biological functions of a protein depend upon its conformation. Any change in conformation may lead to loss of function. The conformation depends upon the sequence of amino acids.

The complex structure of proteins is stabilised by two types of bonds, covalent or strong bonds and non-covalent or weak bonds.

Covalent Bonds

These bonds are relatively strong. These include:

1. Peptide Bonds

These are the basic linkages between two consecutive amino acids (Fig. 5.8). As they are formed between α-amino groups and α-carboxyl groups, they are known as α-peptide bonds. All amino acids present in a protein take part in the formation of peptide bonds.

2. Disulphide Bonds

A disulphide bond is formed between two cysteine residues. The sulphydryl groups of the cysteine residues are linked together (Fig. 5.13).

The bond may be formed between two cysteine residues in the same polypeptide chain or in two different polypeptide chains. In the latter case, the two polypeptide chains will be linked together.

Non-covalent Bonds

These bonds are much weaker than the covalent bonds. But they also contribute to the stability of the structure of proteins. The main non-covalent bonds in proteins are:

1. Hydrogen Bonds

Hydrogen bonds are weak bonds which are formed between two peptide linkages. The peptide linkages may be present in the same polypeptide chain or in two different polypeptide chains. In hydrogen bonds, the hydrogen atom

of the –NH– group present in a peptide bond is shared between nitrogen and oxygen atoms. The nitrogen atom involved in this sharing belongs to one peptide bond, and the oxygen atom belongs to another peptide bond (Fig. 5.14).

Hydrogen bonds are very weak but their contribution to the stability of protein structure is very significant because they are present in very large numbers in protein molecules.

2. Electrostatic Bonds

Electrostatic bonds or salt bonds are formed between two oppositely charged groups in the side chains of amino acids. The side chains of several amino acids contain ionisable groups, e.g. amino groups, carboxyl groups, sulphydryl groups, phenol groups, etc. Such groups may form electrostatic bonds with other groups bearing opposite charges.

3. Hydrophobic Bonds

The side chains of nonpolar amino acids attract each other because of their hydrophobic nature. However, this is only a physical attraction and no chemical bonds are really formed.

These strong and weak bonds are present in large numbers in protein molecules, and are responsible for their complex structure. The structure of proteins can be considered to have four levels of organisation—primary, secondary, tertiary and quaternary. The first three levels of organisation are present in all the proteins. The last is present in many but not all. The important features of

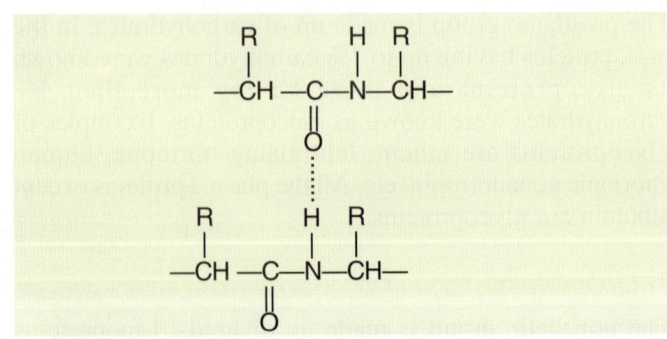

Fig. 5.14: Hydrogen bond between two peptide linkages

different levels of structural organisation of proteins are as follows.

Primary Structure

This is the most fundamental level of structural organisation, and refers to the sequence of amino acids in the polypeptide chain. If one is asked to describe the primary structure of a particular protein, it means one has to describe the sequence of amino acids in that protein. Only peptide bonds are responsible for the formation of the primary structure. Each amino acid takes part in forming peptide bonds. The amino acids present in the polypeptide chain are known as its amino acid residues. Each chain has an N-terminus and a C-terminus. Some polypeptides are cyclic, and have no N- and C-terminus.

The higher levels of structural organisation also depend upon the primary structure. A change in the sequence of amino acids will alter the higher levels of organisation leading to a change in the conformation of the protein molecule. Many genetic diseases, which will be described later, are caused by minor changes in the amino acid sequence of proteins. Such proteins are abnormal in structure as well as function.

Secondary Structure

This is the next higher level of organisation. The polypeptide chain is not straight. It becomes twisted, turned and coiled to form various types of secondary structure, e.g. α-helix, β-pleated sheet, β-bend, etc.

α-Helix

The polypeptide chain is coiled to form a helical structure. The α-helix is produced by formation of hydrogen bonds between peptide linkages three amino acid residues apart. This means that hydrogen bonds are formed between the first and the fourth peptide linkages, between the second and the fifth peptide linkages and so on.

Each peptide linkage in the polypeptide chain participates in hydrogen bonding. There are 3.6 amino acid residues in each turn of the helix. The pitch of the helix (vertical distance per turn) is 0.54 nm. The side chains of the amino acid residues protrude outwards from the centre of the helix (Fig. 5.15). The helix may be right-handed or left-handed. The right-handed helix is more stable. Right-handed α-helix is the commonest secondary structure found in proteins. In myogolobin and haemoglobin, majority of the amino acid residues form a number of α-helical segments.

Some amino acid residues, e.g. proline and hydroxy-proline, tend to disrupt the helix, and produce turns or kinks. The nitrogen atom attached to the α-carbon of proline and hydroxyproline is part of a rigid ring, and lacks the hydrogen atom required to from a hydrogen bond.

β-Pleated Sheets

This is another recurring structural pattern found in many proteins. Portions of a polypeptide chain (or different polypeptide chains) running side by side can be joined by hydrogen bonds, formed between peptide linkages, producing an extended zigzag structure resembling a series of pleats. The portions of the polypeptide chain (or different polypeptide chains) forming the β-pleated sheets may be running in the same direction (N→ C) forming parallel β-pleated sheets or may be running in opposite directions forming anti-parallel β-pleated sheets (Fig. 5.16). Glycine residues promote the formation of β-pleated sheets.

Amyloid proteins, that accumulate in tissues in amyloidosis, are formed from native proteins that have undergone chemical transformations as a result of which most of the protein is converted into β-pleated sheets. Amyloid proteins are relatively insoluble and resistant to degradation. They accumulate in some chronic inflammatory diseases.

β-Bend

The polypeptide chain can turn sharply to form a β-bend or a β-turn. The bend is formed by hydrogen bonding between >NH and >C=O groups of an amino acid residue, n and >C=O and >NH groups of the amino acid residue, $n+3$ (Fig. 5.17).

A given polypeptide chain may possess different types of secondary structure in different regions, i.e. some parts of the chain may form α-helices, other parts may form parallel or anti-parallel β-sheets, and these may be connected by β-turns. Different types of secondary structure are usually shown by simple representations in the structure of proteins. For example, an α-helical region is shown as a coiled ribbon or a cylinder, β-strands (sheets) are shown as broad arrows with the arrow head indicating the N→ C direction. Distinct supersecondary structural motifs are often present in proteins, e.g. helix-turn-helix, β-α-β, β-hairpin, etc. (Fig. 5.18).

Tertiary Structure

The polypeptide chain is folded in complex ways to form different types of secondary structures and super-secondary motifs in different regions of the chain. The folding occurs due to formation of disulphide bonds, hydrogen bonds, electrostatic bonds and hydrophobic bonds. Due to folding, some amino acid residues which are quite distant from each other in the polypeptide chain are brought closer, some residues are buried into the interior of the molecule and some are exposed on the surface of the molecule. The spatial arrangement of amino acid residues forming a specific three-dimensional conformation constitutes the tertiary structure of the protein (Fig. 5.19). As a result of

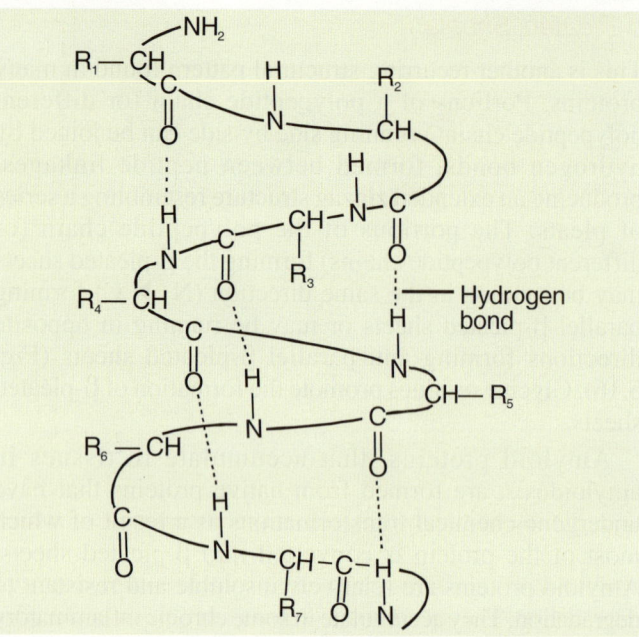

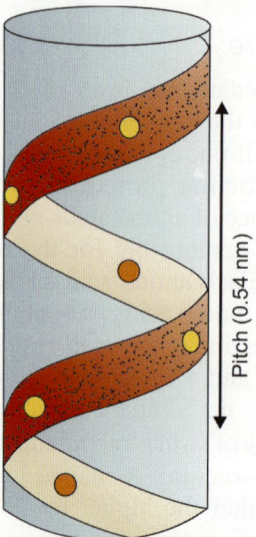

Fig. 5.15: A portion of an α-helix. Hydrogen bonds are formed between the first and the fourth peptide bonds, the second and the fifth peptide bonds and so on. The pitch is 0.54 nm. There are 3.6 amino acid residues in one turn of the helix. The α-helix is often shown as a cylinder

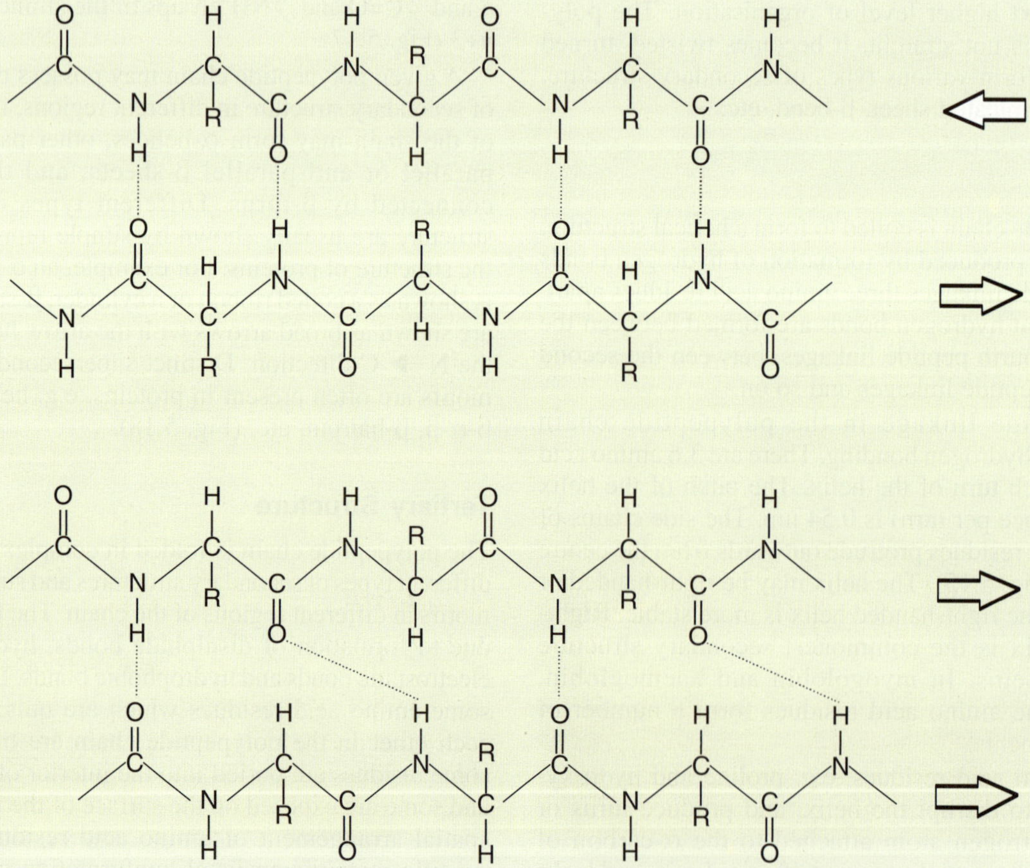

Fig. 5.16: Anti-parallel (above) and parallel (below) β-pleated sheets

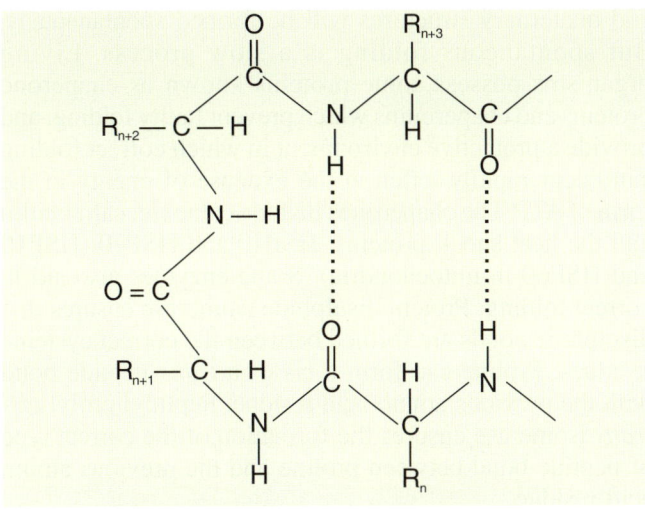

Fig. 5.17: A β-turn in the polypeptide chain

folding, the polypeptide chain acquires a compact three-dimesional conformation. The folding can also produce distinct structural and functional domains. Different secondary structures are present in different segments of the folded polypeptide. For instance, in myoglobin that is made up of 153 amino acid residues, three-fourths of the amino acid residues form eight α-helical segments.

Quaternary Structure

Many proteins are made up of two or more polypeptide chains. Each polypeptide chain is known as a **protomer** a **subunit**. The subunits in such proteins may be similar or dissimilar. The subunits are linked with each other by non-covalent bonds. The structure formed by union of subunits is known as the quaternary structure of the protein.

Some examples of proteins having a quaternary structure are haemoglobin, creatine kinase, lactate dehydrogenase, etc. Haemoglobin is a tetramer made up of two different types of submits. Adult haemoglobin is made up of two α and two β subunits. Creatine kinase is a dimer made up of two different types of subunits, B and M. These subunits

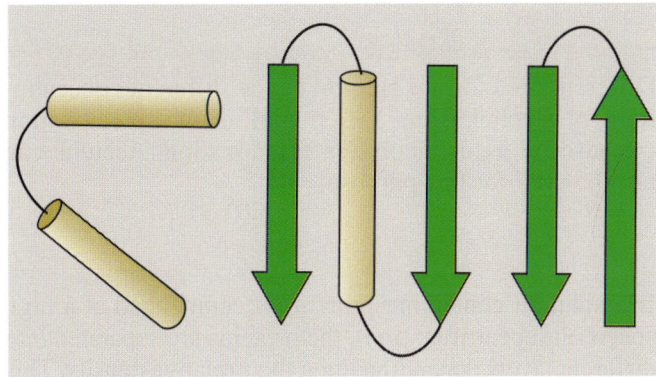

Fig. 5.18: Supersecondary structural motifs in proteins—helix-turn-helix, β-α-β and β-hairpin

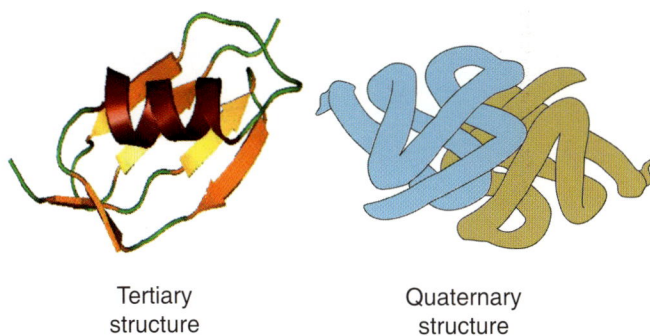

| Tertiary structure | Quaternary structure |

Fig. 5.19: Tertiary and quaternary structure

can combine with each other to form three different creatine kinase dimers (BB, MB and MM). Lactate dehydrogenase is a tetramer. Two different types of subunits, H and M, can combine with each other to form five different lactate dehydrogenase tetramers (HHHH, HHHM, HHMM, HMMM and MMMM). If different polypeptide chains are joined by covalent bonds, e.g. in insulin and immunoglobulins, it is not called quaternary structure.

Disruption of Protein Structure

The normal structure of proteins may be disrupted by physical or chemical agents leading to their denaturation or coagulation. Disruption of structure is associated with loss of function.

Denaturation

Exposure to physical agents, e.g. heat, X-rays, ultraviolet light, high pressure, vigorous shaking, etc. or chemical agents, e.g. acids, alkalis, heavy metals, organic solvents, etc. may disrupt the secondary, tertiary and quaternary structures of proteins. The primary structure remains unaffected. This process is known as denaturation. The denatured protein is less soluble, and is easily precipitated. It is biologically inactive. Sometimes, it is possible to restore the denatured protein to its original structure and function (renaturation) by a reversal of the conditions that led to its denaturation (Fig. 5.20).

Coagulation

When albumins and globulins are heated at their isoelectric pH, they are first denatured. Their subunits are separated and unfolded. The unfolded polypeptide chains are then matted together to form a dense mass known as coagulum. This process is known as coagulation. Coagulation is always irreversible. Milk and egg contain albumin and globulin. These are coagulated on cooking, and become more digestible as the coagulated proteins are hydrolysed more easily than the native proteins.

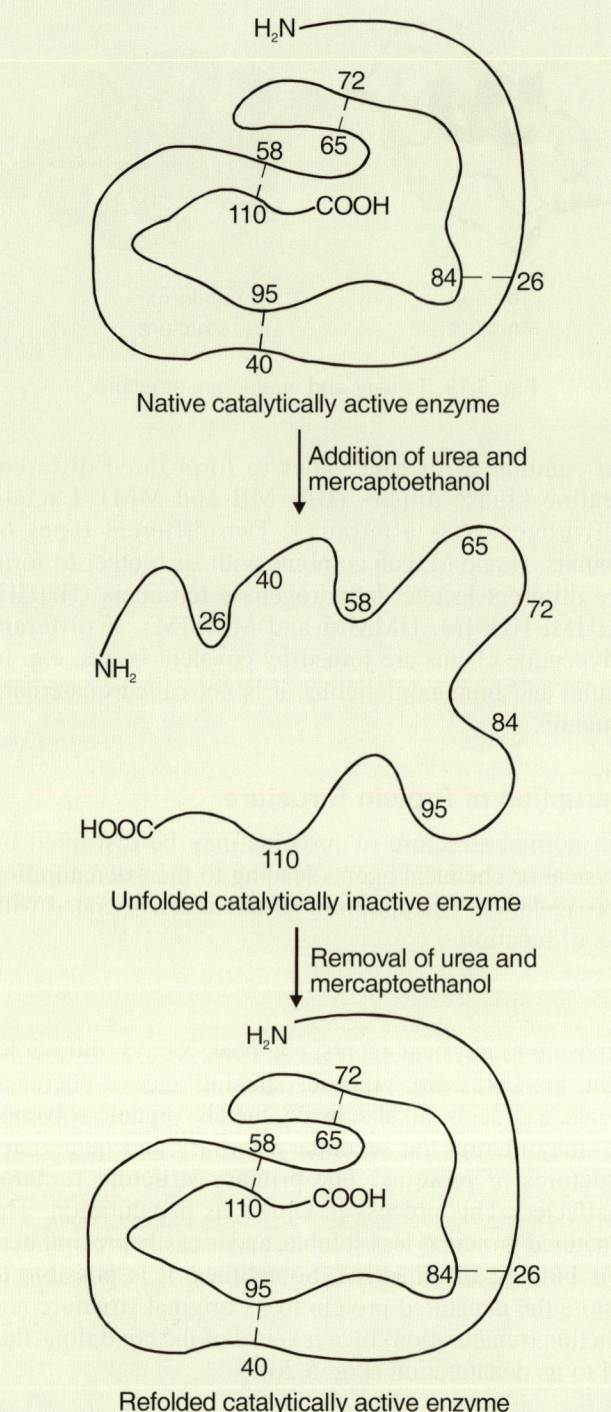

Fig. 5.20: Denaturation of ribonuclease on addition of urea and mercaptoethanol, and its renaturation on removal of urea and mercaptoethanol. The numbers show the positions of cysteine residues which form disulphide bonds in the native state

Chaperones

The higher levels of structural organisation of proteins depend upon primary structure. If the primary structure has been formed correctly, the correct secondary, tertiary and quaternary structures will be formed spontaneously. But spontaneous folding is a slow process. Living organisms possess some proteins known as chaperone proteins and chaperonins which prevent faulty folding, and provide a protective environment in which correct folding can occur rapidly, often at the expense of energy in the form of ATP. The chaperones include calnexin, calreticulin and the heat shock proteins, HSP40 and HSP70 (HSP10 and HSP60 in mitochondria). Some enzymes also aid in correct folding. Protein disulphide isomerase ensures that disulphide bonds are formed between the correct cysteine residues. Proline can form a *cis* or a *trans* peptide bond with the previous amino acid residue. Peptidyl prolyl *cis-trans* isomerase ensures the formation of the correct type of peptide bond between proline and the previous amino acid residue.

Fractionation of Proteins

Biological materials contain a large number of proteins in addition to many non-protein components. Separation of individual proteins from this complex mixture is required many times for academic, diagnostic or therapeutic purposes. Fractionation of proteins is a tedious and time-consuming process. Several techniques of fractionation have to be employed in succession to obtain individual proteins in a pure form. Briefly, the methods for fractionation of proteins include:

1. *Salt Fractionation*

When a mixture of proteins is treated with varying concentrations of salts, different proteins are precipitated at different salt concentrations. This process is known as salting out, and can be used for fractionation of proteins. When a mixture of albumin and globulins is half-saturated with ammonium sulphate, globulins are salted out. The reverse process is known as salting in. For example, if we treat a mixture of two proteins with a particular salt concentration at which one protein is soluble and the other is not, the soluble protein will be dissolved or salted in.

2. *Alcohol Fractionation*

Different proteins are precipitated at different concentrations of alcohol. Thus, differential alcohol precipitation can also be used for protein fractionation. Acetone can also be used for this purpose.

3. *Centrifugation*

If a solution containing proteins is centrifuged at a high speed (ultracentrifugation), the proteins are separated into different layers depending upon their relative density. This technique is frequently used for the separation of lipoproteins present in plasma.

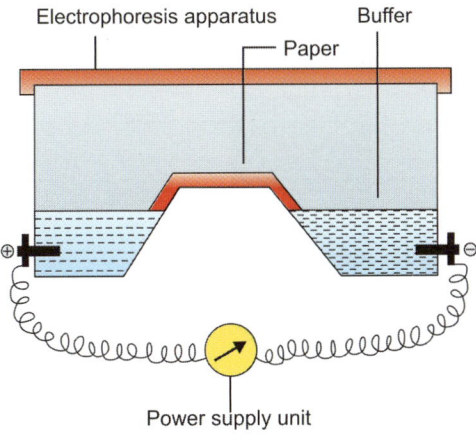

Fig. 5.21: Paper electrophoresis

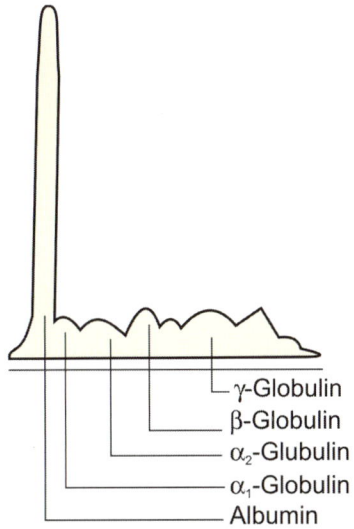

Fig. 5.23: Densitometric recording of serum proteins separated by electrophoresis

4. *Electrophoresis*

Electrophoretic separation is based on the movement of charged particles in an electric field. If the charged particles differ in the number and type of charges, they will move at different rates in an electric field and will form different bands after sometime. Proteins have a number of ionisable groups which differ in number and nature from protein to protein. Therefore, if a mixture of proteins is placed in an electric field, the different proteins will migrate at different speeds and will be separated after sometime. The bands can be visualised and quantitated by staining them with suitable staining agents.

Several types of electrophoresis have been developed. The support media, on which the sample is applied, may be paper, cellulose acetate, agar gel, starch gel, polyacrylamide gel, etc. The supporting medium can be horizontal or vertical. Different buffers are used to maintain the pH as the ionisation of proteins may be altered by a change in the pH.

High voltage electrophoresis can be used for the separation of amino acids. In this technique, a high voltage (2,000 to 5,000 volts) is applied for a short period.

5. *Chromatography*

Chromatography can be used for the separation of proteins, amino acids, lipids, carbohydrates and several other classes of compounds. Basically, a chromatographic system consists of a stationary phase and a mobile phase. The mobile phase (liquid or gas) moves over the stationary phase (solid or liquid). When a mixture of several substances is subjected to chromatography, the components of the mixture are distributed between the stationary phase and the mobile phase depending upon their relative affinities towards the two phases. The distribution generally depends upon two factors—adsorptive affinity and solubility. Accordingly, chromatography can be broadly divided into two types—adsorption chromatography and partition chromatography.

In adsorption chromatography, the stationary phase is an adsorbent, e.g. charcoal, alumina, silica gel, etc. This can be spread over a glass or plastic plate or filled into a column. When the adsorbent is applied over a plate in a thin layer, the technique is known as thin-layer adsorption chromatography. The sample is then applied on the plate which is kept vertically in a glass tank. The mobile phase (liquid) is allowed to flow over the plate in an upward (ascending chromatography) or downward (descending chromatography) direction. Different components of the mixture will move with the mobile phase at different rates depending upon their relative affinities towards the adsorbent. After sometime, they will be separated into different spots on the plate. These can be stained and visualised or quantitated. When the adsorbent is packed into a column, it is known as column chromatography. The sample is layered over the column. The mobile phase is then allowed to flow through the column. The different components of the mixture emerge from the lower end of the column at different times depending upon their relative

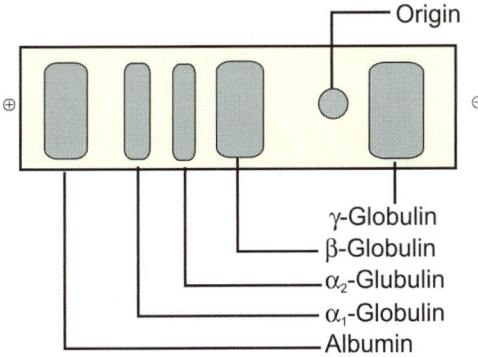

Fig. 5.22: Serum proteins separated by electrophoresis

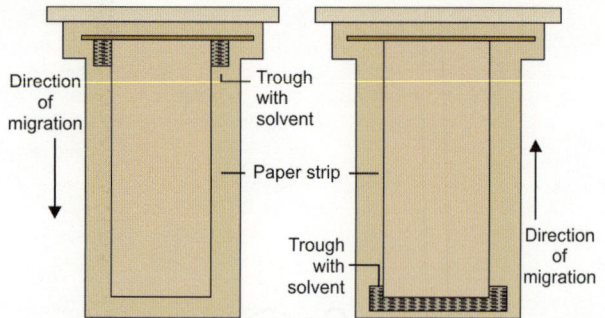

Fig. 5.24: Descending (left) and ascending (right) paper chromatography

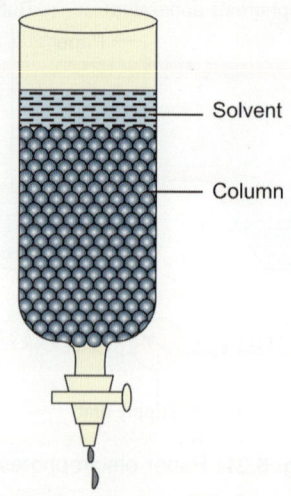

Fig. 5.26: Column chromatography

affinities for the adsorbent. These can be collected in different containers for identification and quantitation.

In partition chromatography, the stationary phase is a liquid supported on a solid medium. In a common form of partition chromatography, called paper chromatography, the support medium is paper. A film of water molecules forms on paper and acts as the stationary phase. The mobile phase is a solvent, generally nonpolar. Different components of the mixture migrate with the mobile phase at different rates depending upon their relative solubilities in the mobile phase and the stationary phase. After sometime, the components are separated forming distinct spots which can be visualised by drying the paper and spraying it with a suitable staining agent. The ratio of the distance travelled by a component to that travelled by the solvent (mobile phase) is known as the Rf value of the component. Rf values are useful in the identification of the compounds.

$$Rf = \frac{\text{Distance travelled by the solute}}{\text{Distance travelled by the solvent}}$$

FUNCTIONS OF PROTEINS

As mentioned earlier, proteins perform a wide variety of functions. Human beings synthesise thousands of different proteins. Each protein has a unique conformation suited to its biological function. Function depends upon structure. A

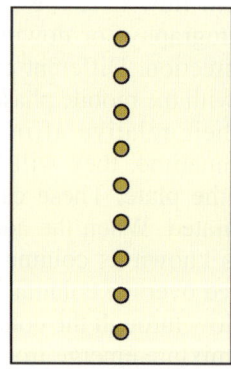

Fig. 5.25: Stained paper chromatogram showing spots

small change in the primary structure of a protein can alter its conformation resulting in a decrease in or loss of function. Thousands of inherited diseases occur because of synthesis of abnormal proteins, many of which are fatal and many others lead to severe clinical abnormalities. This underlines the functional importance of proteins. Depending upon their functions, proteins can be divided into:

1. Catalytic Proteins

One of the most important functions of proteins is to serve as biological catalysts, i.e. enzymes. Except for some ribozymes (RNA enzymes), all enzymes are proteins. Biochemical reactions can occur at a significant rate only in the presence of enzymes. Most enzymes have a unique substrate site to which only one particular substrate can bind. Certain amino acid residues (or cofactors or coenzymes) are located strategically to catalyse the reaction. We will come across examples of enzymes in Chapter 7.

2. Hormones

Hormones play an important role in intercellular communication, and regulate a number of biochemical and physiological activities. Many hormones are chemically proteins. A specific conformation helps them to find and bind to their receptors on the target cells. Examples of protein hormones will be found in Chapter 17.

3. Structural Proteins

Quantitatively, the structural proteins constitute the largest functional group of proteins. Structural proteins are present both inside and outside the cells. Inside the cells, they form the cytoskeleton of the cells. Outside the cells, they are present in the connective tissue. Cytoskeletal proteins include actin, tubulins, keratins, etc. Connective tissue proteins include collagen, elastin, keratin, fibronectin, etc.

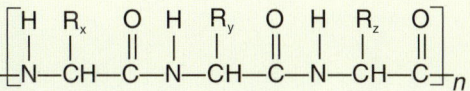

Fig. 5.27: The repeating tripeptide unit of collagen which forms one turn of the helix. R_x is always glycine, about 10% of R_z are proline and another 10% hydroxyproline. Several R_z residues are lysine and hydroxylysine

Collagen is the most abundant protein in mammals, constituting about one-fourth of the total protein content. There are different types of collagen, type I through type XIX, encoded by different genes.

Glycine is the most abundant amino acid in collagen, followed by proline and hydroxyproline (Fig. 5.27). Lysine and hydroxylysine are also present in significant amount. Some of the hydroxylysine residues are glycosylated. Some of the lysine and hydroxylysine residues undergo oxidative deamination at the ε-carbon with the result that the ε-amino group is converted into an aldehyde group. Two such aldehyde groups may undergo aldol condensation or may form Schiff bases with the ε-amino groups of unmodified lysine and hydroxylysine residues (Fig. 5.28). Collagen is a triple helix made up of three polypeptide chains. Each polypeptide chain is coiled into a **left-handed helix** in which three amino acid residues are present in each turn. Three polypeptide chains are intertwined to form a **right-handed triple helix** (Fig. 5.29).

The coiling of three left-handed helices into a right-handed triple helix gives immense tensile strength to collagen. The tensile strength is further increased by cross-links between the three polypeptide chains, and between different triple helices running parallel to each other. Lysine and hydroxylysine residues take part in cross-linking.

Collagen is initially synthesised as a precursor in fibroblasts. The precursor undergoes extensive post-translational modifications to form mature collagen. The newly-synthesised polypeptide chains have a signal sequence which is removed in the lumen of the endoplasmic reticulum. Several proline and lysine residues are hydroxylated by prolyl hydroxylase and lysyl hydroxylase respectively. Three polypeptide chains form a triple helix

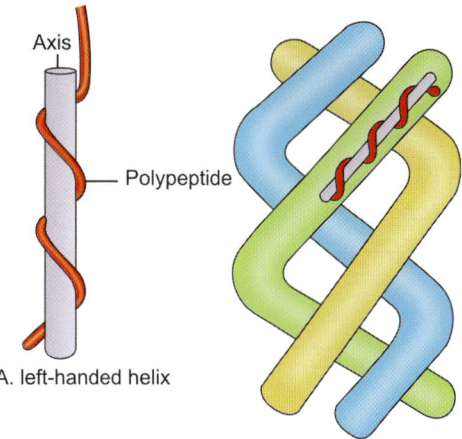

Fig. 5.29: A portion of a collagen molecule. A: A single polypeptide chain coiled into a left-handed helix. B: Three polypeptide chains coiled into a right-handed triple helix.

(procollagen), which is transferred to the Golgi apparatus. Procollagen is glycosylated by addition of glucose or glucosyl-galactose to the –OH groups of some hydroxylysine residues in the Golgi apparatus. The glycosylated procollagen is secreted from the cells. It contains some extra amino acids (propeptides) at the amino and the carboxy terminals of the polypeptide chains. These propeptides are not coiled into a triple helix, and are removed after secretion converting procollagen into tropocollagen. Oxidative deamination of some lysine and hydroxylysine residues at the ε-carbon is catalysed by lysyl oxidase, a copper-containing enzyme. This is followed by cross-linking by aldol condensation or formation of Schiff bases converting tropocollagen into collagen.

Abnormal collagens may be formed due to mutations or nutritional deficiencies. Genetic defects leading to the formation of abnormal collagens may involve the genes encoding collagens or the genes encoding enzymes involved in post-translational modifications of procollagens (e.g. different types of **Ehlers-Danlos syndrome** in which joints are hypermobile, skin is hyperelastic and tissues are fragile). In **scurvy**, hydroxylation of proline and lysine residues of procollagens is impaired as vitamin C is required in this reaction. In **Menkes disease**, which causes severe copper deficiency, oxidative deamination of ε-amino groups of lysine and hydroxylysine residues is impaired as the enzyme, lysyl oxidase catalysing this reaction requires copper. This leads to defective cross-linking. Defective cross-linking may also occur due to binding of some metabolites, e.g. homocysteine and homogentisic acid, to collagen when these metabolites are present in high concentrations in some inherited diseases.

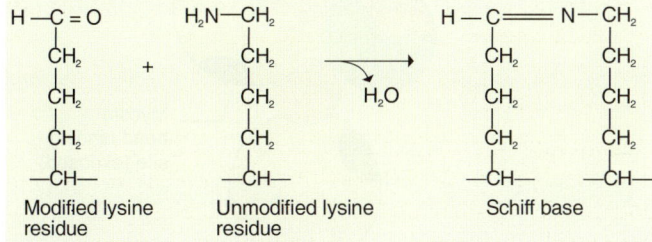

Fig. 5.28: Formation of a Schiff base between a modified lysine residue and a lysine residue that has not undergone oxidative deamination at the ε-carbon atom

4. Membrane Transport Proteins

Some compounds are transported in or out of cells by active transport or facilitated diffusion. Proteins are components

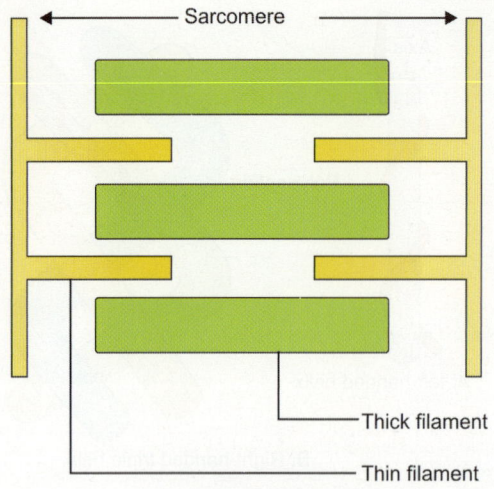

Fig. 5.30: Sarcomere

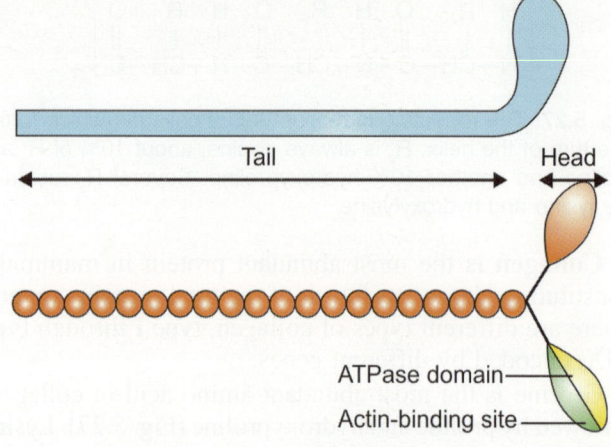

Fig. 5.32: Myosin

of active transport systems as well as facilitated diffusion. Examples are sodium glucose transporter (SGLT1), glucose transporters (GLUTs), etc.

5. Membrane Channels

Membranes possess specific channels for inward or outward movement of some ions, e.g. calcium channel, sodium-potassium channel, chloride channel, etc. Chemically, these channels are proteins.

6. Contractile Proteins

Muscle contraction occurs because of movement of contractile proteins. The contractile proteins are **actin** and **myosin**. Skeletal muscles contain thin filaments and thick filaments (Fig. 5.30).

Thin filaments are made up of actin fibres, tropomyosin and troponin (Fig. 5.31). Thick filaments are made up of myosin, which consists of a long double-helical tail and a globular head. The globular head has an actin-binding site and an ATPase domain (Fig. 5.32). The ATPase domain binds and hydrolyses ATP into ADP and Pi. Hydrolysis of ATP provides the energy for muscle contraction. Actin molecules also have a site for binding myosin head. In the relaxed state, the binding sites on two neighbouring actin molecules are masked by tropomyosin. Troponin, which is a trimer of troponin I, troponin T and troponin C, is attached to tropomyosin.

Muscle contraction begins with release of Ca^{++} from sarcoplasmic reticulum. Binding of four calcium ions to troponin C produces a conformational change that shifts tropomyosin in such a way that the myosin head-binding sites on actin are exposed (Fig. 5.33). Myosin heads form cross-bridges with the binding sites on actin. Swiveling of myosin heads pulls the actin fibres inwards into the sarcomere. The myosin heads dissociate from the binding sites and go back to the initial position to form cross-bridges with other binding sites on actin (Fig. 5.34). A repetition of the cycle leads to further shifting of actin fibre. This cycle is repeated again and again resulting in contraction of the muscle.

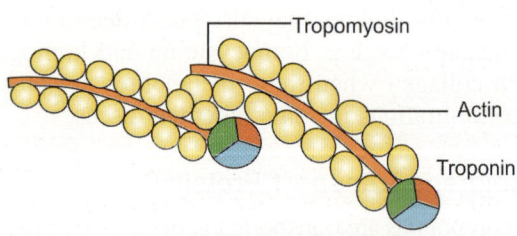

Fig. 5.31: Thin filament

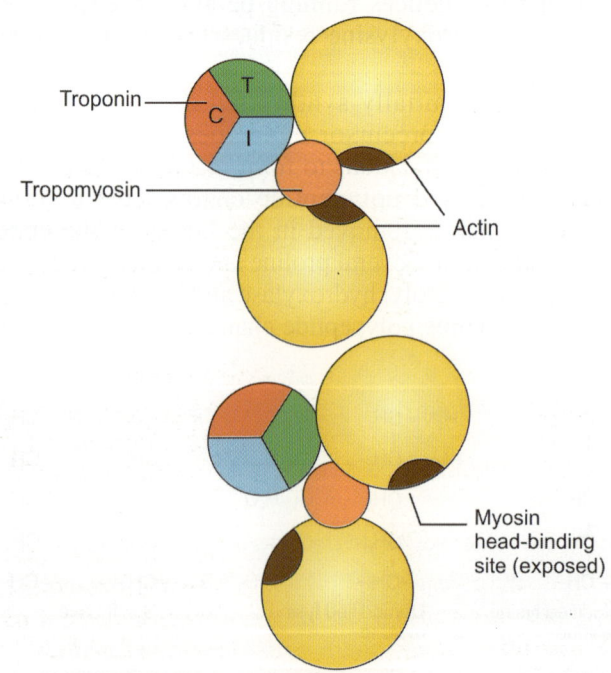

Fig. 5.33: Conformational change in thin filament after binding of Ca^{++} to troponin C

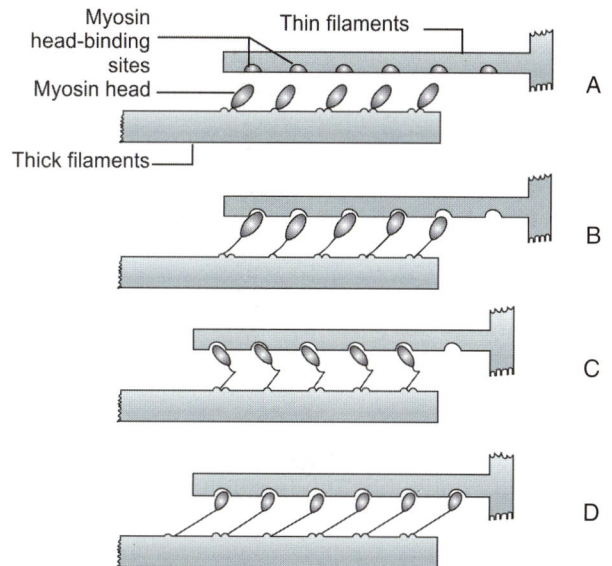

Fig. 5.34: Sliding of thin filaments along thick filaments. A. Myosin head-binding sites on actin concealed. B. Myosin head-binding sites revealed and cross-bridges formed between myosin heads and actin. C. Thin filament pulled in due to swivelling of myosin heads. D. Myosin heads swivel back to form cross-bridges with other sites on actin

7. Receptors

Whether the hormones are proteins, amino acid derivatives or steroids, their receptors are always proteins. Each receptor has a specific hormone-binding domain that binds a particular hormone, and a signal domain that generates a signal inside the target cell. Apart from hormone receptors, cells possess receptors for several other ligands, e.g. transferrin receptor, LDL receptor, T cell receptor, etc.

8. Signal Transducers

On binding of a ligand to its receptor on the cell membrane, signal transducers carry the signal to the effectors inside the cell. Gs-proteins, Gi-proteins, and transducin are examples of proteins that act as signal transducers.

9. Storage Proteins

Some nutrients are stored in the body in association with some storage proteins. For example, ferritin and haemosiderin store iron, cellular retinol-binding protein stores retinol and transcobalamin I stores vitamin B_{12}.

10. Carrier Proteins

Several compounds which are not soluble or are poorly soluble in water require carrier proteins to transport them in circulation. Examples of carrier proteins include haemoglobin, transferrin, lipoproteins, transcobalamins, thyroxine-binding globulin, corticosteroid-binding globulin, retinol-binding protein, albumin, etc.

11. Antibodies

Antibodies (immunoglobulins) are proteins that protect us against foreign antigens. Each antibody has a specific antigen-binding site that recognises and binds a particular antigen, and an effector domain that performs the effector function required to inactivate or destroy the antigen. Details of antibody structure and function will be seen in Chapter 19.

12. Complement Proteins

Complement system consists of a group of proteins present in plasma that aid the immune system. Complement proteins are normally present as inactive proenzymes that are converted into active enzymes by a cascade of reactions culminating in destruction of the cells harbouring an antigen. A detailed description of complement system can be seen in Chapter 19.

13. Coagulation Factors

Coagulation of blood is a process by which an insoluble clot is formed that seals an injured blood vessel and checks bleeding. Except Factors III and IV, all the coagulation factors are proteins. Coagulation occurs by a cascade of reactions in which inactive proenzymes are converted into active enzymes in a specific sequence.

14. Lubricant and Protective Proteins

Mucin is a protein present in mucous secretions that acts as a lubricant, and also protects the mucosa.

PLASMA PROTEINS

Plasma is blood minus the cells. Many solutes are present in plasma, the most abundant of which are proteins. The total protein content of plasma is 6–8 gm/dl. Plasma contains a large number of proteins. Some of these are present in very minute amounts, e.g. protein hormones on their way to target cells and intracellular enzymes that have leaked into circulation due to wear and tear of cells. These are not considered as plasma proteins. Some other proteins are present in significant concentrations and perform their functions in plasma. These are called plasma proteins. Some of their functions are of a general nature, e.g. maintenance of pH and maintenance of colloid osmotic pressure. Some functions are of a specialised nature and are performed by specific proteins, e.g. transport of hormones, vitamins, minerals, lipids, bilirubin, etc. general defence against foreign invaders, specific defence against foreign antigens, coagulation of blood, fibrinolysis, etc.

Plasma proteins can be separated by salt fractionation, alcohol fractionation, electrophoresis, etc. Electrophoresis separates plasma proteins into albumin, α_1-globulins, α_2-globulins, β-globulins, γ-globulins and fibrinogen. By more sensitive techniques, the β-globulins can be separated into β_1- and β_2- globulins. Each globulin fraction comprises a number of proteins. All the plasma proteins except γ-globulins are synthesised in liver. The γ-globulins are synthesised in and secreted by plasma cells.

1. Albumin

Albumin is the most abundant protein in plasma. Its concentration is 3.5 to 5.5 gm/dl. It is responsible for 75% of the colloid osmotic pressure of plasma. It consists of a single polypeptide chain made up of 585 amino acids. Its molecular weight is 69,000. It is a vehicle for transporting amino acids from liver to extrahepatic tissues. It is also a carrier of free fatty acids, calcium, copper, unconjugated bilirubin, lipophilic hormones, etc. Some drugs, e.g. aspirin, phenytoin, dicoumarol, sulphonamides, etc. also bind to albulmin.

Hypoalbuminaemia can occur in liver diseases due to decreased synthesis of albumin and in renal diseases due to loss of albumin in urine. Severe dietary deficiency of proteins (kwashiorkor) can also cause hypoalbuminaemia. The resulting decrease in colloid osmotic pressure of plasma can cause oedema.

Prealbumin is another protein that can bind all the ligands that albumin can bind. It is smaller than albumin and moves ahead of albumin on electrophoresis. Its concentration is much lower than that of albumin.

2. α_1-Globulins

α_1-Globulins comprise several proteins, e.g. α_1-antitrypsin, α_1-acid glycoprotein (orosomucoid), α_1-fetoprotein, α-lipoprotein (high density lipoprotein or HDL), thyroxine-binding globulin (TBG), corticosteroid-binding globulin (CBG), retinol-binding protein (RBP), etc. HDL, TBG, CBG and RBP are carrier proteins, and will be discussed in later chapters.

α_1-Antitrypsin (now called α_1-antiproteinase) is an inhibitor of serine proteases, e.g. trypsin, elastase, etc. An important function of α_1-antitrypsin is to prevent destruction of elastin in lungs by elastase released from neutrophils. Small amounts of elastase are released continuously due to normal destruction of neutrophils. Much larger amounts are released in pulmonary infection due to accumulation of neutrophils at the site of infection. α_1-Antitrypsin binds to elastase and prevents its proteolytic action. An inherited deficiency of α_1-antitrypsin results in unchecked action of elastase on elastin. Destruction of elastin decreases the elasticity of lungs resulting in emphysema. Smokers with α_1-antitrypsin deficiency are particularly prone to emphysema as cigarette smoke converts a critical methionine residue of α_1-antitrypsin into methionine sulphoxide preventing its binding to elastase.

α_1-**Acid glycoprotein** belongs to a group of proteins called acute phase proteins (or reactants) released in acute infections. Their release is induced by some interleukins

secreted by macrophages and T lymphocytes. They help the immune system and the innate defense system in fighting against the infectious agent or in clearing up the debris from the site of infection or in preventing damage to healthy tissue. α_1-Antitrypsin is also an acute phase protein.

α_1-**Fetoprotein** (AFP) is synthesised in foetal life but not after birth. However, it is synthesised in certain cancers as the cancer cells revert to the undifferentiated type and begin to synthesise embryonic and foetal proteins. Therefore, α_1-fetoprotein is used as a tumour (cancer) marker.

3. α_2-Globulins

α_2-Globulins include ceruloplasmin, haptoglobin, α_2-macroglobulin, etc.

Ceruloplasmin is a copper-containing protein. About 90% of the copper present in plasma is tightly bound to ceruloplasmin. The rest is loosely bound to albumin. Ceruloplasmin was believed to be a copper carrier in the past but as the copper bound to ceruloplasmin is not released easily, the carrier function is performed by albumin. Ceruloplasmin possesses ferroxidase activity. Its real function perhaps is to oxidise ferrous iron to the ferric form. It is also an acute phase protein.

Haptoglobin is also an acute phase protein. Another important function of haptoglobin depends upon its ability to bind free haemoglobin.

Haemoglobin released into plasma due to rupture of erythrocytes can easily pass through the glomeruli. This can result in clogging of tubular lumen and loss of iron from the body. Haptoglobin binds free haemoglobin. The combined size of the two is too big to pass through the glomerular membrane.Thus, binding of haemoglobin to haptoglobin prevents leakage of haemoglobin into glomerular filtrate and loss of iron.

α_2-**Macroglobulin** is a general protease inhibitor. It prevents intravascular coagulation of blood by inhibiting the protease activity of coagulation factors.

4. β-Globulins

β-Globulins include haemopexin, transferrin, C-reactive protein, β-lipoprotein (low density lipoprotein or LDL) and the complement components C1q and C3. Transferrin, LDL and the complement components will be discussed in later chapters.

Haemopexin binds free haem. If haem enters the plasma, it is freely filtered by the glomeruli. This can lead to loss of iron from the body. By binding haem, haemopexin prevents the glomerular filtration of haem and loss of iron.

C-reactive protein (CRP) is so named because it reacts with the C polysaccharide present in the capsule of pneumococci. It is an acute phase protein, and can stimulate the classic complement cascade upon entry of a pathogen in the body.

5. γ-Globulins

γ-Globulins are antibodies. They are also known as immunoglobulins as they perform an immune function. They are discussed in detail in Chapter 19.

6. Fibrinogen

Fibrinogen is one of the coagulation factors. During coagulation, it is converted into fibrin. Several molecules of fibrin aggregate to form the clot. Fibrinogen is also an acute phase protein.

EXERCISE

1. Classify proteins giving examples. Describe the functions performed by proteins.

2. Describe the structural organisation of proteins. Explain denaturation and renaturation.

3. Describe the methods for fractionation of proteins.

4. Write short notes on:
   a. Essential amino acids
   b. Isoelectric pH
   c. α-Helix
   d. Physiologically active peptides
   e. Coagulation of proteins
   f. Chaperone proteins
   g. Electrophoresis
   h. Partition chromatography
   i. Collagen
   j. Plasma proteins

5. Write 'true' or 'false':
   a. Proteins are synthesised from L-amino acids only.
   b. Non-essential amino acids are not required for protein synthesis.
   c. Proline and hydroxyproline are aromatic amino acids.
   d. Taurine and γ-aminobutyric acid act as neurotransmitters.
   e. All amino acids can form zwitterions.
   f. In Sanger's reaction, the carboxyl group of the C-terminal amino acid is tagged with 1-fluoro-2,4-dinitrobenzene.
   g. Edman's reagent can be used to determine the amino acid sequence of proteins.
   h. Glutathione is gamma-glutamyl-cysteinyl-glycine.
   i. Proline residues play an important role in the formation of α-helix.
   j. Quaternary structure is essential for the functioning of every protein.
   k. All proteins are coagulated when they are heated at their isoelectric pH.
   l. Collagen is a right-handed triple helix.
   m. Abnormal collagen is formed in Ehlers-Danlos syndrome.
   n. Plasma proteins are synthesised in liver.
   o. α_1-Antitrypsin prevents the destruction of collagen.

6. Fill in the blanks:
   a. .... is an amino acid having no asymmetric carbon atom.
   b. .... and .... are dicarboxylic amino acids.
   c. .... and .... are imino acids.
   d. .... converts angiotensinogen into angiotensin I.
   e. Angiotensin converting enzyme converts .... into ....
   f. The sequence of amino acids in a protein is known as its .... structure.
   g. .... and .... are contractile proteins.
   h. .... is the most abundant protein in mammals.

i. .... is the most abundant amino acid in collagen.

j. Collagen is synthesised in ....

k. All plasma proteins except .... are synthesised in liver.

l. .... is responsible for 75% of the colloid osmotic pressure of plasma.

m. .... prevents destruction of elastin by elastase in lungs.

n. Haptoglobin binds free .... present in plasma.

ANSWERS TO SHORT QUESTIONS

5. a. True
   b. False
   c. False
   d. True
   e. True
   f. False
   g. True
   h. True
   i. False
   j. False
   k. False
   l. True
   m. True
   n. False
   o. False

6. a. Glycine
   b. Aspartate, glutamate
   c. Proline, hydroxyproline
   d. Renin
   e. Angiotensin I, angiotensin II
   f. Primary
   g. Actin, myosin
   h. Collagen
   i. Glycine
   j. Fibroblasts
   k. γ-Globulins
   l. Albumin
   m. α_1-Antitrypsin
   n. Haemoglobin

Chemistry of Nucleotides and Nucleic Acids

Nucleic acids are present in all living organisms. They are known as information molecules. Genetic information is present in most of the organisms in deoxyribonucleic acid (DNA) and in some viruses in ribonucleic acid (RNA). Nucleic acids store information and transmit information from progenitors to progeny, and from a parent cell to daughter cells. This information is used to synthesise proteins. Nucleic acids are made up of nucleotides.

NUCLEOTIDES

Nucleotides are low molecular weight, nitrogenous, intracellular compounds. They are present in all living organisms, and perform some very important functions. The main functions performed by nucleotides are:

Functions

1. Nucleotides are the monomeric units of nucleic acids, i.e. ribonucleic acid (RNA) and deoxyribonucleic acid (DNA). They are required for the synthesis of nucleic acids.
2. Some of them, e.g. adenosine triphosphate (ATP), serve as sources of energy in energy-requiring activities. ATP is described as the energy currency of the living cells. It is formed during exergonic (energy-releasing) reactions, and is utilised during endergonic (energy-consuming) reactions.
3. Some of them, e.g. cyclic adenosine monophosphate (cAMP) and cyclic guanosine monophosphate (cGMP), are important regulatory compounds which control a variety of biochemical and physiological processes by acting as second messengers for some hormones.
4. Many nucleotides serve as coenzymes, e.g. flavin adenine dinucleotide (FAD), nicotinamide adenine dinucleotide (NAD) and nicotinamide adenine dinucleotide phosphate (NADP).
5. Some of them occur as intermediate compounds in various metabolic pathways, e.g. uridine disphosphate glucose (UDP-glucose), uridine diphosphate galactose (UDP-galactose), uridine diphosphate glucuronic acid (UDP-glucuronic acid), cytidine diphosphate diacylglycerol (CDP-diacylglycerol), cytidine diphosphate choline (CDP-choline), etc.
6. Some of them act as allosteric regulators of a variety of allosteric enzymes.

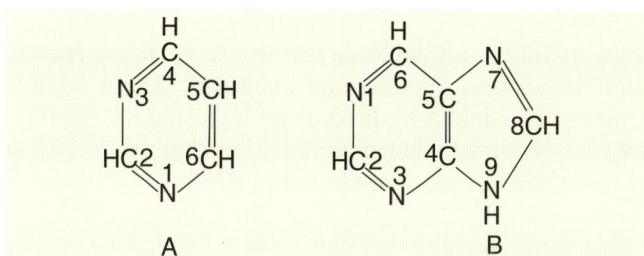

Fig. 6.1: Pyrimidine (A) and purine (B) nuclei

Chemistry

Nucleotides, also known as mononucleotides, are made up of three components—a nitrogenous base, a sugar and phosphoric acid. The nitrogenous base combines with a sugar to form a nucleoside. The nucleoside combines with phosphoric acid to form a nucleotide.

Nitrogenous Bases

Two types of bases are found in nucleotides – pyrimidine bases and purine bases. These are the derivatives of pyrimidine and purine respectively (Fig. 6.1).

Three major pyrimidine bases are found in nucleotides– cytosine, uracil and thymine (Fig. 6.2).

Two major purine bases found in nucleotides are adenine and guanine. Two other purine bases, hypoxanthine and xanthine are the metabolites of adenine and guanine which are ultimately converted into uric acid. Uric acid is the end product of purine catabolism (Fig. 6.3).

Some purine bases, formed by methylation of xanthine, are found in plants, and possess pharmacological properties. These include theophylline (1,3-dimethyl-xanthine), theobromine (3,7-dimethylxanthine) and caffeine (1,3,7-trimethylxanthine). These occur in tea, cocoa and coffee respectively.

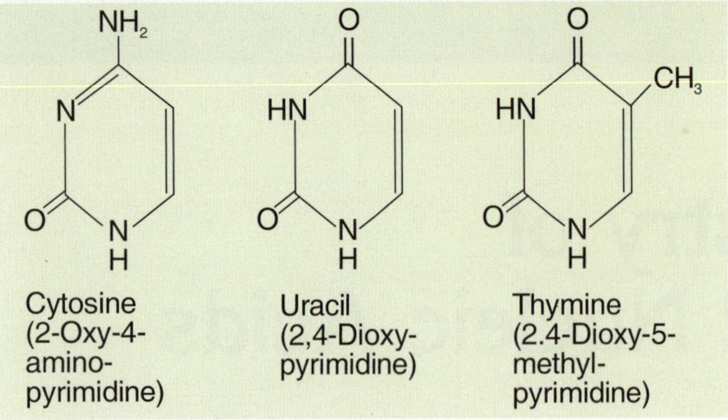

Fig. 6.2: Pyrimidine bases

Cytosine (2-Oxy-4-amino-pyrimidine)

Uracil (2,4-Dioxy-pyrimidine)

Thymine (2.4-Dioxy-5-methyl-pyrimidine)

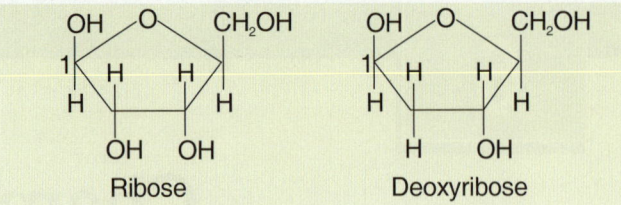

Fig. 6.4: Sugars found in nucleotides and nucleic acids

Besides the five major pyrimidine and purine bases, some minor or unusual bases are also found in the nucleic acids of viruses, bacteria and mammals. These include 5-methylcytosine, 5-hydroxymethylcytosine, N^6-methyladenine, N^6-dimethyladenine and N^7-methylguanine. Most of these unusual bases are found in RNA.

Sugars

Two pentose sugars are found in nucleotides - ribose and deoxyribose (Fig. 6.4).

The sugar is linked to a pyrimidine or a purine base to form a nucleoside. A carbon-nitrogen bond is formed between the sugar and the base. In case of pyrimidines, the bond is formed between carbon atom 1 of the sugar and nitrogen atom 1 of the base. In case of purines, the bond is formed between carbon atom 1 of the sugar and nitrogen atom 9 of the base (Fig. 6.5).

The *anti* conformation in which the base and the sugar are on the opposite sides of the C–N bond is found more commonly than the *syn* conformation in which the base and the sugar are on the same side of the C–N bond. The nucleosides containing ribose are:

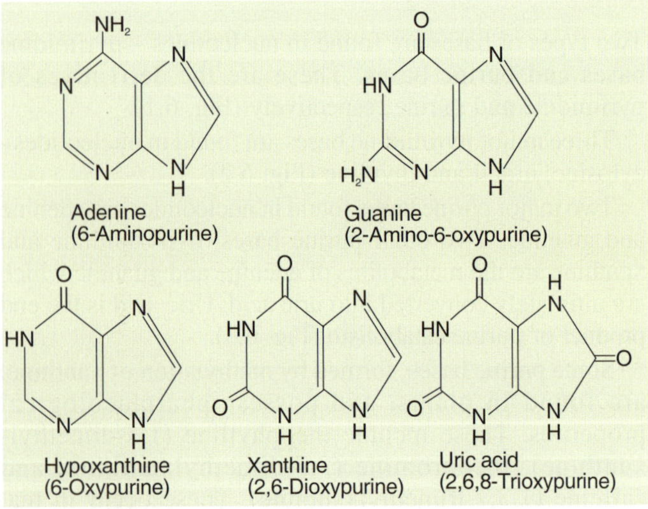

1. Cytidine (cytosine + ribose)
2. Uridine (uracil + ribose)
3. Adenosine (adenine + ribose)
4. Guanosine (guanine + ribose)

The nucleosides containing deoxyribose are:
1. Deoxycytidine (cytosine + deoxyribose)
2. Deoxythymidine (thymine + deoxyribose)
3. Deoxyadenosine (adenine + deoxyribose)
4. Deoxyguanosine (guanine + deoxyribose)

Phosphoric Acid

The nucleosides combine with phosphoric acid (H_3PO_4) to form nucleotides (Fig. 6.6). One of the –OH groups of the sugar portion of nucleoside is esterified with phosphoric acid in nucleotides.

The phosphate group is generally attached to carbon atom 3 or 5 of the sugar. To avoid confusion between the numbering of various atoms in the base and the carbon atoms of the sugar, those of the latter are numbered 1', 2', 3', etc. The prime mark on the numeral shows that we are referring to the carbon atoms of the sugar.

Abbreviations

A single-letter abbreviation is commonly used for ribonucleosides. Adenosine, guanosine, cytidine and uridine are abbreviated as A, G, C and U respectively. The abbreviations for deoxyadenosine, deoxyguanosine, deoxycytidine and deoxythymidine are dA, dG, dC and dT respectively. A single phosphate group, attached to the

Adenine (6-Aminopurine)

Guanine (2-Amino-6-oxypurine)

Hypoxanthine (6-Oxypurine)

Xanthine (2,6-Dioxypurine)

Uric acid (2,6,8-Trioxypurine)

Fig. 6.3: Purine bases and their metabolites

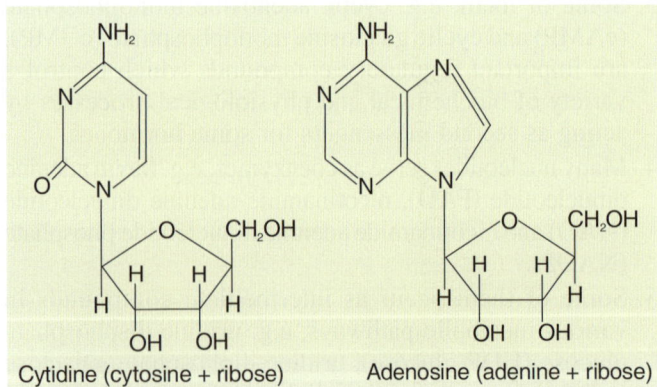

Cytidine (cytosine + ribose)

Adenosine (adenine + ribose)

Fig. 6.5: Ribonucleosides of cytosine and adenin

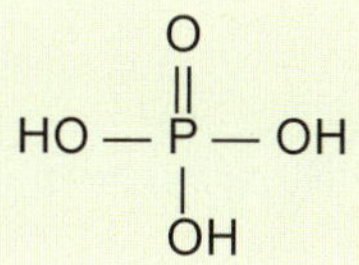

Fig. 6.6: Phosphoric acid

sugar portion of the nucleoside, is represented by the letters MP. Thus, the abbreviations for adenosine monophosphate, guanosine monophosphate, cytidine monophosphate and uridine monophosphate are AMP, GMP, CMP and UMP respectively. These compounds are ribonucleotides. In deoxyribonucleotides, the letter 'd' precedes the abbreviations.

When the phosphate group is attached to carbon atom 5 of the sugar, its position is not indicated in the abbreviation. Thus, AMP means adenosine-5'-monophosphate and so on. When the phosphate group is attached to a carbon atom other than carbon atom 5 of the sugar, its position is indicated by an appropriate numeral, e.g. A-3'-MP (adenosine-3'-monophosphate), G-3'-MP (guanosine-3'-monophosphate), etc (Fig 6.7).

Sometimes, more than one phosphate groups are attached to the nucleoside. The first phosphate group is attached to the sugar portion of the nucleoside by an ester linkage. The subsequent phosphate groups are attached to the preceding ones by acid anhydride bonds. When two phosphate groups are attached to a nucleoside, they are denoted by the letters DP (diphosphate) following the abbreviation for the nucleoside, e.g. ADP (adenosine-5'-diphosphate) When three phosphate groups are attached to a nucleoside, they are denoted by the letters TP (triphosphate), e.g. ATP (adenosine-5'-triphosphate).

Some Important Nucleotides

Besides occurring as constituents of RNA and DNA, many nucleotides occur as such in the body, and perform important functions. Some important nucleotides are the following:

Adenine Derivatives

AMP, ADP and ATP are the nucleotides containing adenine (Fig. 6.8). ADP and ATP are described as high-energy phosphates. Hydrolytic removal of the terminal phosphate of ADP and the last two phosphates of ATP liberates a large amount of energy. Therefore, these two nucleotides can be used as sources of energy in energy-consuming reactions. During biological oxidation, energy is captured in the form of ATP by phosphorylation of ADP.

Another important nucleotide derived from adenine is adenosine-3',5'-monophosphate (Fig. 6.9), also called cyclic AMP (cAMP). Cyclic AMP is formed by the action of adenylate cyclase on ATP. Cyclic AMP can be converted into AMP by another enzyme, cAMP phosphodiesterase. cAMP mediates the actions of several hormones at the cellular level.

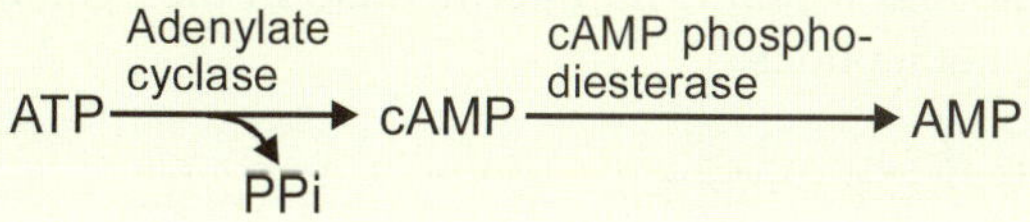

Guanine Derivatives

The guanine-containing nucleotides are GMP, GDP, GTP and cyclic GMP. GDP and GTP are high-energy phosphates just like ADP and ATP, and participate in some energy-transfer reactions. Cyclic GMP is the analogue of cyclic AMP. It is a second messenger for some hormones, and is involved in the process of vision. It is formed by the action of guanylate cyclase, and is degraded by cGMP phosphodiesterase.

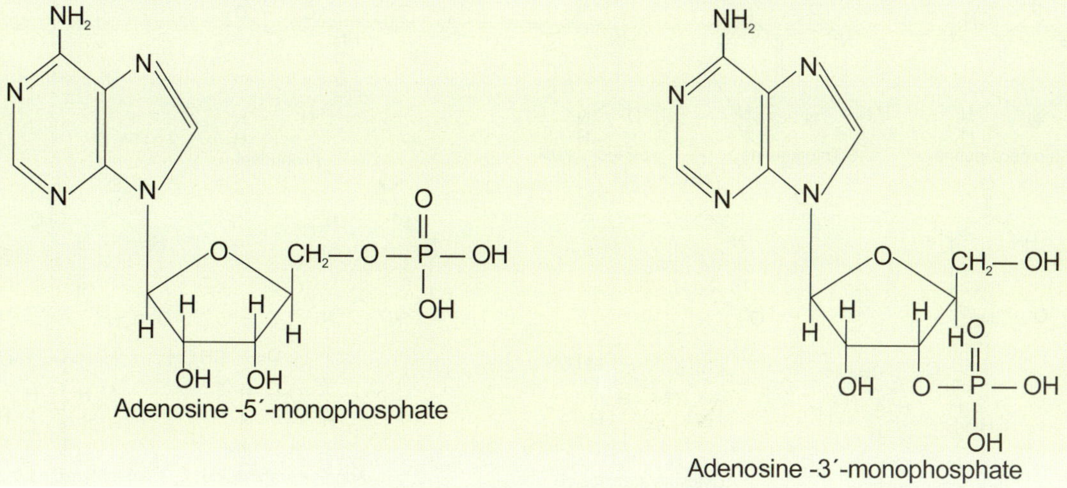

Adenosine -5′-monophosphate

Adenosine -3′-monophosphate

Fig. 6.7: Ribonucleotides of adenine

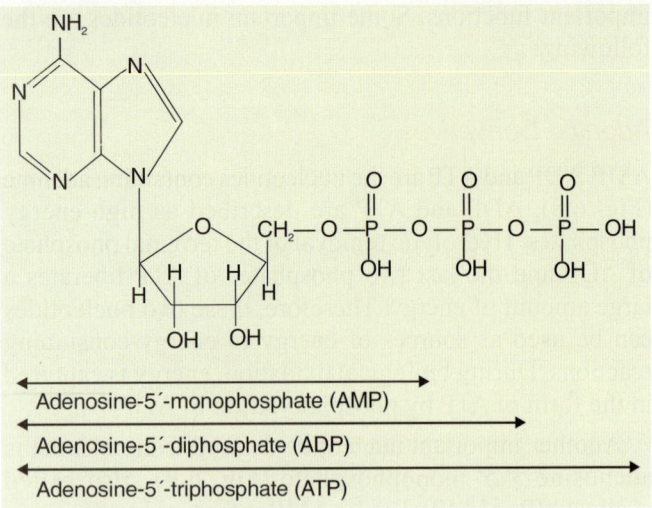

Adenosine-5′-monophosphate (AMP)

Adenosine-5′-diphosphate (ADP)

Adenosine-5′-triphosphate (ATP)

Fig. 6.8: Adenosine mono-, di- and tri-phosphate

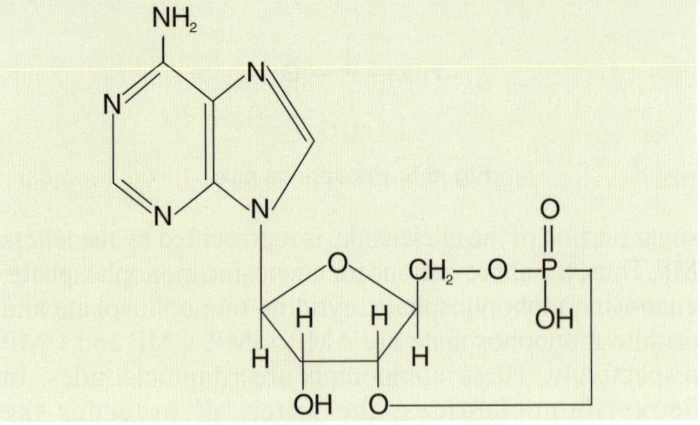

Hypoxanthine Derivatives

Hypoxanthine and ribose form a nucleoside, inosine. Inosine monophosphate (IMP) is the nucleotide formed from inosine which is an intermediate in the synthesis of purine nucleotides.

Cytosine Derivatives

CMP, CDP and CTP are the nucleotides formed from cytosine. CDP and CTP are high-energy phosphates. Derivatives of CDP, e.g. CDP-diacylglycerol and CDP-choline, are intermediates in some pathways of lipid metabolism.

Uracil Derivatives

UMP, UDP and UTP are the uracil-containing nucleotides. The last two are the high-energy analogues of ADP and

Fig. 6.9: Cyclic AMP (cAMP)

ATP respectively. Some derivatives of UDP, e.g. UDP-glucose, UDP-galactose and UDP-glucuronic acid, are intermediates in some pathways of carbohydrate metabolism.

Vitamin Derivatives

Most water-soluble vitamins perform their biochemical functions in the form of coenzymes. Many of these coenzymes are nucleotides containing adenine, ribose, phosphate and some other groups. Examples are flavin adenine dinucleotide (FAD), nicotinamide adenine dinucleotide (NAD), nicotinamide adenine dinucleotide phosphate (NADP), etc.

Synthetic Derivatives

Some synthetic nucleosides and purine and pyrimidine bases are important pharmacological agents (Fig. 6.10).

Cell division entails replication of cellular DNA which requires a ready supply of nucleotides. If substitutions are made in the structures of purine or pyrimidine bases or

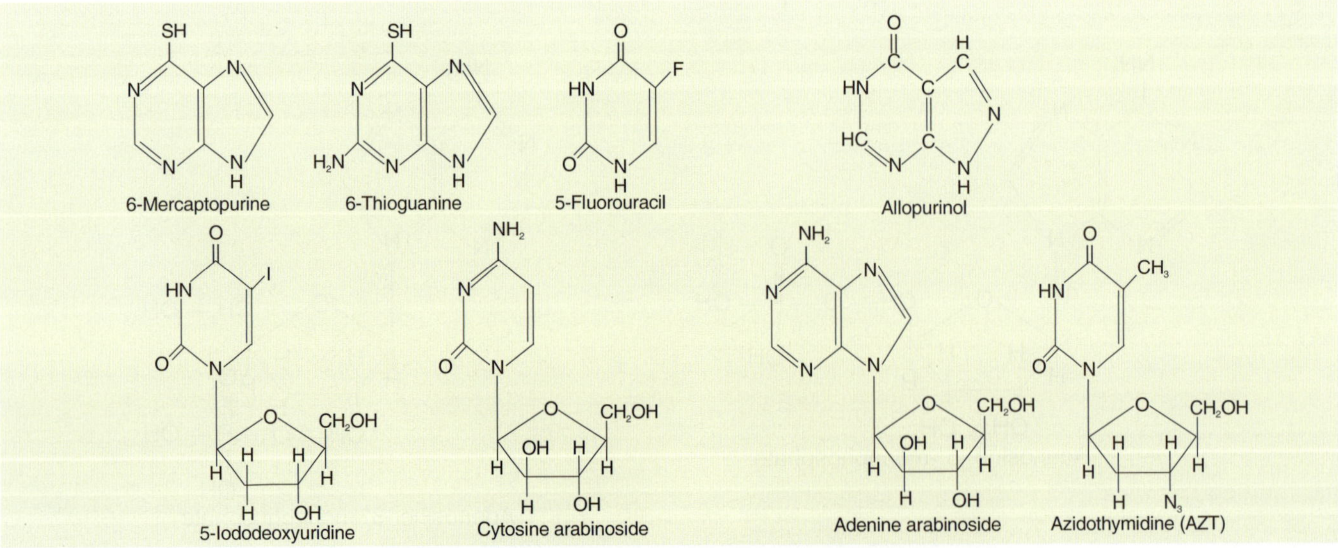

Fig. 6.10: Synthetic bases and nucleosides used as drugs

the sugar portion of the nucleosides, and the substituted bases or nucleosides are given to a subject, they will be incorporated in the nucleic acids. However, DNA containing these abnormal bases or sugars can not be replicated, and this prevents cell division. Therefore, several substituted bases and nucleosides are used as anti-cancer drugs to prevent the uncontrolled proliferation of cells. Many others are being evaluated or used as antiviral drugs to check the multiplication of viruses. Examples of synthetic bases and nucleosides used as anti-cancer drugs include 6-mercaptopurine, 6-thioguanine, 5-fluorouracil, 5-iododeoxyuridine, cytosine arabinoside, adenine arabinoside, etc. Azidothymidine is used in the treatment of AIDS. Allopurinol, a structural analogue of hypo-xanthine, is used in the treatment of gout.

NUCLEIC ACIDS

Nucleic acids are macromolecules made up of a large number of mononucleotides (nucleotides). There are two types of nucleic acids – deoxyribonucleic acid (DNA) and ribonucleic acid (RNA). The former is a polymer of deoxyribonucleotides, and the latter of ribonucleotides. DNA is mainly present in the nuclei of the cells. RNA is mainly extranuclear.

DEOXYRIBONUCLEIC ACID (DNA)

DNA is the repository of genetic information. The earliest evidence about the role of DNA in transmission of genetic information was obtained by Avery, MacLeod and McCarty (1944). They carried out their experiments on two types of pneumococci. One type is encapsulated, forms smooth colonies, and is pathogenic. The other type is non-encapsulated, forms rough colonies, and is non-pathogenic. Each type produces its own kind of offspring. Avery and his associates extracted nuclear material from the encapsulated pneumococci and introduced it into the non-encapsulated pneumococci. As a result, the daughter cells acquired capsules, and became pathogenic. Thus, it was proved that genetic information is present in the nucleus. Since nucleus contains DNA, RNA and proteins, Avery et al treated the nuclear matter with enzymes that hydrolyse DNA or RNA or proteins. Hydrolysis of DNA destroyed the transforming activity of nuclear matter but hydrolysis of RNA or proteins did not.Therefore, Avery et al concluded that genetic information was present in DNA.

Some researchers still speculated that genetic information might be present in nuclear proteins and not in DNA. This doubt was cleared by Hershey and Chase in 1952. They conducted their experiments on T_2 bacteriophage, a virus that infects the bacterium, *E.coli*, and multiplies inside it. When a large number of progeny viruses are formed, the bacterial cell wall ruptures releasing the virus particles. T_2 bacteriophage is a DNA virus made up of a protein coat surrounding the DNA. Hershey and

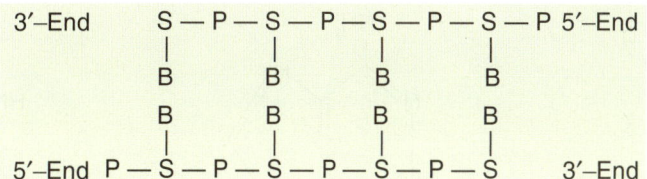

Fig. 6.11: A schematic representation of anti-parallel strands (B, S and P represent base, sugar and phosphate respectively)

Chase labeled the viral proteins with ^{35}S and DNA with ^{32}P. The phage was allowed to infect *E.coli*. It was seen that ^{32}P was present inside the *E.coli* while ^{35}S remained outside the bacterial cell. This showed that when the virus infected the bacterium, only the viral DNA entered the bacterial cell and not the proteins. Since proteins surrounded the new virus particles, DNA must have directed the synthesis of viral proteins. This established the role of DNA as the genetic material.

For the transmission of genetic information from a parent cell to daughter cells, the DNA of the daughter cells should be an exact replica of the DNA of the parent cell. Chargaff (1950) discovered that the number of adenine residues is always equal to the number of thymine residues, and the number of guanine residues is always equal to that of cytosine residues in a molecule of DNA. Wilkins and Franklin carried out extensive X-ray crystallographic studies on DNA and showed that DNA has a helical structure.

Structure

On the basis of the observations referred to above and their own X-ray diffraction studies, Watson and Crick (1953) proposed a model of the DNA molecule. According to this model, DNA is a double-stranded molecule. Each strand is a polymer of mononucleotides. Each strand possesses a polarity. It has a 3'-end at which the –OH group attached to carbon atom 3 of the sugar is unesterified. The other end is the 5'-end at which the –OH group attached to carbon atom 5 of the sugar is unesterified. The two strands are anti-parallel, i.e. they are parallel but run in opposite directions (Fig. 6.11).

Four bases – adenine, guanine, cytosine and thymine – are present in these nucleotides. The sugar is deoxyribose. The successive nucleotides are linked by 3',5'-phospho-diester bonds (Fig. 6.12).

The strands are held together by hydrogen bonds between their purine and pyrimidine bases. Adenine is paired with thymine. Guanine is paired with cytosine. This is known as the **base-pairing rule**. This explains why the number of adenine residues is equal to that of thymine residues, and the number of guanine residues is equal to that of cytosine residues. There are two hydrogen bonds between adenine and thymine, and three hydrogen bonds between guanine and cytosine (Figs 6.13 and 6.14).

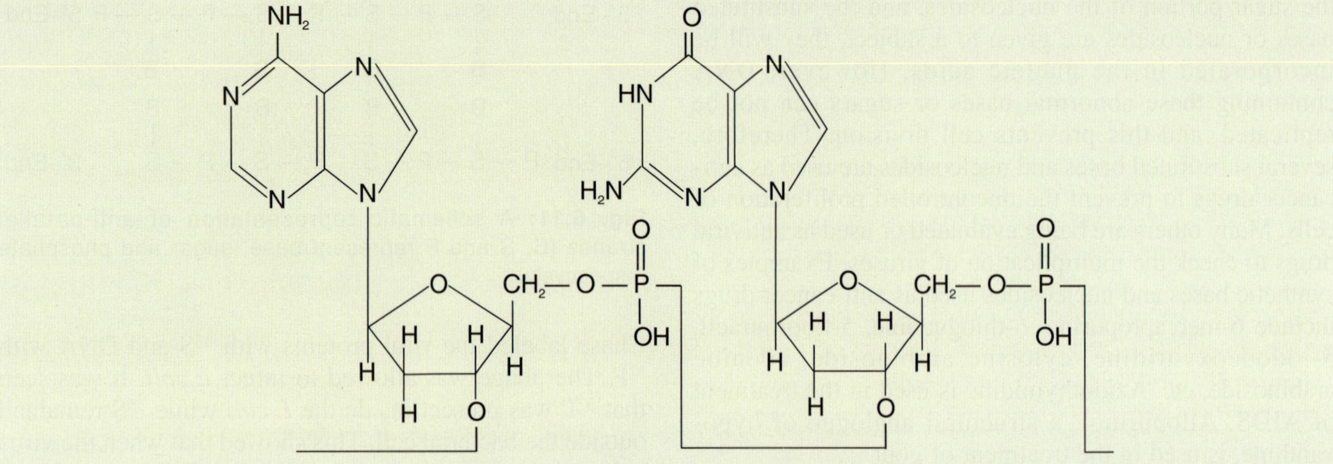

Fig. 6.12: A portion of one strand of DNA

The two strands are not straight. They are twisted around each other to form a double helix. Each turn of the helix contains ten base pairs, and has a pitch (vertical distance per turn) of 3.4 nm. The diameter of the helix is 2 nm. The two strands have opposite polarities, i.e. they run in opposite directions. All the purine and pyrimidine bases present on one strand of the molecule take part in hydrogen bonding with complementary bases on the opposite strand. The bases are present in the interior of the molecule while the sugar and phosphate groups are present on the outer side. The helix is right-handed. Two grooves are seen in the double helix which are termed as the major groove and the minor groove. These grooves are present between the glycosidic bonds on the opposite strands (Fig. 6.15).

After elucidation of the structure of DNA by Watson and Crick, Richard Dickerson found a slightly different structure in DNA crystals. The structure found by him was named as A-DNA, and that described by Watson and

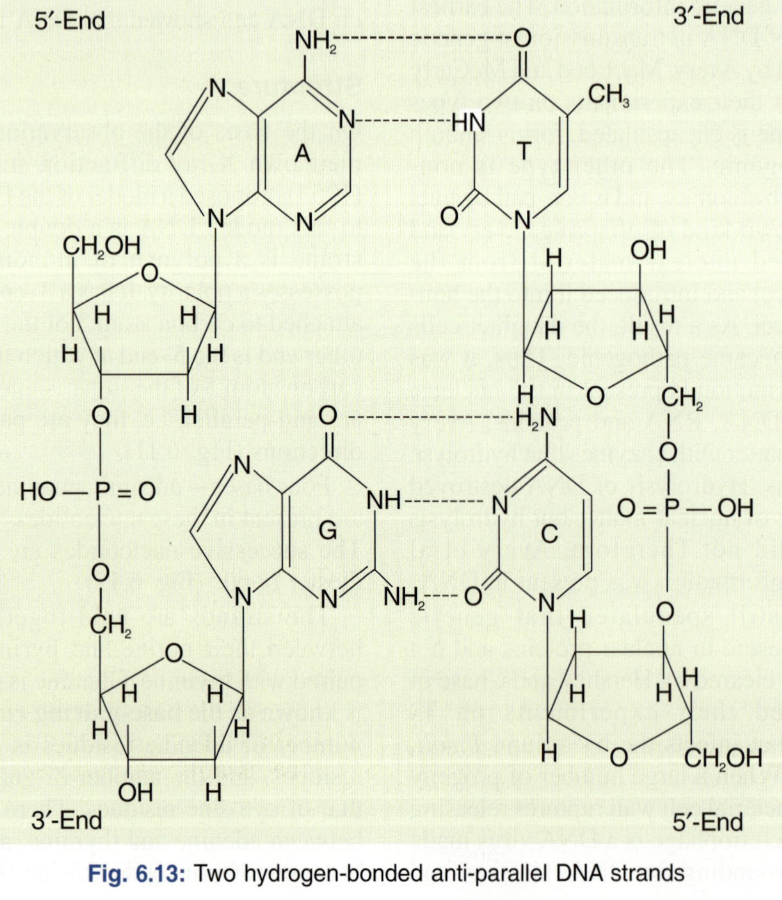

Fig. 6.13: Two hydrogen-bonded anti-parallel DNA strands

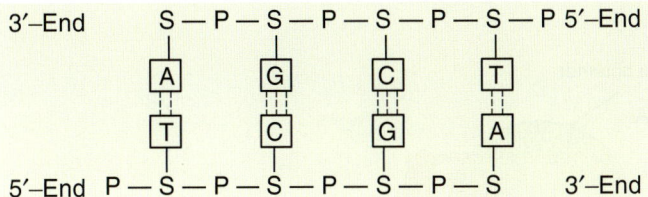

Fig. 6.14: DNA strands (schematic)

Crick as B-DNA. A third type of structure was found by Alexander Rich which was named as Z-DNA. B-DNA is the commonest type of DNA. A-DNA is formed in a less humid environment. Z-DNA is formed when purine and pyrimidine bases alternate in a DNA strand. The structural features of different types of DNA are summarised in Table 6.1.

Genetic information is present on one strand of DNA, known as the sense strand. The other strand, which has a complementary sequence of bases, is known as the anti-sense strand. During replication, the two strands separate, and each serves as a template on which a new strand containing a complementary sequence of bases is synthesised. Thus, the newly-synthesised DNA becomes an exact replica of the original DNA.

The DNA is combined with a nearly equal amount of proteins to form nucleoproteins. The predominant proteins are histones which are of five types – H1, H2A, H2B, H3 and H4. The histones are basic proteins rich in lysine and arginine. These positively charged amino acids interact with negatively charged phosphate groups of DNA. The basic amino acids are present mainly in the N-terminal and C-terminal regions. The inner core of histones contains nonpolar amino acids which form a globular structure. Many non-histone proteins are also associated with DNA in small amounts which have a bearing on various functions like replication and transcription.

Human beings have 23 pairs of chromosomes. Each chromosome consists of a single molecule of double-helical

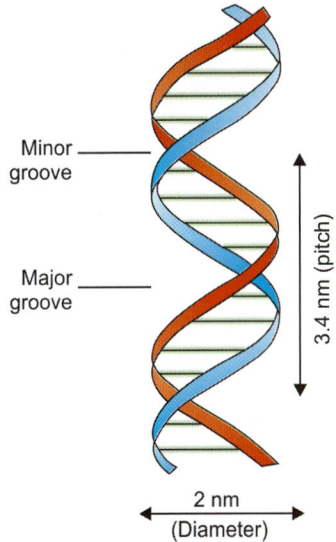

Fig. 6.15: Double-helical DNA

DNA along with several proteins. Two molecules each of histones H2A, H2B, H3 and H4 form an octamer around which DNA is wrapped in two coils to form a nucleosome. A nucleosome associated with histone H1 is called a chromatosome. A series of nucleosomes ("beads on a string") form a polynucleosome. The DNA between two nucleosomes is known as linker DNA. Nucleosomes (10 nm wide) condense to form 30 nm wide nucleofilaments. In this way, the linear DNA becomes highly compact. Even higher compactness is achieved by looping of nucleofilaments. The loops associate with some scaffold proteins to form a chromosome (Fig. 6.16).

Most of the DNA present in a cell is supercoiled (superhelical). In supercoiled DNA, the axis of the double helix is bent and twisted upon itself. In negatively supercoiled DNA, the twists are right-handed. In positively supercoiled DNA, the twists are left-handed. Most of the naturally occurring DNA is negatively supercoiled.

RIBONUCLEIC ACID (RNA)

RNA is also a polymer of mononucleotides. However, it differs from DNA in the following respects:

1. The sugar present in RNA is ribose instead of deoxyribose.
2. The pyrimidine bases are cytosine and uracil instead of cytosine and thymine of DNA. The purine bases are the same as in DNA.
3. The RNA molecule is single-stranded. However, the molecule may be folded upon itself, and hydrogen bonds may be formed between complementary bases on parts of the same strand to give a double-stranded appearance in certain regions of the molecule.
4. The numbers of adenine and guanine residues are not necessarily equal to those of uracil and cytosine residues respectively.
5. Unlike DNA, RNA is hydrolysed by alkalis to form 2',3'-cyclic diesters of mononucleotides.

Table. 6.1: Structural characteristics of A-DNA, B-DNA and Z-DNA

	A-DNA	B-DNA	Z-DNA
Diameter	2.3 nm	2.0 nm	1.8 nm
Rise per base pair	0.25 nm	0.34 nm	0.37 nm
Number of base pairs per turn	11	10	12
Rise per turn(pitch)	2.7 nm	3.4 nm	4.4 nm
Glycosidic bond	*syn*	*anti*	*syn* (purines) *anti* (pyriidines)
Major groove	Narrow	Wide	Flat
Minor groove	Wide	Narrow	Very narrow
Direction of helix	Right-handed	Right-handed	Left-handed

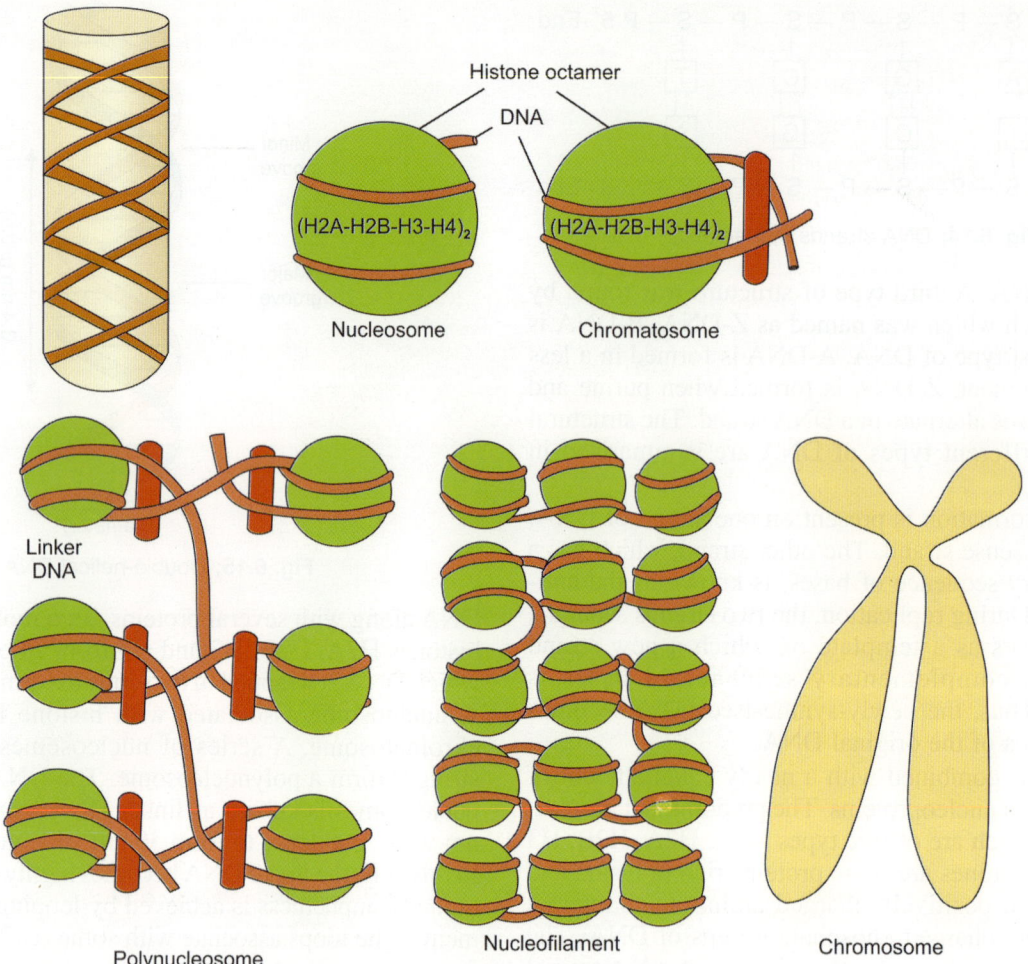

Fig. 6.16: Different levels of structural organisation of DNA ultimately forming a chromosome

There are three types of RNA– messenger RNA (mRNA), transfer RNA (tRNA) and ribosomal RNA (rRNA). Each type performs a specific function, and has a characteristic structure.

Messenger RNA

This type of RNA carries the information (message) from the nucleus to the ribosomes. The genetic information is present on the sense strand of DNA in the form of genes. A gene is a portion of the sense strand having a specific nucleotide sequence that contains coded information for the synthesis of a particular protein. Each mRNA molecule is a transcript of the sense strand of a particular gene. Its nucleotide sequence is complementary to that of the sense strand of the gene, i.e. adenine for thymine, guanine for cytosine, uracil for adenine and cytosine for guanine. At the 5'-end, mRNA possesses a 7-methylguanosine triphosphate cap which helps the protein-synthesising machinery to identify the mRNA. At its 3'-end, there is a poly-A tail made up of several adenylate residues which gives stability to the structure of mRNA.

The messenger RNA molecule is initially synthesised in eukaryotes as a precursor known as heterogeneous nuclear RNA (hnRNA) which is several-fold bigger than the final mRNA molecule, and which is processed to form mRNA.

Transfer RNA

This is made up of about 75 nucleotides, and has a molecular weight of about 25,000. Its function is to transport amino acids from the cytosol to the ribosomes where proteins are synthesised. Proteins are synthesised from 20 amino acids. For each of these amino acids, there is at least one specific tRNA. For some amino acids, there are more than one species of tRNA. But one species of tRNA transports only one specific amino acid and no other. Some intra-strand hydrogen bonds are formed between complementary bases on the same strand giving a clover leaf shape to tRNA. Further folding upon itself gives tRNA an L-shaped tertiary structure (Fig. 6.17).

At the 3'-terminus, the last three nucleotides are: –C–C–A. The amino acid is attached to the terminal adenylate residue. The molecule has three loops (or arms) known respectively as **pseudouridine (ψ) loop, anticodon**

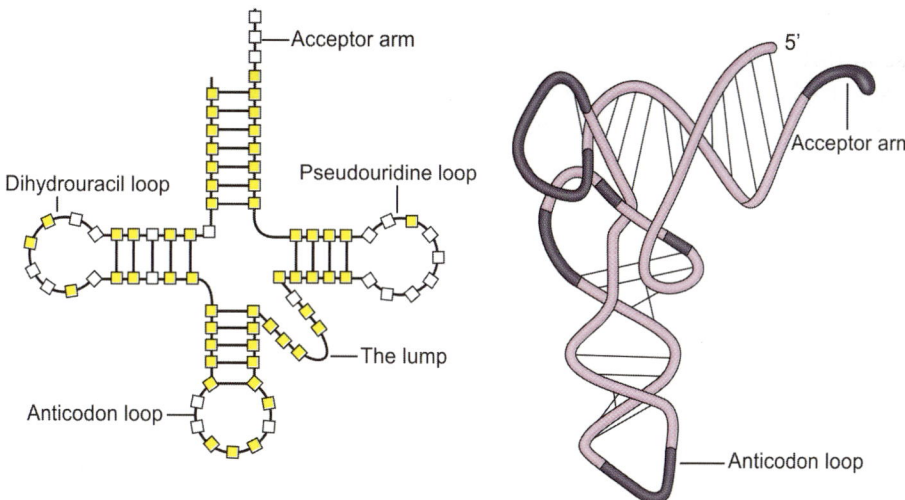

Fig. 6.17: Clover leaf structure of tRNA on left and tertiary structure on right

loop and **dihydrouracil (DHU) loop**. In the ψ loop, a uracil residue is attached to ribose by carbon-carbon linkage rather than carbon-nitrogen linkage. The DHU loop contains a dihydrouracil residue, an unusual pyrimidine base. The anticodon loop contains a triplet of nucleotides which recognises a complementary triplet of nucleotides (codon) on the mRNA.

Ribosomal RNA

This is present in the ribosomes. The ribosomes are made up of two subunits known respectively as the 40S subunit and the 60S subunit in eukaryotes. The 40S subunit is made up of 18S rRNA and about 30 different polypeptides. The 60S subunit is made up of three types of rRNA – 5S rRNA, 5.8S rRNA and 28S rRNA – and about 50 different polypeptides. When proteins are not being synthesised, the two subunits remain separate. At the time of protein synthesis, the two subunits combine to form an 80S unit on which mRNA and tRNAs interact to synthesise a protein. The 5.8S, 18S and 28S rRNAs are formed from a single 45S precursor. The 5S rRNA is formed from a different precursor.

EXERCISE

1. Describe the structural organisation and functions of DNA.

2. Describe the structures and functions of different types of RNA.

3. Write short notes on:
   a. Cyclic AMP
   b. Differences between DNA and RNA
   c. hnRNA
   d. tRNA

4. Write 'true' or 'false':
   a. Cyclic AMP is formed from AMP.
   b. Guanylate cyclase converts GTP into cGMP.
   c. The pyrimidine bases present in DNA are adenine and guanine.
   d. The two strands in DNA are anti-parallel.
   e. The number of adenine bases in DNA is equal to that of thymine bases.
   f. Two hydrogen bonds are formed between cytosine and guanine in DNA.
   g. Z-DNA is formed when purine and pyrimidine bases are present alternately in DNA.
   h. Linker DNA is present between two nucleosomes.
   i. The pyrimidine bases in RNA are cytosine and thymine.
   j. hnRNA is the precursor of mRNA in prokaryotes.

5. Fill in the blanks:
   a. Adenylate cyclase converts .... into ....
   b. A cyclic nucleotide participating in the process of vision is ....

c. The purine bases in DNA are .... and ....

d. The purine base in IMP is ....

e. 7-Methylguanosine triphosphate cap is present at the .... end of ....

f. Poly-A tail is present at the .... end of ....

g. tRNA transports ....from cytosol to ....

h. -CCA is present at the ....end of ....

i. Anticodon loop is present in ....

j. Ribosomes are made up of rRNA and some ....

ANSWERS TO SHORT QUESTIONS

4. a. False
   c. False
   e. True
   g True
   i. False

   b. True
   d. True
   f. False
   h. True
   j. False

5. a. ATP, cAMP
   c. Adenine, guanine
   e. 5', mRNA
   g. Amino acids, ribosomes
   i. tRNA

   b. cGMP
   d. Hypoxanthine
   f. 3', mRNA
   h. 3', tRNA
   j. Proteins

7

Enzymes

A vast multitude of chemical reactions occur in living organisms. These reactions would proceed at extremely low velocities in the absence of catalysts. The common catalysts used in non-living systems, e.g. acids, alkalis, metals are not suitable for living organisms because of their toxicity and lack of specificity. The biological catalysts must be safe as well as specific. They should also be capable of adjusting their catalytic activity according to the ever changing requirements of the organism. All these properties are present in enzymes which are the biological catalysts used by living organisms.

DEFINITION

It is difficult to arrive at an acceptable definition of enzymes. In the past, all enzymes were found to be proteins synthesised by living organisms, and acting within living cells. It was later seen that enzymes could act outside the living cells also. With advances in molecular biology, it is now possible to synthesise genetically engineered enzymes. Thus, the older definitions of enzymes have now outlived their validity. Enzymes may now be defined as protein catalysts that catalyse chemical reactions in biological systems. Even this definition is not entirely correct, as some RNA molecules, called ribozymes, have now been found to catalyse some biochemical reactions.

ENZYME SPECIFICITY

As mentioned earlier, the biological catalysts must be very specific. This is essential for normal functioning of the organism. If a single enzyme catalysed a large number of reactions, it would be impossible to regulate the rates of individual reactions. If a single reaction were to be inhibited at a given time for some reason, all the other reactions catalysed by the same enzyme would also be inhibited. However, this does not happen, as the enzymes are very specific. The degree of specificity may have the following orders:

1. Group Specificity

These enzymes are specific for the chemical group or bond that they act upon but not for the actual substrate (substrates are the molecules on which the enzymes act, and the molecules formed in the reaction are known as products). Group-specific or bond-specific enzymes are frequently present in digestive secretions, and hydrolyse the complex molecules of foodstuffs. For example, pepsin, trypsin and chymotrypsin hydrolyse peptide bonds. But they would hydrolyse the peptide bonds present in any protein. This gives an advantage to the organism in that a large variety of dietary proteins can be digested by a small number of proteolytic enzymes. Other examples include lipases, glycosidases, nucleases, etc.

Some group-specific enzymes have a slightly higher degree of specificity. For example, aminopeptidase and carboxypeptidase split off only the N-terminal and C-terminal amino acids respectively. Endopeptidases hydrolyse the internal peptide bonds (Fig.7.1). Chymotrypsin acts on peptide bonds in which the carboxyl group is contributed by an aromatic amino acid. Amylase is specific for α-1, 4-glycosidic bond.

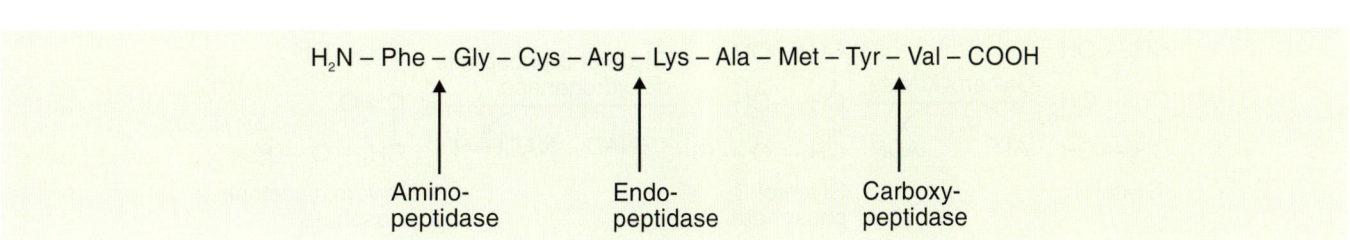

Fig. 7.1: Action of exopeptidases and endopeptidases

65

2. Substrate Specificity

Most of the enzymes are specific not only for a chemical bond or a group but also for the substrate. For example, glucokinase transfers a phosphate group from ATP to C_6 of glucose. Fructokinase transfers a phosphate group from ATP to C_1 of fructose. These are substrate-specific enzymes.

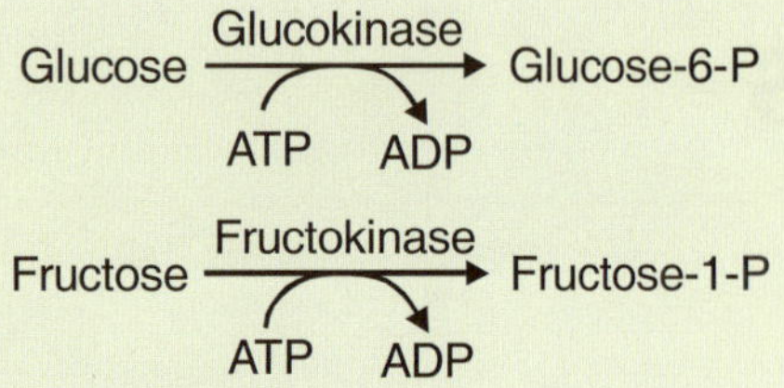

$$\text{Glucose} \xrightarrow[\text{ATP} \quad \text{ADP}]{\text{Glucokinase}} \text{Glucose-6-P}$$

$$\text{Fructose} \xrightarrow[\text{ATP} \quad \text{ADP}]{\text{Fructokinase}} \text{Fructose-1-P}$$

3. Stereospecificity

Many biomolecules exhibit stereoisomerism (and optical isomerism), e.g. carbohydrates and amino acids. Enzymes acting on such substrates are usually specific for a particular stereoisomer. For example, mammalian enzymes acting on carbohydrates are generally specific for D-isomers and those acting on amino acids are generally specific for L-isomers. Exceptions are the racemases which can interconvert the D- and L-isomers of a compound.

COENZYMES AND COFACTORS

Some enzymes require the presence of a non-protein substance for their catalytic activity. If the non-protein substance is organic, it is known as a coenzyme. If it is inorganic, it is known as a cofactor. The coenzyme or the cofactor may be an integral part of the enzyme molecule or its presence may be required during the reaction. The protein portion of an enzyme that requires a coenzyme is called **apoenzyme**. The apoenzyme combines with the coenzyme to form the holoenzyme which is the catalytically active form of the enzyme.

$$\text{Apoenzyme + Coenzyme} \longrightarrow \text{Holoenzyme}$$

The coenzymes generally contain vitamins of B-complex family, e.g. thiamin, riboflavin, niacin, pantothenic acid, pyridoxine, folic acid, vitamin B_{12}, lipoic acid, biotin, etc. Some of these, e.g. lipoic acid and biotin, act as coenzymes by themselves. The others can be converted into coenzymes.

Coenzymes are generally required in group transfer reactions in which a chemical group is transferred from one compound to another, e.g. oxidation-reduction, transamination, phosphorylation, etc. They can be divided into two groups according to the nature of the chemical group that they help to transfer:

A. Coenzymes involved in transfer of hydrogen

1. FMN (Flavin mononucleotide)
2. FAD (Flavin adenine dinucleotide)
3. NAD^+ (Nicotinamide adenine dinucleotide)
4. $NADP^+$ (Nicotinamide adenine dinucleotide phosphate)
5. Lipoic acid
6. Coenzyme Q

B. Coenzymes involved in the transfer of groups other than hydrogen

1. TPP (Thiamin pyrophosphate) or TDP (Thiamin diphosphate)
2. CoA (Coenzyme A)
3. PLP (Pyridoxal phosphate)
4. H_4- Folate (Tetrahydrofolate)
5. Cobamides (B_{12}-coenzymes)
6. Lipoic acid
7. Biotin
8. ATP (Adenosine triphosphate) and similar nucleotides

Role of Coenzymes

The enzyme acts upon its substrate, and converts it into a product.

$$\text{Substrate} \xrightarrow{\text{Enzyme}} \text{Product}$$

The coenzyme may be regarded as a co-substrate or a second substrate in the group transfer reactions. The coenzyme participates in the reaction either as a donor or as an acceptor of the group that is being transferred (Fig. 7.2).

In the first reaction in Fig.7.2, glycerol is the main substrate which is converted by glycerol kinase into glycerol-3-phosphate. The coenzyme ATP acts as a second substrate, and provides the phosphate group. In the second reaction, glycerol-3-phosphate is the main substrate which is oxidised by removal of two hydrogen atoms. The

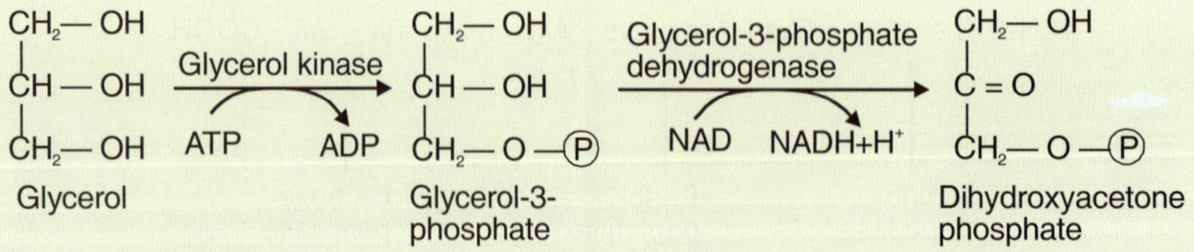

Fig. 7.2: Examples illustrating transfer of phosphate and hydrogen

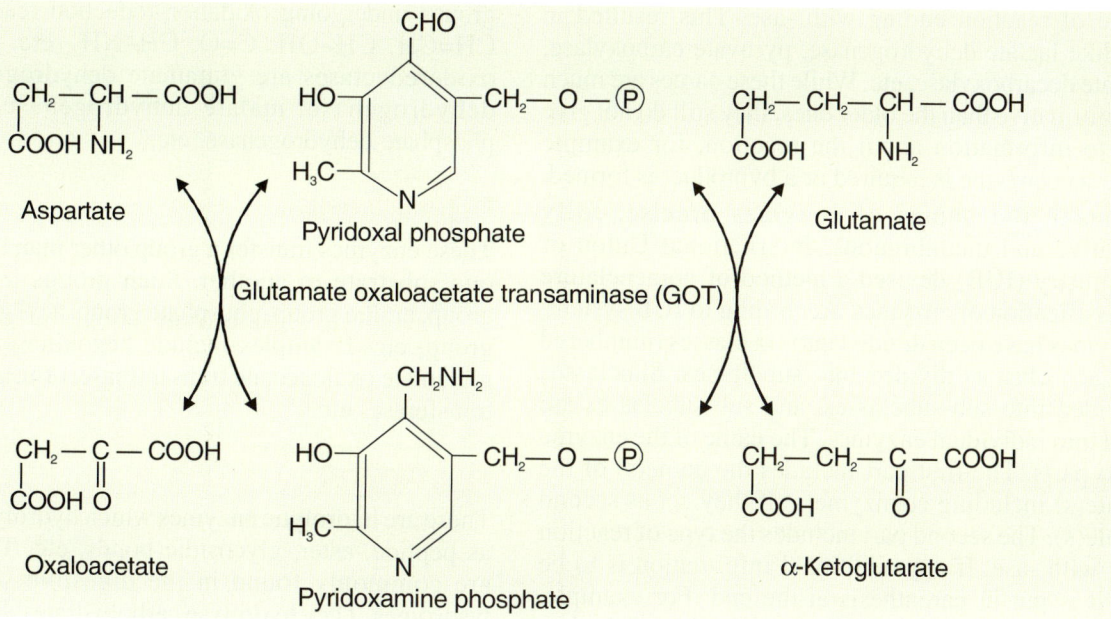

Fig. 7.3: Pyridoxal phosphate as a carrier of amino group in transamination

coenzyme NAD^+ acts as a second substrate, and accepts the hydrogen atoms. The chemical change in the coenzyme is opposite to that in the substrate.

Some coenzymes accept a chemical group from one substrate and donate it to another. Thus, they act only as carriers, and regain their original form at the end of the reaction. Pyridoxal phosphate is an example which acts as a carrier of amino group in transamination reactions.

In the transamination reaction catalysed by glutamate oxaloacetate transaminase (Fig. 7.3), pyridoxal phosphate accepts the amino group from aspartate, and transfers it to α-ketoglutarate. Aspartate is converted into oxaloacetate, and α-ketoglutarate into glutamate. The coenzyme goes back to its original form at the end of the reaction. Though pyridoxal phosphate is a reactant in transamination, the reaction is often shown as:

Aspartate + α-Ketoglutarate

PLP | GOT

Oxaloacetate + Glutamate

Sometimes, the change in the coenzyme is more important than the change in the substrate. For example,

in aerobic glycolysis, glucose is converted into pyruvate, and NAD^+ is reduced in one of the reactions. Reduced NAD^+ transfers its hydrogen atoms to oxygen forming water, and NAD^+ is regenerated. In anaerobic conditions, NAD^+ can not be regenerated due to lack of oxygen. Therefore, an additional reaction occurs in which pyruvate is reduced to lactate, and NADH is oxidised to NAD^+. Here, regeneration of NAD^+ is more important for continuation of glycolysis (Fig. 7.4).

ENZYME NOMENCLATURE AND CLASSIFICATION

The nomenclature of enzymes has undergone many changes over the years. The names assigned to enzymes in the beginning were very vague and uninformative. Some of the earliest names, e.g. pepsin, ptylin, zymase, etc. indicate neither the substrates of the enzymes nor the type of reactions catalysed by them. Later on, a slightly more informative nomenclature was adopted. Suffix -ase was added to the name of the substrate, e.g. lipase, protease, ribonuclease, etc. Still the type of reaction catalysed by the enzyme remained unclear. Nomenclature was modified further, to include the name of the substrate followed by

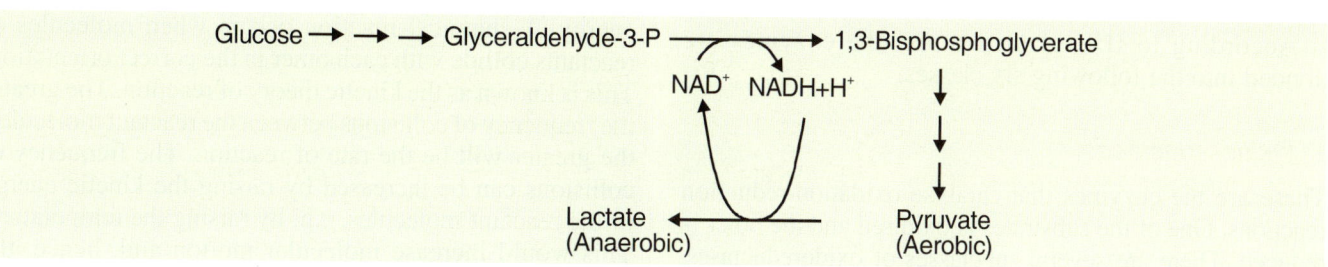

Fig. 7.4: Regeneration of NAD^+ in anaerobic glycolysis

the type of reaction ending with -ase. This resulted in names like lactate dehydrogenase, pyruvate carboxylase, glutamate decarboxylase, etc. While these names are much more informative than the older ones, they still do not give complete information about the reaction, for example whether a coenzyme is required or a byproduct is formed.

To make the names of enzymes precise, fully informative and unambiguous, International Union of Biochemistry (IUB) devised a method of nomenclature and classification of enzymes. According to IUB system, the enzymes have been divided into six classes (numbered 1–6). Each class is divided into subclasses. Subclasses are divided into sub-subclasses, and sub-subclasses are divided into individual enzymes. The name of the enzyme has two parts. The first part includes the name(s) of the substrate(s) including coenzyme(s) if they act as second substrate(s). The second part includes the type of reaction ending with -ase. If any additional information is to be given, it is put in parenthesis at the end. For example, the enzyme having the trivial name glutamate dehydrogenase catalyses the following reaction:

$$\text{L-Glutamate} + \text{NAD(P)}^+ + \text{H}_2\text{O}$$
$$\downarrow$$
$$\alpha\text{-Ketoglutarate} + \text{NAD(P)H} + \text{H}^+ + \text{NH}_3$$

According to IUB system, this enzyme is known as L-glutamate: NAD(P) oxidoreductase (deaminating). This name shows that the enzyme acts on L-glutamate. NAD^+ or $NADP^+$ is required as a co-substrate. The type of reaction is oxidoreduction, i.e. L-glutamate is oxidised and the co-substrate is reduced. The amino group of L-glutamate is released as ammonia. Thus, the name gives complete information about the reaction catalysed by the enzyme.

Moreover, each enzyme has been given a code number (EC) consisting of four digits which, successively, denote the number of the class, subclass, subsubclass and the individual enzyme. The code number of L-glutamate: NAD(P) oxidoreductase (deaminating) is EC 1.4.1.3 which shows that is it the third enzyme of subsubclass 1 of subclass 4 of class 1. The code number gives complete identity of the enzyme. However, trivial names of enzymes are still commonly used because of their brevity and prolonged usage.

According to IUB classification, the enzymes are divided into the following six classes.

1. Oxidoreductases

These are the enzymes that catalyse oxidation-reduction reactions. One of the substrates is oxidised and the other is reduced. There are several subclasses of oxidoreductases, each acting on a particular chemical group. The chemical groups undergoing oxidation-reduction reactions include $CH=CH$, $CH-OH$, $C=O$, $CH-NH_2$, etc. Examples of oxidoreductases are glutamate dehydrogenase, lactate dehydrogenase, malate dehydrogenase, glycerol-3-phosphate dehydrogenase, etc.

2. Transferases

These enzymes transfer a group other than hydrogen from one substrate to another. Such groups include methyl group, amino group, phosphate group, acyl group, glycosyl group, etc. Examples include hexokinase, glucokinase, glutamate oxaloacetate transaminase, ornithine carbamoyl transferase, etc.

3. Hydrolases

These are hydrolytic enzymes which hydrolyse bonds such as peptide, ester, glycosidic bonds, etc. These enzymes are commonly found in the digestive secretions and lysosomes. They hydrolyse carbohydrates, lipids, proteins, etc. Examples are amylase, lipase, pepsin, ribonuclease, sucrase, lactase, maltase, etc.

4. Lyases

These enzymes remove chemical groups from substrates by mechanisms other than hydrolysis. The groups removed may be water, amino group, carboxyl group, etc. Examples include aldolase, enolase, fumarase, etc.

5. Isomerases

These enzymes catalyse interconversion of isomers of a compound. Examples include alanine racemase, triose phosphate isomerase, phosphohexose isomerase, ribose-5-phosphate ketoisomerase, etc.

6. Ligases

These enzymes ligate or bind two compounds together. Since the binding occurs by a covalent bond, a source of energy is required, usually a high-energy phosphate compound. Examples are glutamine synthetase, squalene synthetase, acetyl CoA carboxylase, etc.

Mechanism of Action of Enzymes

At temperatures above absolute zero, i.e. $-273°C$, molecules are in constant motion because of their kinetic energy. A chemical reaction occurs when molecules of reactants collide with each other in the correct orientation. This is known as the kinetic theory of reaction. The greater the frequency of collisions between the reactant molecules, the greater will be the rate of reaction. The frequency of collisions can be increased by raising the kinetic energy of the reactant molecules, e.g. by raising the temperature. This would increase molecular motion and, hence, the frequency of collisions.

The energy level of the reactants has to be raised to a critical level for the reaction to occur. The energy input required to reach this critical level is known as the energy of activation. However, the option of raising the temperature to reach the critical level is not available in living organisms. Enzymes provide an alternate pathway for the reaction. They lower the energy of activation (Fig. 7.5).

Enzyme-Substrate Interaction

The enzyme molecules are usually much larger than their substrates. An enzyme possesses a specific binding site for its substrate(s) known as the substrate site (or the active site). The substrate binds to this site forming an enzyme-substrate (ES) complex (Fig. 7.6). This may bring two substrates in close proximity (bond-forming distance) in the correct orientation so that a bond may be formed between the two.

Sometimes, the binding of a substrate to the enzyme induces a strain in the substrate. Due to this strain, a bond is broken, and the substrate is split into two or more products. Or on binding of two substrates to the enzyme, a chemical group may be transferred from one substrate to another.

The catalytic action of the enzyme may be exerted by cofactors or coenzymes or by some amino acid residues present at the substrate site. Serine, histidine, cysteine and aspartate are some common amino acid residues involved in catalysis.

In carbonic anhydrase, the cofactor (zinc) is placed strategically at the substrate site. The reaction between carbon dioxide and water is catalysed by zinc (Fig. 7.7). In transamination reactions, the coenzyme pyridoxal phosphate, which is tightly bound to the enzyme, is involved in catalysis (Fig. 7.8).

Serine proteases are proteolytic enzymes in which serine residues present at the substrate site catalyse hydrolysis of peptide bonds (Fig. 7.9). Examples of serine proteases are trypsin, chymotrypsin, thrombin, etc.

MODELS OF ENZYME CONFORMATION

In the beginning, it was proposed by Emil Fischer that the conformation of enzymes was rigid, and there was a lock and key type of complementarity between the substrate site on the enzyme and its substrate.

This came to be known as the rigid template model, and adequately explained the specificity of enzymes. However, this model did not agree with certain experimental findings obtained later on. It was seen experimentally that the conformation of the enzyme is not rigid. The conformation changes when the enzyme combines with its substrate.

To explain the difference between the conformation of free enzyme and the enzyme bound to the substrate, Daniel Koshland proposed the induced fit model. According to this model, the conformation of the enzyme is not rigid. Just as with any protein, the conformation of the enzyme can also change. The complementarity between the substrate and the substrate site is not apparent when the enzyme is present in the free form.

When the substrate approaches the enzyme, it induces a change in the conformation of the enzyme as a result of which the substrate site becomes complementary to the substrate (Fig. 7.10). The substrate, then, binds to the enzyme, and is converted into the product. The release of the product restores the enzyme to its original conformation. Koshland's model has become the accepted model of enzyme conformation now.

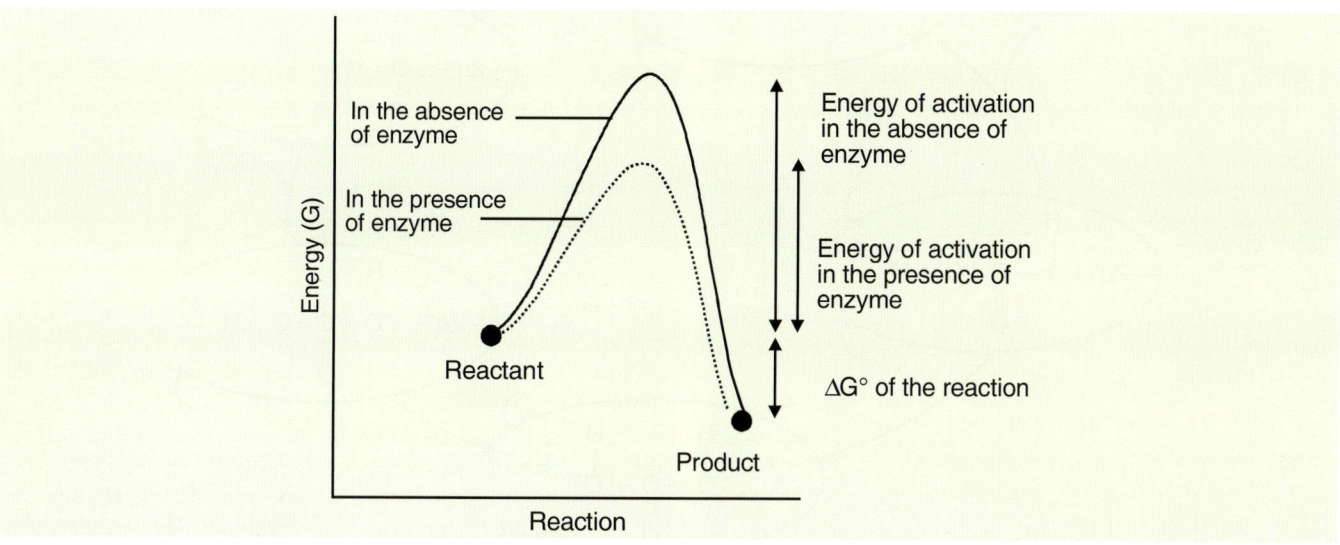

Fig. 7.5: The difference between the energy level of the reactant and the product is the standard free energy change ($\Delta G°$) of the reaction. Enzymes do not change the $\Delta G°$. They lower the energy of activation

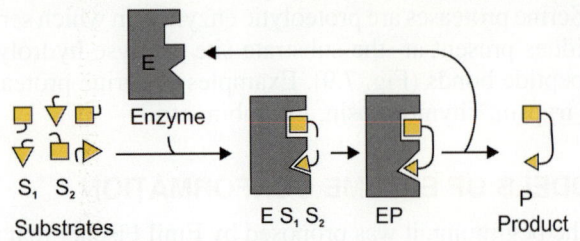

Fig. 7.6: Formation of enzyme-substrate complex is followed by formation of the product, and its release from the enzyme

Allosteric Enzymes

Some enzymes possess a site, in addition to the substrate site, known as the allosteric site. Binding of an allosteric molecule to the allosteric site affects the conformation of the substrate site. Such enzymes are termed as allosteric enzymes. The allosteric molecule (effector or modifier or regulator) may facilitate the conformational change required for substrate binding. Such regulators are known as allosteric activators (positive modifiers). An example is N-acetylglutamate which is an allosteric activator of carbamoyl phosphate synthetase (mitochondrial).

Some allosteric regulators prevent the conformational change required for the binding of the substrate (Fig. 7.11). These are known as allosteric inhibitors (negative modifiers). The enzymes subject to allosteric inhibition are generally present in the beginning of long metabolic pathways. The allosteric inhibitor is generally the product of the pathway. The allosteric enzyme regulates the rate of formation of the product. If the product is not being utilised and accumulates, it inhibits the allosteric enzyme, and further synthesis of the product is stopped. When the concentration of the product decreases, it dissociates from the allosteric enzyme, and the inhibition is relieved.

Factors Affecting the Rates of Enzyme-Catalysed Reactions

1. *Enzyme Concentration*

An enzyme catalyses a reaction by forming the enzyme-substrate complex which dissociates into the enzyme and the product.

$$E + S \rightleftharpoons ES \rightleftharpoons E + P$$

The enzyme may be considered to take part in the reaction as a reactant though it is regenerated in its original form at the end of the reaction. Therefore, the rate of the initial reaction leading to the formation of ES is directly proportional to the product of molar concentrations of E and S.

$$\text{Rate of formation of ES} \propto [E][S]$$

Similarly, the rate of the second reaction leading to the formation of E and P is directly proportional to the molar concentration of ES.

$$\text{Rate of formation of E and P} \propto [ES]$$

Therefore, the rate of formation of the product, i.e. the rate of the overall reaction is proportional to the enzyme concentration provided that enough substrate is available to combine with the enzyme.

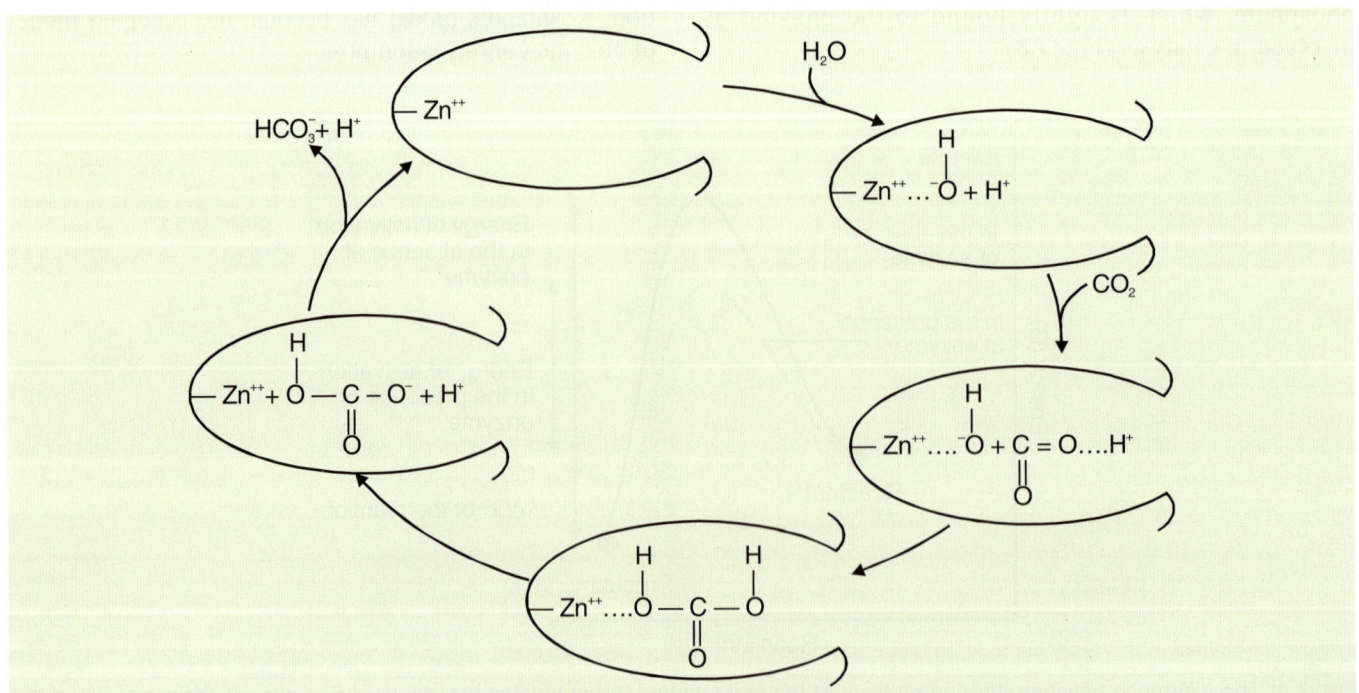

Fig. 7.7: In the reaction between water and carbon dioxide catalysed by carbonic anhydrase, the zinc ion plays the catalytic role

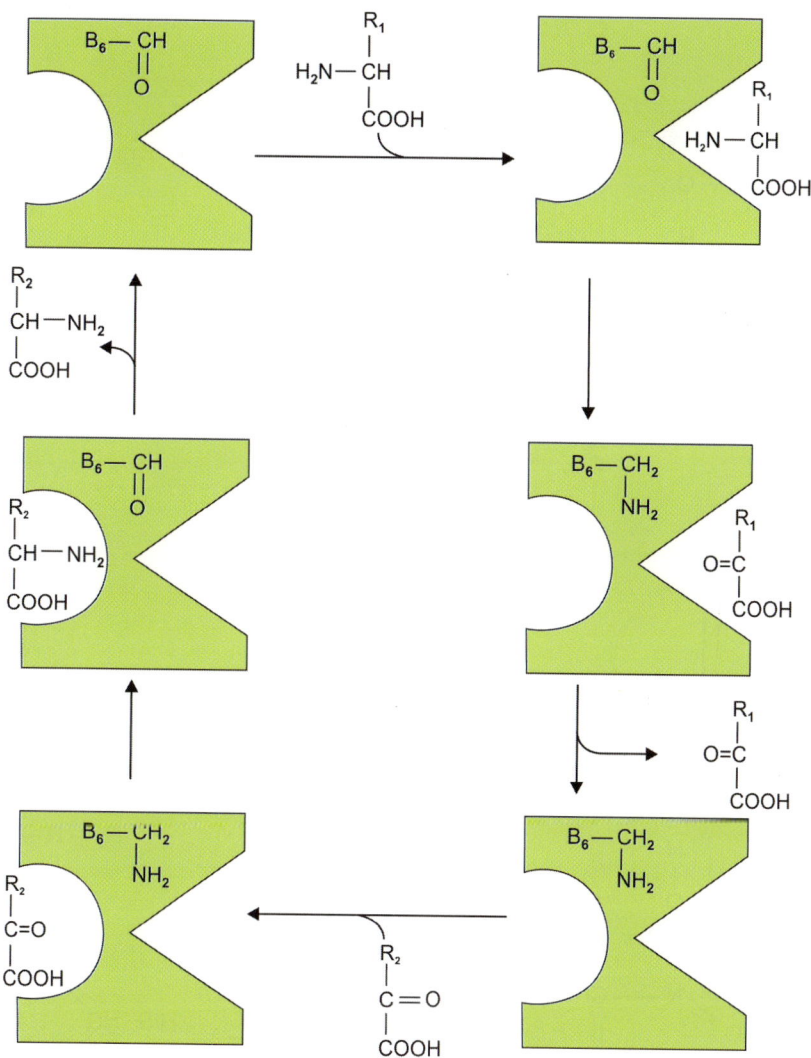

Fig. 7.8: In the transamination reaction between the amino acid and the keto acid, pyridoxal phosphate plays the catalytic role

2. Substrate Concentration

Just as the rate of the reaction is proportional to enzyme concentration, theoretically it should be proportional to substrate concentration also. But this is possible only when enough enzyme is available to bind the substrate. However, the availability of enzymes in the cells is limited whereas the concentration of substrates can vary over a wide range. Therefore, when the substrate concentration rises, initially there is a proportionate increase in the velocity of the reaction. But as the enzyme molecules begin to be saturated with the substrate, the rise in velocity becomes slower. When all the enzyme molecules are saturated with the substrate, no further increase in velocity is possible, and maximum velocity (V_{max}) is reached (Fig. 7.12).

At V_{max}, all the enzyme molecules are saturated with the substrate, and no further increase in velocity is possible even if the substrate concentration goes on increasing. The substrate concentration at which the velocity is half of V_{max} is known as the Michaelis constant (Km) of the enzyme.

The relationship between the velocity of the reaction and the substrate concentration can be expressed by Michaelis-Menten equation, which is:

$$v = \frac{V_{max} \cdot [S]}{Km + [S]}$$

When the substrate concentration is very low, the sum of Km and [S] is nearly equal to Km as [S] is negligible. Therefore, the equation may be rewritten as:

$$v = \frac{V_{max} \cdot [S]}{Km}$$

Since both V_{max} and Km are constant,

$$V \propto [S]$$

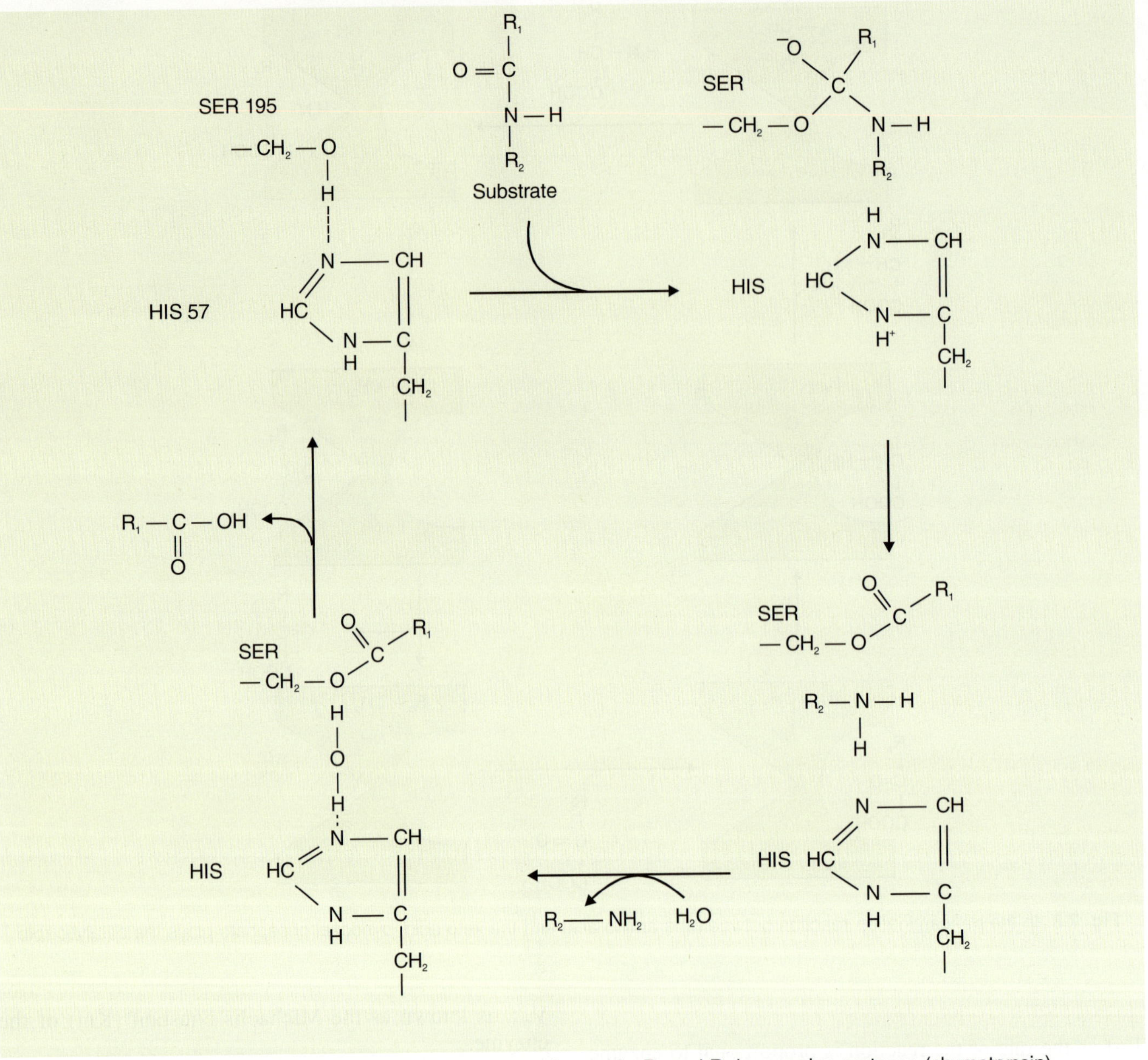

Fig. 7.9: Hydrolysis of the peptide bond between amino acids, R_1 and R_2 by a serine protease (chymotrypsin)

Thus, at very low substrate concentrations, the velocity of the reaction is directly proportional to the substrate concentration.

When the substrate concentration is very high, the sum of Km and [S] is nearly equal to [S] as Km is relatively negligible. Therefore, the equation may be rewritten as:

$$v = \frac{V_{max} \cdot [S]}{[S]}$$

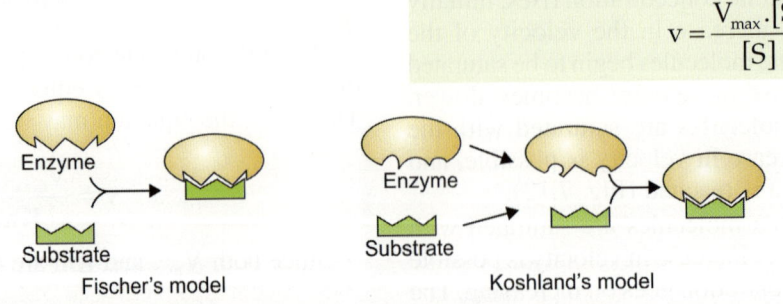

Enzyme

Substrate

Fischer's model

Enzyme

Substrate

Koshland's model

Fig. 7.10: Fischer's rigid template model and Koshland's induced fit model of enzyme conformation

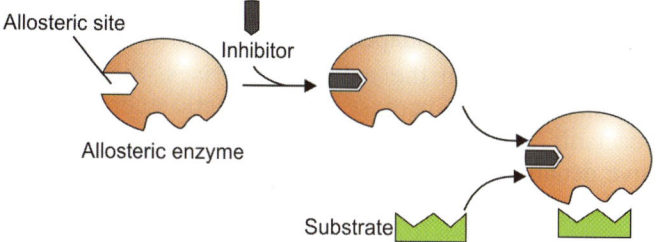

Fig. 7.11: Binding of an allosteric inhibitor to the allosteric site of the enzyme prevents a change in conformation when the substrate approaches the enzyme. The substrate can not bind to the enzyme, and the reaction can not occur

$$\text{or } v = V_{max}$$

Thus, at very high substrate concentrations, the velocity becomes constant and equal to V_{max}.

When the substrate concentration is exactly equal to Km, the sum of Km and [S] may be taken as 2 [S]. The equation may be rewritten as:

$$v = \frac{V_{max} \cdot [S]}{2[S]} = \frac{V_{max}}{2}$$

This shows that when the substrate concentration is exactly equal to Km, the velocity is half of V_{max}. This also proves the definition of Km.

Determination of Km

Every enzyme has got a characteristic Km. Determination of Km is important in the study of enzyme kinetics, for assay of enzyme activity and for evaluation of enzyme inhibitors. Plotting v versus [S] is an inconvenient and cumbersome process as the velocity has to be measured at a large number of substrate concentrations until V_{max} is reached.

A simpler method was devised by Lineweaver and Burk in which velocity is measured at a small number (5-6) of substrate concentrations, and a graph is plotted between the reciprocal of v and the reciprocal of [S], that is, 1/v vs 1/[S]. The 1/v vs 1/[S] plot is known as Lineweaver-Burk plot or double reciprocal plot.

Michaelis-Menten equation is inverted:

$$\frac{1}{v} = \frac{Km + [S]}{V_{max} \cdot [S]}$$

or

$$\frac{1}{v} = \frac{Km}{V_{max} \cdot [S]} + \frac{[S]}{V_{max} \cdot [S]}$$

or

$$\frac{1}{v} = \frac{Km}{V_{max}} \times \frac{1}{[S]} + \frac{1}{V_{max}}$$

This is the equation for a straight line, i.e. y = ax+b where x (x-axis) is 1/[S], y (y-axis) is 1/v, a (slope of the line) is Km/V_{max} and b (y-intercept) is $1/V_{max}$.

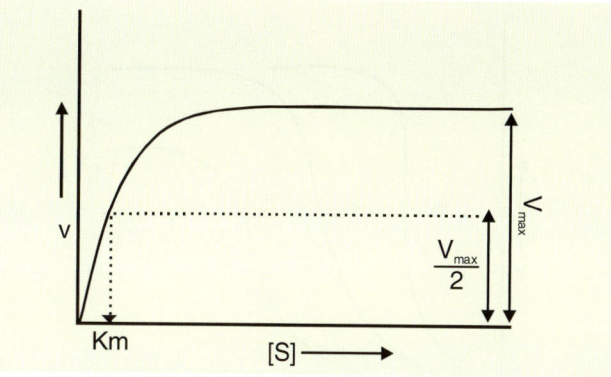

Fig. 7.12: Plot between substrate concentration [S] and velocity [v] of the reaction. Km is the substrate concentration at which the velocity is half of the maximum velocity (V_{max})

At the x-intercept (where the line meets the x-axis), the value of y = 0 (Fig. 7.13). Therefore, at the x-intercept:

$$ax + b = 0$$
$$\text{or} \quad ax = -b$$
$$\text{or} \quad x = -b/a$$

Substituting the values of b and a,

$$x = -\frac{1}{V_{max}} \div \frac{Km}{V_{max}}$$

$$\text{or} \quad x = -\frac{1}{V_{max}} \times \frac{V_{max}}{Km}$$

$$\text{or} \quad x = -\frac{1}{Km}$$

Thus, the x-intercept, i.e. the value of 1/[S] at the x-intercept gives the value of 1/Km, and the reciprocal of this will be the Km.

Allosteric enzymes do not follow Michaelis-Menten equation. The v versus [S] plot of allosteric enzymes is sigmoidal showing co-operative binding of the substrate to the enzyme. Allosteric activators shift the plot to the left, and allosteric inhibitors shift it to the right (Fig. 7.14).

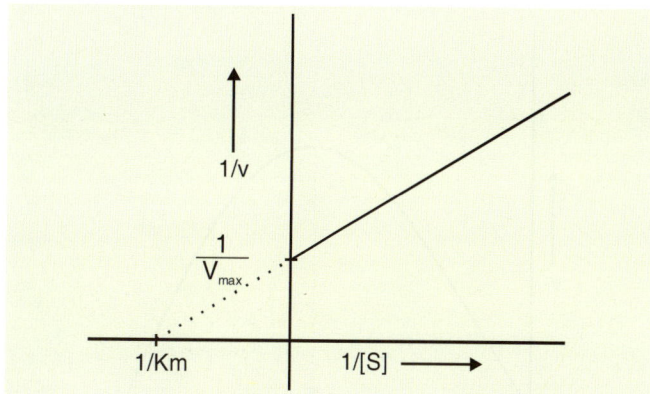

Fig. 7.13: Lineweaver-Burk plot between 1/[S] and 1/v. The x-intercept gives the value of 1/Km, and the y-intercept that of $1/V_{max}$

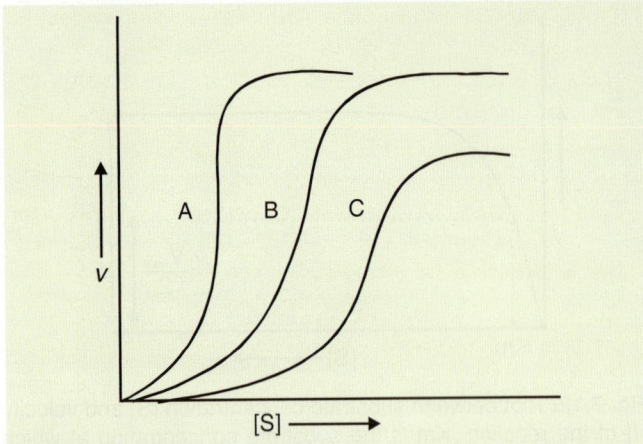

Fig. 7.14: Velocity (v) versus substrate concentration [S] plot of an allosteric enzyme in the absence of an allosteric modifier (B), in the presence of an allosteric activator (A), and in the presence of an allosteric inhibitor (C)

Kinetics of allosteric enzymes follow the Hill equation. S50 (the substrate concentration at which the velocity is half of V_{max}) of allosteric enzymes can be determined from the Hill plot which is plotted between log $v/V_{max}-v$ and log [S].

3. *Coenzyme Concentration*

If a coenzyme is required in the reaction, the concentration of coenzyme can also affect the velocity of the reaction. Some coenzymes are very tightly bound to the apoenzyme, and form an integral part of the holoenzyme molecule. In case of such coenzymes, the effect of coenzyme concentration will be identical to that of the enzyme concentration. Other coenzymes act as co-substrates in the reaction. In such cases, the effect of coenzyme concentration is similar to that of the substrate concentration.

4. *Temperature*

If the velocity of a reaction is measured at different

temperatures, and a curve is plotted between velocity and temperature, a bell-shaped curve is obtained.

Initially, when the temperature rises, the velocity increases due to increase in the kinetic energy of the reactants. A further rise in temperature leads to progressive denaturation of the enzyme, and the velocity begins to decrease until the reaction practically stops when the enzyme is completely denatured. The temperature at which the velocity is the highest is known as the optimum temperature of the enzyme (Fig. 7.15). For all human enzymes, the optimum temperature is 37°C.

In the initial part of the curve, the number of times the velocity increases when the temperature rises by 10°C is known as the temperature coefficient (Q_{10}) of the enzyme. For most of the enzymes, the temperature coefficient is two. This means that the velocity is doubled when the temperatures rises by 10°C.

5. *pH*

If the velocity of the reaction is determined at different pH levels, and the velocity is plotted as a function of pH, a bell-shaped curve is obtained (Fig. 7.16). A change in pH alters the electrical charges on the enzyme molecules, and often on the substrate molecules as well. This may affect the binding of the substrate to the enzyme or the catalytic activity of the enzyme or both. At an optimum pH, the velocity of the reaction is the highest as the electrical charges on the enzyme and the substrate are the most suitable for enzyme-substrate binding and catalysis.

As we move away from the optimum pH, the velocity of the reaction decreases. At extremely low or high pH, the enzyme may be denatured. The optimum pH is different for different enzymes.

Enzyme Inhibition

Catalytic activity of some enzymes can be inhibited by certain chemical compounds. Enzyme inhibition may be of two types – competitive and non-competitive.

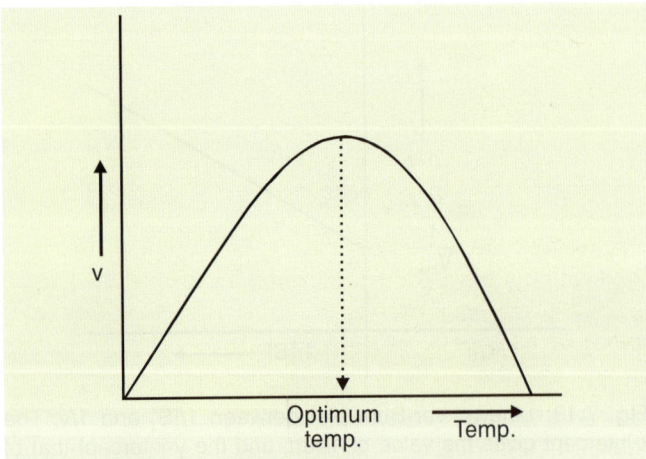

Fig. 7.15: Velocity versus temperature plot

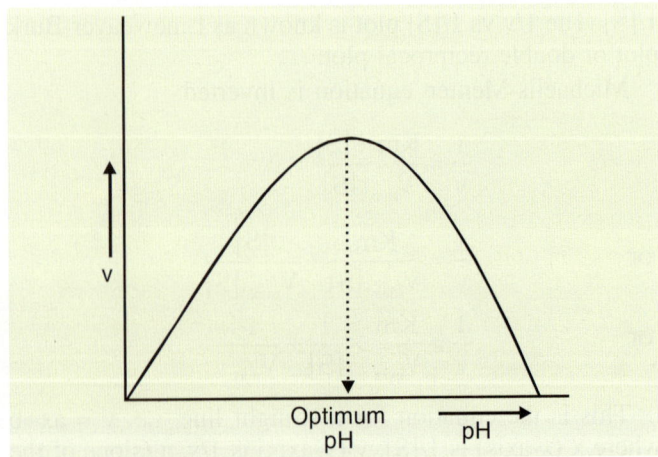

Fig. 7.16: Velocity versus pH plot

Competitive Inhibition

This is also known as substrate-analogue inhibition. The inhibitor has a close structural resemblance with the substrate. Therefore, the inhibitor (I) may bind to the substrate site on the enzyme forming enzyme-inhibitor (EI) complex. However, the inhibitor can not form the product. Thus, in the presence of the inhibitor, the catalytic activity of the enzyme is inhibited.

When the enzyme, the substrate and the inhibitor are present together, there is a competition between the substrate and the inhibitor to bind to the enzyme. That is why this type of inhibition is known as competitive inhibition. Both ES and EI complexes will be formed. But only ES can form the product.

$$E + S + I \rightleftharpoons ES + EI$$
$$\Updownarrow$$
$$E + P$$

The relative amounts of ES and EI complexes depend upon the relative concentrations of the substrate and the inhibitor. If the inhibitor concentration is higher, more EI complex will be formed resulting in decreased formation of the product. If the substrate concentration is higher, more ES complex will be formed, and the inhibition will be of smaller degree. If the substrate concentration is raised to a very high level, the inhibition will be practically relieved.

If a Lineweaver-Burk plot is plotted in the absence and in the presence of the competitive inhibitor, it is seen that the y-intercept ($1/V_{max}$) is the same in both the cases. This means that the competitive inhibitor does not affect the V_{max} which can be attained even in the presence of the inhibitor. However, the apparent Michaelis constant (K'm) is higher (1/ K'm is lower) in the presence of the inhibitor. This means that more substrate is required to reach the half-maximum velocity in the presence of the inhibitor (Fig. 7.17).

The efficacy of a competitive inhibitor can be evaluated by measuring the Km in the presence and in the absence of the inhibitor. The inhibitors that raise the Km to a higher degree are more effective inhibitors. Many competitive inhibitors are used as drugs. Some examples are:

i. Physostigmine and neostigmine resemble acetylcholine in structure, and are competitive inhibitors of acetylcholinesterase. Acetylcholinesterase catalyses breakdown of acetylcholine:

Acetylcholine + H_2O
↓ Acetylcholinesterase
Acetate + Choline

Physostigmine and neostigmine decrease the breakdown of acetylcholine, and are used as drugs when the concentration of acetylcholine needs to be increased, e.g. in myasthenia gravis, an autoimmune disorder in which acetylcholine receptors are decreased in number.

ii. Amethopterin and aminopterin resemble dihydrofolate in structure, and are competitive inhibitors of dihydrofolate reductase which catalyses the reaction:

Dihdrofolate + NADPH + H⁺ →
Tetrahydrofolate + NADP⁺

This reaction is important in the synthesis of purine and thymine nucleotides. Inhibition of this reaction inhibits DNA synthesis, and cell division. Therefore, amethopterin and aminopterin are used to suppress unregulated cell division that occurs in cancer.

iii. Allopurinol is a structural analogue of hypoxanthine. It is a competitive inhibitor of xanthine oxidase which converts hypoxanthine into xanthine, and xanthine into uric acid:

Hypoxanthine → Xanthine → Uric acid

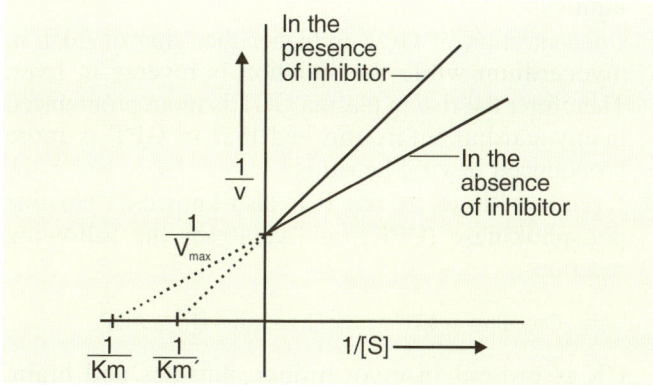

Fig. 7.17: Lineweaver-Burk plot in the absence and in the presence of a competitive inhibitor. The inhibitor increases the apparent Km (K'm) but does not affect the V_{max}

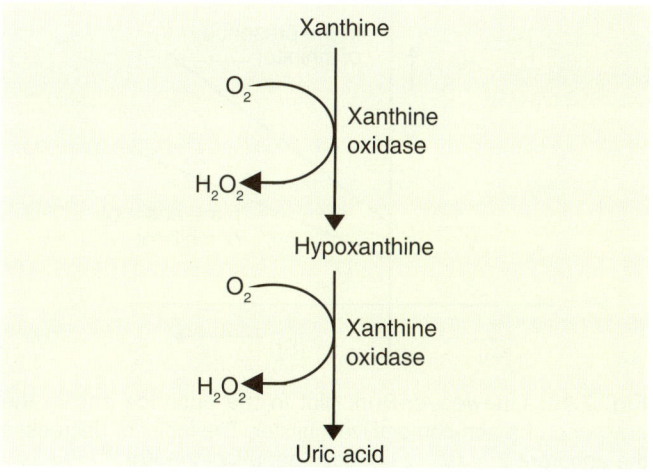

In gout, serum uric acid concentration is raised due to overproduction of uric acid. Allopurinol is used as a drug in gout to decrease serum uric acid concentration by inhibiting the formation of uric acid.

Non-competitive Inhibition

The non-competitive inhibitors have no structural resemblance with the substrate. They do not compete with the substrate for the substrate site on the enzyme. They bind to some other region of the enzyme and render it inactive. Non-competitive inhibition may be reversible or irreversible. Generally it is irreversible. Examples of non-competitive inhibitors include heavy metals, iodoacetamide, p-chloromercuribenzoate, etc.

The Lineweaver-Burk plot shows that the x-intercept remains unchanged while the y-intercept is higher in the presence of a non-competitive inhibitor. This means that the non-competitive inhibitors lower the V_{max} but do not affect the Km (Fig. 7.18).

ENZYMES OF DIAGNOSTIC IMPORTANCE

A large number of enzymes are synthesised in the cells. They are continuously released into circulation in small amounts as a result of the normal wear and tear of cells. They are removed from circulation by degradation or excretion. These enzymes are normally present in circulation in minute concentrations. The circulating enzymes may be divided into two types:

A. Functional Plasma Enzymes or Plasma-specific Enzymes

These enzymes are purposely secreted into circulation to perform specific catalytic functions. These include lipoprotein lipase, blood coagulation factors, complement proteins, etc.

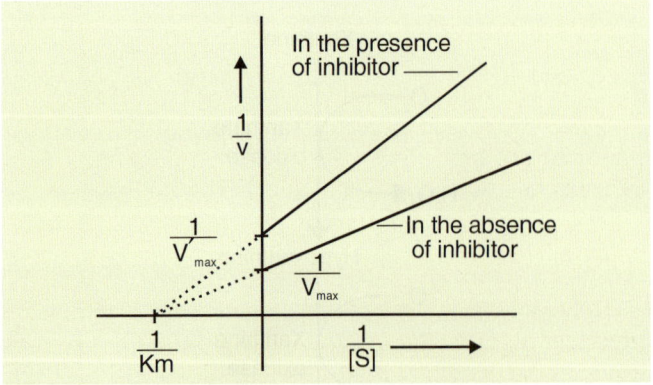

Fig. 7.18: Lineweaver-Burk plot in the absence and in the presence of a non-competitive inhibitor. The inhibitor decreases the apparent V_{max} (V'_{max}) but does not affect the Km

B. Non-functional Plasma Enzymes or Non-plasma-specific Enzymes

These enzymes do not perform their catalytic functions in plasma. These are the intracellular enzymes which enter the circulation when the cells in which they are synthesised disintegrate. When breakdown of cells is occurring at normal rate, these enzymes are present in plasma in very low concentrations. If the rate of destruction of cells increases due to some pathological condition, these enzymes will be released into circulation in large amounts, and their concentrations in plasma will rise many times above normal. If a given enzyme is widely distributed in the tissues, a rise in the plasma level of the enzyme can not pinpoint the tissue which is being destroyed. However, if the enzyme has a selective tissue distribution or if it is present in far higher concentration in some tissues than elsewhere in the body, it can pinpoint the site of the disease. Thus, it is the non-functional plasma enzymes having a selective tissue distribution which can provide information of diagnostic importance. The following plasma enzymes have become established diagnostic tools:

1. **Lactate dehydrogenase (LDH):** This enzyme catalyses the interconversion of pyruvate and lactate. Its tissue distribution is very wide. However, its concen-tration is much higher in myocardium, muscles and liver than in other tissues. Therefore, plasma LDH rises in myocardial infarction, viral hepatitis and muscle injuries. In myocardial infarction, the rise begins 24 hours after the episode of infarction, the peak value is reached in about three days, and the level returns to normal in about a week.

2. **Transaminases:** The two most important transaminases are glutamate oxaloacetate transaminase (GOT) and glutamate pyruvate transaminase (GPT). These are also known as aspartate aminotransferase (AST) and alanine aminotransferase (ALT) respectively. These are present in high concentrations in myocardium, liver and muscles. Therefore, their plasma levels are raised in myocardial infarction, viral hepatitis and muscle injuries.

   Concentration of GOT is higher than that of GPT in myocardium while the situation is reverse in liver. Therefore, the rise in plasma GOT is more pronounced in myocardial infarction and that in GPT is more pronounced in viral hepatitis.

3. **Creatine kinase (CK):** It is also known as creatine phosphokinase (CPK), and catalyses the following reaction:

$$\text{Creatine} + \text{ATP} \rightleftharpoons \text{Creatine} \sim \textcircled{P} + \text{ADP}$$

CK is present in myocardium, muscles and brain. Plasma CK rises in myocardial infarction, myopathies and muscle injuries. Plasma CK is a more specific and early indicator of myocardial infarction than LDH and

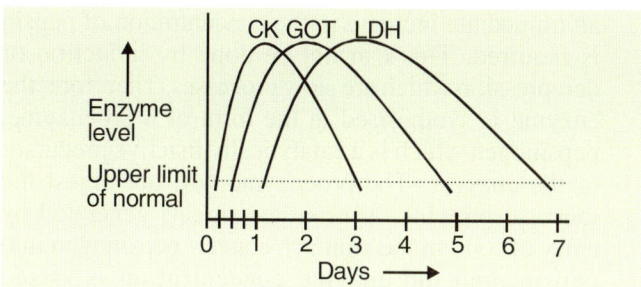

Fig. 7.19: Time course of changes in plasma CK, GOT and LDH after the occurrence of myocardial infarction (O hr)

GOT. It begins to rise within 3–6 hours of occurrence of infarction, reaches its peak in 24 hours, and returns to normal in about three days (Fig. 7.19).

4. **Gamma glutamyl transpeptidase (GGT):** This enzyme catalyses the transfer of the gamma-glutamyl residue of glutathione to other substrates. Its plasma level increases in most of the liver diseases, and is an early indicator of alcoholic hepatitis.

5. **Alkaline phosphatase (ALP):** This is a group of enzymes that hydrolyse organic phosphate esters at an alkaline pH. ALP is released in circulation mainly from bones and liver. Smaller amounts come from intestines and placenta. Liver excretes ALP in bile. The maximum elevation of plasma ALP occurs in obstructive jaundice. Smaller elevations occur in viral hepatitis, rickets, hyperparathyroidism, osteosarcoma, bony metastases, etc.

6. **Acid phosphatase (ACP):** This enzyme hydrolyses organic phosphate esters at an acidic pH. The main source of ACP is the prostate gland. Plasma ACP is elevated in metastatic carcinoma of prostate.

7. **Amylase:** This is a digestive enzyme, synthesised in the pancreas and the parotid gland. Sharp elevation of plasma amylase occurs in acute pancreatitis. A smaller elevation occurs in acute parotitis.

8. **Lipase:** This lipolytic enzyme is released into circulation from the pancreas. Plasma lipase rises in acute pancreatitis.

9. **Ceruloplasmin:** This is a copper-containing protein having ferroxidase activity. It is absent or greatly decreased in plasma in an inherited disorder, Wilson's disease (hepatolenticular degeneration).

ISOENZYMES

Some enzymes exist in multiple molecular forms which catalyse the same reaction but differ slightly from each other in their physical, chemical and immunological properties. These multiple forms of the enzyme are known as its isoenzymes or isozymes. Isoenzymes possess quaternary structure, and are made up of two or more different subunits. The subunits have slightly different primary structures.

The isoenzymes can be separated from each other by electrophoretic, chromatographic or immunochemical techniques. Separation and quantitation of isoenzymes can give information of great diagnostic importance as the tissue distribution of isoenzymes is quite specific. Several enzymes exist in the form of isoenzymes. The following have been found to be of particular diagnostic importance:

1. Lactate Dehydrogenase

Lactate dehydrogenase was the first enzyme shown to exist in the form of five isoenzymes by Markert (1956). The enzyme is a tetramer made up of two types of subunits – H and M. These subunits can form five different tetramers (isoenzymes):

   i. HHHH or LD_1 or LDH_1
  ii. HHHM or LD_2 or LDH_2
 iii. HHMM or LD_3 or LDH_3
 iv. HMMM or LD_4 or LDH_4
  v. MMMM or LD_5 or LDH_5

The LD isoenzymes in plasma can be separated by electrophoresis. The normal pattern of LD isoenzymes is $LD_2 > LD_1 > LD_3 > LD_4 > LD_5$. The predominant isoenzymes in myocardium are LD_1 and LD_2. In myocardial infarction, the rise in LD_1 is greater than that in LD_2. Therefore, plasma LD pattern becomes $LD_1 > LD_2 > LD_3 > LD_4 > LD_5$. The predominant isoenzyme in liver is LD_5 which is raised in viral hepatitis.

2. Creatine Kinase

Creatine kinase is a dimer made up of two types of subunits – B and M. Three different dimers (isoenzymes) can be formed from these two subunits:

   i. BB or CK_1 or CK-BB
  ii. MB or CK_2 or CK-MB
 iii. MM or CK_3 or CK-MM

The major isoenzyme in myocardium is CK-MB. Therefore, elevation of plasma CK-MB is diagnostic of myocardial infarction.

3. Alkaline Phosphatase

Bone, liver, intestine and placenta form different isoenzymes of ALP which can be separated by electrophoresis. The bone isoenzyme is raised in plasma in bone diseases and the liver isoenzyme in liver diseases.

REGULATION OF ENZYMES

All metabolic pathways operating in an organism must be precisely regulated so that there is neither a deficiency of products of the pathways nor wastage of raw materials. As the requirements of the organism keep on changing all the time, the regulatory mechanisms must be responsive to these changes. Very complex mechanisms of metabolic regulation have evolved in higher organisms, and enzymes play a crucial role in the regulatory mechanisms. Basically, the metabolic pathways are regulated either by changing the concentrations of enzymes or by altering the catalytic activity of enzymes. Generally, the regulation involves one or a few "key" enzymes in a pathway. A key enzyme (or regulatory enzyme) may catalyse the rate-limiting step in the pathway or the committed step in the pathway. A rate-limiting step is an early reaction in the pathway, which controls the availability of substrates (intermediates) for the subsequent reactions. The committed step is the earliest irreversible reaction unique to the pathway. Sometimes, the rate-limiting step is also the committed step. The regulatory mechanisms include:

A. Regulation of Enzyme Concentration

Some metabolic pathways are regulated by changing the absolute concentrations of the key enzymes. The rates of the reactions would change accordingly. Concentration of an enzyme may be changed by altering its rate of synthesis or the rate of degradation. Regulation of enzyme synthesis is commoner.

1. Regulation of Enzyme Synthesis

Enzyme synthesis may be regulated by:

i. *Induction*: Certain enzymes, known as inducible enzymes, are synthesised only when they are required and in quantities that are required as opposed to the constitutive enzymes which are always present in the cell. The inducible enzymes are synthesised (induced) when a specific inducer enters the cell. The inducer acts on DNA, and increases the transcription of the gene that encodes the enzyme. The inducer may be the substrate for the enzyme or it may be a gratuitous inducer, i.e. an inducer which is not a substrate for the enzyme. An example is induction of key enzymes of gluconeogenesis by glucocorticoid hormones.

ii. *Repression*: Synthesis of some key enzymes is regulated by repression of transcription of their genes. When a compound, known as corepressor, enters or accumulates in the cell, it combines with a protein, known as aporepressor, which is always present in the cell, to form the repressor molecule which represses the synthesis of the enzyme. The corepressor is generally the product of the pathway. An example is regulation of haem synthesis by δ-aminolevulinic acid synthetase. Haem acts as corepressor, and represses the synthesis of this early enzyme in the pathway. When the product is used up, the repression is relieved, and the enzyme synthesis recommences (derepression).

iii. *Conversion of proenzyme into enzyme*: Sometimes, the concentration of enzymes needs to be increased quickly. For example, when food enters the stomach,

an immediate increase in the concentration of pepsin is required. This can not be done by induction or derepression which are slow processes. Therefore, the enzyme is synthesised in the form of a proenzyme, pepsinogen which is a catalytically inactive precursor of the enzyme. The proenzyme will not digest the mucosal proteins. Appropriate signals generated by entry of food in the stomach convert pepsinogen into pepsin, and the enzyme concentration is raised quickly.

2. Regulation of Enzyme Degradation

Enzyme concentration may also be altered by increasing or decreasing its breakdown. This is not a commonly used mechanism in higher organisms. However, in starvation when the nutrients need to be used very economically, the concentration of some of the enzymes, e.g. tryptophan pyrrolase, is increased by decreasing the rate of breakdown of the enzymes.

B. Regulation of Catalytic Activity of Enzymes

In this case, the concentration of the enzyme remains unchanged but its catalytic activity is increased or decreased according to the requirement.

The catalytic activity may be altered by allosteric regulation or by covalent modification of the enzyme.

1. Allosteric Regulation

This regulatory mechanism is used in some long metabolic pathways in which a substrate is converted into a product by a series of reactions, each catalysed by a specific enzyme. The earliest functionally irreversible reaction in the pathway is catalysed by an allosteric enzyme. Usually, the product of the pathway is the allosteric inhibitor of this enzyme (Fig. 7.20). When the product accumulates, it inhibits the allosteric enzyme. When the product is used up, the inhibition is relieved. In this way, the rate of synthesis of the product is regulated according to the rate of utilisation of the product. Some enzymes are regulated by positive allosteric modulation (activation) and some by negative allosteric modulation (inhibition). Some are subject to positive as well as negative allosteric regulation. In some pathways having a number of irreversible steps, allosteric regulation may occur at a number of sites. In branched pathways also, in which a number of products

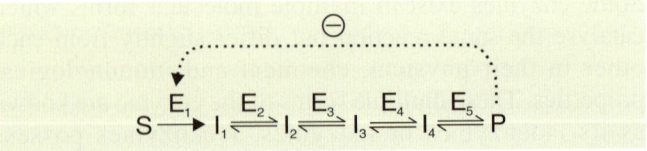

Fig. 7.20: A hypothetical pathway in which the enzyme, E_1 catalysing the earliest functionally irreversible reaction, is an allosteric enzyme, and the product, P is its allosteric inhibitor

are formed from a single substrate, allosteric regulation occurs at a number of sites. Some examples of allosteric regulation are:

i. Carbamoyl phosphate synthetase I (mitochondrial) is allosterically activated by N-acetylglutamate.

ii. Asparate transcarbamoylase, an early enzyme in de novo synthesis of pyrimidine nucleotides, is allosterically inhibited by cytidine triphosphate, a product of the pathway.

iii. Phosphofructokinase-1, which catalyses one of the functionally irreversible reactions in the glycolytic pathway, is subject to allosteric activation by AMP and allosteric inhibition by ATP.

2. Covalent Modification

The enzymes regulated by covalent modification can exist in two forms. The two forms of the enzyme can be converted into each other by a covalent modification of the enzyme molecule. The most common covalent modification is the addition or removal of a phosphate group.

The phosphate group is usually added to or removed from a serine residue in the enzyme molecule. A protein kinase transfers a phosphate group from ATP to the enzyme, and a protein phosphatase removes the phosphate group from the enzyme (Fig. 7.21).

One of the forms of the enzyme, either phosphorylated or dephosphorylated, is active and the other is inactive. Whether the enzyme will be active or inactive at a given time depends upon the relative activities of protein kinase and protein phosphatase which are usually controlled by hormones through second messengers. An example is glycogen synthetase, which is active in the dephosphorylated form and inactive in the phosphorylated form.

In some cases, the enzyme may be regulated by several mechanisms. For example, acetyl CoA carboxylase, which regulates de novo synthesis of fatty acids, is subject to induction, repression, allosteric regulation and covalent modification.

ASSAY OF ENZYMES

Measurement of enzyme levels in biological fluids, e.g. plasma, is often required for diagnostic purposes. However,

the usual analytical methods can not be used to measure enzyme concentrations because of the very low concentrations of the enzymes, and the need to isolate an enzyme from a mixture of a large number of other proteins. Therefore, enzyme concentrations are measured indirectly. The velocity of the reaction catalysed by the given enzyme is measured in such conditions that the rate of the reaction is proportional to the enzyme concentration.

During the reaction, the temperature is kept constant by carrying out the reaction in a fixed-temperature water-bath or an incubator. The optimum pH is maintained with the help of a suitable buffer. The substrate concentration is kept very high. Under such conditions, the rate of the reaction will be proportional to the enzyme concentration.

The rate of the reaction can be measured by determining the rate of disappearance of the substrate or rate of appearance of the product. In endpoint methods, the reaction is carried out for a fixed period, and the initial and the final concentrations of either the substrate or the product are measured. In kinetic methods, the concentration of the substrate or the product is measured at regular intervals for a brief period. The result in either case is expressed in arbitrary units of enzyme activity, e.g. International Units, Somogyi Units, King-Armstrong Units, etc rather than enzyme concentration.

ENZYMES AS LABORATORY TOOLS

Many enzymes are used as tools in diagnostic and research laboratories:

1. Glucose oxidase and peroxidase are routinely used for measurement of glucose concentration. Hexokinase and glucose-6-phosphate dehydrogenase are used in another method for measurement of glucose concentration.

2. Cholesterol esterase, cholesterol oxidase and peroxidase are used for measuring cholesterol concentrations.

3. Lipase, glycerol kinase, glycerol phosphate oxidase and peroxidase are used for measuring triglyceride concentration.

4. Urease is used for measurement of urea concentration.

5. Uricase is used for measuring uric acid concentration.

6. Peroxidase and alkaline phosphatase are used to label antibodies in ELISA.

7. A number of enzymes are used in recombinant DNA technology, e.g. restriction endonucleases, DNA ligase, terminal transferase, S1 nuclease, reverse transcriptase, Taq polymerase, etc.

ENZYMES AS DRUGS

Some human, animal, plant and microbial enzymes are used as drugs also:

1. Streptokinase, urokinase and tissue plasminogen activator are used as thrombolytic drugs to clear blockage of blood vessels, e.g. in myocardial infarction.

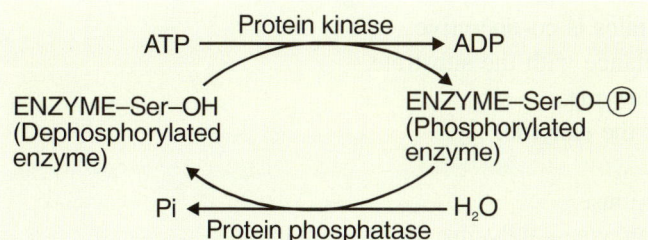

Fig. 7.21: Covalent modification of an enzyme by phosphorylation-dephosphorylation

2. Asparaginase is used in the chemotherapy of leukaemia. Leukaemic cells are deficient in asparagine synthetase, and depend upon pre-formed asparagine. Asparaginase converts asparagine into aspartate and deprives leukaemic cells of this essential nutrient. However, asparaginase is used as a last resort drug only as remissions produced by it are not long-lasting.

3. Some digestive enzymes, e.g. diastase, papain, pepsin, chymotrypsin, etc are used to aid digestion but their use is limited.

EXERCISE

1. Define enzymes. Discuss the factors affecting the velocity of enzyme-catalysed reactions.

2. Classify enzymes giving two examples from each class. Explain the mechanism of action of enzymes.

3. Discuss the diagnostic importance of enzymes and isoenzymes.

4. Explain the role of enzymes in metabolic regulation. Give one example of each regulatory mechanism.

5. Write short notes on:
   a. Enzyme specificity
   b. Coenzymes
   c. Koshland model
   d. Allosteric enzymes
   e. Michaelis constant
   f. Competitive inhibition
   g. Isoenzymes
   h. Repression-derepression

6. Write 'true' or 'false':
   a. Chemically, all the enzymes are proteins.
   b. Pepsin is a group-specific enzyme.
   c. A coenzyme combines with a proenzyme to form the holoenzyme.
   d. Enzymes lower the energy of activation.
   e. Km of an enzyme can be determined from Lineweaver-Burk plot.
   f. Kinetics of all enzymes follow the Michaelis-Menten equation.
   g. Competitive inhibitors lower the V_{max} but do not affect the Km.
   h. Competitive inhibition can be relieved by raising the substrate concentration.
   i. Creatine kinase is an early indicator of myocardial infarction.
   j. Serum acid phosphatase is raised in obstructive jaundice.
   k. Constitutive enzymes are always present in the cell.
   l. Catalytic activity of inducible enzymes is increased by inducers.
   m. Repressor is made up of aporepressor and corepressor.
   n. Pepsinogen is a proenzyme.
   o. Allosteric regulators increase or decrease the catalytic activity of allosteric enzymes.

7. Fill in the blanks:
   a. RNA molecules having catalytic activity are known as ....
   b. An apoenzyme combines with a coenzyme to form the ....
   c. Transferases transfer a chemical group other than .... from one susbtrate to another.
   d. .... constant is the substrate concentration at which the velocity is half of V_{max}.
   e. Kinetics of allosteric enzymes follow the .... equation.
   f. The velocity versus substrate concentration plot of .... enzymes is sigmoidal.
   g. The binding of .... enzymes and their substrates is co-operative.
   h. A ....inhibitor has a close structural resemblance with the substrate.
   i. Competitive inhibitors raise the .... of the enzyme.
   j. Non-competitive inhibitors lower the .... of the enzyme.
   k. Amethopterin is a competitive inhibitor of ....
   l. .... is a competitive inhibitor of xanthine oxidase.
   m. .... are the multiple molecular forms of an enzyme catalysing the same reaction.
   n. .... is the major isoenzyme of creatine kinase in myocardium.
   o. A committed step is the earliest .... reaction unique to the pathway.

ANSWERS TO SHORT QUESTIONS

6. a. False
   b. True
   c. False
   d. True
   e. True
   f. False
   g. False
   h. True
   i. True
   j. False
   k. True
   l. False
   m. True
   n. True
   o. True

7. a. Ribozymes
   b. Holoenzyme
   c. Hydrogen
   d. Michaelis
   e. Hill
   f. Allosteric
   g. Allosteric
   h. Competitive
   i. Km
   j. V_{max}
   k. Dihydrofolate reductase
   l. Allopurinol
   m. Isoenzymes
   n. CK-MB or CK_2
   o. Irreversible

8

Bio-energetics and Oxidative Phosphorylation

We require energy for various activities, e.g. muscle contraction, nerve conduction, synthetic reactions, active transport, etc. The ultimate source of energy is the food that we consume. Carbohydrates, lipids and proteins present in food provide us energy. These complex molecules present in food are digested in the gastro-intestinal tract to yield smaller molecules, e.g. mono-saccharides, fatty acids and amino acids. These, in turn, are oxidised in various catabolic pathways. Their carbon atoms are oxidised to carbon dioxide while the hydrogen atoms are transferred to coenzymes, e.g. NAD^+, FMN, FAD, etc. The reduced coenzymes transfer the hydrogen atoms to the mitochondrial respiratory chain wherein these are oxidised to water. The energy released during this oxidation is used to phosphorylate adenosine diphosphate (ADP) to adenosine triphosphate (ATP). This oxidation coupled with phosphorylation of ADP is known as oxidative phosphorylation. Oxidative phosphorylation, thus, is the mechanism by which the energy present in various nutrients is captured in an easily utilisable form.

High-energy Phosphates

The energy released during the oxidation of mono-saccharides, fatty acids and amino acids may not be required immediately. Therefore, there must be some way of storing the energy so that it may be readily available when needed. The energy released during catabolism is captured in the form of a group of compounds known as "high-energy phosphates". The most important member

of this group is ATP (Fig. 8.1). Hydrolysis of ATP into ADP and Pi liberates 7.3 kcal of energy per mol. Similarly, hydrolysis of ADP into AMP and Pi also releases nearly the same amount of energy. However, hydrolysis of AMP into adenosine and Pi liberates much less energy (3.4 kcal/mol). This difference is because of the nature of bonds by which phosphate is attached. The third phosphate is attached to the second, and the second to the first, by acid anhydride bond. The first phosphate is attached to ribose by an ester bond. Hydrolysis of acid anhydride bonds releases much more energy than the hydrolysis of ester bonds. Lipmann suggested a curved line (~) to denote a high-energy bond. Thus, ATP may be represented as:

Adenosine —Ⓟ~Ⓟ~Ⓟ

The organic phosphates which liberate 6 kcal/mol or more on hydrolysis of the phosphate group are known as high-energy phosphates. Besides ATP and the related nucleotides, these include phosphoenol pyruvate, carbamoyl phosphate, 1,3-biphosphoglycerate, creatine phosphate, etc. Those organic phosphates which release less than 6 kcal/mol on hydrolysis of the phosphate group are known as low-energy phosphates. These include AMP, glucose-6-phosphate, glucose-1-phosphate, fructose-6-phosphate, glycerol-3-phosphate, etc. (Table 8.1).

The compounds having ΔG_o above that of ATP can transfer their phosphate group to ADP forming ATP. The compounds having ΔG_o below that of ATP can not transfer their phosphate groups to ADP. On the contrary, ATP can

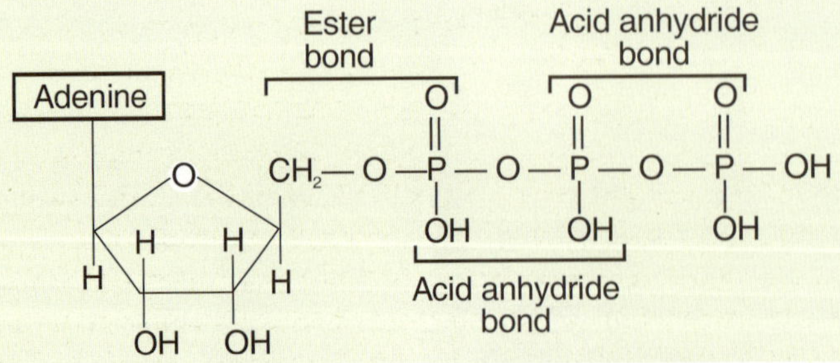

Fig. 8.1: Bonding of the three phosphate groups in ATP

Table. 8.1: Standard free energy (ΔG_o) of hydrolysis of some physiologically important phosphorylated compounds (kcal/mol)[*]

Compound	ΔG_o	Compound	ΔG_o
Phosphoenol pyruvate	– 14.8	AMP ($\rightarrow$Adenosine + Pi)	– 3.4
Carbamoyl phosphate	–12.3	Glucose-1-phosphate	– 5.0
1,3-Biphosphoglycerate	– 11.8	Fructose-6-phosphate	– 3.8
Creatine phosphate	– 10.3	Glucose-6-phosphate	– 3.3
ATP ($\rightarrow$ADP + Pi)	– 7.3	Glycerol-3-phosphate	–2.2

[*] These are the values of ΔG_o obtained in standard laboratory conditions of 1M reactant concentration at pH 7.0 at 25°C. The values obtained in living cells ($\Delta G'_o$) are different as the reactant concentrations, pH and temperature in living cells are different.

transfer a phosphate group to glucose, fructose, glycerol, etc. forming their respective phosphates. Therefore, ATP has been described as the energy currency of the cells which can capture energy from exergonic (energy-releasing) reactions, and can transfer it to endergonic (energy-consuming) reactions. Moreover, cells store energy in the form of ATP which can be drawn upon whenever energy is required.

Besides high-energy phosphates, some sulphur compounds having thioester bonds are also high-energy compounds. In acetyl CoA, succinyl CoA, acyl CoA, etc. CoA is attached by a high-energy thioester bond.

Oxidation and Reduction

Oxidation was defined in the past as addition of oxygen to or removal of hydrogen from a substance. The reverse was termed as reduction. These definitions have now been supplanted by a more comprehensive concept. Oxidation is now defined as removal of electrons and reduction as addition of electrons. The electron being removed or added may be a free electron or it may be associated with a proton as in a hydrogen atom.

$$Fe^{++} \underset{\text{Reduction of Fe}^{+++}}{\overset{\text{Oxidation of Fe}^{++}}{\rightleftharpoons}} Fe^{+++} + e^- \text{ (electron)}$$

$$AH_2 + NAD^+ \underset{\text{Reduction of A}}{\overset{\text{Oxidation of AH}_2}{\rightleftharpoons}} A + NADH + H^+$$

$$AH_2 + FAD \underset{\text{Reduction of A}}{\overset{\text{Oxidation of AH}_2}{\rightleftharpoons}} A + FADH_2$$

Our earliest concepts of oxidation in living beings (biological oxidation) originated from the work of Lavoisier who proposed that respiration in animals is an oxidative process in which atmospheric oxygen is used to oxidise carbon atoms to carbon dioxide. Pasteur showed later that the presence of oxygen is not essential for oxidation, and that living organisms can oxidise substrates even in the absence of oxygen. Wieland proposed that

biological oxidation occurred by dehydrogenation of activated substrates. With the discovery of cytochromes by Keilin, it became clear that the substrates are dehydrogenated, and the reducing equivalents (H or e⁻) are taken up by cytochromes to be finally transferred to oxygen in the presence of cytochrome oxidase (Warburg's enzyme) to be converted into water.

The enzymes and coenzymes concerned with the removal of reducing equivalents from the substrates and their transfer to oxygen are present in the inner mitochondrial membrane in an ordered sequence. This sequence of carriers of reducing equivalents is known as the electron transfer chain (ETC) or respiratory chain. The sequence of carriers in the respiratory chain is:

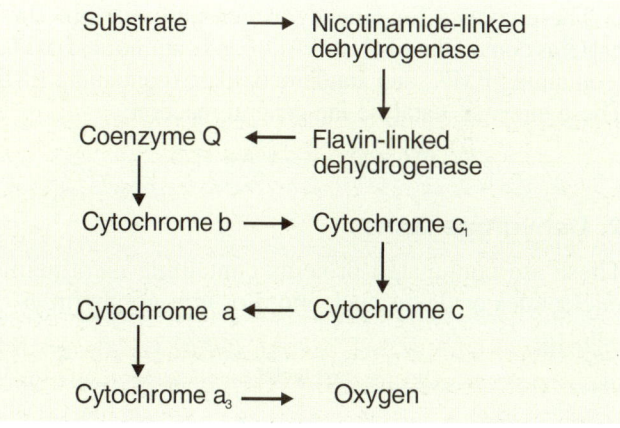

Redox Potential

A reactant which can undergo reduction and oxidation can exist in the reduced form and the oxidised form. The reduced and the oxidised forms of the reactant constitute a redox couple. Every redox couple has a redox potential which is a measure of the affinity of the reactant for electrons. A redox couple having a high redox potential has a high affinity for electrons, and can readily accept electrons from a redox couple having a lower redox potential. The redox potential of a reactant can be measured in the laboratory. The reduced and the oxidised forms of the reactant at 1M concentration each are taken in a sample cell. A 1M solution of hydrogen ions in equilibrium with hydrogen gas is taken in a reference cell. The two are connected by an agar bridge through which electrons can flow. Electrodes dipping in each solution are connected to a voltmeter. The potential difference between the two solutions is the redox potential of the reactant (Fig. 8.2).

For biological systems, the redox potential (E_o) is measured at pH 7.0, and is denoted by E'_o. The components of the respiratory chain are arranged in the order of increasing redox potential. The electrons move from a relatively electronegative component to a relatively electropositive component at every site. E'_o of major components of the respiratory chain is shown in Table 8.2.

ENZYMES CONCERNED WITH BIOLOGICAL OXIDATION

The enzymes concerned with biological oxidation are oxidoreductases. They can be sub-divided into:

1. Oxidases

These enzymes remove hydrogen from a substrate and transfer it to oxygen forming water or hydrogen peroxide. The enzymes forming water are metalloenzymes that usually contain copper, e.g. cytochrome oxidase and tyrosinase. The general reaction catalysed by these enzymes is:

$$AH_2 + \tfrac{1}{2} O_2 \longrightarrow A + H_2O$$

The enzymes forming hydrogen peroxide are flavoproteins containing FMN or FAD, e.g. L-amino acid oxidase (containing FMN) and xanthine oxidase (containing FAD). These enzymes catalyse the general reaction:

$$AH_2 + O_2 \longrightarrow A + H_2O_2$$

2. Dehydrogenases

These are conjugated proteins containing nicotinamide nucleotides or flavin nucleotides or iron-porphyrin as the

Table 8.2: Redox potential (E'_o) of carriers in the respiratory chain

Redox couple	E'_o (volts)	Redox couple	E'_o (volts)
$2H^+ - H_2$	−0.42	Cyt c_1 (Fe^{+++}) - Cyt c_1 (Fe^{++})	+0.22
$NAD^+ - NADH$	−0.32	Cyt c (Fe^{+++}) - Cyt c (Fe^{++})	+0.25
$FAD - FADH_2$	−0.22	Cyt a (Fe^{+++}) - Cyt a (Fe^{++})	+0.29
Cyt b(Fe^{+++})- Cyt b(Fe^{++})	−0.08	Cyt a_3 (Fe^{+++}) - Cyt a_3 (Fe^{++})	+0.38
$CoQ - CoQH_2$	+0.04	$\tfrac{1}{2} O_2 - H_2O$	+0.82

prosthetic group. They remove hydrogen from a substrate, and transfer it to another substrate. The prosthetic group acts as carrier of hydrogen atoms.

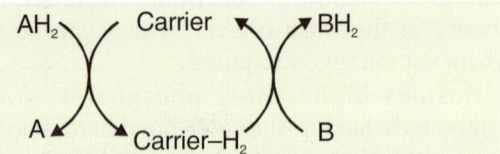

Examples of dehydrogenases are:

a. Those containing NAD: Lactate dehydrogenase, malate dehydrogenase, etc.

b. Those containing NADP: Glucose-6-phosphate dehydrogenase, 6-phosphogluconate dehydrogenase, etc.

c. Those containing flavin nucleotides: Succinate dehydrogenase, acyl CoA dehydrogenase, etc.

d. Those containing iron-porphyrin: Cytochrome a, cytochrome b, etc.

3. Hydroperoxidases

These enzymes convert hydrogen peroxide into water, and protect the tissues against the toxic effects of hydrogen peroxide. These include:

a. Peroxidase: It catalyses the reaction:

$$H_2O_2 + AH_2 \longrightarrow A + 2 H_2O$$

b. Catalase: It catalyses the reaction:

$$2 H_2O_2 \longrightarrow O_2 + 2 H_2O$$

4. Oxygenases

These enzymes incorporate oxygen into a substrate. They can be sub-divided into:

Di-oxygenases

They catalyse the incorporation of both the atoms of oxygen molecule into the substrate.

$$A + O_2 \longrightarrow AO_2$$

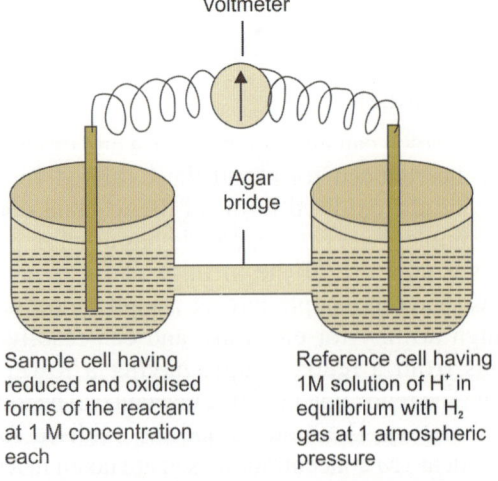

Voltmeter

Agar bridge

Sample cell having reduced and oxidised forms of the reactant at 1 M concentration each

Reference cell having 1M solution of H$^+$ in equilibrium with H$_2$ gas at 1 atmospheric pressure

Fig. 8.2: Measurement of redox potential

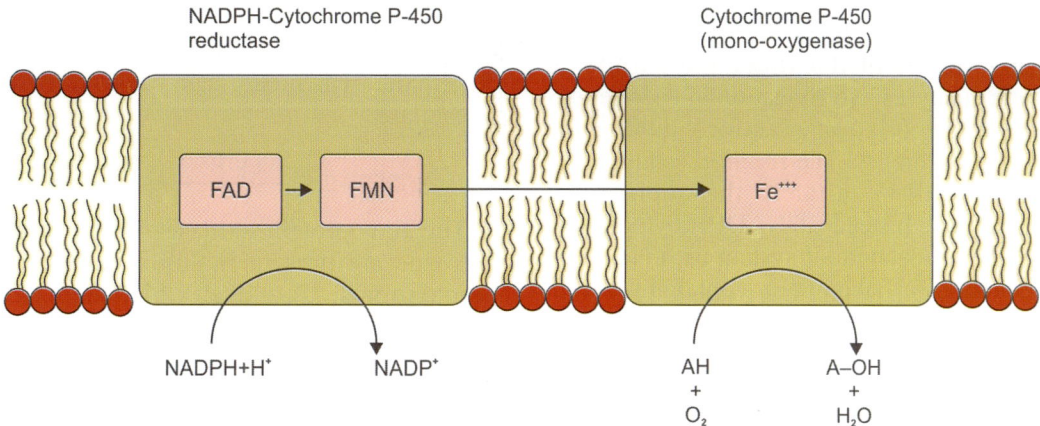

Fig. 8.3: Microsomal hydroxylase system

Examples include homogentisate oxidase and tryptophan pyrrolase.

Mono-oxygenases

They incorporate one atom of the oxygen molecule into the substrate. The other atom of oxygen oxidises another reduced substrate to water:

$$AH + O_2 + BH_2 \longrightarrow A-OH + B + H_2O$$

These enzymes are also known as hydroxylases or mixed function oxidases. They are used to metabolise xenobiotics (foreign compounds), for example drugs like morphine, phenobarbitone, rifampicin, etc. They also catalyse hydroxylation of endogenous substrates, e.g.

phenylalanine, tryptophan, steroids, cholecalciferol, etc. Two slightly different hydroxylase systems are present in microsomes and mitochondria.

Microsomal Hydroxylase System

The complete system required for hydroxylation of xenobiotics and some steroids is present in the microsomes, and is known as the microsomal hydroxylase system. The system consists of cytochrome P450 (CYP) which possesses mono-oxygenase activity, NADPH, NADPH: Cytochrome P450 reductase (a flavoprotein containing FAD and FMN) and molecular oxygen (Fig. 8.3). In some hydroxylation reactions, cytochrome b_5 is also required. A typical microsomal hydroxylation reaction is shown in Fig. 8.4.

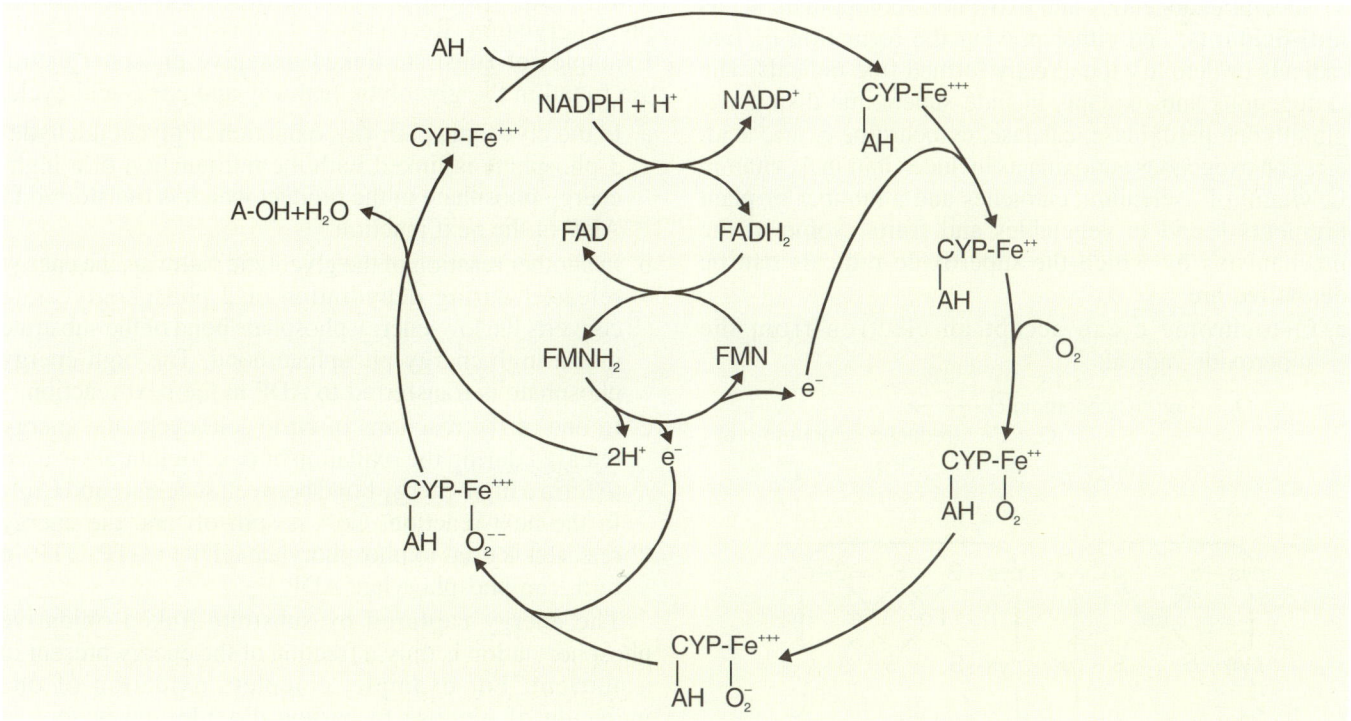

Fig. 8.4: Microsomal hydroxylation of a substrate, AH

Mitochondrial Hydroxylase System

This system is present in the inner membrane of mitochondria, and catalyses hydroxylation of endogenous substrates, e.g. hydroxylation reactions during the synthesis of steroid hormones. The reaction catalysed by this system is basically similar to the microsomal hydroxylation reaction. Instead of NADPH:cytochrome P450 reductase, the mitochondrial system uses NADPH: adrenodoxin reductase (a flavoprotein containing FAD). The reducing equivalents accepted by FAD are transferred to cytochrome P450 via adrenodoxin (iron-sulphur protein). Adrenodoxin possesses an iron-sulphur centre having catalytic activity (Fig. 8.5).

Metabolism of Superoxide Radicals

Hydrogen peroxide is continuously formed in the body by the action of flavoprotein oxidases. It was believed in the past that the toxicity of molecular oxygen is solely due to its conversion into hydrogen peroxide. It was shown later that toxic effects of oxygen are also due to its conversion into free radicals or superoxide radicals (O_2^-). Free radicals, once formed, can start a chain reaction forming more free radicals. These highly reactive radicals can damage nucleic acids, proteins and lipids, specially unsaturated fatty acids. Several diseases are now believed to occur due to damage caused by free radicals. Superoxide radicals can be formed due to incomplete oxidation of reduced flavoprotein oxidases.

$$FpH_2 + O_2 \longrightarrow FpH + H^+ + O_2^-$$

Several endogenous and exogenous compounds act as **anti-oxidants**, and either prevent the formation of free radicals or detoxify the already formed free radicals. The endogenous anti-oxidants include superoxide dismutase, glutathione peroxidase, catalase, cytochrome c, uric acid, etc. The exogenous antioxidants include vitamin A, vitamin C, vitamin E, selenium, carotenes and a number of plant pigments found in vegetables and fruits. Some of the mechanisms by which the superoxide radicals can be detoxified are:

a. Cytochrome c can accept an electron from the superoxide radical:

$$O_2^- + Fe^{+++} \text{ (Cytochrome c)} \longrightarrow$$
$$O_2 + Fe^{++} \text{ (reduced cytochrome c)}$$

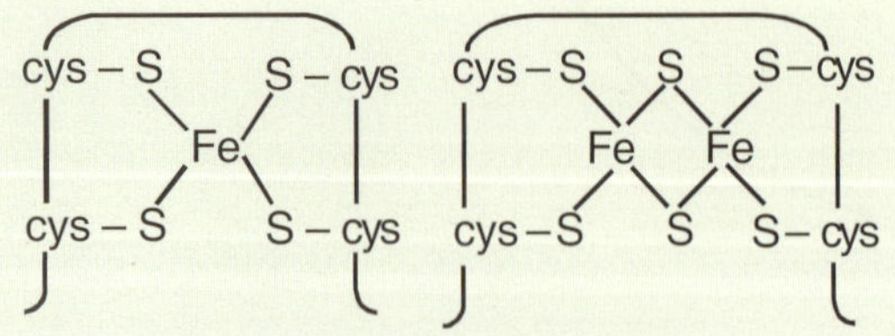

Fig. 8.5: Iron-sulphur centres

b. Superoxide dismutase, a widely distributed metallo-enzyme, can convert superoxide radicals into hydrogen peroxide which can, then, be converted into water by catalase:

$$2O_2^- + 2H^+ \xrightarrow{\text{Superoxide dismutase}} H_2O_2 + O_2$$

The flavoprotein oxidases which produce hydrogen peroxide are present in sub-cellular organelles called peroxisomes. Catalase, which detoxifies hydrogen peroxide, is also present in peroxisomes. This protects the cell against the toxic effects of hydrogen peroxide. Peroxisomes are congenitally absent in Zellweger's syndrome resulting in extensive damage to brain, liver and kidneys.

OXIDATIVE PHOSPHORYLATION

Oxidative phosphorylation is the process by which the energy released during the oxidation of energy-rich substrates is used to phosphorylate ADP. Oxidative phosphorylation can occur at the substrate level or at the level of the respiratory chain. In the former case, oxidation of the substrate is linked with formation of a high-energy bond in the product which, in turn, is used to convert ADP into ATP. In the latter case, ADP is phosphorylated when the reducing equivalents removed from various substrates are oxidised in the respiratory chain.

Oxidative Phosphorylation at the Substrate Level

This is also known as substrate-linked oxidative phosphorylation. Respiratory chain is not involved here. Examples of substrate-linked oxidative phosphorylation are found in the glycolytic pathway and citric acid cycle.

a. In the glycolytic pathway, oxidation of glyceraldehyde-3-phosphate is linked with the introduction of a high-energy phosphate in the product which is transferred to ADP in the next reaction.

b. In another reaction of the glycolytic pathway, the energy released during dehydration of 2-phosphoglycerate converts the low-energy phosphate bond of the substrate into a high-energy phosphate bond. The high-energy phosphate is transferred to ADP in the next reaction.

c. In one of the reactions of citric acid cycle, the energy released during the oxidation of α-ketoglutarate is used to form a high-energy bond between succinate and CoA. In the next reaction, CoA is split off and the energy released is used to phosphorylate GDP to GTP. GTP, in turn, can phosphorylate ADP.

The energy captured by substrate-linked oxidative phosphorylation is only a fraction of the energy present in a nutrient. For example, complete oxidation of one molecule of glucose to carbon dioxide and water via glycolysis and citric acid cycle phosphorylates 38

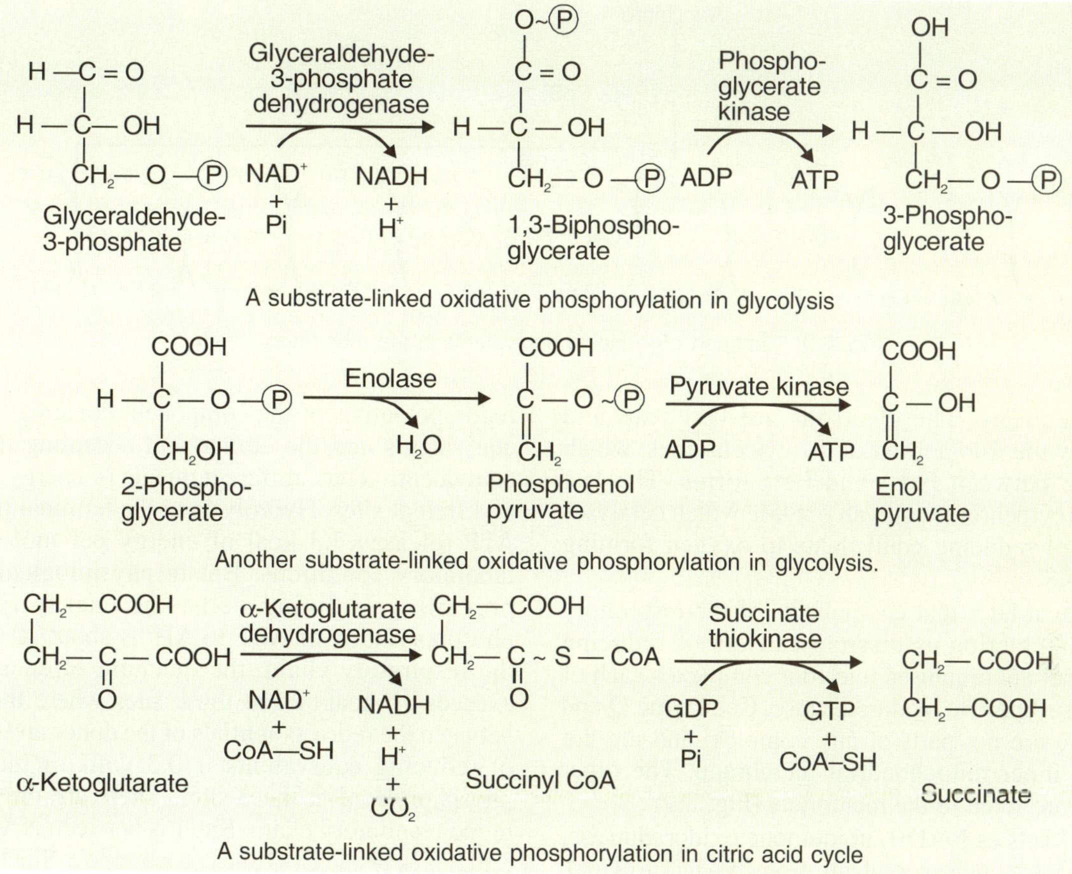

Fig. 8.6: Some examples of substrate-linked oxidative phosphorylation

molecules of ADP. Of these, only six are phosphorylated at the substrate level. The rest of the energy is captured by oxidative phosphorylation at the level of the respiratory chain.

Oxidative Phosphorylation at the Level of Respiratory Chain

Energy-rich nutrients like glucose, fatty acids and amino acids are oxidised stepwise by a series of reactions in various metabolic pathways. In many reactions, reducing equivalents are removed from the substrates, and are taken up by coenzymes like NAD and FAD. The reduced coenzymes transfer the reducing equivalents to respiratory chain. Oxidation of reducing equivalents in the respiratory chain is coupled with phosphorylation of ADP to ATP. This is the most important mechanism for capturing the energy present in various nutrients. As the respiratory chain is located in the **mitochondria**, the mitochondria have been described as the power house of the cells.

Most of the substrates transfer the reducing equivalents to NAD which, in turn, transfers the reducing equivalents to a flavoprotein containing FMN and iron-sulphur (FeS) centre. The reduced flavoprotein transfers the reducing equivalents to coenzyme Q (ubiquinone). Coenzyme Q is a fat-soluble compound resembling vitamin K in structure.

It contains 6–10 isoprenoid units ($n = 6$–10), and can be reduced to ubiquinol (Fig. 8.7).

Reduced coenzyme Q transfers the reducing equivalents to cytochrome b which is associated with iron-sulphur protein. The subsequent carriers, cytochromes c_1, c and a, are typical iron-porphyrin proteins which differ from each other in their protein portions and the nature of the side chains attached to the porphyrin nucleus. The cytochromes

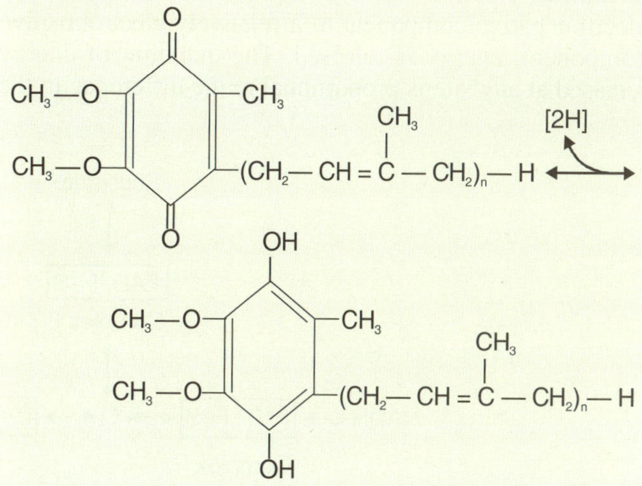

Fig. 8.7: Oxidised and reduced forms of coenzyme Q

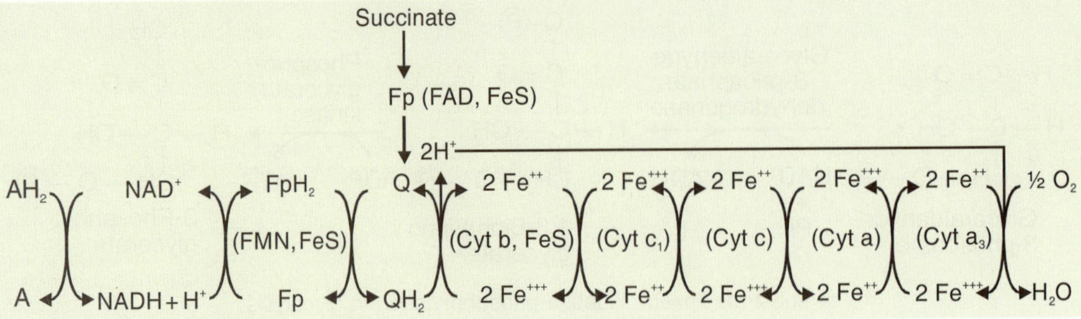

Succinate

↓

Fp (FAD, FeS)

↓ 2H⁺

AH_2 NAD⁺ FpH_2 Q 2 Fe⁺⁺ 2 Fe⁺⁺⁺ 2 Fe⁺⁺ 2 Fe⁺⁺⁺ 2 Fe⁺⁺ ½ O_2

(FMN, FeS) (Cyt b, FeS) (Cyt c_1) (Cyt c) (Cyt a) (Cyt a_3)

A NADH + H⁺ Fp QH_2 2 Fe⁺⁺⁺ 2 Fe⁺⁺ 2 Fe⁺⁺⁺ 2 Fe⁺⁺ 2 Fe⁺⁺⁺ H_2O

Fig. 8.8: Transport of reducing equivalents in the respiratory chain

transport electrons. The electrons are taken up and transferred by the iron portion of the cytochromes, which can oscillate between Fe⁺⁺⁺ and Fe⁺⁺ forms. The last cytochrome (cytochrome a_3) is an oxidase which catalyses the transfer of reducing equivalents to oxygen forming water (Fig. 8.8).

It was shown later that components of the respiratory chain do not function as discrete carriers of reducing equivalents but are organised into four complexes each of which acts as a specific oxidoreductase. Coenzyme Q and cytochrome c are not parts of any complex, and are not fixed in the inner mitochondrial membrane. The other components are fixed in the membrane (Fig. 8.9).

Complex I acts as NADH: ubiquinone oxidoreductase, and transfers reducing equivalents from NADH to CoQ. Complex II acts as succinate: ubiquinone oxidoreductase, and transfers reducing equivalents from succinate to CoQ. Complex III acts as ubiquinol: ferricytochrome c oxidoreductase, and transfers reducing equivalents from reduced CoQ to cytochrome c. Complex IV acts as ferrocytochrome c: oxygen oxidoreductase, and transfers reducing equivalents from reduced cytochrome c to oxygen.

The proximal end of the respiratory chain has a negative redox potential while the distal end has a positive redox potential. As the electrons move from a relatively electronegative component to a relatively electropositive component, energy is released. The quantum of energy released at any site is proportional to the difference in the redox potentials of the component donating the reducing equivalents and the component accepting the reducing equivalents. Thus, different quanta of energy are released at different sites. Hydrolysis of the terminal phosphate of ATP releases 7.3 kcal of energy per mol in standard laboratory conditions. But in physiological conditions prevailing in living cells, the energy required for phosphorylation of ADP to ATP is about 10 kcal/mol. In the respiratory chain, the quantum of energy released exceeds 10 kcal/mol at those sites where the difference between the redox potentials of the donor and the acceptor of reducing equivalents is 0.3 volts or more. ADP is phosphorylated at these sites. There are three such sites in the respiratory chain. Site I is between NAD and CoQ. Site II is between CoQ and cytochrome c. Site III is between cytochrome c and oxygen. These sites correspond to complexes I, III and IV respectively in the respiratory chain.

All the substrates undergoing dehydrogenation do not transfer the reducing equivalents to NAD. Reducing equivalents are accepted by a carrier having a redox potential just above that of the substrate. The substrates that transfer reducing equivalents to NAD, e.g. isocitrate, malate, glutamate, etc. can phosphorylate three molecules of ADP. The substrates that transfer reducing equivalents to FAD phosphorylate only two molecules of ADP as Site I is bypassed, e.g. succinate, glycerol-3-phosphate, acyl CoA, etc.

The ratio of ADP molecules phosphorylated to the number of oxygen atoms reduced is known as P:O ratio.

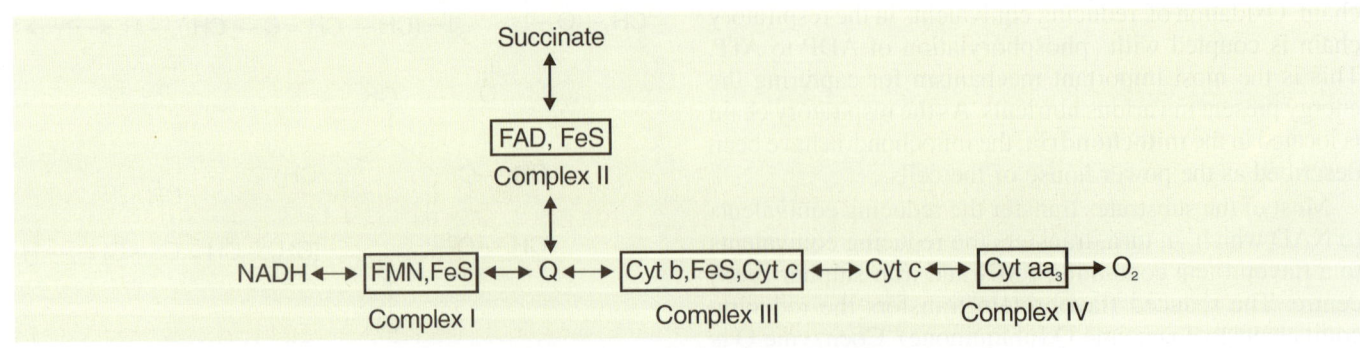

Fig. 8.9: Complexes I, II, III and IV in the respiratory chain

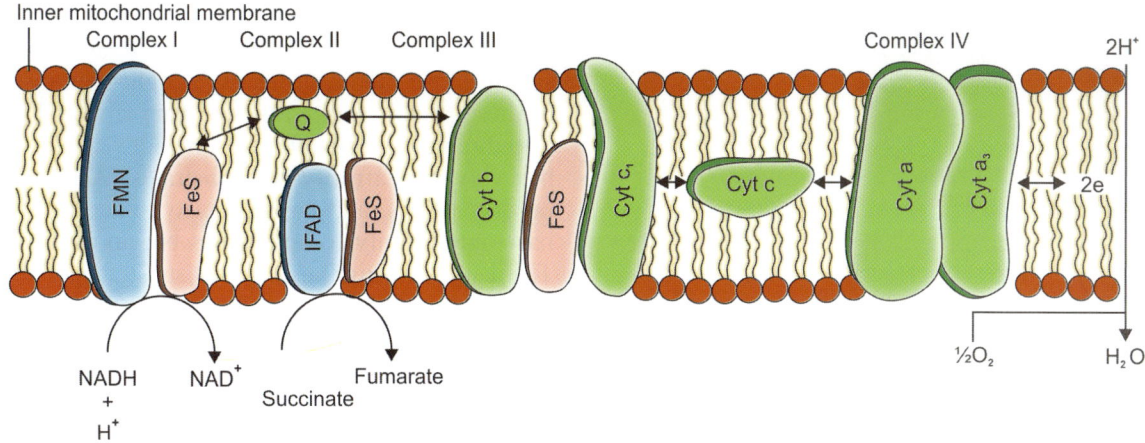

Fig. 8.10: Transport of reducing equivalents by complexes I, II, III and IV in the respiratory chain

The P:O ratio is three when the reducing equivalents are accepted by NAD, and is two when the reducing equivalents are accepted by FAD.

MECHANISM OF OXIDATIVE PHOSPHORYLATION

While the association between the oxidation of reducing equivalents and phosphorylation of ADP in the respiratory chain is known for a long time, the exact mechanism by which these two processes are coupled is emerging only now. Several hypotheses have been advanced to explain the mechanism of this coupling of which the chemiosmotic hypothesis is the most plausible.

Chemiosmotic Hypothesis

According to the chemiosmotic hypothesis proposed by Mitchell, the energy released during the transport of electrons in the respiratory chain is used to actively eject the hydrogen ions (H^+) or protons from the matrix through the inner mitochondrial membrane which is otherwise impermeable to hydrogen ions. This ejection establishes an electrochemical gradient across the membrane. The concentration of hydrogen ions on the outer side becomes higher as compared to the inner side. The outer side also becomes electropositive as compared to the inner side. This electrochemical gradient increases up to a certain limit. When this limit is reached, the hydrogen ions re-enter the matrix releasing energy. This energy is used to activate a membrane-bound enzyme, vectorial ATP synthetase which converts ADP and Pi into ATP. The complexes I, III and IV in the respiratory chain act as proton pumps ejecting hydrogen ions from the mitochondrial matrix to the intermembrane space (Figs 8.10 and 8.11).

Efraim Racker showed by electron microscopy that vectorial ATP synthetase is made up of F_o and F_1 components. F_o component is embedded in the inner mitochondrial membrane while the F_1 component projects into the matrix (Fig. 8.12). F_o acts as a channel for the passage of hydrogen ions. F_1 component possesses ATP synthetase activity, which is switched on when the hydrogen ions pass through the F_o component. The F_o-F_1 complex is also known as complex V of the respiratory chain. If the F_o component is removed, the F_1 component acts as ATPase rather than ATP synthetase.

John Walker deciphered the genes encoding the F_o and F_1 components. The F_o component is made up of a, b and c subunits. The F_1 component is made up of α, β, γ, δ and ϵ subunits and has the composition, $\alpha_3\beta_3\gamma\delta\epsilon$ (Fig. 8.13). The subunits of F_o and F_1 components of vectorial ATP synthetase are encoded by a cluster of genes called the unc operon. These genes are present in mitochondrial DNA (mitochondrial DNA also encodes 11 other polypeptides which are components of respiratory chain).

According to the mechanism of phosphorylation envisaged in the chemiosmotic hypothesis, when hydrogen ions flow back into the matrix, two hydrogen ions combine

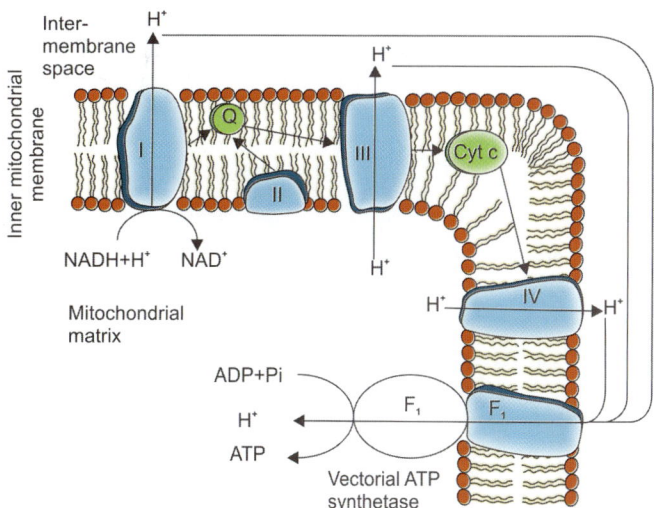

Fig. 8.11: Complexes I, III and IV eject protons. Re-entry of protons into the matrix activates vectorial ATP synthetase which phosphorylates ADP to ATP

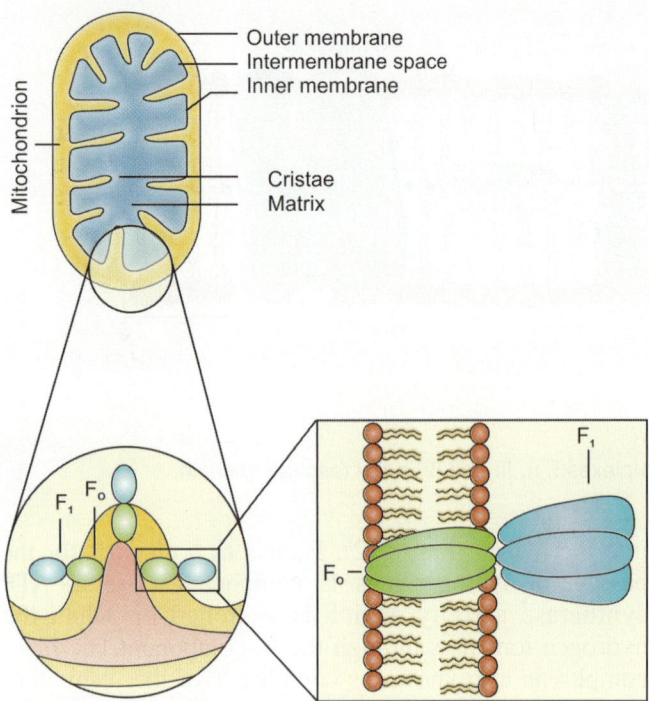

Fig. 8.12: The inner mitochondrial membrane is folded into cristae. F_o component of vectorial ATP synthetase is embedded in the inner mitochondrial membrane. The F_1 component projects into the matrix

with two electrons and one oxygen atom of inorganic phosphate forming water and converting inorganic phosphate into a highly reactive form which readily combines with ADP by a high-energy bond (Fig. 8.14).

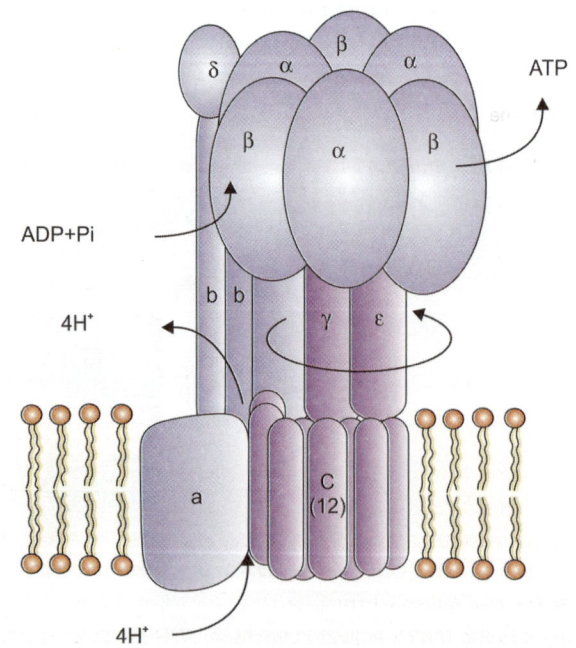

Fig. 8.13: Subunits of F_O and F_1 components of ATP synthetase

Paul Boyer has proposed that the F_1 complex has three catalytic sites having specific conformations – O (open) site, L (loose-binding) site and T (tight-binding) site. Each of these sites is formed by one pair of α and β subunits. The three conformations are interconvertible. The O site has very low affinity for substrates (ADP and Pi) and product (ATP), and has no catalytic activity. The L site has some affinity for substrates but no catalytic activity. The T site has high affinity for substrates, and possesses catalytic activity.

In the absence of an electrochemical gradient, equal amounts of ATP and ADP and Pi are bound to the T and L sites, respectively. According to the **binding-change mechanism** proposed by Boyer, the energy released during the influx of hydrogen ions causes rotation of the γ subunit in steps of 120°. This rotation converts the T site into O site, the O site into L site and the L site into T site. Conversion of T site into O site releases the bound ATP. Conversion of L site into T site converts the bound ADP and Pi into ATP as the T site possesses ATP synthetase activity. Another pair of ADP and Pi enters the new L site, and the cycle is repeated (Fig. 8.15).

There is strong experimental evidence in support of chemiosmotic hypothesis. Building up of H^+ gradient is the basic premise of the hypothesis. It has been shown experimentally that if H^+ gradient is created artificially by bathing intact mitochondria in a fluid having a relatively high H^+ concentration as compared to the mitochondrial matrix, phosphorylation occurs even in the absence of oxidation. The hypothesis envisages a membrane-bound vectorial ATP synthetase. It has been shown that disruption of the mitochondrial membrane leads to loss of ATP synthetase activity. The $P:H^+$ and $H^+:O$ ratios of various substrates are also in agreement with the experimental evidence. Thus, the chemiosmotic hypothesis has now become the accepted theory to explain the mechanism of oxidative phosphorylation in the respiratory chain.

Inhibitors and Uncouplers of Oxidative Phosphorylation

Certain agents are known to inhibit oxidative phosphorylation at specific sites in the respiratory chain. Amobarbitone, rotenone and piericidin A which inhibit oxidative phosphorylation at site I have now been shown to inhibit the oxidoreductase activity of complex I. Dimercaprol and antimycin inhibit the oxidoreductase activity of complex III. Hydrogen sulphide, carbon monoxide and cyanide inhibit the oxidoreductase activity of complex IV. When oxidation is inhibited, phosphorylation also can not occur.

Oligomycin inhibits oxidative phosphorylation at all the sites. It has been shown to bind to, and inhibit, F_o component of ATP synthetase. In fact, the subscript 'o' derives from the tendency of this component to bind oligomycin.

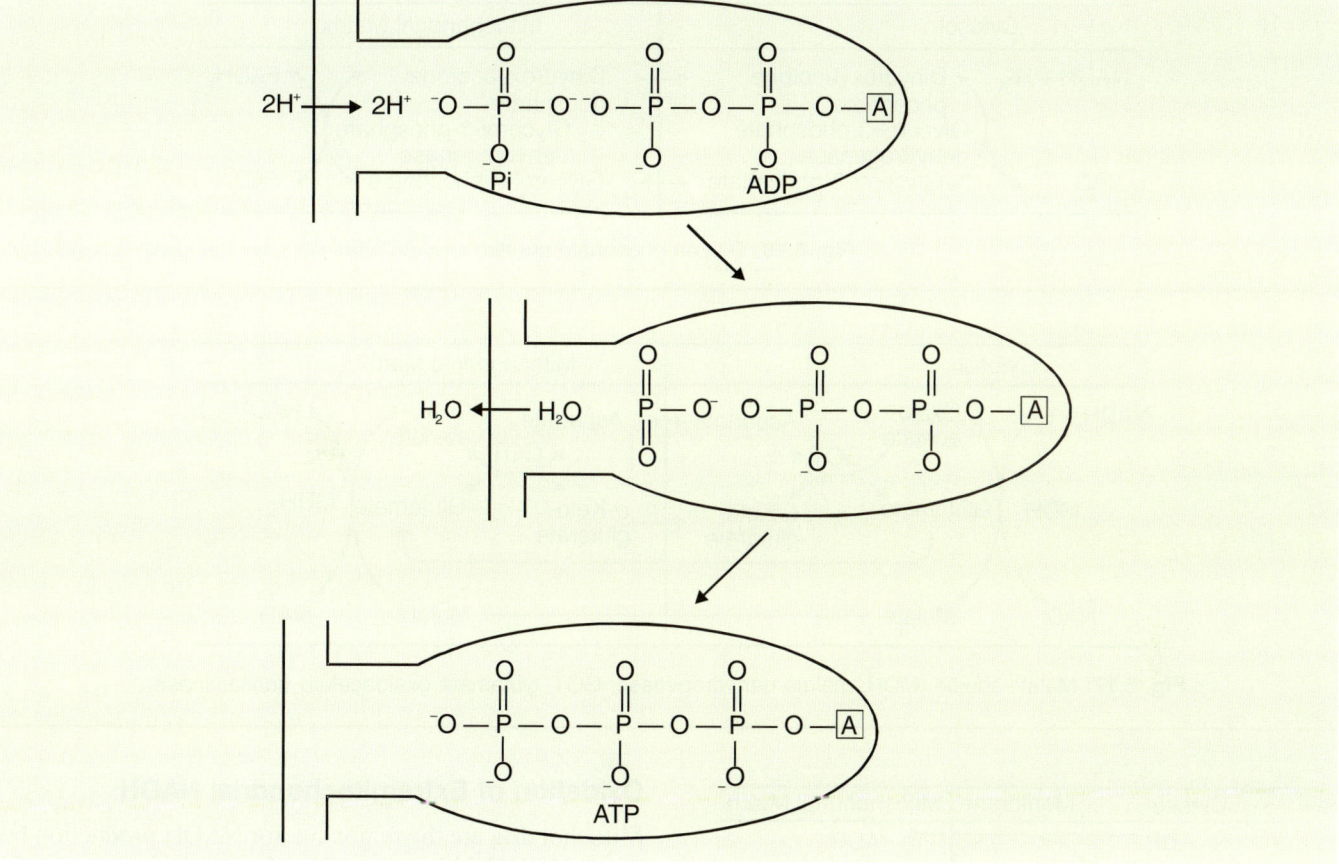

Fig. 8.14: Synthesis of ATP from ADP and Pi on the catalytic site of F_1 component of vectorial ATP synthetase

Certain agents, e.g. dinitrophenol, dinitrocresol and dicoumarol, uncouple oxidation and phosphorylation. In their presence, phosphorylation is inhibited but oxidation goes on. It has been shown that they make the inner mitochondrial membrane freely permeable to hydrogen ions. This does not allow the electrochemical gradient to build up and, therefore, ATP cannot be synthesised even though oxidation is going on.

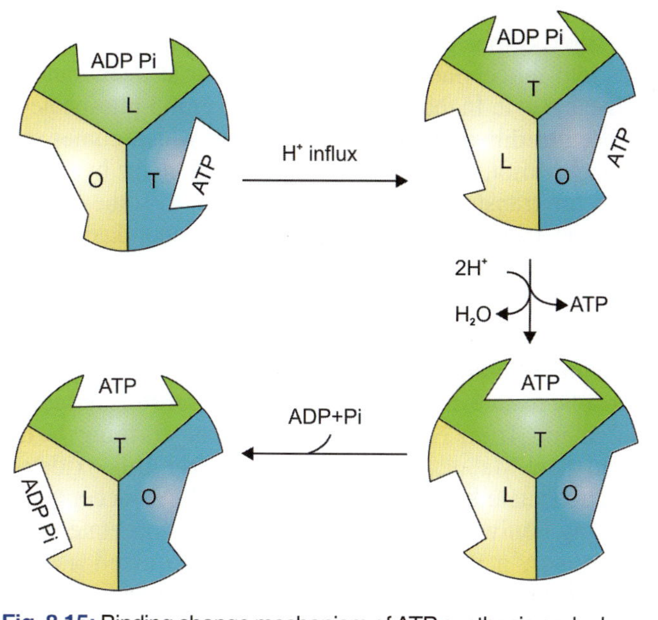

Thermogenin, a protein present in brown adipose tissue, also uncouples oxidation and phosphorylation by acting as a channel for re-entry of hydrogen ions so that the hydrogen ions gradient cannot build up. Brown adipose tissue is rich in mitochondia and cytochromes. Oxidation occurring in brown adipose tissue without generation of ATP results in production of heat. Brown adipose tissue is present in significant amount in infancy and decreases with age. It is also present in large amount in hibernating animals, and helps in maintaining their body temperature.

Regulation of Oxidative Phosphorylation

Oxidative phosphorylation in the respiratory chain results in consumption of oxygen. This is also known as tissue respiration. Under the usual physiological conditions when oxidisable substrates and oxygen are available, the rate of tissue respiration is regulated mainly by the concentration of ADP. Increased utilisation of ATP raises the concentration of ADP which increases tissue respiration resulting in increased conversion of ADP into ATP.

Fig. 8.15: Binding change mechanism of ATP synthesis and release

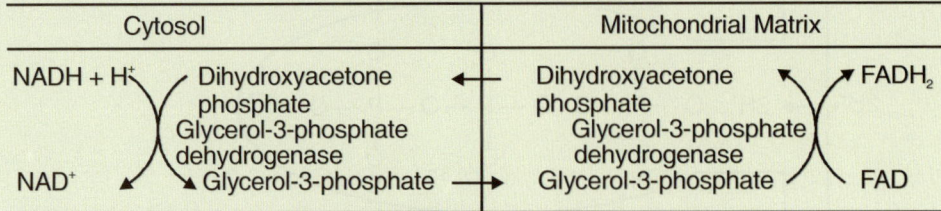

Fig. 8.16: Glycerophosphate shuttle

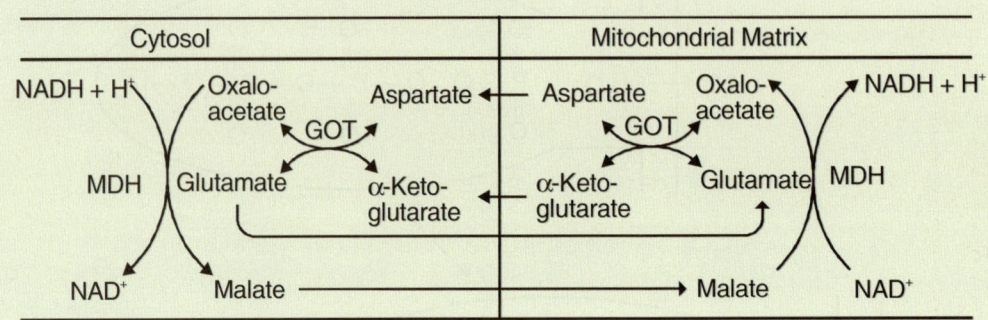

Fig. 8.17: Malate shuttle (MDH, malate dehydrogenase; GOT, glutamate oxaloacetate transaminase)

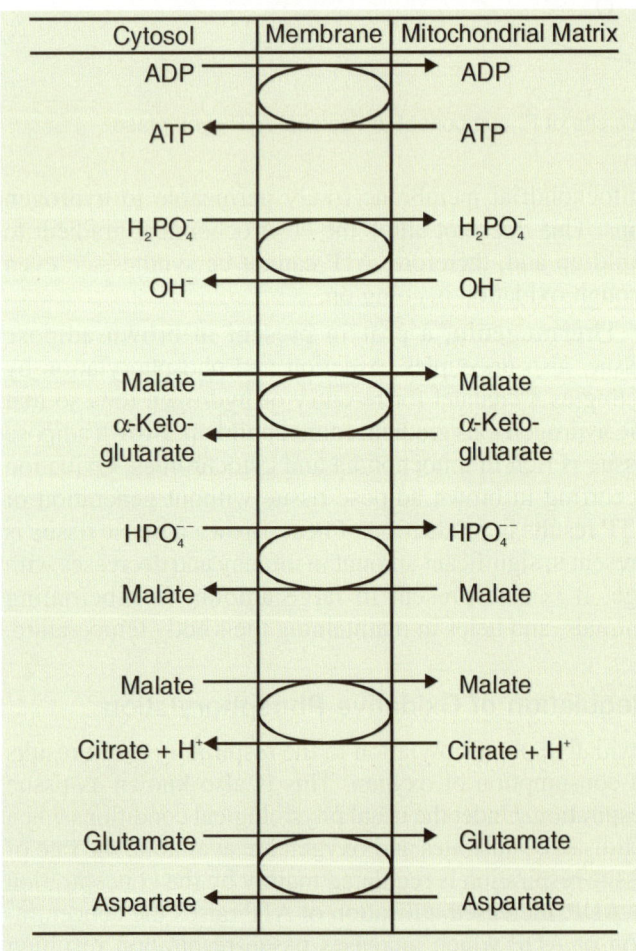

Fig. 8.18: Some mitochondrial antiports

Oxidation of Extramitochondrial NADH

Mitochondria are the major site for NADH production but some NADH is produced in the cytosol also. As the mitochondrial membrane is not permeable to NADH, special mechanisms are required to transport NADH from cytosol into mitochondria. Glycerophosphate shuttle and malate shuttle are two important mechanisms for transferring cytosolic NADH into mitochondria.

Glycerophosphate Shuttle

In this mechanism, cytosolic NADH is used to reduce dihydroxyacetone phosphate to glycerol-3-phosphate which goes into mitochondria as the mitochondrial membrane is permeable to it. In the mitochondria, glycerol-3-phosphate is oxidised to dihydroxyacetone phosphate which comes out into the cytosol. In the mitochondrial reaction, the hydrogen atoms are transferred to FAD. This leads to some loss of energy as only two ADP molecules are phosphorylated when $FADH_2$ is oxidised in the respiratory chain (Fig. 8.16).

Malate Shuttle

This mechanism is quantitatively more significant. Cytosolic malate dehydrogenase (MDH) transfers reducing equivalents from NADH to oxaloacetate forming NAD and malate. Malate goes into mitochondria. It is oxidised to oxaloacetate by mitochondrial MDH. NAD accepts the reducing equivalents. For transporting oxaloacetate back to cytosol, a special mechanism is required as the mitochondrial membrane is impermeable to it. Mitochondrial glutamate oxaloacetate transaminase (GOT) transfers an amino group from glutamate to oxaloacetate forming α-ketoglutarate and aspartate which come out of the mitochondria. These are converted into glutamate and oxaloacetate by cytosolic GOT. Glutamate goes back into mitochondria. The net result is that the cytosolic NADH is converted into NAD, and the mitochondrial NAD is converted into NADH (Fig. 8.17).

Transport Across Mitochondrial Membrane

The mitochondrial membrane is selectively permeable. Small uncharged molecules and monocarboxylic acids can pass through the membrane easily but special transport mechanisms are required to transport dicarboxylic acids, tricarboxylic acids and amino acids as the membrane is not permeable to these.

These transport mechanisms may operate as symports (two compounds passing through the membrane in the same direction) or as antiports (two compounds passing through the membrane in opposite directions). Transport of pyruvate and H^+ into mitochondria is an example of a symport.

Some important antiports are shown in Fig. 8.18.

EXERCISE

1. Describe the enzymes concerned with biological oxidation.

2. Explain the chemiosmotic theory of oxidative phosphorylation.

3. Write short notes on:
   a. High-energy phosphates
   b. Redox potential
   c. Microsomal hydroxylase system
   d. Superoxide radicals
   e. Substrate-linked oxidative phosphorylation
   f. Respiratory chain
   g. Vectorial ATP synthetase
   h. Binding change mechanism
   i. Malate shuttle

4. Write 'true' or 'false':
   a. ATP has two high-energy bonds.
   b. Low-energy phosphates can transfer their phosphate group to ADP.
   c. Respiratory chain is present in the outer membrane of mitochondria.
   d. The components of the respiratory chain are arranged in the increasing order of redox potential.
   e. Cytochrome P450 is the last cytochrome in the respiratory chain.
   f. Mitochondrial hydroxylase system hydroxylates some endogenous substrates.
   g. Hydrogen peroxide is produced and degraded in peroxisomes.
   h. Hydrogen peroxide is formed by the action of flavoproteins.
   i. Peroxisomes are congenitally absent in Zellweger's syndrome.
   j. The P:O ratio is three when the reducing equivalents enter the respiratory from $FADH_2$.
   k. The unc operon encodes some endogenous uncouplers of oxidative phosphorylation.
   l. ATP synthetase activity is present in the F_o component of vectorial ATP synthetase.
   m. F_o component of vectorial ATP synthetase is so named because of its tendency to bind oxygen.
   n. O, L and T sites are present in F_1 component of vectorial ATP synthetase.
   o. Uncouplers of oxidative phosphorylation make the inner mitochondrial membrane freely permeable to hydrogen ions.

5. Fill in the blanks:
   a. .... is described as the energy currency of the cells.
   b. Respiratory chain is present in the .... mitochondrial membrane.
   c. Redox potential is a measure of the affinity of a redox couple for ....
   d. Enzymes that incorporate oxygen into a substrate are known as ....

e. Adrenodoxin is a component of .... hydroxylase system.

f. Hydrogen peroxide is formed and degraded in subcellular organelles known as ....

g. .... are described as the power house of the cells.

h. The prosthetic group in cytochromes is ....

i. All the carriers in the respiratory chain except ....and .... are present in the form of complexes.

j. Except ....and ...., all the components of electron transfer chain are fixed in the inner mitochondrial membrane.

k. There are .... sites of phosphorylation in the respiratory chain.

l. The complexes ...., ... and .... in the respiratory chain act as proton pumps.

m. Vectorial ATP synthetase is made up of .... and .... components.

n. ....component of vectorial ATP synthetase acts as a channel for hydrogen ions.

o. .... component of vectorial ATP synthetase possesses ATP synthetase activity.

ANSWERS TO SHORT QUESTIONS

4. a. True
   b. False
   c. False
   d. True
   e. False
   f. True
   g. True
   h. True
   i. True
   j. False
   k. False
   l. False
   m. False
   n. True
   o. True

5. a. ATP
   b. Inner
   c. Electrons
   d. Oxygenases
   e. Mitochondrial
   f. Peroxisomes
   g. Mitochondria
   h. Iron-porphyrin
   i. Coenzyme Q, cytochrome c
   j. Coenzyme Q, cytochrome c
   k. Three
   l. I, III, IV
   m. F_o, F_1
   n. F_o
   o. F_1

Citric Acid Cycle

Citric acid cycle is a metabolic pathway in which acetyl CoA, obtained from diverse sources, is oxidised. Intermediates of this pathway can also be used to synthesise a variety of compounds. It is a cyclic pathway. It is also known as Krebs cycle or tricarboxylic acid cycle or central oxidative pathway. Enzymes of this pathway are located in the mitochondria. The pathway is present in all the cells having mitochondria.

The cycle begins with the condensation of acetyl CoA, a two-carbon compound, with oxaloacetate, a four-carbon compound, to form a six-carbon compound, citrate. By a series of reactions, citrate is reconverted into oxaloacetate. Two carbon atoms are removed as carbon dioxide in these reactions. A number of reducing equivalents are also removed which are oxidised to water in the respiratory chain.

Sources of Oxaloacetate

There is no net utilisation of oxaloacetate in citric acid cycle as it is regenerated at the end. However, if the overall rate of reactions is to be increased, the concentration of intermediates of the cycle has to be raised. Reactions which lead to net entry of intermediates into the cycle are known as **anaplerotic reactions**. An important anaplerotic reaction is the synthesis of oxaloacetate from pyruvate. The reaction is catalysed by pyruvate carboxylase. Biotin

is required as a coenzyme. ATP provides energy for the formation of the covalent bond. Pyruvate carboxylase is an allosteric enzyme which is activated by acetyl CoA.

$$CH_3 - \overset{\displaystyle O}{\overset{\displaystyle \|}{C}} - COOH + CO_2 + ATP$$
Pyruvate

Biotin | Pyruvate carboxylase

$$O = C - COOH$$
$$|$$
$$CH_2 - COOH + ADP + Pi$$
Oxaloacetate

Oxaloacetate may also be formed by a transamination reaction between aspartate and α-ketoglutarate. However, this reaction is not anaplerotic as one intermediate of citric acid cycle, oxaloacetate is formed at the expense of another, α-ketoglutarate (Fig. 9.2).

Sources of Acetyl CoA

Acetyl CoA occupies a unique place in metabolism as it can be formed from glucose, fatty acids and amino acids. Glucose, lactate and some amino acids, e.g. glycine, alanine, serine, threonine, cysteine, tryptophan and hydroxyproline, can be converted into pyruvate which, in turn, can be converted into acetyl CoA. End product of fatty acid oxidation is acetyl CoA. Ketone bodies are also converted into acetyl CoA before their eventual oxidation.

Oxidative Decarboxylation of Pyruvate

While fatty acids and ketone bodies are directly converted into acetyl CoA, the conversion of glucose, lactate and amino acids mentioned above into acetyl CoA occurs via pyruvate. Pyruvate is converted into acetyl CoA by oxidative decarboxylation. Oxidative decarboxylation occurs by a series of reactions catalysed by three enzymes in the presence of five coenzymes. The enzymes are

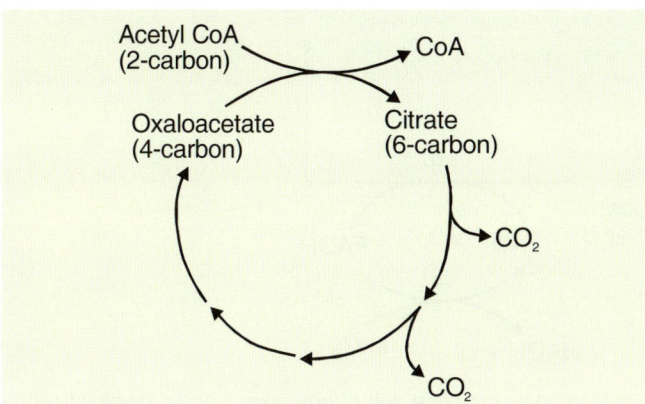

Fig. 9.1: An overview of citric acid cycle

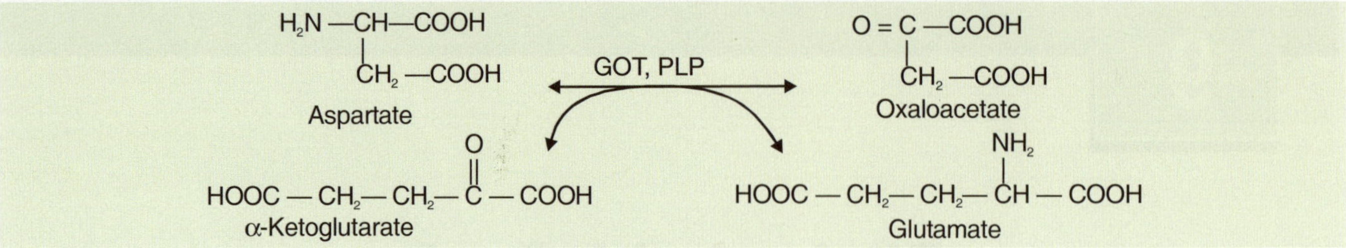

H2N—CH—COOH
CH2—COOH
Aspartate
GOT, PLP
O = C—COOH
CH2—COOH
Oxaloacetate
HOOC — CH2— CH2— C — COOH
α-Ketoglutarate
NH2
HOOC — CH2— CH2— CH — COOH
Glutamate

Fig. 9.2: Formation of oxaloacetate from aspartate

pyruvate dehydrogenase, dihydrolipoyl acetyltransferase and dihydrolipoyl dehydrogenase which are tightly bound together to form the pyruvate dehydrogenase complex. In *E.coli,* the complex is made up of 24 polypeptide chains having pyruvate dehydrogenase activity, 24 polypeptide chains having dihydrolipoyl acetyltransferase activity and 12 polypeptide chains having dihydrolipoyl dehydrogenase activity. In other species, the numbers of polypeptide chains are different. The coenzymes required by the complex are thiamin pyrophosphate (TPP), lipoic acid, coenzyme A (CoA), FAD and NAD. The reactions occur in mitochondria (Fig. 9.3).

The net reaction catalysed by pyruvate dehydrogenase complex can be summed up as:

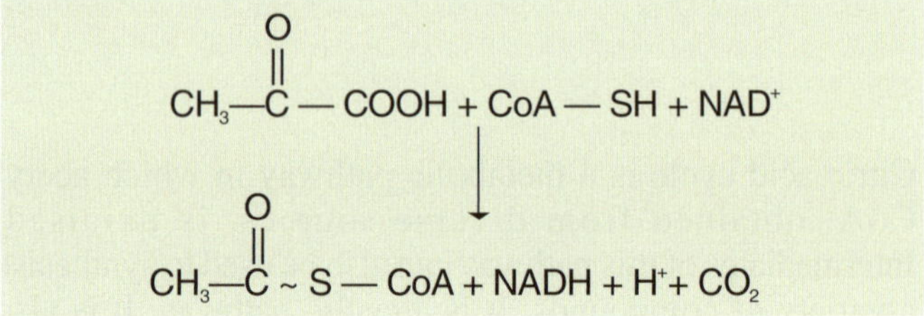

CH3—C — COOH + CoA — SH + NAD+
CH3—C ~ S — CoA + NADH + H+ + CO2

Fate of Acetyl CoA

A major fate of acetyl CoA is its oxidation in the citric acid cycle. This produces a large amount of energy in the form of ATP. But when the supply of energy is abundant, acetyl CoA is used to synthesise fatty acids.

CH3— C — COOH
Pyruvate
R—H
Thiamin pyrophosphate
CH3— C — COOH
CO2
CH3— C — H
CoA – SH
Coenzyme A
CH3 — C ~ S SH
S-Acetyl lipoic acid
S — S
Oxidised lipoic acid
CH3— C ~ S — CoA
Acetyl CoA
SH SH
Reduced lipoic acid
FAD
FADH2
NADH + H+
NAD+

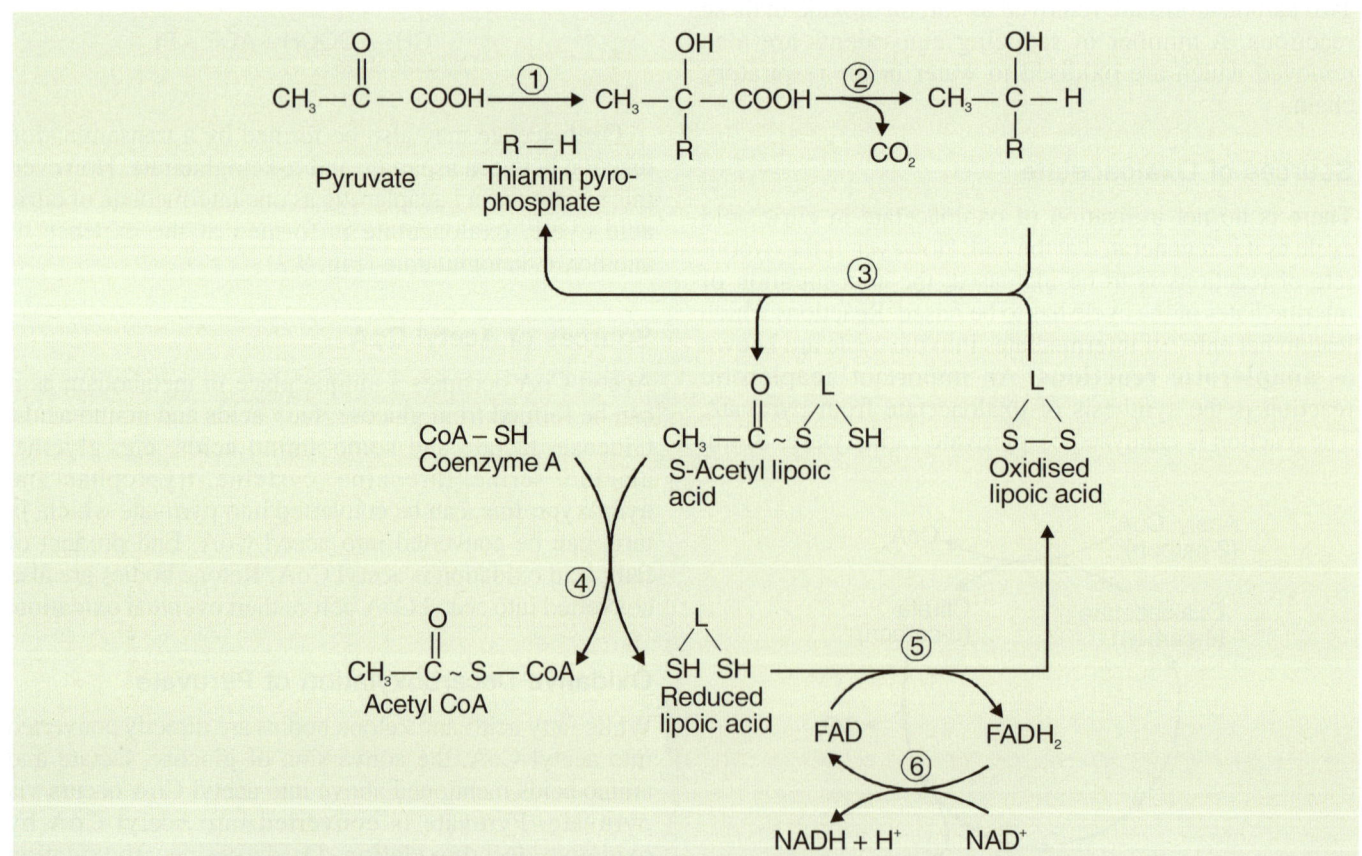

Fig. 9.3: Oxidative decarboxylation of pyruvate. Reactions 1 and 2 are catalysed by pyruvate dehydrogenase, 3 and 4 by dihydrolipoyl acetyltransferase, and 5 and 6 by dihydrolipoyl dehydrogenase

Small amounts are used for the synthesis of cholesterol, steroid hormones, vitamin D and ketone bodies, and for various acetylation reactions.

Reactions of Citric Acid Cycle

1. In the first reaction of the cycle, acetyl CoA reacts with oxaloacetate in the presence of citrate synthetase to form citrate and CoA. The high-energy thioester bond of acetyl CoA is broken releasing free energy which ensures that the reaction proceeds in the forward direction only.

$$O = C - COOH$$
$$\quad\quad |$$
$$\quad\quad CH_2 - COOH$$
$$\quad\quad \text{Oxaloacetate}$$
$$\quad\quad O$$
$$\quad\quad ||$$
$$H_2O + CH_3 - C \sim S - CoA$$
$$\quad\quad \text{Acetyl CoA}$$

Citrate synthetase

CoA — SH

$$CH_2 - COOH$$
$$\quad |$$
$$HO - C - COOH$$
$$\quad |$$
$$CH_2 - COOH$$
$$\quad \text{Citrate}$$

2. Aconitase removes a molecule of water from citrate converting it into *cis*-aconitate. This reaction is inhibited by fluoroacetate.

$$CH_2 - COOH \qquad\qquad CH_2 - COOH$$
$$\quad | \qquad\qquad\qquad\qquad\qquad |$$
$$HO - C - COOH \xrightarrow{\text{Aconitase}} C - COOH$$
$$\quad | \qquad\qquad\qquad\qquad\qquad ||$$
$$CH_2 - COOH \quad H_2O \quad CH - COOH$$
$$\quad \text{Citrate} \qquad\qquad\qquad \textit{cis}\text{-Aconitate}$$

3. Aconitase, then, adds a water molecule to *cis*-aconitate. The net result of this and the preceding reaction is that the position of the –OH group is shifted, and citrate is converted into isocitrate.

$$CH_2 - COOH \qquad\qquad CH_2 - COOH$$
$$\quad | \qquad\quad \text{Aconitase} \qquad\qquad |$$
$$C - COOH \xleftrightarrow{\quad\quad\quad} CH - COOH$$
$$\quad || \qquad\qquad\qquad\qquad\qquad |$$
$$CH - COOH \quad H_2O \quad HO - CH - COOH$$
$$\textit{cis}\text{-Aconitate} \qquad\qquad \text{Isocitrate}$$

4. Isocitrate is dehydrogenated to oxalosuccinate by isocitrate dehydrogenase. Isocitrate dehydrogenase is present in mitochondria as well as cytosol. The mitochondrial enzyme of citric acid cycle uses NAD as an acceptor of reducing equivalents while the cytosolic enzyme uses NADP.

$$CH_2 - COOH$$
$$\quad |$$
$$CH - COOH$$
$$\quad |$$
$$HO - CH - COOH$$
$$\quad \text{Isocitrate}$$

NAD^+

Isocitrate dehydrogenase

$NADH + H^+$

$$CH_2 - COOH$$
$$\quad |$$
$$CH - COOH$$
$$\quad |$$
$$O = C - COOH$$
$$\quad \text{Oxalosuccinate}$$

5. Oxalosuccinate is a transient intermediate which is decarboxylated to α-ketoglutarate by isocitrate dehydrogenase. This is the first reaction of the cycle in which a carbon atom is removed.

$$CH_2 - COOH$$
$$\quad |$$
$$CH - COOH$$
$$\quad |$$
$$O - C \quad COOH$$
$$\quad \text{Oxalosuccinate}$$

CO_2 — Isocitrate dehydrogenase, Mn^{++}

$$CH_2 - COOH$$
$$\quad |$$
$$CH_2$$
$$\quad |$$
$$O = C - COOH$$
$$\quad \text{α-Ketoglutarate}$$

6. α-Ketoglutarate undergoes oxidative decarboxylation to succinyl CoA. This reaction is analogous to the oxidative decarboxylation of pyruvate to acetyl CoA.

$$CH_2 - COOH$$
$$\quad |$$
$$CH_2$$
$$\quad |$$
$$O = C - COOH$$
$$\quad \text{α-Ketoglutarate}$$

$CoA - SH + NAD^+$ ⟩ α-Ketoglutarate dehydrogenase complex

$CO_2 + NADH + H^+$

$$CH_2 - COOH$$
$$\quad |$$
$$CH_2$$
$$\quad |$$
$$O = C \sim S - CoA$$
$$\quad \text{Succinyl CoA}$$

The reaction is catalysed by α-ketoglutarate dehydrogenase complex which is made up of α-ketoglutarate dehydrogenase, dihydrolipoyl acetyltransferase and dihydrolipoyl dehydrogenase. Thiamin pyrophosphate, lipoic acid, CoA, FAD and NAD are required as coenzymes. The net reaction may be described as above. This is the second reaction of the cycle in which a carbon atom is removed. This is also an example of substrate-linked oxidative phosphorylation. Energy released during oxidation of α-ketoglutarate is used to form a high-energy thioester bond in the product of the reaction. In the subseqent reaction, this energy is used to convert GDP into GTP. The reaction is physiologically irreversible. Arsentite inhibits this reaction by forming a stable complex with lipoic acid.

7. Succinate thiokinase (succinyl CoA synthetase) splits succinyl CoA into succinate and CoA. The energy released in the reaction is used to phosphorylate GDP to GTP. GTP can transfer a high-energy phosphate to ADP forming ATP.

$$
\begin{array}{c}
CH_2-COOH \\
| \\
CH_2 \\
| \\
O=C\sim S-CoA \\
\textbf{Succinyl CoA}
\end{array}
$$

GDP + Pi ⟶ ⟶ Succinate thiokinase
GTP + CoA—SH ⟵

$$
\begin{array}{c}
CH_2-COOH \\
| \\
CH_2-COOH \\
\textbf{Succinate}
\end{array}
$$

8. Succinate is a four-carbon dicarboxylic acid which is converted into another four-carbon dicarboxylic acid, oxaloacetate by a series of reactions. First, succinate dehydrogenase, a flavoprotein, transfers two hydrogen atoms from succinate to FAD. Succinate is converted into fumarate.

$$
\begin{array}{c}
CH_2-COOH \\
| \\
CH_2-COOH \\
\textbf{Succinate}
\end{array}
$$

FAD ⟶ Succinate dehydrogenase
FADH$_2$ ⟵

$$
\begin{array}{c}
H-C-COOH \\
\| \\
HOOC-C-H \\
\textbf{Fumarate}
\end{array}
$$

9. Fumarate is hydrated to L-malate. The reaction is catalysed by fumarase.

$$
\begin{array}{c}
H-C-COOH \\
\| \\
HOOC-C-H \\
\textbf{Fumarate}
\end{array}
$$

H$_2$O ⟶ Fumarase

$$
\begin{array}{c}
HO-CH-COOH \\
| \\
CH_2-COOH \\
\textbf{L-Malate}
\end{array}
$$

10. L-Malate is dehydrogenated to oxaloacetate by malate dehydrogenase. NAD accepts the reducing equivalents. Thus, oxaloacetate is regenerated and acetyl CoA is oxidised. However, the two carbon atoms that are removed as carbon dioxide are not actually derived from acetyl CoA. These are derived from oxaloacetate, and the two incoming carbon atoms from acetyl CoA appear in the new molecule of oxaloacetate which is formed at the end of the cycle. Oxaloacetate formed at the end of the last reaction reacts with another molecule of acetyl CoA to start a new cycle.

$$
\begin{array}{c}
HO-CH-COOH \\
| \\
CH_2-COOH \\
\textbf{L-Malate}
\end{array}
$$

NAD$^+$ ⟶ Malate dehydrogenase
NADH + H$^+$ ⟵

$$
\begin{array}{c}
O=C-COOH \\
| \\
CH_2-COOH \\
\textbf{Oxaloacetate}
\end{array}
$$

The net changes occurring in one revolution of the cycle may be summed up as:

$$
\begin{array}{c}
O \\
\| \\
CH_3-C\sim S-CoA + 2\,H_2O + 3\,NAD^+ + FAD + GDP + Pi \\
\downarrow \\
CoA-SH + 2\,CO_2 + 3\,NADH + 3H^+ + FADH_2 + GTP
\end{array}
$$

The reactions of the cycle are summarised in Fig. 9.4.

ENERGETICS

During complete oxidation of one molecule of acetyl CoA in citric acid cycle, three molecules of NAD and one molecule of FAD are reduced. These are oxidised in the respiratory chain. Oxidation of three molecules of NADH will phosphorylate nine molecules of ADP to ATP. Oxidation of one molecule of FADH$_2$ will phosphorylate two molecules of ADP to ATP. Thus, 11 ATP equivalents are formed by oxidative phosphorylation in the respiratory chain per molecule of acetyl CoA oxidised. One high-energy phosphate bond is formed by substrate-linked

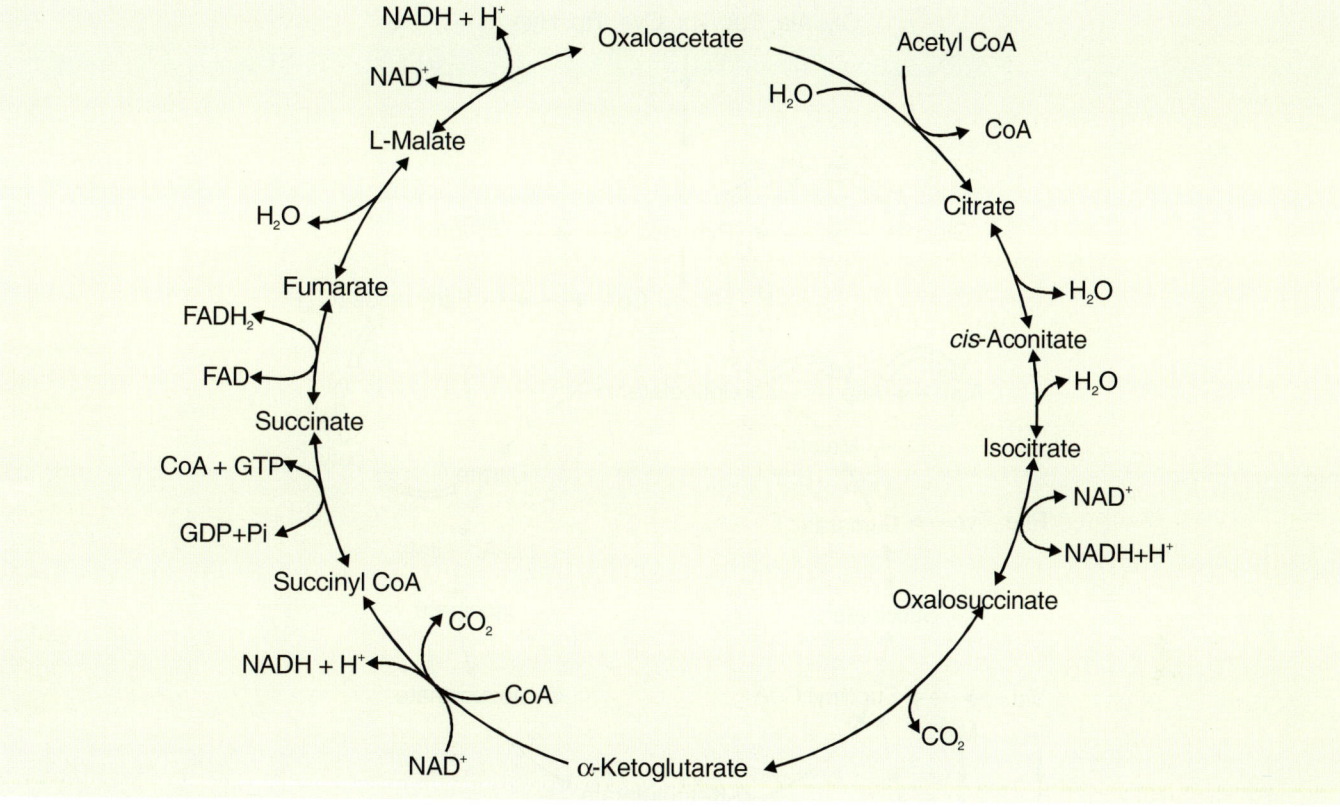

Fig. 9.4: Citric acid cycle

oxidative phosphorylation in the form of GTP which, in turn, can convert ADP into ATP. Therefore, 12 high-energy phosphate bonds or ATP equivalents are formed on complete oxidation of one molecule of acetyl CoA in citric acid cycle and respiratory chain (Table 9.1).

One molecule of NAD is reduced during oxidative decarboxylation of pyruvate into acetyl CoA. This will form three ATP equivalents when it is oxidised in the respiratory chain. Therefore, the energy yield from complete oxidation of one molecule of pyruvate is 15 ATP equivalents.

Importance of Citric Acid Cycle

1. Citric acid cycle is the final catabolic pathway for carbohydrates, lipids and proteins. All carbohydrates

can be converted into glucose. Glucose is converted into pyruvate in the glycolytic pathway which can enter citric acid cycle after its conversion into acetyl CoA. Oxidation of fatty acids directly produces acetyl CoA which is oxidised in the citric acid cycle. Glycerol released from lipids can be converted into pyruvate in the glycolytic pathway (Glycerol $\rightarrow$ Glycerol-3-phosphate $\rightarrow$ Dihydroxyacetone phosphate $\rightarrow$ $\rightarrow$ Pyruvate). Many amino acids are converted into pyruvate as mentioned earlier. These can enter the cycle as acetyl CoA. Glutamate can be converted into α-ketoglutarate. Thus, glutamate and other amino acids that can be converted into glutamate, e.g. glutamine, arginine, histidine and proline, can enter the cycle as α-ketoglutarate. Valine, isoleucine and methionine can enter as succinyl CoA. A part of the carbon skeleton of

Table 9.1: Energy captured during oxidation of one molecule of acetyl CoA in citric acid cycle and respiratory chain		
Reaction	Change in conezyme	Energy captured as ATP equivalents
Isocitrate to oxaloacetate	NAD$^+$ $\rightarrow$ NADH	3 ATP equivalents
α-Ketoglutarate to succinyl CoA	NAD$^+$ $\rightarrow$ NADH	3 ATP equivalents
Malate to oxaloacetate	NAD$^+$ $\rightarrow$ NADH	3 ATP equivalents
Succinate to fumarate	FAD $\rightarrow$ FADH$_2$	2 ATP equivalents
Succinyl CoA to succinate	GDP $\rightarrow$ GTP	1 ATP equivalent
	Net gain	12 ATP equivalents

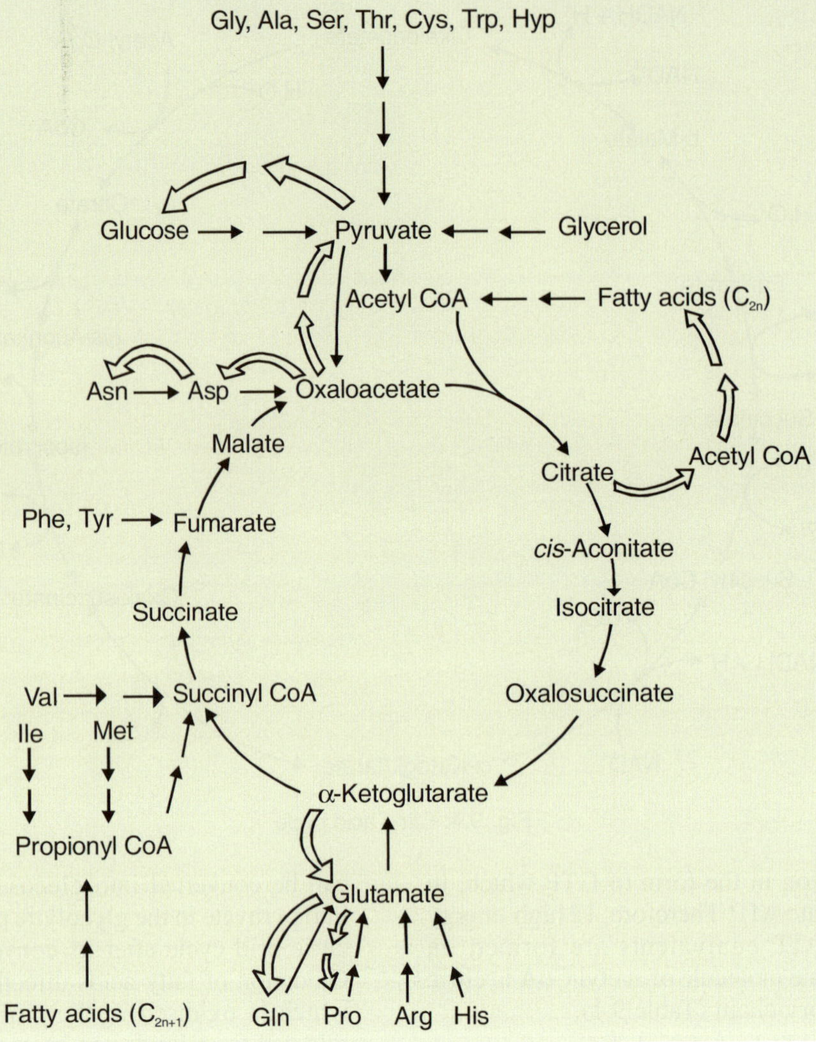

Gly, Ala, Ser, Thr, Cys, Trp, Hyp

Glucose → → Pyruvate ← ← Glycerol

Acetyl CoA ← ← Fatty acids (C_{2n})

Asn → Asp → Oxaloacetate

Malate

Citrate   Acetyl CoA

Phe, Tyr → Fumarate

cis-Aconitate

Succinate

Isocitrate

Val →   → Succinyl CoA

Ile   Met

Oxalosuccinate

α-Ketoglutarate

Propionyl CoA

Glutamate

Fatty acids (C_{2n+1})   Gln Pro Arg His

Fig. 9.5: Amphibolic nature of citric acid cycle. Glucose, fatty acids and amino acids can enter at different points, and can be synthesised from the intermediates of the cycle

phenylalanine and tyrosine is converted into fumarate. Asparagine and aspartate can enter the cycle as oxaloacetate.

2. Many intermediates of citric acid cycle can be used to synthesise glucose, fatty acids and amino acids (Fig. 9.5). Therefore, this cycle plays an important role in the interconversion of these compounds. Since this pathway is catabolic as well as anabolic, it is said to be an **amphibolic** pathway.

All intermediates of the cycle can serve as substrates for the synthesis of glucose by gluconeogenesis. Some intermediates can be transaminated to amino acids, e.g. α-ketoglutarate to glutamate and oxaloacetate to aspartate. Some other amino acids can be formed from these two. Citrate can provide acetyl CoA, the building block for fatty acid synthesis. For fatty acid synthesis, citrate leaves the mitochondria, and is cleaved into acetyl CoA and oxaloacetate in the cytosol.

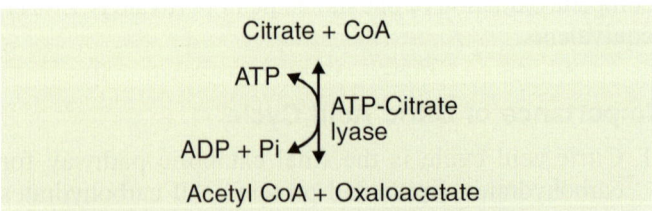

Citrate + CoA

ATP

ATP-Citrate lyase

ADP + Pi

Acetyl CoA + Oxaloacetate

3. One of the most important functions of citric acid cycle is to capture the energy present in carbohydrates, lipids and proteins in the form of ATP when these fuels are oxidised in the citric acid cycle and the respiratory chain.

Regulation

Since the major function of citric acid cycle is to provide energy, the overall rate of reactions is regulated by the availability of energy in the cell as indicated by concentrations of ATP and ADP. In addition, citrate synthetase, isocitrate dehydrogenase and α-ketoglutarate

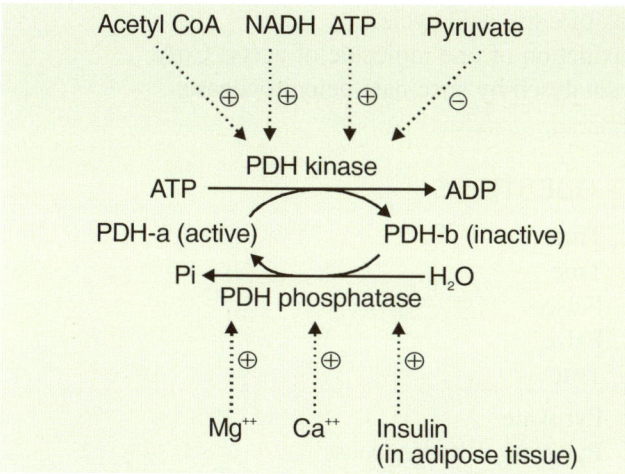

Fig. 9.6: Regulation of pyruvate dehydrogenase (PDH)

citric acid cycle reactions is regulated mainly by the availability of acetyl CoA which, in turn, is regulated by pyruvate dehydrogenase complex. This enzyme complex is regulated by allosteric mechanism as well as covalent modification. Of the three components of the complex, dihydrolipoyl acetyltransferase and dihydrolipoyl dehydrogenase are allosteric enzymes which are inhibited by acetyl CoA and NADH respectively. The third component, pyruvate dehydrogenase (PDH) is regulated by covalent modification. PDH-a (active) is phosphorylated to PDH-b (inactive) by PDH kinase. PDH kinase is allostericaliy activated by acetyl CoA, NADH and ATP. It is allosterically inhibited by pyruvate. PDH-b is dephosphorylated to PDH-a by PDH phosphatase. PDH phosphatase is activated by Ca^{++} and Mg^{++} (in adipose tissue, it is activated by insulin). Thus, high concentrations of acetyl CoA, NADH and ATP convert active PDH into its inactive form, and decrease the conversion of pyruvate into acetyl CoA. This, in turn, decreases the rate of citric acid cycle reactions. A high concentration of pyruvate has the opposite effect. In adipose tissue, insulin promotes the conversion of inactive PDH into active PDH by activating PDH phosphatase. This increases the oxidative decarboxylation of pyruvate into acetyl CoA.

dehydrogenase are allosteric enzymes. They are activated by Ca^{++}. Citrate synthetase is inhibited by ATP and fatty acyl CoA. Isocitrate dehydrogenase is inhibited by ATP and NADH. α-Ketoglutarate dehydrogenase is inhibited by succinyl CoA and NADH.

In brain, acetyl CoA is formed mainly from pyruvate which, in turn, is formed from glucose. The fate of acetyl CoA is its oxidation in the citric acid cycle. The rate of

EXERCISE

1. Describe the reactions and energetics of citric acid cycle. What are the sources of oxaloacetate and acetyl CoA?
2. Explain the importance and regulation of citric acid cycle.
3. Write short notes on:
   a. Oxidative decarboxylation   b. Anaplerotic reactions
4. Write 'true' or 'false':
   a. Citric acid cycle is located in the cytosol.
   b. Two carbon atoms enter the citric acid cycle in the form of acetyl CoA.
   c. Formation of oxaloacetate from aspartate is an anaplerotic reaction.
   d. Acetyl CoA can be formed by oxidative decarboxylation of pyruvate.
   e. Pyruvate dehydrogenase complex is made up of five enzymes.
   f. Pyruvate dehydrogenase complex requires three coenzymes.
   g. Nine ATP equivalents are formed on complete oxidation of one molecule of acetyl CoA.
   h. Twelve ATP equivalents are formed on complete oxidation of one molecule of pyruvate.
   i. Citric acid cycle is an amphibolic pathway.
   j. Pyruvate dehydrogenase is regulated by covalent modification.
5. Fill in the blanks:
   a. Enzymes of Krebs cycle are located in the ....
   b. Formation of oxaloacetate from .... is an anaplerotic reaction.
   c. .... is formed by oxidative decarboxylation of pyruvate.
   d. Pyruvate dehydrogenase, dihydrolipoyl acetyltransferase and dihydrolipoyl dehydrogenase constitute the .... complex.
   e. A five-carbon intermediate in citric acid cycle is ....
   f. GTP is formed in citric acid cycle in the reaction catalysed by ....

g. ....is required as a coenzyme in three reactions of citric acid cycle.

h. ....ATP equivalents are formed on complete oxidation of one molecule of acetyl CoA.

i. .... is required as a coenzyme in the reaction catalysed by succinate dehydrogenase.

j. Citrate is cleaved into acetyl CoA and oxaloacetate by ....

ANSWERS TO SHORT QUESTIONS

4. a. False
   c. False
   e. False
   g. False
   i. True

   b. True
   d. True
   f. False
   h. False
   j. True

5. a. Mitochondria
   c. Acetyl CoA
   e. α-Ketoglutarate
   g. NAD
   i. FAD

   b. Pyruvate
   d. Pyruvate dehydrogenase
   f. Succinate thiokinase
   h. Twelve
   j. ATP-citrate lyase

Metabolism of Carbohydrates

Carbohydrates constitute the largest component of an ordinary diet. One of the most important functions of carbohydrates is to provide energy. Some tissues, e.g. brain and erythrocytes, are dependent almost exclusively on glucose as a source of energy. Moreover, glucose is the only fuel which can be oxidised under anaerobic conditions. Therefore, during prolonged exercise, even muscles can obtain energy only from glucose. Besides providing energy, carbohydrates perform some other functions also. Some carbohydrates are used as structural constituents of tissues. Ribose and deoxyribose are used to synthesise nucleotides and nucleic acids. Some carbohydrates form the prosthetic group of hormones, immunoglobulins, blood group substances, etc.

DIGESTION

Carbohydrates are mostly consumed in diet as poly-saccharides, e.g. starch, glycogen, cellulose, etc. Small amount of disaccharides and monosaccharides, e.g. sucrose, lactose, fructose, glucose, etc. are also present in food. Since only monosaccharides can be absorbed from the intestine, the larger carbohydrates are hydrolysed into monosaccharides during the course of digestion. Cellulose cannot be digested in human beings but its presence in food is important because it stimulates peristalsis and helps in bowel movement.

Among the digestive juices, saliva, pancreatic juice and the intestinal secretion contain enzymes capable of digesting carbohydrates. Saliva contains amylase which can hydrolyse starch and glycogen but the contribution of salivary amylase in the digestion of carbohydrates is not significant as food stays in the mouth for a very short period, and soon after it reaches the stomach, the salivary amylase becomes inactive in the acid environment of stomach.

Digestion of carbohydrates really begins in the small intestine. **Pancreatic amylase** (α-amylase) hydrolyses the internal α-1,4-glycosidic bonds of starch and glycogen at an alkaline pH forming maltose, isomaltose and maltotriose. The enzyme does not act on the terminal α-1, 4-glycosidic bonds and the α-1,6-glycosidic bonds present at the branch points (Fig. 10.1).

Intestinal secretion contains various disaccharidases which hydrolyse disaccharides into monosaccharides. **Maltase** hydrolyses maltose and maltotriose into glucose. **Isomaltase** (α-1,6-glucosidase) hydrolyses isomaltose into glucose. **Sucrase** (invertase) hydrolyses sucrose into glucose and fructose.

Lactase hydrolyses lactose into glucose and galactose (hereditary lactase deficiency in children or acquired lactase deficiency in adults can cause lactose intolerance). Thus, the major products of digestion of carbohydrates are glucose, fructose and galactose. Small amounts of mannose, ribose, xylose, etc. may also be present in food.

ABSORPTION

Monosaccharides are absorbed mainly in the small intestine. The purpose of absorption is to transfer the products of digestion from the lumen of the intestine– where, technically speaking, they are still outside the body– into circulation from where they can be taken up and utilised by the tissues. The monosaccharides are absorbed from the lumen of the intestine into the mucosal cells of the intestine from where they are delivered into portal circulation.

There are two mechanisms for the absorption of monosaccharides from the intestine – active transport and facilitated diffusion. The monosaccharides having pyranose ring structure with a methyl or a substituted methyl group on carbon 5, and an –OH group on carbon 2 having the same configuration as in D-glucopyranose are absorbed by active transport. Such monosaccharides are glucose and galactose. Other monosaccharides are absorbed by facilitated diffusion.

Active Transport

Active transport occurs against concentration gradient. Energy is spent for moving the compound from a lower concentration to a higher concentration. A carrier (a protein molecule) is required for active transport, and the process is saturable.

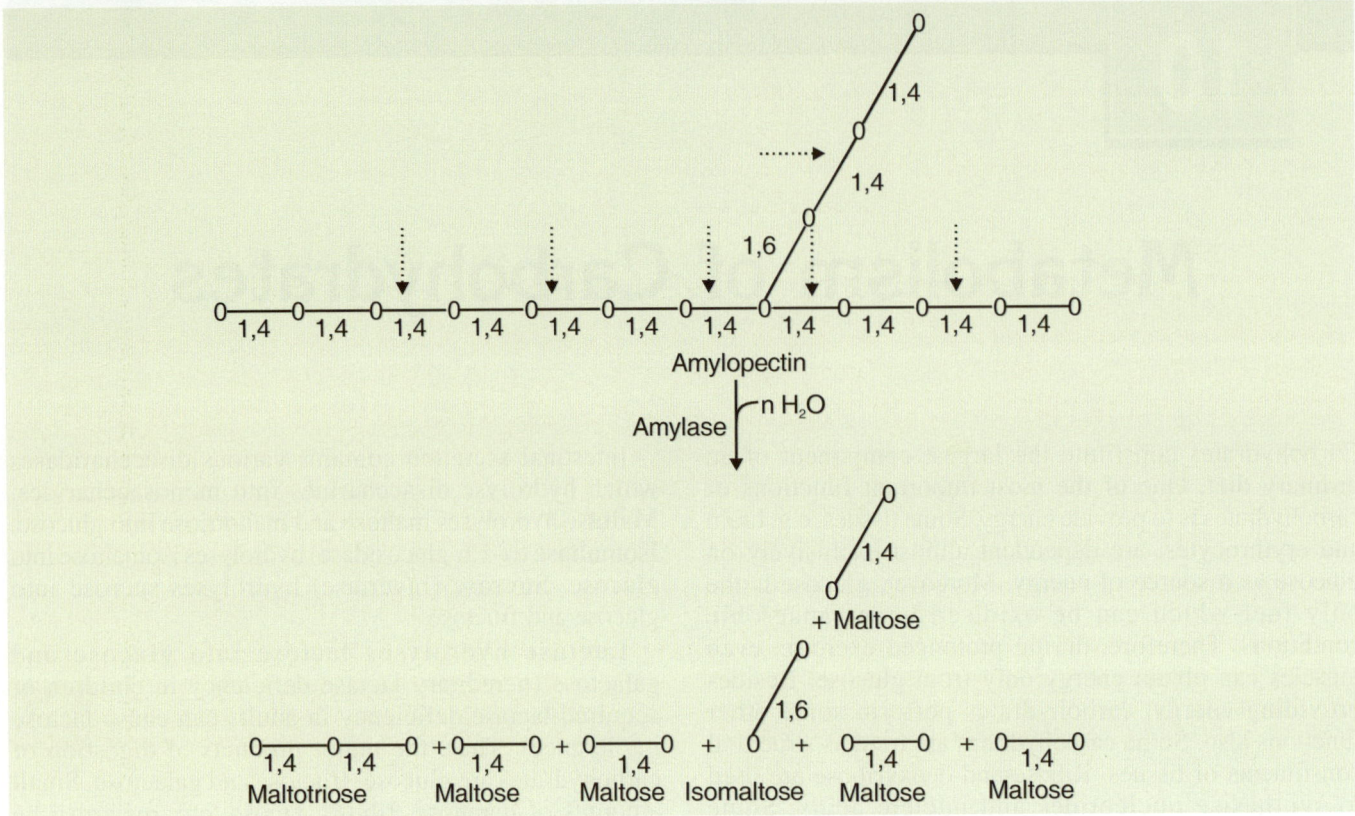

Fig. 10.1: Hydrolysis of amylopectin by amylase. Broken arrows indicate the glycosidic bonds attacked by amylase

Glucose is absorbed actively from the intestinal lumen into the mucosal cells by **Sodium Glucose Transporter** (SGLT 1). This protein, present in the cell membrane, has two binding sites–one for sodium and the other for glucose. Sodium and glucose, present in the lumen, bind to SGLT 1. As the concentration of sodium in the intestinal lumen is much higher than in the mucosal cells, sodium is transported into the mucosal cells down its concentration gradient. At the same time, glucose is transported into the mucosal cells against its concentration gradient. However, a rise in sodium concentration in intracellular fluid is physiologically intolerable. To keep the intracellular sodium concentration low, sodium is actively pumped out of the cell against its concentration gradient. For every three sodium ions pumped out, two potassium ions move into the cell. Ejection of sodium against its concentration gradient requires energy which is provided by hydrolysis of ATP into ADP and Pi. Hydrolysis of ATP is catalysed by membrane-bound **Na^+, K^+-exchanging ATPase** (or Na^+, K^+-ATPase). Thus, energy is really spent to maintain sodium homeostasis which is disturbed during the transport of glucose into the mucosal cells. The system that ejects sodium ions in exchange for potassium ions is also known as **sodium pump** or sodium-potassium pump. Galactose is absorbed similarly by SGLT 1. The transport is disrupted by ouabain which inhibits the sodium pump, and by phlorhizin which displaces sodium from the carrier.

Facilitated Diffusion

Fructose is absorbed by facilitated diffusion from a higher concentration (in the intestinal lumen) to a lower concentration (in the mucosal cells). The carrier involved in this transport is **GLUT 5** which is present on the luminal side of the cell membrane of mucosal cells. Another transporter, **GLUT 2**, is present on the contraluminal side of cell membrane which can transport glucose, galactose and fructose across the membrane by facilitated diffusion. When the concentration of these monosaccharides increases in the mucosal cells following absorption, they are transported into capillaries by GLUT2 down their concentration gradient (Fig. 10.2).

The monosaccharides released from intestinal mucosa into capillaries are taken by portal veins to liver which is the first destination of the dietary carbohydrates after digestion and absorption. All pathways of carbohydrate metabolism are present in liver. Glucose and galactose/fructose can be converted into each other in liver. Excess glucose can be stored in liver as glycogen. Non-carbohydrates can be converted into glucose in liver, and glucose is also released from liver into systemic circulation.

Different tissues take up glucose from circulation for their metabolic requirements with the help of specific Glucose Transporters (GLUTs). Some important features

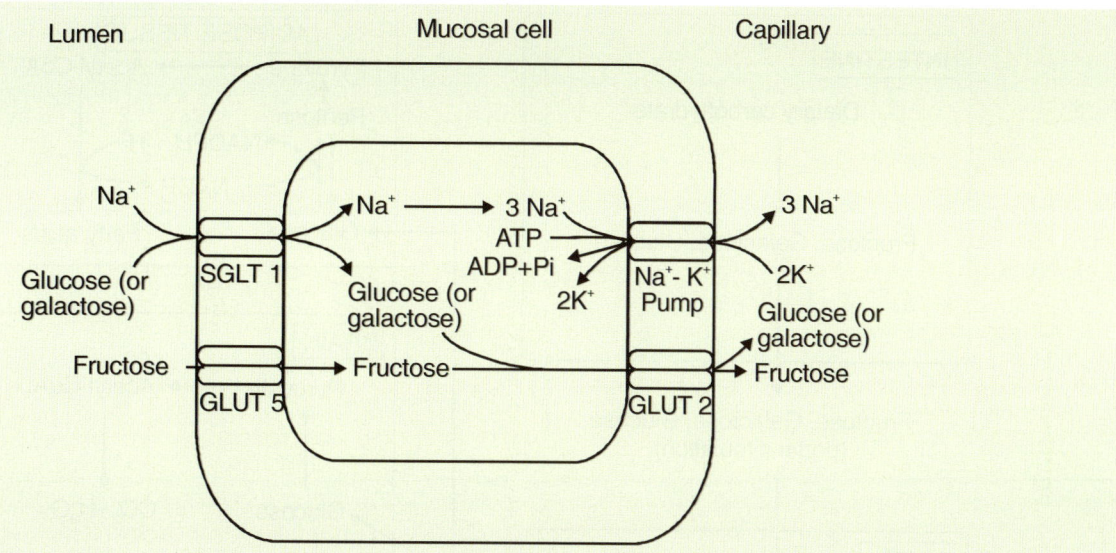

Fig. 10.2: Active uptake of glucose and galactose by SGLT 1 and facilitated diffusion of fructose by GLUT 5 from the lumen of the intestine into the mucosal cell is followed by ejection of Na⁺ by Na⁺-K⁺ pump and facilitated diffusion of glucose, galactose and fructose by GLUT 2 into the capillaries

of GLUTs are summarised in Table 10.1. Inter-organ flow of glucose and its metabolites, and some important pathways of carbohydrate metabolism in different tissues are depicted in Fig. 10.3.

MAJOR PATHWAYS OF CARBOHYDRATE METABOLISM

The main pathways for metabolism of carbohydrates are:

1. Glycolysis: This is the main pathway for oxidation of glucose. The end product is pyruvate or lactate.
2. Hexose monophosphate shunt: This is another pathway for oxidation of glucose. Pentoses are formed as intermediates in this pathway.
3. Glycogenesis: Glucose is converted into glycogen for storage by this pathway.
4. Glycogenolysis: Stored glycogen is broken down by this pathway. In muscles, glycogenolysis is immediately followed by glycolysis.
5. Gluconeogenesis: Glucose is synthesised from non-carbohydrates by this pathway.
6. Uronic acid pathway: Glucuronic acid is synthesised from glucose in this pathway.

GLYCOLYSIS

Glycolysis or Embden-Meyerhof pathway is the main pathway for oxidation of glucose. Enzymes of this pathway are present in cytosol of nearly all the cells. Oxidation of one molecule of glucose produces two molecules of pyruvate or lactate.

In aerobic conditions, i.e. when the supply of oxygen is adequate, the end product of glycolysis is pyruvate. During

	Location	Specificity	Energy dependence	Insulin dependence
		Table 10.1: Salient features of glucose transporters		
SGLT 1	Luminal side of enterocytes and renal tubular cells	Glucose and galactose	Yes	No
GLUT 1	Erythrocytes	Glucose	No	No
GLUT 2	Contraluminal side of enterocytes, liver and renal tubular cells	Glucose, galactose and fructose	No	No
GLUT 3	Brain	Glucose	No	No
GLUT 4	Adipocytes, muscles and myocardium	Glucose	No	Yes*
GLUT 5	Luminal side of enterocytes and liver	Fructose	No	No

* Insulin causes translocation of GLUT 4 from the cytosol to the cell membrane.

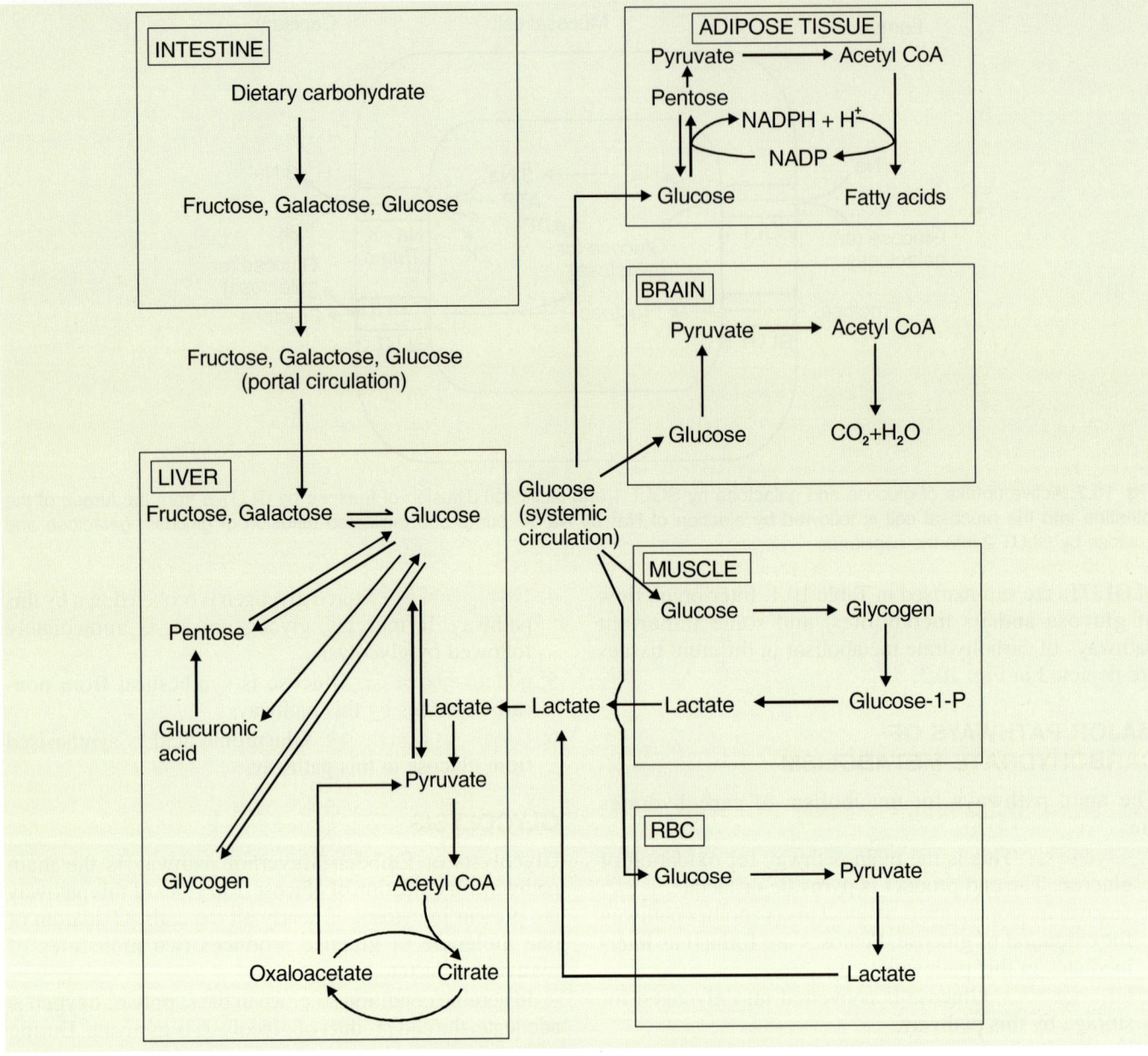

Fig. 10.3: Inter-organ flow and major pathways of carbohydrate metabolism in different tissues

the conversion of glucose into pyruvate, one molecule of NAD is reduced per molecule of pyruvate formed. The reduced NAD is reoxidised in the respiratory chain by molecular oxygen. Thus, a continuous supply of NAD is assured for continuation of glycolysis. However, the reduced NAD cannot be reoxidised under anaerobic conditions due to lack of oxygen. When all the available NAD is reduced, glycolysis will stop. To prevent this, pyruvate is reduced to lactate. This reaction is coupled with oxidation of NADH to NAD. Thus, conversion of pyruvate into lactate under anaerobic conditions ensures a steady supply of NAD so that glycolysis can continue. When the conditions become aerobic again, lactate is oxidised to pyruvate which is either converted into glucose

or is oxidised in the citric acid cycle after its conversion into acetyl CoA. The glycolytic reactions may be divided into three phases:

1. Priming or preparatory phase,
2. Splitting phase, and
3. Oxidative phase.

In the priming phase, glucose is prepared for splitting and oxidation by its conversion into fructose 1,6-biphosphate at the expense of two high-energy bonds of ATP. In the splitting phase, fructose-1,6-biphosphate is cleaved into two triose phosphates, glyceraldehyde-3-phosphate and dihydroxyacetone phosphate. Dihydroxy-acetone phosphate is isomerised to glyceraldehyde-3-phosphate. Thus, two molecules of glyceraldehyde-3-

phosphate are formed from each molecule of fructose-1,6-biphosphate. In the oxidative phase, each molecule of glyceraldehyde-3-phosphate is oxidised to pyruvate liberating energy. During anaerobic conditions, the product of glycolysis is lactate which is formed by reduction of pyruvate.

The reactions of the priming phase are as follows:

a. Glucose is phosphorylated to glucose-6-phosphate by hexokinase or glucokinase. The phosphate group is provided by ATP. As some free energy is liberated during this reaction, the reaction is functionally irreversible.

Hexokinase is a widely distributed enzyme. It can phosphorylate all hexoses, and has a low Km. It can act even when the intracellular concentration of glucose is low as during fasting condition. It is subject to allosteric regulation.

Glucokinase is an inducible enzyme present only in liver and β-cells in the islets of Langerhans. It is induced by insulin in liver and by glucose in the β-cells. It can act only on glucose, and has a high Km. It acts only when the intracellular glucose concentration is high as after a meal.

Conversion of glucose into glucose-6-phosphate is important for two reasons. Firstly, after glucose has been converted into glucose-6-phosphate, it cannot leave the cell as glucose transporters can transport only free glucose and not glucose-6-phosphate. Secondly, glucose enters most of the metabolic pathways, e.g. glycolysis, hexose monophosphate shunt, glycogenesis, uronic acid pathway, etc. in the form of glucose-6-phosphate.

Glycolysis can begin with glycogen also. Glycogenolysis results in the liberation of glucose-1-phosphate which can be isomerised to glucose-6-phosphate by phosphoglucomutase. This would conserve one high-energy phosphate bond required for the conversion of glucose into glucose-6-phosphate.

b. Glucose-6-phosphate is isomerised to fructose-6-phosphate by phosphohexose isomerase.

c. Fructose-6-phosphate is phosphorylated to fructose-1,6-biphosphate. The phosphate group is provided by ATP. This reaction is catalysed by phosphofructokinase-1 (PFK-1). The reaction is functionally irreversible due to release of free energy. The reactions of the priming phase are depicted in Fig.10.4.

The second phase begins now in which fructose-6-phosphate is converted into two molecules of glyceraldehyde-3-phosphate.

a. In the first reaction of this phase, aldolase splits fructose-1,6-biphosphate into two triose phosphates which are glyceraldehyde-3-phosphate and dihydroxyacetone phosphate.

b. In the next reaction, dihydroxyacetone phosphate is isomerised to glyceraldehyde-3-phosphate by phosphotriose isomerase.

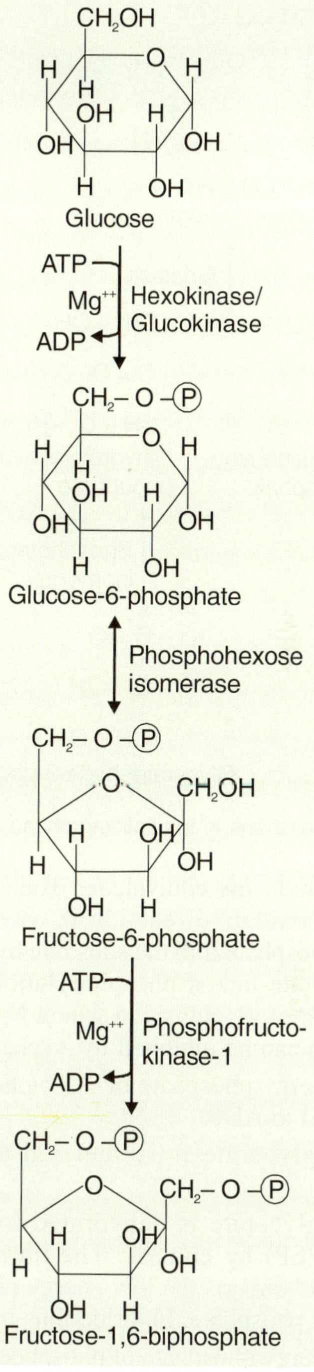

Fig. 10.4: Reactions in the priming phase of glycolysis

Thus, two molecules of glyceraldehyde-3-phosphate are formed from one molecule of glucose. The reactions are shown in Fig.10.5.

The third phase of glycolysis, the oxidation phase, begins now in which glyceraldehyde-3-phosphate is oxidised to pyruvate. The reactions are shown in Fig.10.6.

a. Glyceraldehyde-3-phosphate dehydrogenase oxidises glyceraldehyde-3-phosphate, NAD acting as the

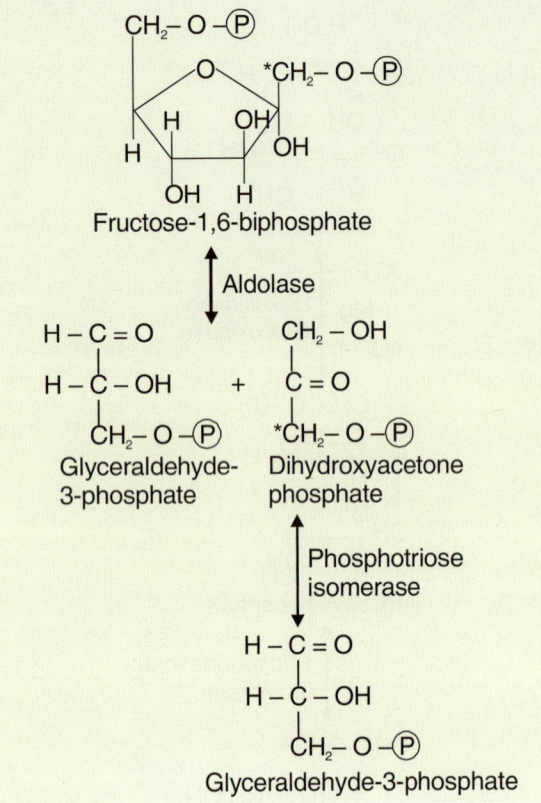

Fig. 10.5: Reactions in the splitting phase of glycolysis

acceptor of reducing equivalents. The energy released during this oxidative reaction is used to introduce inorganic phosphate into the substrate by a high-energy bond (substrate-linked phosphorylation). This is the only reaction of glycolysis in which NAD is reduced. The reaction can be inhibited by arsenate.

b. The high-energy phosphate of 1,3-biphosphoglycerate is transferred to ADP.

c. 3-Phosphoglycerate is isomerised to 2-phosphoglycerate.

d. 2-Phosphoglycerate is dehydrated to phosphoenol pyruvate (PEP) by enolase. The intramolecular re-arrangement converts the low-energy phosphate into a high-energy phosphate. Fluoride ions inhibit enolase.

e. The high-energy phosphate of phosphoenol pyruvate is transferred to ADP. The reaction is functionally irreversible.

Pyruvate is the end product of aerobic glycolysis. It is converted into acetyl CoA which is oxidised in the citric acid cycle.

f. A further reaction occurs in anaerobic conditions. Pyruvate is reduced to lactate and NADH is oxidised to NAD which is required for the oxidation of glyceraldehyde-3-phosphate.

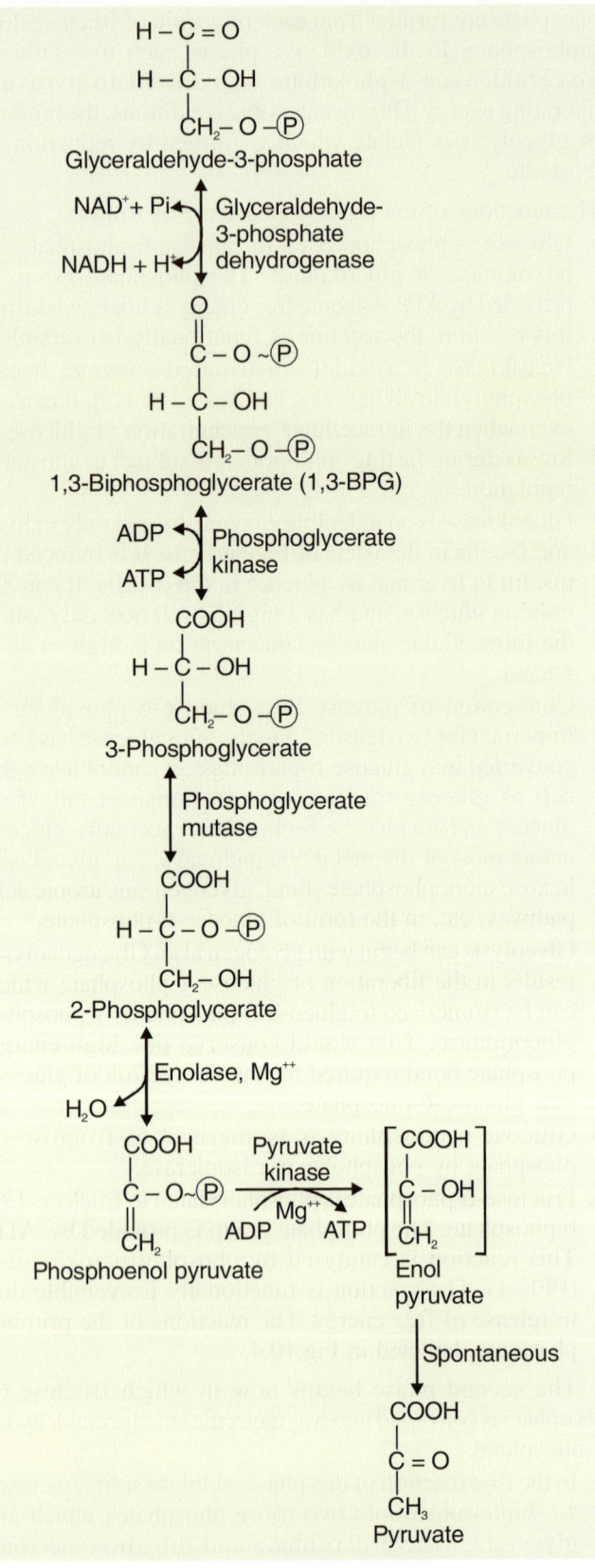

Fig. 10.6: Reactions in the oxidative phase of aerobic glycolysis

$$
\begin{array}{c}
\text{COOH} \\
| \\
\text{C} = \text{O} \\
| \\
\text{CH}_3 \\
\text{Pyruvate}
\end{array}
$$

NADH + H⁺

Lactate
dehydrogenase

NAD⁺

$$
\begin{array}{c}
\text{COOH} \\
| \\
\text{HO} - \text{C} - \text{H} \\
| \\
\text{CH}_3 \\
\text{L-Lactate}
\end{array}
$$

Anaerobic glycolysis occurs in muscles during exercise when oxygen utilisation outstrips the supply. It also occurs in cells lacking mitochondria, e.g. erythrocytes, corneal cells and lens cells. When the conditions become aerobic again, lactate is converted into pyruvate again, and can be oxidised as described earlier in citric acid cycle (Fig. 10.7).

In erythrocytes, an alternate intermediate of glycolysis, 2,3-biphosphoglycerate (2,3-BPG), is also formed from 1,3-biphosphoglycerate. 2,3-Biphosphoglycerate has an important function in RBCs because it helps in the release of oxygen from oxyhaemoglobin. No ATP is formed when 2,3-biphosphoglycerate is converted into 3-phosphoglycerate (Fig.10.8).

Energetics

When one molecule of glucose is oxidised in the glycolytic pathway, two high-energy phosphate bonds of ATP are utilised. One high-energy phosphate bond is used to convert glucose into glucose-6-phosphate and another to convert fructose-6-phosphate into fructose-1,6-biphosphate.

Two molecules of glyceraldehyde-3-phosphate are formed from one molecule of fructose-1,6-biphosphate. Oxidation of glyceraldehyde-3-phosphate to 1,3-biphosphoglycerate reduces one NAD molecule to NADH which will form three ATP equivalents on oxidation in the respiratory chain. One ADP is phosphorylated to ATP when 1,3-biphosphoglycerate is converted into 3 phosphoglycerate, and another when phosphoenol pyruvate is converted into pyruvate. Thus, five ATP equivalents are formed from oxidation of one molecule of glyceraldehyde-3-phosphate to pyruvate, and ten from the oxidation of two molecules. When we subtract the initial utilisation of two ATP equivalents in the priming phase, the net gain of energy is eight ATP equivalents from each molecule of glucose oxidised to pyruvate by aerobic glycolysis.

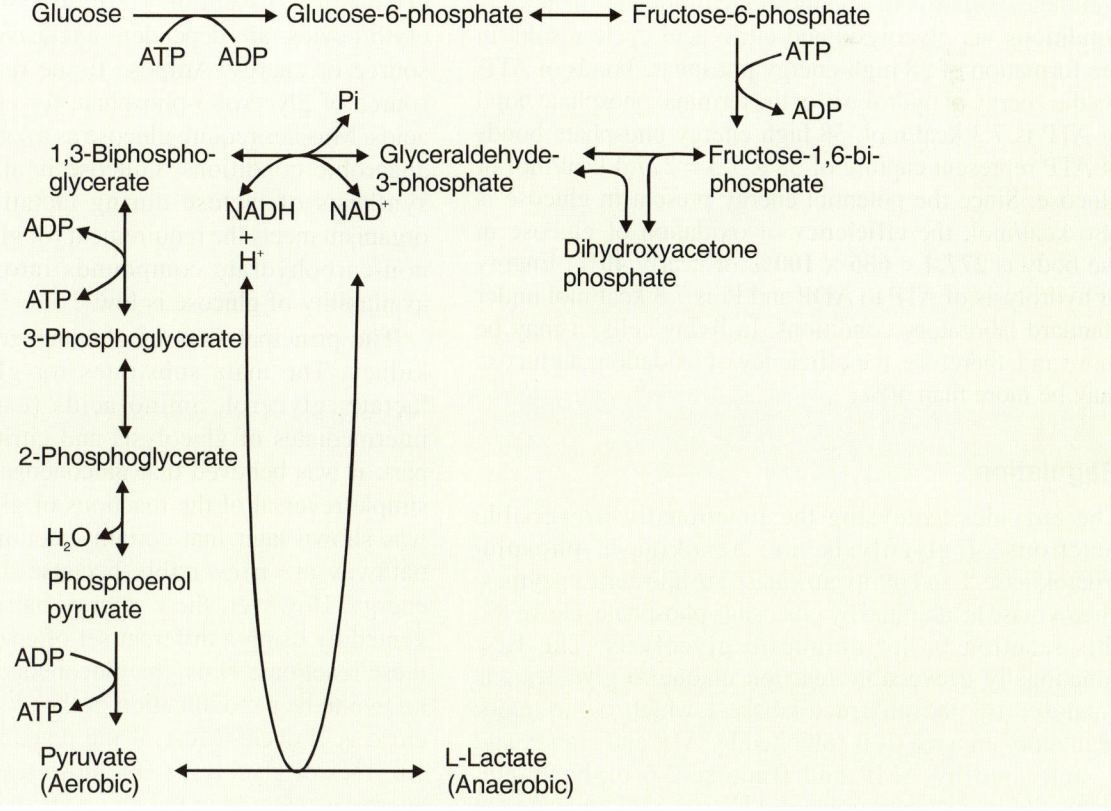

Fig. 10.7: An outline of glycolysis

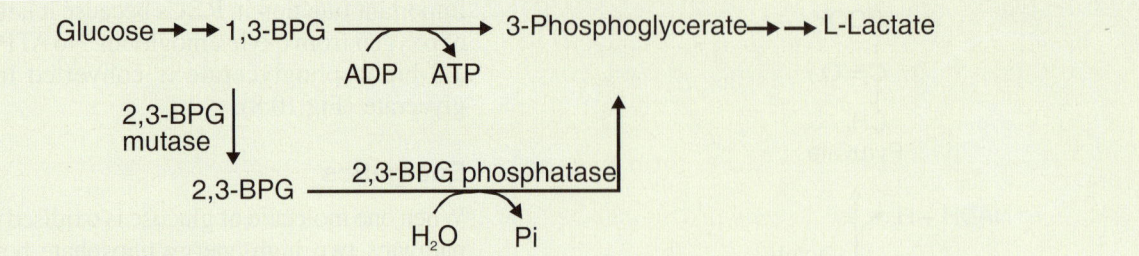

Fig. 10.8: 2,3-Biphosphoglycerate (BPG) shunt (Rapaport-Leubering cycle) in erythrocytes

NADH cannot be oxidised in the respiratory chain in the absence of oxygen. Therefore, the energy which could be captured from oxidation of NADH in the respiratory chain would not be captured in anaerobic conditions. Instead, oxidation of NADH to NAD is coupled with reduction of pyruvate to lactate in anaerobic conditions. Therefore, the net gain of energy is only two ATP equivalents when one molecule of glucose is converted into lactate by anaerobic glycolysis.

In aerobic conditions, further oxidation of each pyruvate molecule to acetyl CoA and oxidation of acetyl CoA to carbon dioxide and water in citric acid cycle and respiratory chain will form 15 ATP equivalents. Thus, eight ATP equivalents are formed from oxidation of one molecule of glucose to two molecules of pyruvate, and 30 ATP equivalents are formed from oxidation of two molecules of pyruvate to carbon dioxide and water. So, complete oxidation of one molecule of glucose in aerobic conditions via glycolysis and citric acid cycle results in the formation of 38 high-energy phosphate bonds of ATP. As the energy of hydrolysis of the terminal phosphate bond of ATP is 7.3 kcal/mol, 38 high-energy phosphate bonds of ATP represent capture of $38 \times 7.3 = 277.4$ kcal/mol of glucose. Since the potential energy present in glucose is 686 kcal/mol, the **efficiency** of oxidation of glucose in the body is $\mathbf{277.4 \div 686 \times 100\%}$ or nearly **40%**. Energy of hydrolysis of ATP to ADP and Pi is 7.3 kcal/mol under standard laboratory conditions. In living cells, it may be more and, therefore, the efficiency of oxidation of glucose may be more than 40%.

Regulation

The enzymes catalysing the functionally irreversible reactions of glycolysis, i.e. hexokinase, phospho fructokinase-1 and pyruvate kinase are allosteric enzymes. Hexokinase is inhibited by glucose-6-phosphate. However, this reaction is not unique to glycolysis. The first functionally irreversible reaction unique to glycolysis is catalysed by phosphofructokinase-1 which is the major regulatory enzyme. It is inhibited by ATP and citrate, and is activated by AMP and fructose-2,6-biphosphate. Intracellular concentrations of ATP and AMP indicate the energy status of the cell. Abundance of energy indicated by a high ATP concentration decreases glycolysis. Lack of energy indicated by a high AMP concentration increases glycolysis.

Pyruvate kinase is inhibited by ATP and alanine, and is activated by fructose-1,6-biphosphate. Glucokinase, in liver, is induced by insulin. It is activated by fructose-1-phosphate and inhibited by fructose-6-phosphate.

GLUCONEOGENESIS

Synthesis of glucose from non-carbohydrate sources is termed as gluconeogenesis. Gluconeogenesis occurs mainly when the availability of dietary carbohydrates is low, as during fasting or when carbohydrates cannot be metabolised, e.g. in diabetes mellitus. Though the energy requirements of the organism can be met by lipids, provision of a certain amount of carbohydrate to the organism is essential. Certain tissues, e.g. brain and erythrocytes, are dependent exclusively on glucose as a source of energy. Adipose tissue requires glucose as a source of glycerol-3-phosphate for esterification of fatty acids. Muscles require glucose as a source of energy under anaerobic conditions. Glucose is also required for the synthesis of lactose during lactation. Therefore, the organism meets the requirement for glucose by converting non-carbohydrate compounds into glucose when the availability of glucose is low.

The principal sites of gluconeogenesis are liver and kidney. The main substrates for gluconeogenesis are lactate, glycerol, amino acids (except leucine), and intermediates of glycolysis and citric acid cycle. In the past, it was believed that gluconeogenesis occurred by a simple reversal of the reactions of glycolytic pathway. It was shown later that certain reactions of the glycolytic pathway are irreversible because of liberation of free energy. However, these energy barriers can be circumvented by using a different set of enzymes for catalysing these reactions. Thus, the gluconeogenic pathway is now known to be a modification of the glycolytic pathway and citric acid cycle. Most of the reactions are catalysed by enzymes of glycolysis. But those reactions in which free energy is released in the glycolytic pathway are catalysed by different enzymes.

Energy Barriers

Free energy is released in the following reactions of the glycolytic pathway which constitute energy barriers:

1. Conversion of glucose into glucose-6-phosphate.
2. Conversion of fructose-6-phosphate into fructose-1,6-biphosphate.
3. Conversion of phosphoenol pyruvate into pyruvate.

Bypassing Energy Barriers

The irreversible glycolytic reactions are catalysed by the following enzymes in the gluconeogenic pathway:

1. Conversion of glucose-6-phosphate into glucose is catalysed by **glucose-6-phosphatase**.
2. Conversion of fructose-1,6-biphosphate into fructose-6-phosphate is catalysed by **fructose-1,6-biphosphatase**.
3. Conversion of pyruvate into phosphoenol pyruvate takes place through two reactions. First, pyruvate enters the mitochondria and is converted into oxaloacetate by **pyruvate carboxylase**. Oxaloacetate comes out of mitochondria with the help of the malate shuttle. It is converted into phosphoenol pyruvate by **phosphoenol pyruvate (PEP) carboxykinase**. The phosphate group is provided by GTP (Fig. 10.9).

These four enzymes are the **key enzymes** of gluconeogenesis (or gluconeogenic enzymes).

The substrates for gluconeogenesis enter the pathway at different stages. Glycerol is converted into dihydroxyacetone phosphate which can gluconeogenesis (Fig. 10.10). Lactate is a major substrate for gluconeogenesis and is used via Cori cycle.

Cori Cycle

Anaerobic glycolysis in muscles results in the production of lactate which cannot be converted into glucose, as gluconeogenesis does not occur in muscles. Lactate is released into circulation. It is taken up by liver, and is converted into glucose by gluconeogenesis. Glucose can be transported again to muscles (Fig. 10.11). Similarly, pyruvate formed in muscles can be used via glucose alanine cycle.

Glucose-alanine Cycle

Pyruvate formed in muscles by aerobic glycolysis is transported to liver after its transamination to alanine. This

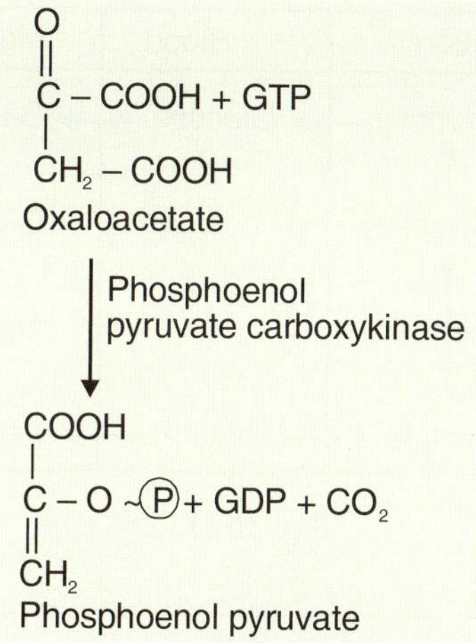

Fig. 10.9: Synthesis of phosphoenolpyruvate

not only transports pyruvate but also transports the α-amino groups of amino acids to liver which is the major site for urea synthesis. In liver, alanine transfers its amino group to α-ketoglutarate. Alanine is converted into pyruvate, and α-ketoglutarate is converted into glutamate. Amino group of glutamate is used to synthesise urea. Pyruvate is converted into glucose by gluconeogenesis which is released into circulation and can go back to liver (Fig. 10.12).

The sequence of reactions leading to the synthesis of glucose from pyruvate and the role of gluconeogenic enzymes are shown in Fig. 10.13.

Intermediates of glycolysis enter the pathway directly at the stages where they are formed. Intermediates of citric acid cycle are converted into oxaloacetate which is a substrate for gluconeogenesis. Gluconeogenic amino acids are converted into pyruvate or various intermediates of citric acid cycle (Fig. 10.14).

Regulation

Regulation of gluconeogenesis is **long-term** as well as **short-term**. Long-term regulation occurs through **induction** and **repression**. Synthesis of the key enzymes of gluconeogenesis, i.e. pyruvate carboxylase, PEP carboxykinase, fructose-1,6-biphosphatase and glucose-6-phosphatase is induced by **glucocorticoids** and is repressed by **insulin**.

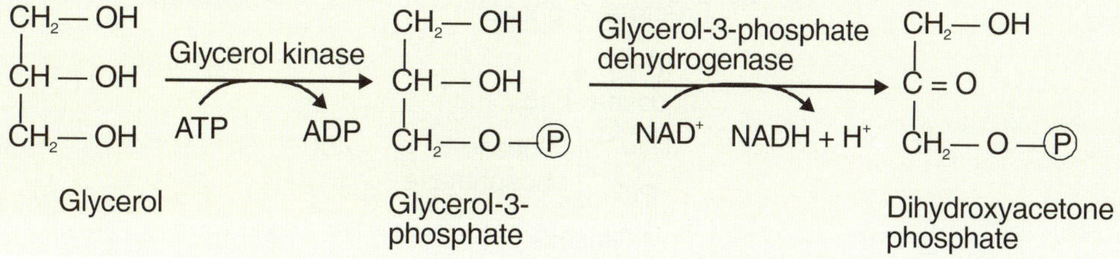

Fig. 10.10: Glycerol can enter gluconeogenesis via dihydroxyacetone phosphate

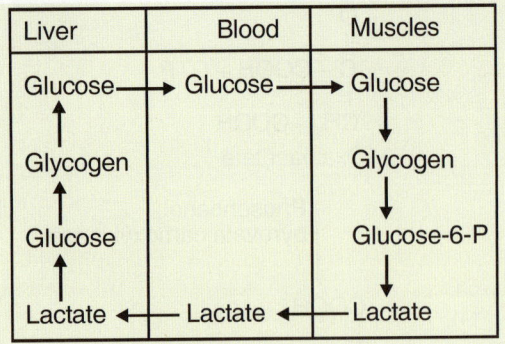

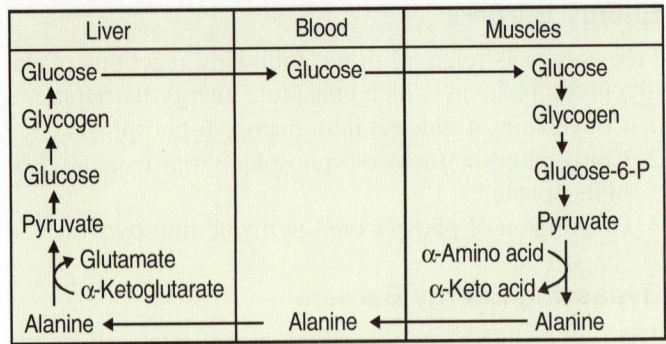

Fig. 10.11: Cori cycle   **Fig. 10.12:** Glucose-alanine cycle

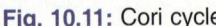

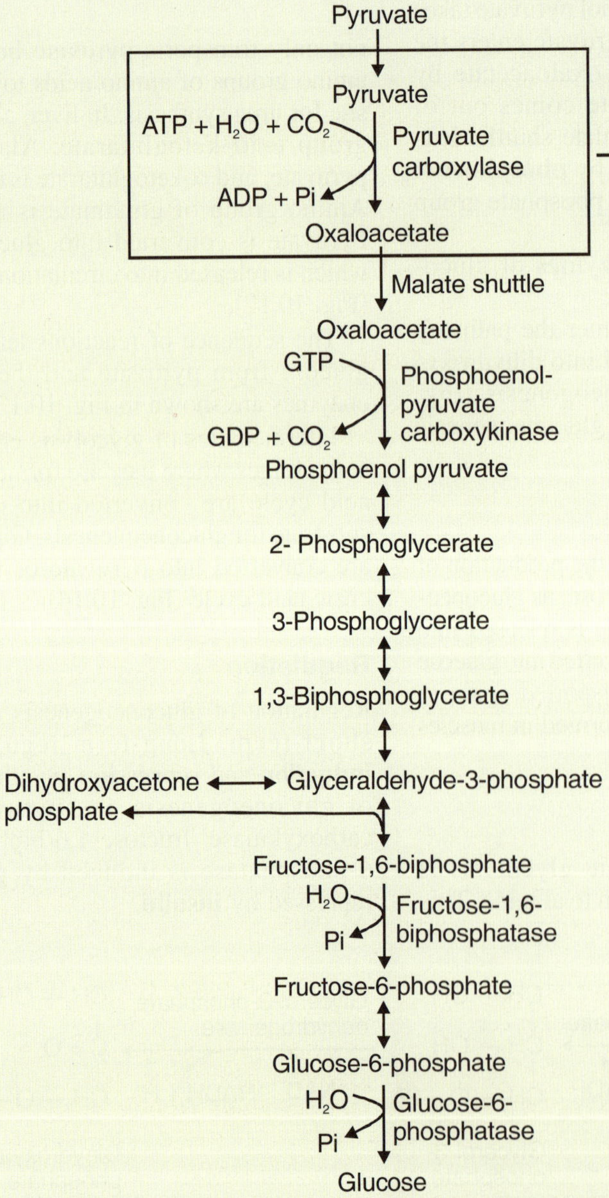

Fig. 10.13: Synthesis of glucose from pyruvate

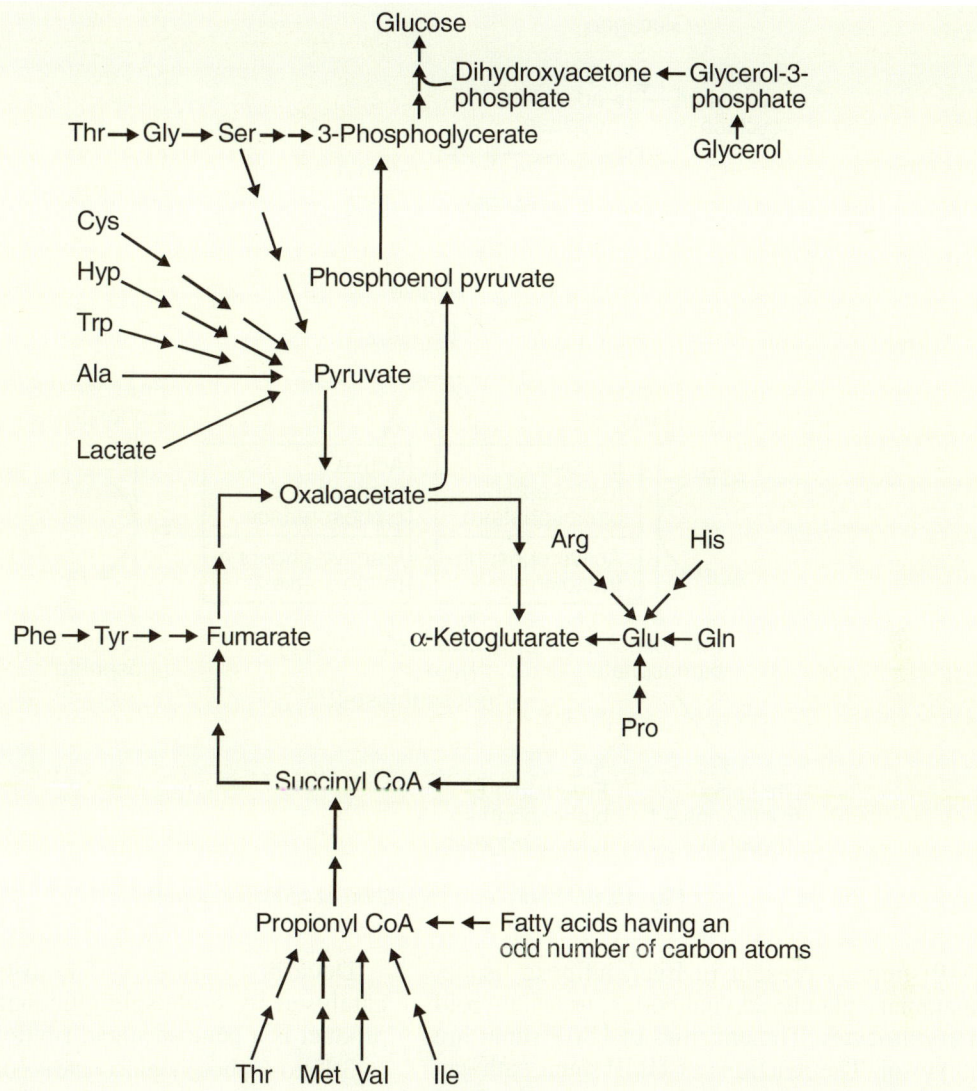

Fig. 10.14: Points of entry of different substrates in the gluconeogenic pathway

Short-term regulation occurs by **covalent modification** and **allosteric mechanism**, and the major regulator is **glucagon** which regulates the phosphorylation of a **bifunctional** enzyme possessing fructose-2,6-biphosphatase and phosphofructokinase-2 activities.

When glucagon is not being secreted, as after a meal, phosphofructokinase-2 is active converting fructose-6-phosphate into fructose-2,6-biphosphate which increases glycolysis by activating phosphofructokinase-1, and decreases gluconeogenesis by inhibiting fructose-1,6-biphosphatase. The reverse occurs after secretion of glucagon. Short-term regulation of gluconeogenesis and glycolysis is **reciprocal** (Fig. 10.15).

HEXOSE MONOPHOSPHATE SHUNT (HMP SHUNT)

This is another pathway for oxidation of glucose. It is also known as pentose phosphate pathway, phosphogluconate oxidative pathway or direct oxidative pathway. Oxidation of glucose occurs in the absence of oxygen. The reducing equivalents are taken up by NADP. Unlike reduced NAD, reduced NADP cannot be oxidised in the respiratory chain. It is used mainly for reductive synthesis, i.e. synthetic reactions in which reducing equivalents are required. Decarboxylation of the hexose monophosphate produces a pentose monophosphate, ribulose-5-phosphate which can be isomerised to ribose-5-phosphate. Deoxyribose can be formed from ribose. Thus, HMP shunt provides ribose and deoxyribose for the synthesis of nucleic acids.

Unutilised ribulose-5-phosphate can be reconverted into glucose-6-phosphate. When six molecules of glucose-6-phosphate are oxidised in the HMP shunt, six molecules of CO_2 are formed, 12 molecules of NADP are reduced, and six molecules of pentose phosphate are produced. The six pentose phosphate molecules can be rearranged to form five molecules of glucose-6-phosphate.

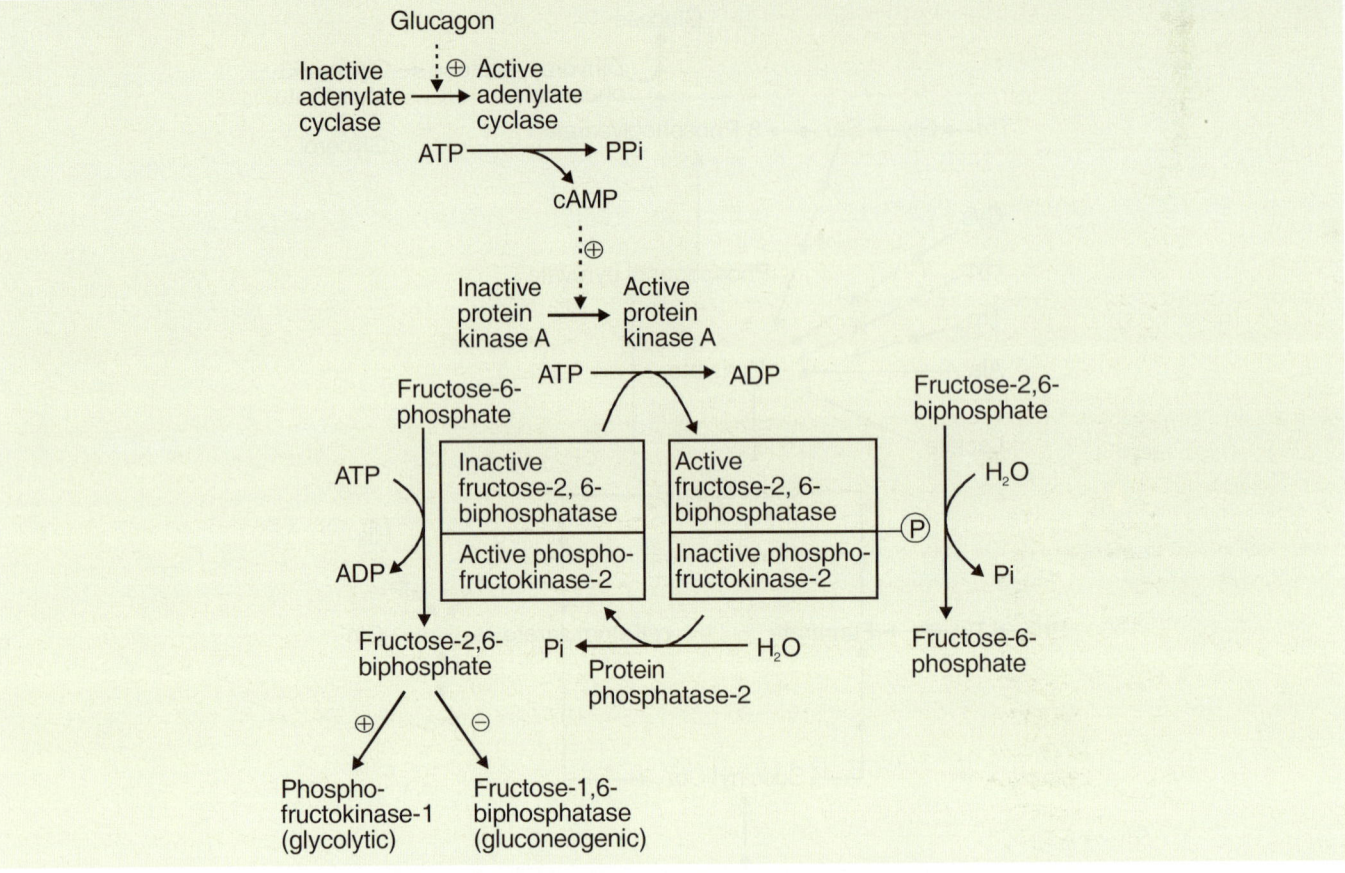

Fig. 10.15: Short-term regulation of gluconeogenesis

The HMP shunt is present in liver, adipose tissue, lactating mammary glands, adrenal cortex, testes, thyroid gland and erythrocytes. The enzymes of HMP shunt are present in cytosol. The reactions of HMP shunt pathway may be divided into three phases: (i) oxidation of hexose monophosphate, (ii) decarboxylation and (iii) regeneration of hexose monophosphate (the second and third phase may also be collectively called as the non-oxidative phase).

In the first phase, two pairs of reducing equivalents are removed from glucose-6-phosphate forming 3-keto-6-phosphogluconate (Fig. 10.16). The reactions are as follows:

a. Glucose-6-phosphate is reduced to 6-phosphogluconolactone by glucose-6-phosphate dehydrogenase (G6PD) and Mg^{++} or Ca^{++}. The reducing equivalents are accepted by NADP. G6PD is inhibited by some drugs, e.g. sulphonamides and quinacrine.

b. Gluconolactone hydrolase adds a molecule of water to 6-phosphogluconolactone to convert it into a straight chain phosphorylated derivative of gluconate, 6-phosphogluconate. The enzyme requires a divalent cation, e.g. Mg^{++} or Mn^{++} or Ca^{++} as a cofactor.

c. Two reducing equivalents are removed from 6-phosphogluconate and are transferred to NADP by 6-phosphogluconate dehydrogenase. This enzyme also requires Mg^{++} or Mn^{++} or Ca^{++} as a cofactor.

Decarboxylation of 3-keto-6-phosphogluconate is catalysed by 6-phosphogluconate dehydrogenase. The product is a pentose sugar, ribulose-5-phosphate.

3-Keto-6-phosphogluconate is only a transient intermediate in the conversion of 6-phosphogluconate into ribulose-5-phosphate. Some of the ribulose-5-phosphate molecules are isomerised to ribose-5-phosphate. The reaction is catalysed by ribose-5-phosphate ketoisomerase. Some ribulose-5-phosphate molecules are epimerised by ribulose-5-phosphate epimerase to xylulose-5-phosphate (Fig. 10.17).

The third phase begins now. In this phase, unutilised ribulose-5-phosphate is reconverted into glucose-6-phosphate. One molecule of ribose-5-phosphate and two molecules of xylulose-5-phosphate, formed from three molecules of ribulose-5-phosphate, react with each other to form two molecules of fructose-6-phosphate and one molecule of glyceraldehyde-3-phosphate. The reactions occur as follows and are shown in Fig. 10.18.

a. Transketolase transfers a 2-carbon glycolaldehyde moiety from xylulose-5-phosphate to ribose-5-phosphate in the presence of thiamin pyrophosphate and Mg^{++} to form sedoheptulose-7-phosphate and glyceraldehyde-3-phosphate.

b. A 3-carbon dihydroxyacetone moiety is transferred from sedoheptulose-7-phosphate to glyceraldehyde-3-

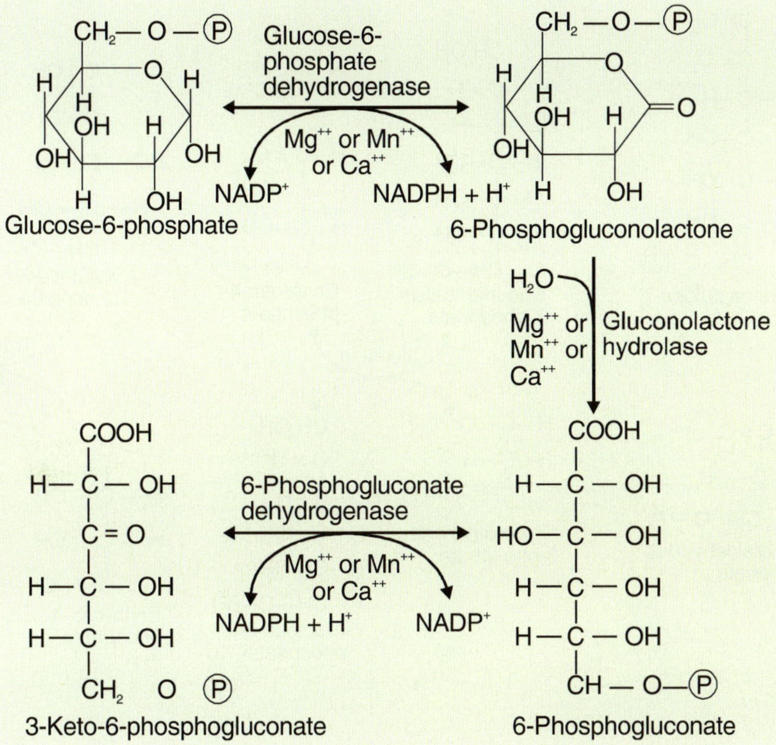

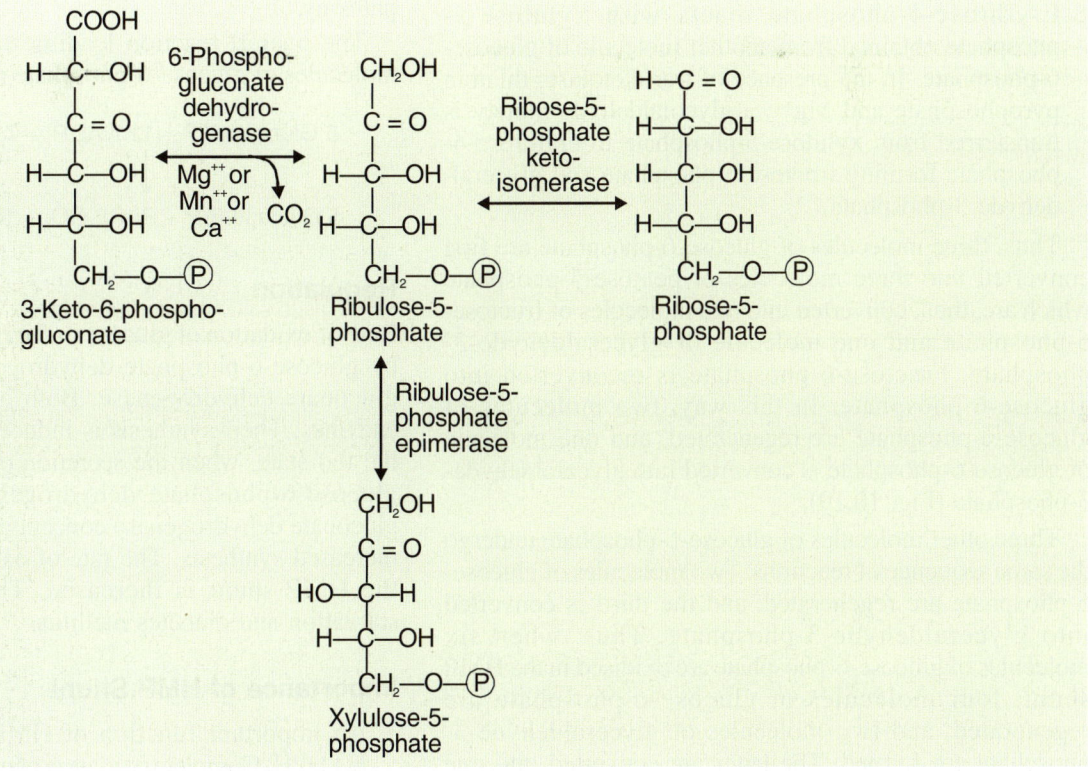

Fig. 10.16: Oxidative phase of hexose monophosphate shunt

Fig. 10.17: Decarboxylation of 3-keto-6-phosphogluconate and isomerisation of ribulose-5-phosphate to ribose-5-phosphate and xylulose-5-phosphate

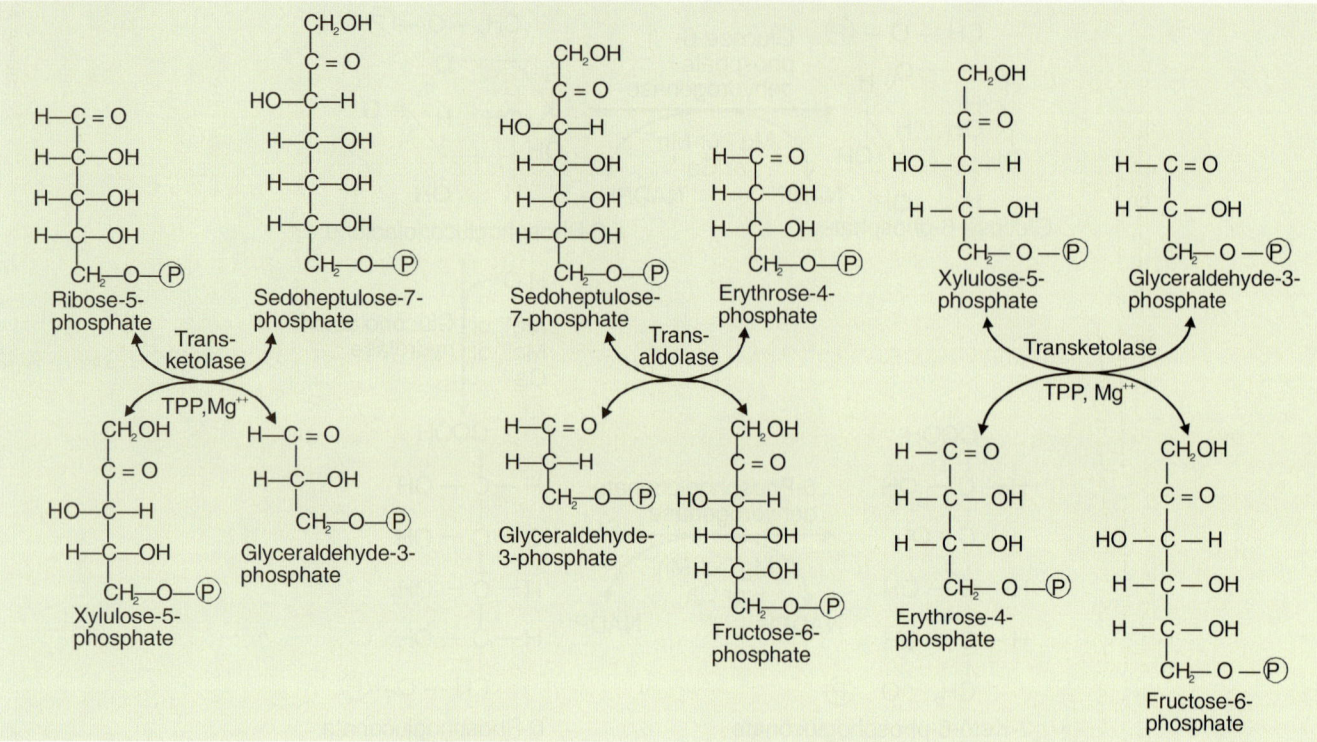

Fig. 10.18: Three molecules of pentose phosphate are converted into two molecules of hexose phosphate and one molecule of triose phosphate

phosphate to form fructose-6-phosphate and erythrose-4-phosphate. This reaction is catalysed by transaldolase.

c. Erythrose-4-phosphate reacts with xylulose-5-phosphate obtained from another molecule of glucose-6-phosphate. In the presence of transketolase, thiamin pyrophosphate and Mg++, a glycolaldehyde moiety is transferred from xylulose-5-phosphate to erythrose-4-phosphate forming fructose-6-phosphate and glyceraldehyde-3-phosphate.

Thus, three molecules of glucose-6-phosphate are first converted into three molecules of pentose-5-phosphate which are, then, converted into two molecules of fructose-6-phosphate and one molecule of glyceraldehyde-3-phosphate. Fructose-6-phosphate is reconverted into glucose-6-phosphate. In this way, two molecules of glucose-6-phosphate are regenerated, and one molecule of glucose-6-phosphate is converted into glyceraldehyde-3-phosphate (Fig. 10.19).

Three other molecules of glucose-6-phosphate undergo the same sequence of reactions. Two molecules of glucose-6-phosphate are regenerated, and the third is converted into glyceraldehyde-3-phosphate. Thus, when six molecules of glucose-6-phosphate are oxidised in the HMP shunt, four molecules of glucose-6-phosphate are regenerated, and two molecules of glyceraldehyde-3-phosphate are formed. The latter are converted into one molecule of glucose-6-phosphate (Fig. 10.20). Conversion of fructose-1,6-biphosphate into fructose-6-phosphate is

catalysed by fructose-1,6-biphosphatase. The other reactions are catalysed by the enzymes of glycolytic pathway.

The overall reaction leading to the oxidation of six molecules of glucose-6-phosphate may be summed up as:

$$6 \text{ Glucose-6-P} + 12 \text{ NADP}^+ + 7 \text{ H}_2\text{O}$$
$$\downarrow$$
$$5 \text{ Glucose-6-P} + \text{Pi} + 6 \text{ CO}_2 + 12 \text{ NADPH} + 12 \text{ H}^+$$

Regulation

Rate of oxidation of glucose in the HMP shunt is regulated by glucose-6-phosphate dehydrogenase and 6-phosphogluconate dehydrogenase. Both of these are inducible enzymes. Their synthesis is induced by insulin. Thus, in the fed state, when the secretion of insulin is increased, glucose-6-phosphate dehydrogenase and 6-phosphogluconate dehydrogenase concentrations are raised due to increased synthesis. The rate of oxidation of glucose via the HMP shunt is increased. The reverse occurs in starvation and diabetes mellitus.

Importance of HMP Shunt

1. An important function of HMP shunt is to provide NADPH. Complete oxidation of one molecule of glucose in HMP shunt produces 12 molecules of NADPH. These are used mainly for the synthesis of fatty acids and, to a

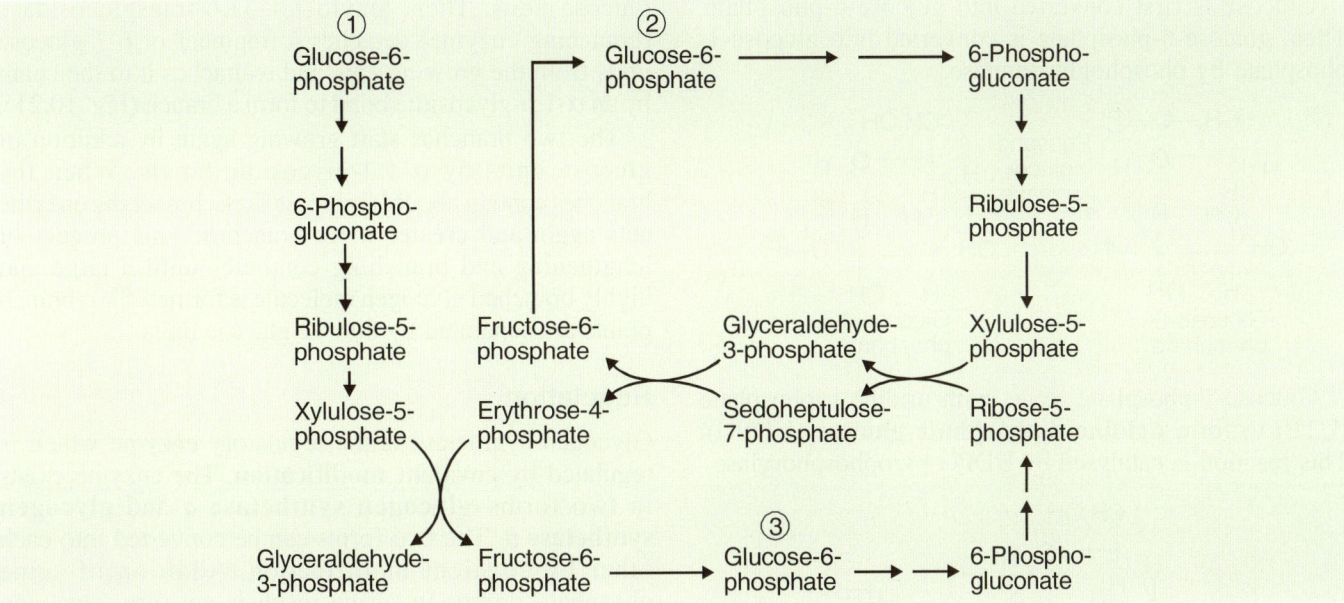

Fig. 10.19: Out of three molecules of glucose-6-phosphate entering the hexose monophosphate shunt, two are regenerated and one is converted into glyceraldehyde-3-phosphate

smaller extent, for the synthesis of cholesterol, steroid hormones, some amino acids, nucleotides, etc. HMP shunt is highly active in tissues synthesising these compounds.

2. Production of NADPH in erythrocytes is necessary to restore the level of reduced glutathione which is oxidised while detoxifying hydrogen peroxide and free radicals. This prevents premature destruction of erythrocytes.

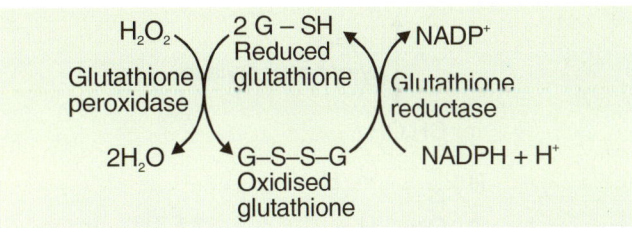

In hereditary glucose-6-phosphate dehydrogenase deficiency, haemolysis occurs due to decreased production of NADPH, specially on administration of drugs like quinacrine and primaquin which generate free radicals in erythrocytes.

3. Ribose-5-phosphate, an intermediate of HMP shunt, is used for synthesising nucleotides and nucleic acids.

GLYCOGENESIS

Synthesis of glycogen is known as glycogenesis. Glycogenesis is a mechanism by which excess glucose can be stored in the tissues, to be utilised when the supply of glucose is scarce. Glycogenesis occurs in almost all the tissues, but the predominant sites for storage of glycogen are liver and muscles. After a meal rich in carbohydrate, glycogenesis occurs rapidly in liver and muscles. The glycogen content of liver may go up to 5% and that of muscles up to 1% of wet tissue weight. Glycogenesis occurs in the cytosol.

Glycogen is a macromolecule made up of a large number of glucose units. Glycogenesis begins with a small glycogen molecule known as a **glycogen primer**. The core of the primer is made up of a protein, **glycogenin** to which a glucose molecule is attached via a tyrosine residue. Successive glucose units are added to the primer until a large glycogen molecule is formed.

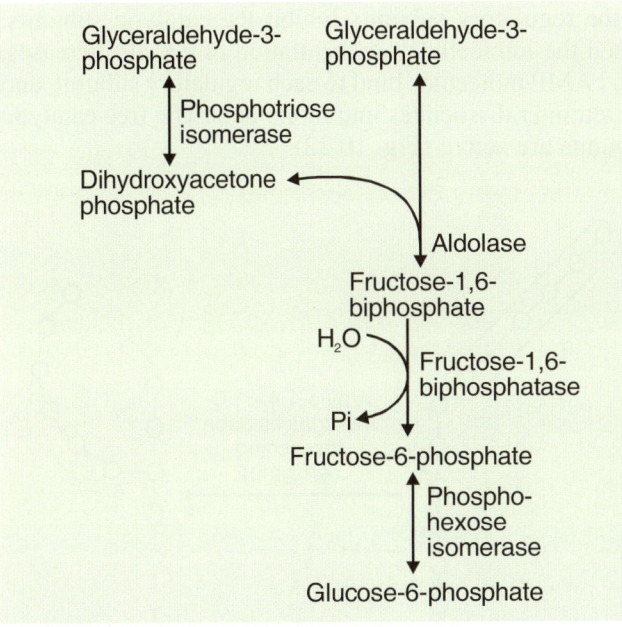

Fig. 10.20: Two molecules of glyceraldehyde-3-phosphate are converted into one molecule of glucose-6-phosphate

Glucose is first converted into glucose-6-phosphate. Then, glucose-6-phosphate is converted into glucose-1-phosphate by phosphoglucomutase.

CH₂—O—(P) → Phospho-gluco-mutase → CH₂OH

Glucose-6-phosphate   Glucose-1-phosphate

Glucose-1-phosphate reacts with uridine triphosphate (UTP) to form **uridine diphosphate glucose** (UDPG). This reaction is catalysed by UDPG pyrophosphorylase.

CH₂OH ... Glucose-1-phosphate   + UTP

↕ UDPG pyrophosphorylase

CH₂OH ... UDPG   + PPi

Inorganic pyrophosphate is hydrolysed into inorganic phosphate. As free energy is released, the reaction is functionally irreversible.

$$PPi + H_2O \xrightarrow{\text{Inorganic pyrophosphatase}} 2\,Pi$$

UDPG reacts with glycogen primer. UDP is released and glucose is added to the glycogen primer. Thus, if the glycogen primer had **n** glucose units before the reaction, it would have **n + 1** glucose units after the reaction. C_1 of the new glucose unit forms a glycosidic bond with C_4 of the last glucose unit on the non-reducing end of the glycogen primer. The reaction is catalysed by **glycogen synthetase**.

$$UDPG + (Glucose)_n$$
↓ Glycogen synthetase
$$UDP + (Glucose)_{n+1}$$

This process of addition of glucose units to the glycogen primer continues until the chain contains about eleven glucose units. Then, amylo-1,4→1,6-transglucosidase (branching enzyme) detaches a fragment of 6-7 glucose units from the growing end, and reattaches it to the chain by an α-1,6-glycosidic bond to form a branch (Fig. 10.21).

The two branches start growing again by addition of glucose units by α-1,4-glycosidic bonds. When the branches contain about 11 glucose units, branching enzyme acts again and creates more branches. This process of lengthening and branching continues until a large and highly branched glycogen molecule is formed. Two branch points are separated by 8 to 12 glucose units.

Regulation

Glycogen synthetase is the regulatory enzyme which is regulated by **covalent modification**. The enzyme exists in two forms–**glycogen synthetase a** and **glycogen synthetase b**. The two forms can be converted into each other by covalent modification. Addition of some phosphate groups to serine residues converts glycogen synthetase a into glycogen synthetase b. Removal of the phosphate groups converts glycogen synthetase b into glycogen synthetase a. The dephosphorylated glycogen synthetase a is the active form of the enzyme. The phosphorylated glycogen synthetase b is the inactive form.

Phosphorylation of glycogen synthetase a is catalysed by **cAMP-dependent protein kinase (protein kinase A)**. Dephosphorylation of glycogen synthetase b is catalysed by **protein phosphatase-1**. The relative activities of protein kinase A and protein phosphatase-1 determine the amount of active glycogen synthetase in a cell.

Protein kinase A is a tetramer made up of two identical **regulatory (R) subunits** and two identical **catalytic (C) subunits**. The tetrameric form of the enzyme is inactive as the regulatory subunits inhibit the catalytic subunits. When the intracellular concentration of cAMP increases, two cAMP molecules bind to each regulatory subunit, and the tetramer dissociates into monomers. The free catalytic subunits are active (Fig. 10.22).

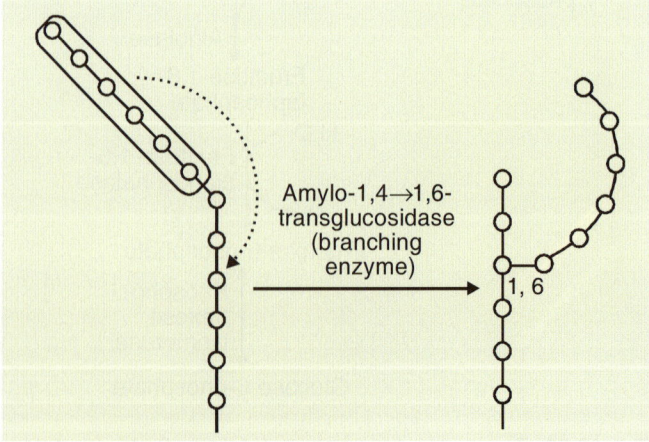

Amylo-1,4→1,6-transglucosidase (branching enzyme)

1, 6

Fig. 10.21: Creation of a branch in glycogen

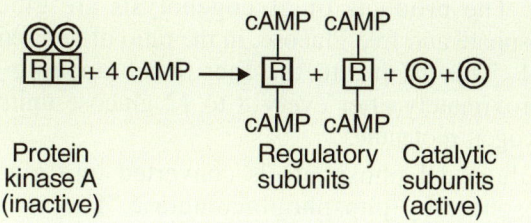

Fig. 10.22: Activation of protein kinase A

Active protein kinase A phosphorylates the active glycogen synthetase *a* to convert it into inactive glycogen synthetase *b*. It also phosphorylates a protein known as **inhibitor-1**.

The phosphorylated form of inhibitor-1 inhibits protein phosphatase-1 thereby inhibiting the conversion of glycogen synthetase *b* into glycogen synthetase *a*. Thus, active protein kinase A increases the conversion of active glycogen synthetase into its inactive form and, at the same time, decreases the conversion of inactive glycogen synthetase into active glycogen synthetase. The net result is a decrease in the rate of glycogenesis. The reverse occurs when the concentration of cAMP is low. The rate of glycogenesis is increased. Thus, the rate of glycogenesis is regulated by the intracellular concentration of cAMP.

Since the intracellular concentration of cAMP in muscles and liver is governed by the hormones, **epinephrine, glucagon** and **insulin**, the ultimate regulators of glycogenesis are these three hormones. Epinephrine and glucagon, which increase the concentration of cAMP, decrease the rate of glycogenesis. Insulin, which decreases the concentration of cAMP, increases the rate of glycogenesis. In muscles, the rate of glycogenesis is regulated mainly by epinephrine and insulin, and in liver by glucagon and insulin (Fig. 10.23).

GLYCOGENOLYSIS

Breakdown of glycogen is known as glycogenolysis. Glycogenolysis is not a reversal of glycogenesis but is a separate pathway having its own enzymes. Glycogenolysis occurs in all the tissues in which glycogen is stored. The major sites of glycogenolysis are liver and muscles in which large amounts of glycogen are stored. The main purpose of hepatic glycogenolysis is to maintain the blood glucose concentration within the normal range. When blood glucose level decreases, glycogenolysis occurs in liver. Glucose is released into circulation, and blood glucose level is restored. In muscles, glycogenolysis occurs mainly to provide energy for muscle contraction.

The key enzyme responsible for glycogenolysis is **phosphorylase** (glycogen phosphorylase) which catalyses the phosphorolytic removal of glucose (as glucose-1-phosphate) from glycogen. This enzyme hydrolyses the terminal **α-1,4-glycosidic bonds** at the non-reducing ends of the glycogen molecule. Presence of a large number of branches in the glycogen molecule facilitates rapid glycogenolysis as the terminal glucose units on all the branches can be split off simultaneously. The energy present in the glycosidic bond is conserved by incorporating a phosphate group into the liberated glucose molecule.

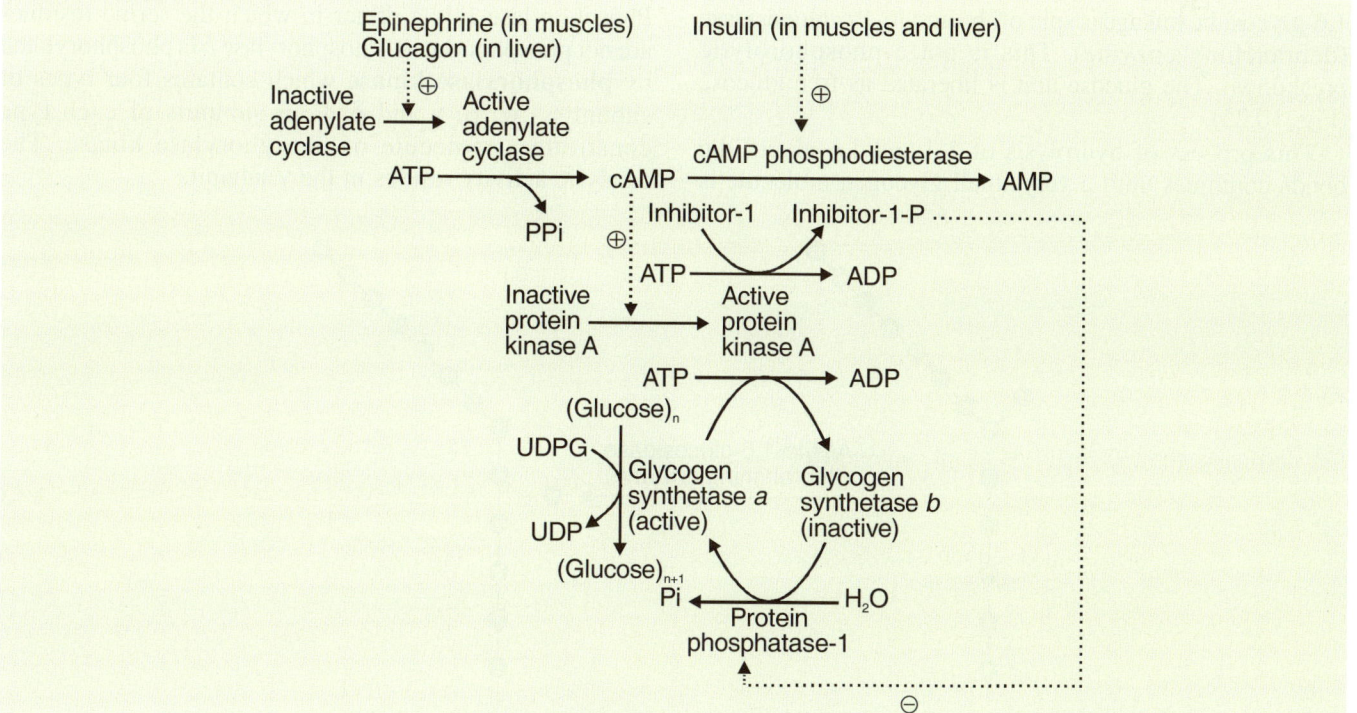

Fig. 10.23: Regulation of glycogenesis

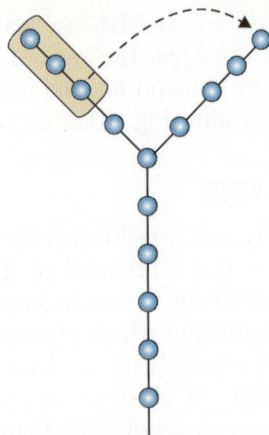

Fig. 10.24: Transfer of a trisaccharide unit from one branch to another

$$(Glucose)_n + Pi$$
$$\downarrow \text{Phosphorylase}$$
$$(Glucose)_{n-1} + \text{Glucose-1-phosphate}$$

This process of stepwise removal of glucose units from each branch continues until only four glucose units are left distal to the branch points. The molecule so formed is known as limit dextrin. After the formation of limit dextrin, oligo-(α-1,4$\rightarrow$$\alpha$-1,4)-glucan transferase transfers a trisaccharide from one branch to another so that one branch has now got seven glucose units distal to the branch point and the other has got only one glucose unit linked to the main chain by α-1,6-glycosidic bond.

The single glucose unit attached to the main chain by 1,6-glycosidic linkage is split off by amylo-1,6-glucosidase (debranching enzyme). This is not a phosphorolytic breakdown. The glucose unit is liberated as free glucose (Fig. 10.25).

This process of hydrolysis of 1,4-and 1,6-glycosidic bonds continues until a very small glycogen molecule is left. The products of glycogenolysis are glucose-1-phosphate and free glucose, in the ratio of approximately 10:1. This is due to the fact that branching occurs approximately after every 8 to 12 glucose units in the glycogen molecule.

Glucose-1-phosphate is converted into glucose-6-phosphate by phosphoglucomutase. The reaction is reversible as described earlier. Many tissues, with the notable exception of muscle, possess glucose-6-phosphatase which splits off inorganic phosphate from glucose-6-phosphate and liberates free glucose.

Thus, the end product of glycogenolysis is glucose in most tissues, e.g. liver, kidney, intestine, etc. In muscle, the major end product is glucose-6-phosphate. Since glycogenolysis occurs in muscles only when energy is required for muscle contraction, glucose-6-phosphate directly enters the glycolytic pathway, and is broken down to lactate as the conditions during muscle contraction are usually anaerobic.

Regulation

The regulatory enzyme is phosphorylase. It occurs in two forms–**phosphorylase *a*** (phosphophosphorylase) and **phosphorylase *b*** (dephosphophosphorylase). Phosphorylase *a* is the active form of the enzyme while phosphorylase *b* is inactive. The liver and muscle enzymes are slightly different from each other. In muscle, phosphorylase *a* is a dimer, made up of two identical subunits. Each subunit contains one molecule of pyridoxal phosphate. Each subunit has got a serine residue which is phosphorylated. Phosphorylase *b* is a dimer in which the serine residues are not phosphorylated. Phosphorylase *b* is phosphorylated by **phosphorylase kinase** which contains four types of subunits - α, β, γ and δ. Four subunits of each type constitute a molecule of phosphorylase kinase. The catalytic activity resides in the γ subunit.

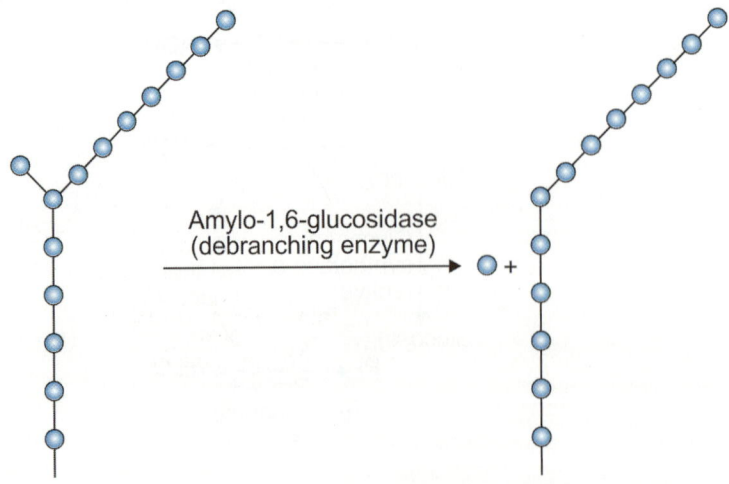

Fig. 10.25: Removal of the glucose unit linked by α-1,6-glycosidic bond

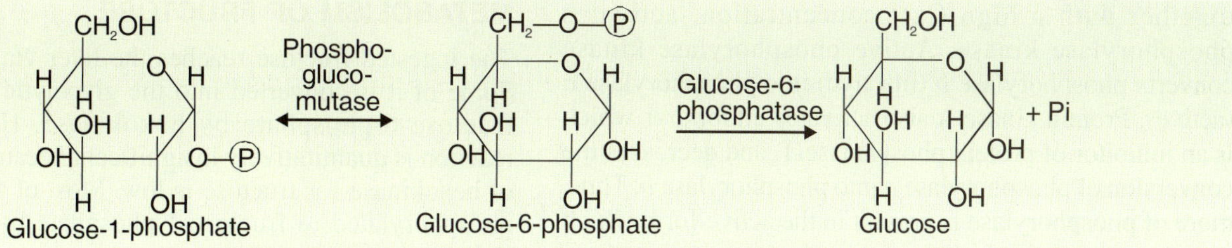

Glucose-1-phosphate — Phosphogluco-mutase ⟷ **Glucose-6-phosphate** — Glucose-6-phosphatase → **Glucose** + Pi

Fig. 10.26: Conversion of glucose-1-phosphate into glucose

Phosphorylase kinase can exist in an inactive form (phosphorylase kinase b) and an active form (phosphorylase kinase a). In the inactive form, the α and β subunits are not phosphorylated, and δ subunits lack Ca^{++}. When Ca^{++} concentration increases in muscles, four calcium ions are bound to each δ subunit, and the enzyme becomes partially active. The Ca^{++}– bound δ subunit is identical to troponin C and calmodulin. Calmodulin is a ubiquitous calcium modulating protein. Increase in cAMP concentration activates **protein kinase A**. Active protein kinase A phosphorylates α and β subunits which makes the enzyme

fully active. This protein kinase is the same which phosphorylates glycogen synthetase a and inhibitor-1.

Active phosphorylase kinase phosphorylates phosphorylase b, and converts it into active phosphorylase a. Phosphorylase a is dephosphorylated to phosphorylase b by protein phosphatase-1, the same enzyme which dephosphorylates glycogen synthetase b.

Binding of **epinephrine** to specific receptors on the cell membrane of muscles activates adenylate cyclase. Intracellular concentration of cAMP increases which activates protein kinase A. Active protein kinase A,

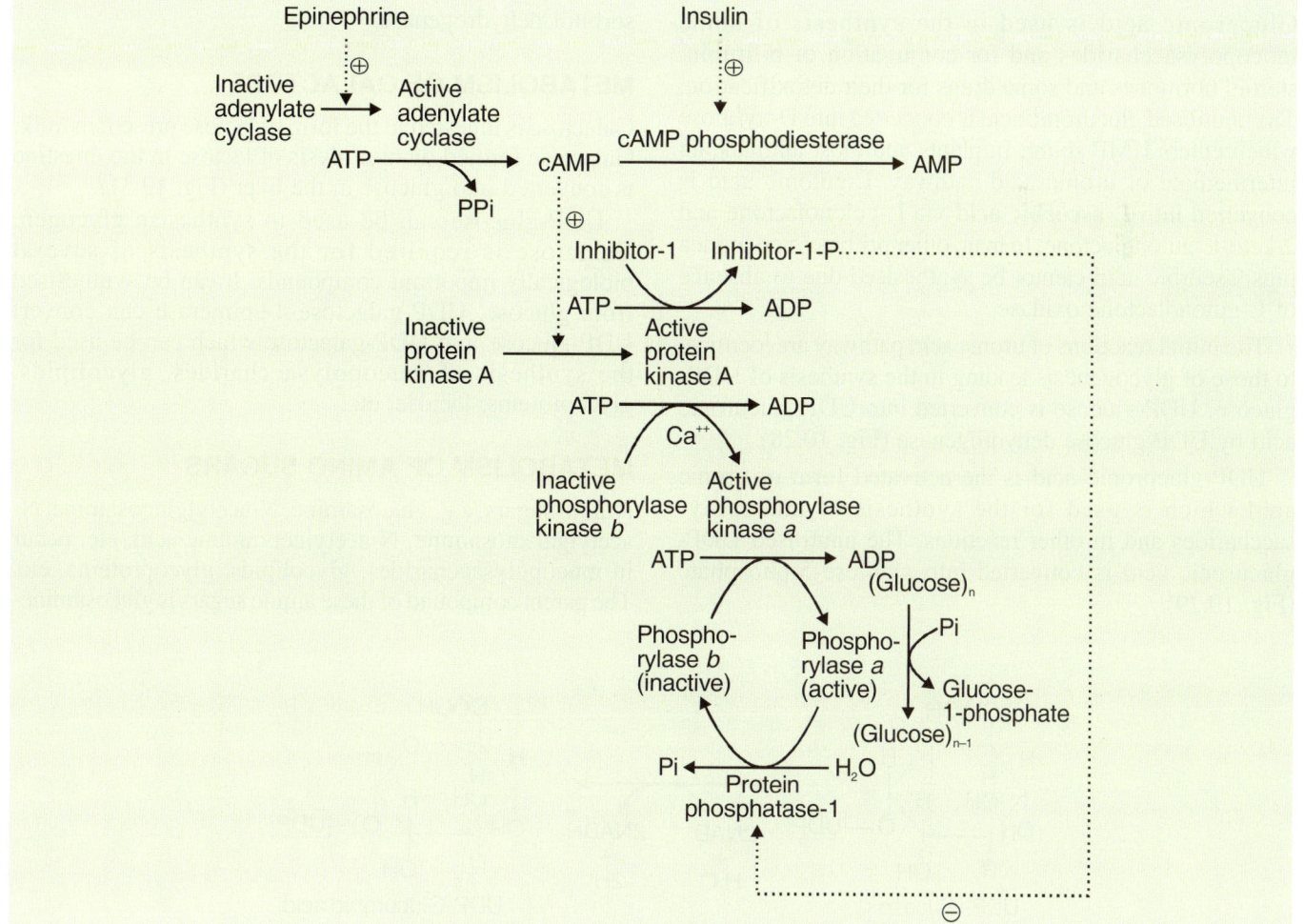

Fig. 10.27: Regulation of glycogenolysis in muscles

together with a high Ca^{++} concentration, activates phosphorylase kinase. Active phosphorylase kinase converts phosphorylase *b* (inactive) into phosphorylase *a* (active). Protein kinase A also activates inhibitor-1 which is an inhibitor of protein phosphatase-1, and decreases the conversion of phosphorylase *a* into phosphorylase *b*. Thus, more of phosphorylase is present in the active form which increases the rate of glycogenolysis. At the same time, there is a decrease in the rate of glycogenesis because the active protein kinase A converts active glycogen synthetase into its inactive form. The reverse occurs when **insulin** secretion is raised, as after a meal. There is a decrease in cAMP concentration. More of phosphorylase is present in inactive form, and more of glycogen synthetase in active form. Therefore, the rate of glycogenolysis is decreased, and the rate of glycogenesis is increased.

Hepatic glycogenolysis is regulated in a similar way but the main hormone increasing the rate of hepatic glycogenolysis is **glucagon**.

URONIC ACID PATHWAY

This pathway forms glucuronic acid from glucose. Glucuronic acid is used in the synthesis of some mucopolysaccharides and for conjugation of bilirubin, steroid hormones and some drugs for their detoxification. The unutilised glucuronic acid is converted into D-xylulose which enters HMP shunt. In plants and most animals, an intermediate of uronic acid pathway, L-gulonic acid is converted into **L-ascorbic acid** via L-gulonolactone and 2-keto-L-gulonolactone. In man, other primates and guinea pigs, ascorbic acid cannot be synthesised due to absence of L-gulonolactone oxidase.

The initial reactions of uronic acid pathway are identical to those of glycogenesis leading to the synthesis of UDP-glucose. UDP-glucose is converted into UDP-glucuronic acid by UDP-glucose dehydrogenase (Fig. 10.28).

UDP-glucuronic acid is the activated form of uronic acid which is used for the synthesis of mucopoly-saccharides and in other reactions. The unutilised UDP-glucuronic acid is converted into xylulose-5-phosphate (Fig. 10.29).

METABOLISM OF FRUCTOSE

The ingested fructose reaches the liver via portal blood. Some of it is converted into the glycolytic intermediate, fructose-6-phosphate by hexokinase. However, this reaction is quantitatively insignificant because the affinity of hexokinase for fructose is low. Most of the fructose is phosphorylated to fructose-1-phosphate by fructokinase in liver.

Fructose-1-phosphate can neither be converted into fructose-6-phosphate nor into fructose-1,6-biphosphate. It is split into glyceraldehyde and dihydroxyacetone phosphate by aldolase B present in liver. Glyceraldehyde is phosphorylated by triokinase (Fig. 10.30).

Glyceraldehyde-3-phosphate and dihydroxyacetone phosphate may be converted into glucose via the gluconeogenic pathway or may be oxidised via the glycolytic pathway.

Fructose is required as a source of energy by **spermatozoa**. Fructose is synthesised from glucose in **seminal vesicles**, and is secreted into seminal plasma. The highest concentration of fructose among biological fluids is found in seminal plasma. Fructose is synthesised from glucose by the sequential actions of aldose reductase and sorbitol dehydrogenase.

METABOLISM OF GALACTOSE

Galactose is ingested in the form of lactose present in milk. Galactose formed by hydrolysis of lactose in the intestine is converted into glucose in the liver (Fig. 10.31).

UDP-glucose can be used to synthesise glycogen. Galactose is required for the synthesis of several biologically important compounds. It can be synthesised from glucose. UDP-galactose-4-epimerase can convert UDP-glucose into UDP-galactose which can be used for the synthesis of mucopolysaccharides, glycolipids, glycoproteins, lactose, etc.

METABOLISM OF AMINO SUGARS

Amino sugars, e.g. glucosamine, N-acetylglucosamine, N-acetylgalactosamine, N-acetylneuraminic acid, etc. occur in mucopolysaccharides, glycolipids, glycoproteins, etc. The parent compound of these amino sugars is glucosamine-

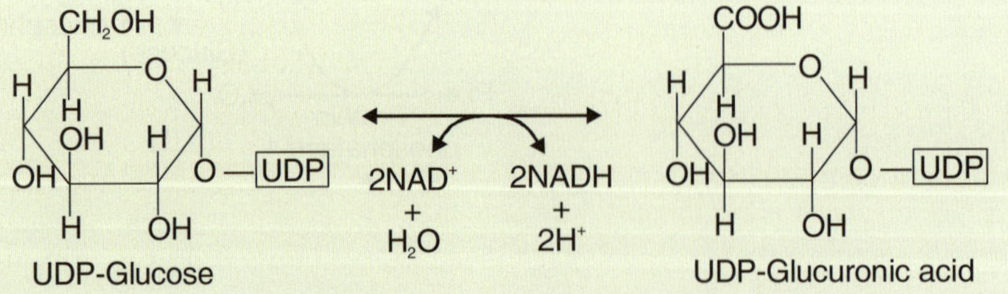

Fig. 10.28: Formation of UDP-glucuronic acid

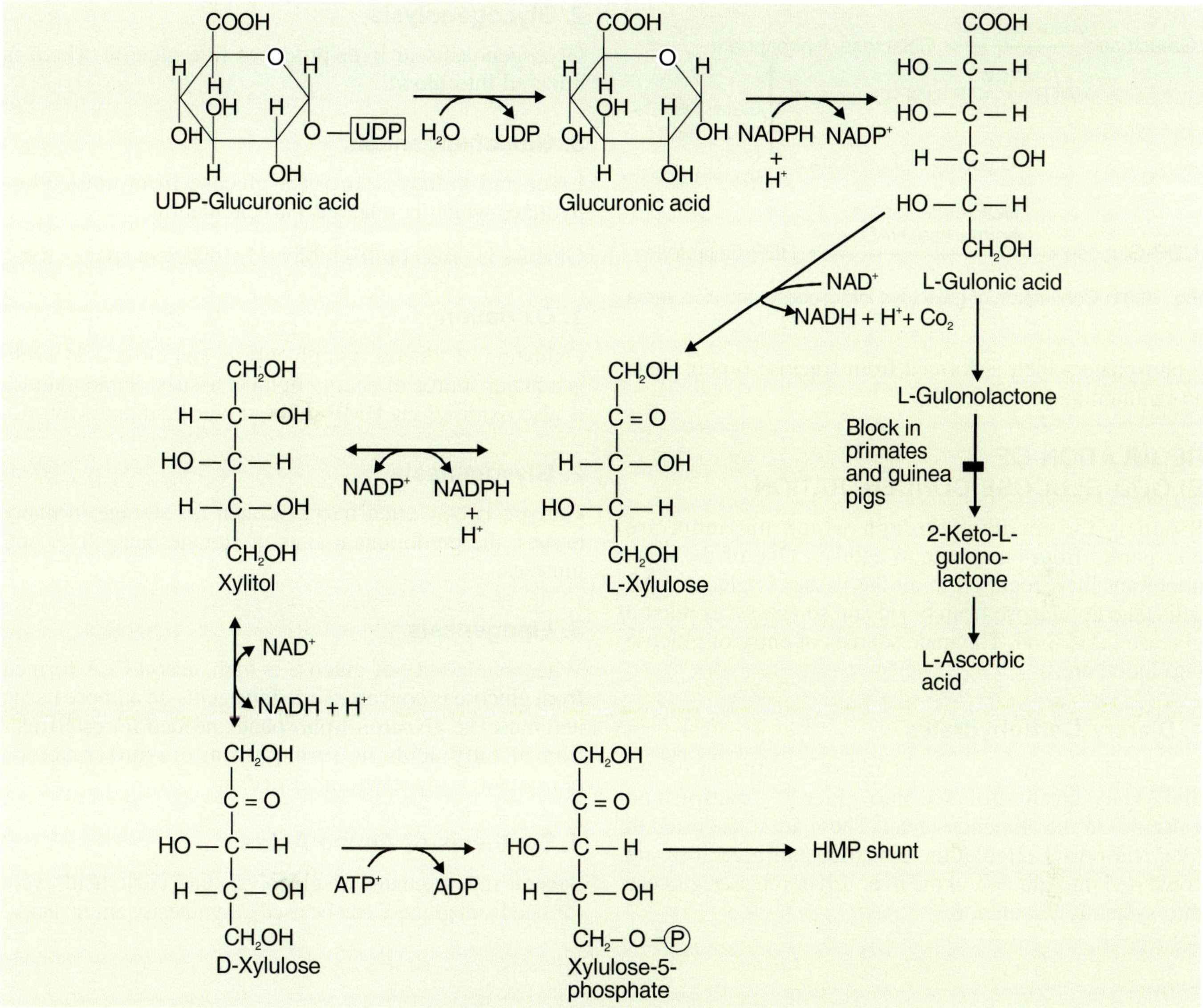

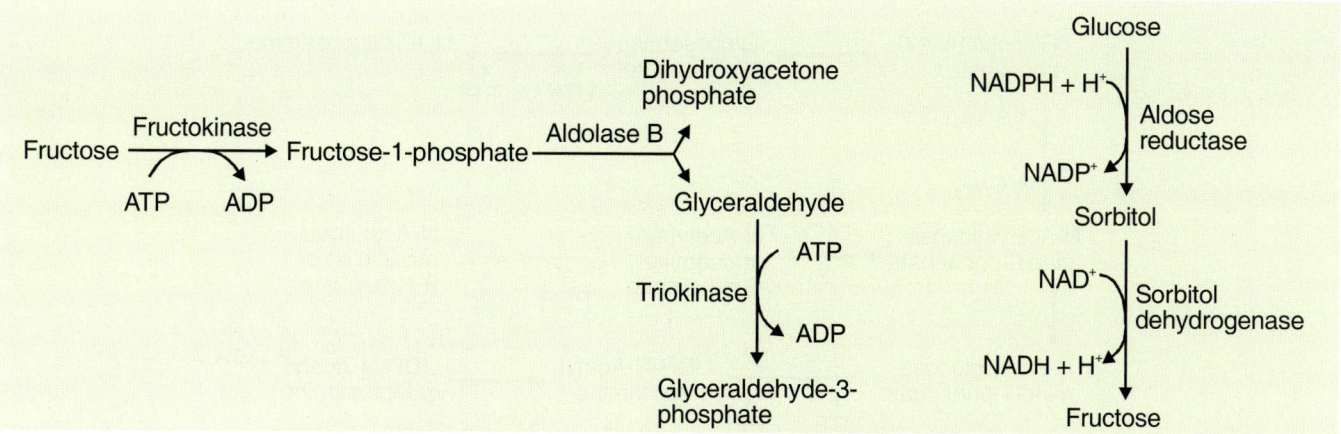

Fig. 10.29: Metabolism of UDP-glucuronic acid

Fig. 10.30: Catabolism of fructose (left) and synthesis (right)

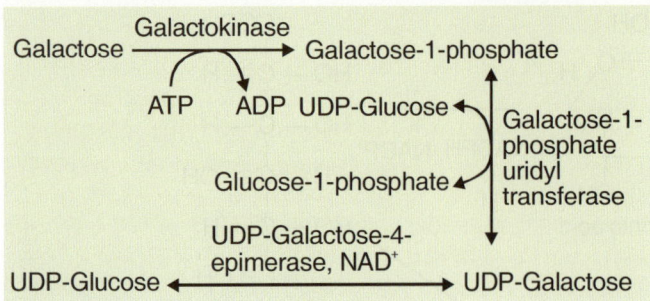

Fig. 10.31: Conversion of galactose into glucose and vice versa

6-phosphate which is formed from fructose-6-phosphate and glutamine (Fig. 10.32).

REGULATION OF BLOOD GLUCOSE CONCENTRATION

Blood is the medium through which nutrients are transported from one tissue to another. One of the most important fuels required in all the tissues is glucose. All cells take up glucose from blood and some tissues release glucose into blood. The main sources of entry of glucose into blood are:

1. Dietary Carbohydrates

Carbohydrates are the most abundant constituent of our diet. They are hydrolysed into glucose, fructose and galactose in the alimentary tract. These are transported to liver via portal circulation. Fructose and galactose are converted into glucose in the liver. Liver releases glucose into systemic circulation.

2. Glycogenolysis

Glycogenolysis in liver produces free glucose which is released into blood.

3. Gluconeogenesis

Liver and kidneys can form glucose from non-carbohydrates which is released into circulation.

Glucose is taken up from blood by different tissues for:

1. Oxidation

Oxidation of glucose via glycolysis and citric acid cycle is a major source of energy in most tissues. Some glucose is also oxidised via HMP shunt, uronic acid pathway, etc.

2. Glycogenesis

Glucose is converted into glycogen for storage in many tissues, the predominant sites of storage being liver and muscles.

3. Lipogenesis

When availability of glucose is high, acetyl CoA formed from glucose is converted into fatty acids. In adipose tissue and muscles, glycerol-3-phosphate, needed for esterification of fatty acids, is formed from dihydroxyacetone phosphate, a glycolytic intermediate.

4. Synthesis of Amino Acids

Several intermediates of glycolysis and citric acid cycle formed from glucose can be used to synthesise amino acids.

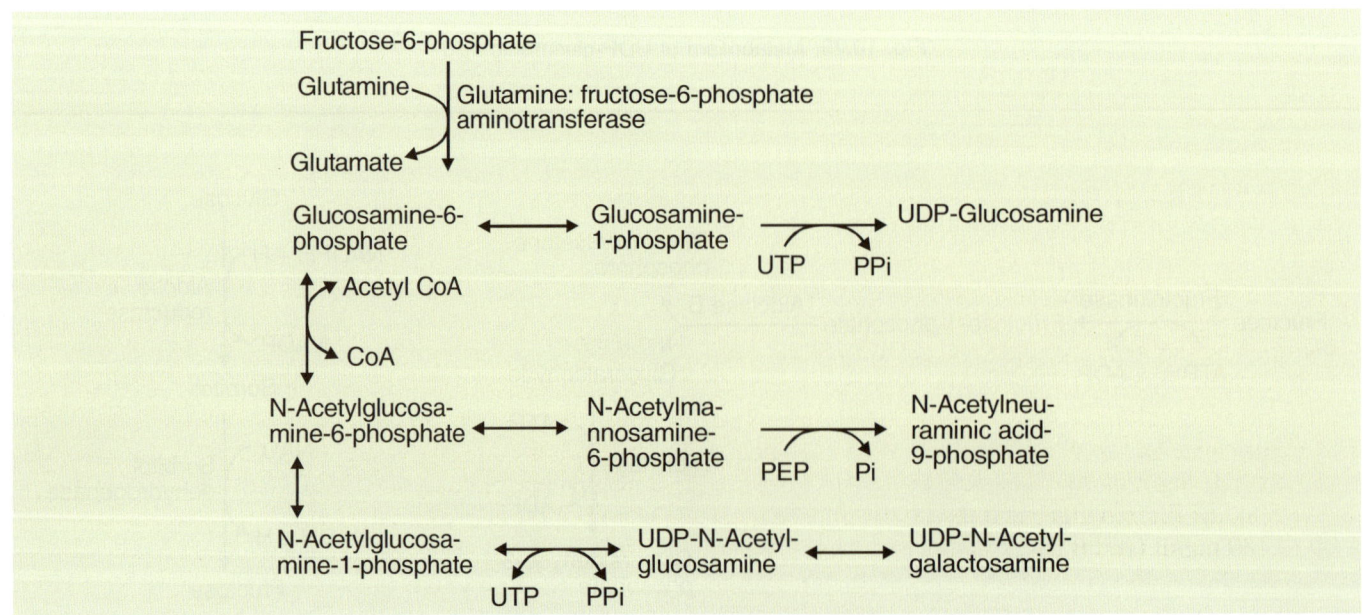

Fig. 10.32: Synthesis of amino sugars

5. Synthesis of Other Compounds

Several other compounds, e.g. lactose, ribose, muco-polysaccharides, glycolipids, glycoproteins, etc. are synthesised from glucose or its metabolites.

In spite of continuous entry of glucose into circulation and its continuous removal, blood glucose concentration is maintained within a narrow range. Blood glucose concentration is 60 to 100 mg/dl in the fasting state. It may go up to 130 to 140 mg/dl after a meal but is brought back to the fasting (post-absorptive) level within a few hours. A decrease in blood glucose level (**hypoglycaemia**) can deprive the tissues, especially brain, of an essential fuel. An increase in blood glucose level (**hyperglycaemia**) can disturb osmotic balance, acid-base balance and fluid and electrolyte balance of body fluids. Therefore, elaborate regulatory mechanisms have evolved to maintain the blood glucose level within the normal range. Liver, kidneys and several endocrine glands are involved in the regulation of blood glucose concentration.

ROLE OF LIVER

Liver is a key organ as far as metabolism is concerned. Pathways for synthesis and oxidation of carbohydrates, lipids, amino acids, purines, pyrimidines, etc. are all present in liver. Liver cells can take up and release glucose. Uptake of glucose by liver depends upon the blood glucose level. When the blood glucose level is high, hepatic uptake of glucose increases, and pathways which utilise glucose, e.g. glycolysis, HMP shunt, glycogenesis, lipogenesis, etc. become active. When the blood glucose level is low, the pathways which produce glucose, e.g. glycogenolysis, gluconeogenesis, etc. become active, and glucose is released into blood. Thus, liver helps in maintaining the blood glucose level by uptake and utilisation or production and release of glucose according to the ever-changing needs.

ROLE OF KIDNEYS

Role of kidneys in the maintenance of blood glucose level is relatively minor. When blood passes through the kidneys, all the glucose present in plasma enters the glomerular filtrate. Practically all the filtered glucose is reabsorbed by tubular cells and is returned to blood, and a loss of glucose in urine is prevented. Tubular reabsorption of glucose is a saturable process. The maximum capacity for tubular reabsorption of glucose (Tm_G) is 350 mg/minute. This capacity is sufficient to reabsorb all the filtered glucose if the blood glucose level is up to 180 mg/dl (**renal threshold for glucose**). When the blood glucose level exceeds 180 mg/dl, the excess glucose is excreted in urine to prevent a precipitous rise in blood glucose concentration.

ROLE OF ENDOCRINES

Hormonal regulation is the most important mechanism for regulation of blood glucose level. Several hormones, e.g. growth hormone, thyroid hormones, glucocorticoids, epinephrine and glucagon, raise the blood glucose level, and are known as **hyperglycaemic** or **diabetogenic hormones**. Insulin decreases the blood glucose level, and is known as a **hypoglycaemic** or **antidiabetogenic** hormone. These hormones affect the blood glucose level by influencing the cellular uptake of glucose and/or utilisation or production of glucose by different metabolic pathways.

Growth Hormone

This anterior pituitary hormone decreases glucose uptake and glycolysis in extrahepatic tissues such as muscles. It increases lipolysis in adipose tissue. The fatty acids released from adipose tissue are used as fuel, and the need for utilisation of glucose is decreased. Therefore, the blood glucose level is raised.

Thyroid Hormones

The thyroid hormones increase the intestinal absorption of glucose, and increase the secretion of growth hormone from anterior pituitary.

Glucocorticoids

Glucocorticoids increase gluconeogenesis by inducing the synthesis of gluconeogenic enzymes. They decrease the uptake of glucose and glycolysis in muscles and adipose tissue.

Epinephrine

Epinephrine increases glycogenolysis and decreases glycogenesis mainly in muscles and, to a smaller extent, in liver.

Glucagon

Glucagon increases glycogenolysis and decreases glycogenesis in liver. It also increases gluconeogenesis.

Insulin

Insulin increases glucose uptake in muscles and adipose tissue. It increases glycolysis, HMP shunt and glyco-genesis. It decreases glycogenolysis and gluconeogenesis. It also increases the synthesis of lipids from glucose. The overall result is a decrease in the blood glucose level.

When the blood glucose level is decreased, for example in a fasting condition, the secretion of hyperglycaemic hormones increases, and the blood glucose level is raised. When the blood glucose level is increased, for example after a meal, the secretion of insulin increases which lowers the blood glucose level. The blood glucose level is, thus, maintained within the normal range (*see* Chapter 17).

The regulatory mechanisms may fail in some pathological conditions resulting in hyperglycaemia or hypoglycaemia. Hyperglycaemia is more common, and is mostly due to deficient secretion of insulin or decreased responsiveness to insulin resulting in **diabetes mellitus**. Less common causes are hyperpituitarism, hyperthyroidism, Cushing's syndrome, etc. Hypoglycaemia is most frequently due to an accidental over administration of insulin to a diabetic patient. Less common causes are Addison's disease, severe liver disease, etc.

Diabetes mellitus is the most common disorder of blood glucose regulation (*see* Chapter 17). Most diabetic cases can be diagnosed by measuring fasting blood glucose level. But if the results are not conclusive, glucose tolerance test (GTT) may be performed to confirm the diagnosis.

Glucose Tolerance Test

Glucose tolerance test may be done orally or intravenously. The oral test is preferred. In the oral test, a blood sample is collected after an overnight fast and, then, glucose dissolved in water is given to the subject orally in the dose of **1.5 gm/kg** of body weight subject to a maximum of **75 gm**. Blood samples (post-glucose load) are collected 30, 60, 90 and 120 minutes after the ingestion of glucose. Blood glucose concentration is measured in each sample. Any urine passed during the period is qualitatively examined for the presence of glucose.

In normal subjects, the fasting blood glucose is within the normal range, blood glucose rises to 130 to 140 mg/dl an hour after ingestion of glucose, and returns to the fasting level within two hours of glucose ingestion. Glucose is not present in any urine sample. In diabetic subjects, fasting blood glucose is often above normal, the rise in blood glucose after glucose ingestion is excessive and blood glucose does not return to the fasting level in two hours. One or more urine samples may contain glucose (Fig. 10.33).

The full glucose tolerance test is not required in most of the suspected cases of diabetes mellitus. A shortened version is usually enough in which only the fasting blood glucose and 120-minute post-glucose load blood glucose are measured. According to the recently revised criteria of World Health Organization (WHO), diagnosis of diabetes mellitus is confirmed if any of the following is seen:

a. Fasting plasma glucose is above **126 mg/dl** on two occasions.

b. 120-Minute post-glucose load plasma glucose is above **200 mg/dl** on one occasion.

c. Fasting plasma glucose is above **126 mg/dl** and the 120-minute post-glucose load plasma glucose is above **200 mg/dl** on the same occasion.

Once a diagnosis of diabetes mellitus is made and treatment instituted, blood glucose measurements are required to monitor the adequacy of control of diabetes. However, post-glucose load blood glucose is not required for monitoring purposes. Generally, fasting blood glucose and 120-minute post-prandial (post-meal) blood glucose are measured for monitoring. The post-prandial (PP) blood glucose is measured two hours after breakfast or lunch when the level is likely to be at its peak. For monitoring long-term control, glycosylated haemoglobin can be measured.

Full glucose tolerance test is required for the diagnosis of **alimentary glycosuria** and **renal glycosuria**. In alimentary glycosuria, fasting and 120-minute post-glucose load blood glucose levels are normal but the peak in between exceeds the renal threshold for glucose. In renal glycosuria, the renal threshold is lowered leading to excretion of glucose in urine even though the blood glucose values remain below 180 mg/dl. The oral glucose tolerance test becomes invalid if the intestinal absorption is impaired. In such cases, intravenous glucose tolerance test may be done. The principle is the same. In a fasting condition, glucose is given intravenously in the dose of 0.5 gm/kg of body weight as a 20% solution infused at a uniform rate over a period of 30 minutes. Blood samples are collected before glucose infusion and one, two, three and four hours after the infusion. Glucose concentration is measured in each blood sample.

In normal subjects, fasting blood glucose is within the normal range, the level may go up to 250 mg/dl after glucose infusion, falls below the fasting level at two hours, and returns to normal in three to four hours. In diabetic subjects, the fasting blood glucose level may be high, the rise in blood glucose after glucose infusion is excessive, and the return to the fasting level is delayed.

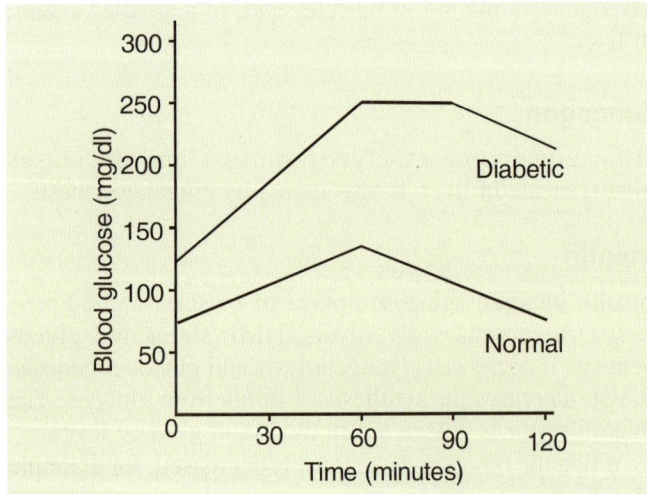

Fig. 10.33: Glucose tolerance test in a normal and a diabetic individual

Glycosylated Haemoglobin

In diabetic patients, blood glucose level has to be monitored from time to time to see whether the control of diabetes is adequate as good control can prevent or delay the development of complications. However, blood glucose measurement gives information about control of diabetes at the time of testing only. Whether the control has been adequate during the past few weeks can be assessed by measuring HbA_{1c} (glycosylated or glycated haemoglobin). Glucose combines spontaneously and irreversibly with haemoglobin to form glycosylated haemoglobin. The degree of glycosylation depends upon the blood glucose level and the lifespan of erythrocytes. Glucose can combine with the α-amino groups of the polypeptide chains and also with the ϵ-amino groups of the various lysine residues. The product formed by the union of glucose with the amino terminus of the β-polypeptide chains is known as HbA_{1C}. HbA_{1C} can be separated by ion-exchange chromatography or electrophoresis. In normal subjects, HbA_{1C} comprises 4–6% of the total haemoglobin. In diabetics, the degree of glycosylation is higher depending upon the blood glucose level over the preceding **6–8 weeks**. Therefore, long-term control of diabetes can be monitored by measuring glycosylated haemoglobin every two months.

INBORN ERRORS OF CARBOHYDRATE METABOLISM

Certain diseases occur due to inherited defects in the enzymes involved in the metabolism of carbohydrates. These diseases are known as inborn errors of carbohydrate metabolism. The affected enzyme may be catalytically inactive or may have decreased catalytic activity. As a result, the reaction catalysed by the enzyme will not occur or its velocity will decrease. Some important inborn errors of carbohydrate metabolism are the following:

Glycogen Storage Diseases (Glycogenosis)

This is a group of diseases in which the synthesis or breakdown of glycogen is impaired. Abnormally excessive amounts of glycogen accumulate in the affected tissues. The accumulated glycogen may be normal or abnormal in structure. The inheritance of these disorders is autosomal recessive.

Hypoglycaemia and muscular weakness generally occur due to decreased availability of glucose. In some of the diseases, ketosis can also occur. The affected organs may be enlarged or even damaged due to excessive deposition of glycogen. Glycogen storage diseases are classified into:

Type I (von Gierke disease)

This is due to absence or severe deficiency of glucose-6-phosphatase in liver and kidneys. The final reaction of glycogenolysis, i.e. conversion of glucose-6-phosphate into glucose does not occur.

Fasting hypoglycaemia, lactic acidosis, hyperlipidaemia, enlargement of liver and retardation of growth are the usual clinical abnormalities. Hyperuricaemia and gout can also occur around puberty. Nasogastric infusion of glucose in infancy and frequent feeding of raw cornstarch in childhood can prevent episodes of hypoglycaemia.

Type II (Pompe's disease)

Lysosomal α-1,4-glucosidase is deficient. Glycogen accumulates in lysosomes, principally in skeletal and cardiac muscles. There is progressive muscular weakness, hypotonia, cardiomegaly and congestive heart failure. Serum CK, GOT and LDH may be elevated. Involvement of respiratory muscles may cause difficulties in ventilation. No effective treatment is known.

Type III (Cori's disease)

Amylo-1,6-glucosidase (debranching enzyme) is absent. The distribution is generalised. Glycogenolysis stops at the branch points. The product of glycogenolysis is, therefore, limit dextrin which is deposited in excessive quantities. This disease is also known as limit dextrinosis. Clinical features include hypoglycaemia, hepatomegaly, muscle weakness, muscle atrophy and retardation of growth. Nasogastric glucose infusion and feeding of cornstarch can prevent hypoglycaemia.

Type IV (Andersen's disease)

Amylo-1,4 $\rightarrow$ 1,6-transglucosidase (branching enzyme) is deficient. A glycogen having very few branches, resembling amylopectin, accumulates in the affected tissues. The disease is also known as amylopectinosis. The defect is present usually in liver leading to hepatomegaly, cirrhosis of liver, growth retardation and hepatic failure. In some patients, muscles may also be affected leading to hypotonia, muscle weakness and muscle atrophy. No effective treatment is known.

Type V (McArdle's disease)

Phosphorylase is deficient in muscles. Glycogen accumulates in muscles. The disease usually manifests in adulthood with exercise intolerance and cramps on exercise. Serum creatine kinase is elevated, specially after physical activity. Myoglobinuria can occur after strenuous exercise. Avoiding strenuous exercise prevents the symptoms.

Type VI (Her's disease)

Phosphorylase is deficient in liver. Glycogen accumulates in liver. Hypoglycaemia and hepatomegaly are the usual clinical abnormalities. Frequent feeding of carbohydrates prevents the symptoms. The condition improves with age.

Type VII (Tarui disease)

Phosphofructokinase is deficient in muscles. Phosphofructokinase is a glycolytic enzyme. But glycogenolysis is linked with glycolysis in muscles. Glycogenolysis occurs when energy is required for muscle contraction, and is immediately followed by glycolysis. Therefore, decreased glycolysis leads to decreased glycogenolysis as well.

Phosphofructokinase consists of isoenzymes containing M (muscle), L (liver) and P (platelet) subunits. The M subunit is defective in Tarui disease. The muscle isoenzyme is made up of M subunits only. The erythrocyte isoenzyme is made up of M and L subunits. Therefore, the genetic defect leads to severe deficiency of phosphofructokinase in muscles and a moderate deficiency in erythrocytes.

The clinical features include easy fatigability and cramps on exercise. Severe exercise may cause myoglobinuria. Exercise after a carbohydrate-rich meal causes more severe symptoms as the unutilised glucose inhibits lipolysis, and the muscles are deprived of glucose as well as fatty acids. Some degree of haemolysis is usually present because of phosphofructokinase deficiency in erythrocytes. Avoiding vigorous exercise prevents muscle pain.

Type VIII

Phosphorylase kinase is deficient in liver. Hypoglycaemia can occur due to decreased glycogenolysis in liver. Frequent feeding of carbohydrates prevents the symptoms.

Congenital Galactosaemia

Galactose-1-phosphate uridyl transferase is absent from liver. Galactose ingested as milk lactose cannot be converted into glucose. Galactose concentration in blood increases after ingestion of milk, and galactose is excreted in urine. Clinical abnormalities are wide-ranging and varied. They appear soon after birth and may include vomiting, hypoglycaemia, hepatomegaly, jaundice, cirrhosis of liver, growth retardation, convulsions, premature cataract and mental retardation. Diagnosis should be made as soon after birth as possible. Galactose should be excluded from diet. This will prevent most of the clinical abnormalities. If treatment is delayed, the damage to brain and liver becomes irreversible.

Galactokinase Deficiency

This is relatively rare. Galactosaemia and galactosuria occur after ingestion of milk. Premature cataract is the main clinical abnormality. Early diagnosis and exclusion of galactose from diet leads to improvement.

Essential Fructosuria

Fructokinase is absent from liver. Dietary fructose cannot be metabolised, and is excreted in urine. This is a harmless condition.

Hereditary Fructose Intolerance

Aldolase B is absent from liver. Dietary fructose is converted into fructose-1-phosphate which cannot be metabolised further. Hypoglycaemia and liver damage occur after continued intake of fructose. Exclusion of fructose and sucrose from diet can prevent the clinical abnormalities.

Essential Pentosuria

This disease is common in Jews. L-Xylulose reductase is absent. This enzyme converts L-xylulose into xylitol which is, then, converted into D-xylulose. Dietary L-xylulose is excreted in urine. This is a harmless condition.

EXERCISE

1. Describe the digestion and absorption of carbohydrates. What is the cause of lactose intolerance?

2. Describe glycolysis and its regulation. Explain the energetics of aerobic and anaerobic glycolysis.

3. Describe gluconeogenesis. Explain the reciprocal regulation of gluconeogenesis and glycolysis.

4. Describe hexose monophosphate shunt and its importance.

5. Discuss the regulation of blood glucose concentration.

6. Discuss the regulation of glycogenesis and glycogenolysis. What is the purpose of glycogenolysis in liver and in muscles?

7. Write short notes on:
   a. GLUTs
   b. Cori cycle
   c. Glucose-alanine cycle
   d. BPG shunt
   e. Importance of galactose
   f. Glucose tolerance test
   g. Renal glycosuria
   h. Glycosylated haemoglobin
   i. Glycogen storage diseases
   j. Congenital galactosaemia

8. Write 'true' or 'false':
   a. Hereditary fructose intolerance is caused by a deficiency of phosphofructokinase-1.
   b. Insulin decreases gluconeogenesis.
   c. 2,3-Biphosphoglycerate is formed from 1,3-biphosphoglycerate in erythrocytes.
   d. McArdle's disease is caused by deficiency of hepatic phosphorylase.
   e. Phosphofructokinase-1 is one of the regulatory enzymes in glycolysis.
   f. Transaldolase requires thiamin pyrophosphate as a coenzyme.
   g. Two ATP equivalents are formed when one glucose molecule is converted into lactate.
   h. Anaerobic glycolysis occurs in erythrocytes in venous blood due to decreased availability of oxygen.
   i. BPG shunt is present in erythrocytes.
   j. Complete oxidation of one molecule of glucose under aerobic condition yields 38 ATP equivalents.
   k. Glucokinase is present in liver and β-cells in the islets of Langerhans.
   l. Hexokinase has a higher Km than glucokinase.
   m. Fluoride ions inhibit enolase.
   n. Glucocorticoids repress the synthesis of gluconeogenic enzymes.
   o. Short-term regulation of gluconeogenesis and glycolysis is reciprocal.
   p. The enzymes of HMP shunt are present in cytosol.
   q. Insulin increases glycogenesis and decreases glycogenolysis.
   r. Insulin increases the uptake of glucose in muscles and adipose tissue.
   s. Glycosylated haemoglobin is useful in monitoring the short-term control of diabetes mellitus.
   t. Congenital galactosaemia is due to absence of galactose-1-phosphate uridyl transferase ....

9. Fill in the blanks:
   a. Amylase hydrolyses .... bonds of starch and glycogen.
   b. SGLT1 has binding sites for .... and ....
   c. Insulin causes the translocation of GLUT4 from cytosol to cell membrane in .... and ....
   d. Glucose is phosphorylated by .... in the fasting state.
   e. Glycolysis is anaerobic in erythrocytes as erythrocytes lack ....
   f. The first functionally irreversible reaction unique to glycolysis is catalysed by ....
   g. No ATP is formed when glycolysis occurs via .... shunt.
   h. .... and .... are allosteric inhibitors of phosphofructokinase-1.
   i. Fructose-2,6-biphosphate is formed by the action of ....
   j. Fructose-2,6- biphosphate activates ....
   k. The coenzymes required in HMP shunt are .... and ....
   l. .... is a protein which forms the core of glycogen primer.
   m. Protein kinase A is activated when the intracellular concentration of .... increases.
   n. Protein kinase A is made up of two .... subunits and two .... subunits.
   o. Muscles can not form glucose from glycogen as they lack ....
   p. Fructose-1-phosphate is split into glyceraldehyde and dihydroxyacetone phosphate by ....
   q. Aldose reductase converts glucose into ....
   r. Renal threshold for glucose is ....
   s. .... is an antidiabetogenic hormone.
   t. The main clinical abnormality in galactokinase deficiency is ....

ANSWERS TO SHORT QUESTIONS

8. a. False b. True
   c. True d. False
   e. True f. False
   g. True h. False
   i. True j. True
   k. True l. False

m. True

o. True

q. True

s. False

9. a. α-1,4-glycosidic

c. Muscles, adipocytes

e. Mitochondria

g. BPG

i. Phosphofructokinase-2

k. NADP, TPP

m. cAMP

o. Glucose-6-phosphatase

q. Sorbitol

s. Insulin

n. False

p. True

r. True

t. True

b. Sodium, glucose/galactose

d. Hexokinase

f. Phosphofructokinase-1

h. ATP, citrate

j. Phosphofructokinase-1

l. Glycogenin

n. Regulatory, catalytic

p. Aldolase B

r. 180 mg/dl

t. Premature cataract

Metabolism of Lipids

Lipids constitute an important source of energy. Even carbohydrates, when available in abundance, are converted into lipids. Some amino acids can also be converted into lipids. Unlike carbohydrates and proteins, lipids can be stored in the body in large quantities, and constitute an important reservoir of energy. In an average person, about 80% of the stored energy is in the form of lipids. The major **storage** form of lipids is triglycerides (triacylglycerols). The triglycerides are stored in **fat depots** which include subcutaneous fat, peri-renal fat, mesentery, omentum, intermuscular connective tissue, etc. Triglycerides are stored in specialised cells called **adipocytes**. Triglyceride molecules coalesce to form globules which may occupy most of the space in adipocytes. A tissue rich in adipocytes is known as **adipose tissue**.

Fat depots are metabolically dynamic. There is a continuous exchange of lipids between fat depots and blood. Stored triglycerides are hydrolysed into fatty acids and glycerol which are released into circulation. Fatty acids are taken up by various tissues which require them as a source of energy or for synthesising phospholipids, glycolipids etc. Glycerol is mostly taken up by liver where it is converted into glycerol-3-phosphate. Glycerol-3-phosphate is converted into dihydroxyacetone phosphate, which can be oxidised in the glycolytic pathway or can be converted into glucose by gluconeogenesis. Circulating fatty acids, coming from diet or endogenous synthesis, are taken up by adipose tissue, and are converted into triglycerides. Glycerol-3-phosphate required for the synthesis of triglycerides comes from glucose. Dihydroxy-acetone phosphate formed from glucose in the glycolytic pathway is converted into glycerol-3-phosphate.

Glycerol formed from hydrolysis of triglycerides in the adipose tissue cannot be used for synthesis of triglycerides as **glycerol kinase** which converts glycerol into glycerol-3-phosphate is not present in adipose tissue.

DIGESTION AND ABSORPTION

The major dietary lipids are triglycerides, phospholipids, esterified cholesterol and the fat-soluble vitamins. Triglycerides, phospholipids and esterified cholesterol have to be hydrolysed before their absorption from the alimentary tract. The fat-soluble vitamins are absorbed along with the dietary lipids. The digestive juices which participate in the digestion of lipids are saliva, pancreatic juice and succus entericus. Bile also plays an important role in digestion and absorption of lipids.

Saliva contains a lipase which is secreted by the dorsal surface of tongue. Though food stays in the oral cavity for a very short period, **salivary lipase** remains active even in the acidic environment of stomach. It acts preferentially on the ester bond at position 3. Triglycerides containing short-chain fatty acids are particularly susceptible to the action of salivary lipase. Thus, salivary lipase converts triglycerides into diglycerides and free fatty acids which are mostly short-chain fatty acids.

Pancreatic juice also contains a lipase which is far more powerful than salivary lipase. **Pancreatic lipase** can easily hydrolyse the ester bonds at positions 1 and 3 but the ester bond at position 2 is resistant to the action of pancreatic lipase. Thus, pancreatic lipase converts triglycerides into 2-monoacylglycerol and free fatty acids. Pancreatic lipase requires **co-lipase** (a protein present in pancreatic juice) and **phospholipids** to become active. Bile salts are also required for its activity. Pancreatic juice also contains phospholipase A_2 and cholesterol esterase. Phospholipase A_2 hydrolyses the ester bond at position 2 of glycerophos-pholipids. Cholesterol esterase hydrolyses the ester bond of esterified cholesterol, and converts it into cholesterol.

Succus entericus contains a phospholipase which catalyses the complete hydrolysis of phospholipids.

Bile does not contain any digestive enzyme but still plays a vital role in the digestion and absorption of lipids.

$$CH_2-OH \qquad\qquad CH_2-OH$$
$$| \qquad\qquad\qquad Glycerol\text{-}3\text{-} \qquad |$$
$$C=O \qquad\qquad phosphate \qquad CH-OH$$
$$| \qquad\qquad dehydrogenase \qquad |$$
$$CH_2-O-\textcircled{P} \qquad\qquad\qquad CH_2-O-\textcircled{P}$$

Dihydroxy-acetone phosphate | NADH + H$^+$ | NAD$^+$ | Glycerol-3-phosphate

It contains bile salts (sodium and potassium salts of glycocholic acid and taurocholic acid) which are very efficienct **emulsifying agents**. Bile salts lower the surface tension of water, and break up the lipids into small droplets. The surface area of these droplets is very large, which facilitates the action of enzymes. Moreover, the emulsified lipids can be absorbed easily.

Glycerol, cholesterol, fatty acids and some monoglycerides, produced in the lumen of the intestine from hydrolysis of larger lipid molecules, are passively absorbed into the mucosal cells of the small intestine. Glycerol and short-chain fatty acids enter the portal circulation, and are transported to liver. Other products of digestion are recombined in the mucosal cells to form triglycerides, esterified cholesterol and phospholipids. These are combined with a small amount of some specific proteins to form **chylomicrons**, a type of lipoproteins. The chylomicrons enter the lymphatic vessels (lacteals), and ultimately reach the systemic circulation via thoracic duct. The plasma appears milky after a meal due to the presence of chylomicrons. The lipids present in chylomicrons are taken up by the various extrahepatic tissues in which enzymes of metabolic pathways involving lipids are present.

OXIDATION OF FATTY ACIDS

Oxidation of fatty acids occurs in the matrix of the mitochondria where the enzymes required for oxidation of fatty acids are present in close vicinity of the respiratory chain. However, the fatty acids have to be activated before they can be oxidised. Activation involves union of the fatty acids with CoA, catalysed by thiokinase. ATP provides the energy for this reaction.

$$R-CH_2-CH_2-\underset{\substack{\| \\ O}}{C}-OH + CoA-SH$$
Fatty acid

ATP
AMP + PPi — Thiokinase

$$R-CH_2-CH_2-\underset{\substack{\| \\ O}}{C}\sim S-CoA$$
Acyl CoA

Though the activation reaction is reversible, immediate hydrolysis of PPi makes the backward reaction impossible.

Existence of several different thiokinases has been reported, each of which is specific for fatty acids of a particular chain length. A thiokinase acting on short-chain fatty acids is present in mitochondria. But thiokinases acting on medium-chain and long-chain fatty acids are present on the outer mitochondrial membrane and on microsomes. Therefore, long-chain and medium-chain fatty acids are activated outside the mitochondria and, then, transported into the mitochondria for oxidation. Since the inner mitochondrial membrane is not permeable to medium-chain and long-chain fatty acids, a special transport mechanism is required for transporting them into mitochondria. The key component of this transport system is **carnitine** (β-hydroxy-γ-trimethyl ammonium butyrate). This can react with acyl CoA to form acylcarnitine.

$$H_3C-\underset{\substack{| \\ CH_3}}{\overset{\substack{CH_3 \\ |}}{N^+}}-CH_2-\underset{\substack{| \\ OH}}{CH}-CH_2-COOH$$
Carnitine

$$R-\underset{\substack{\| \\ O}}{C}\sim S-CoA$$
Acyl CoA

CoA—SH
CoA

$$H_3C-\underset{\substack{| \\ CH_3}}{\overset{\substack{CH_3 \\ |}}{N^+}}-CH_2-\underset{\substack{| \\ O-C-R \\ \| \\ O}}{CH}-CH_2-COOH$$
Acylcarnitine

On the outer surface of inner mitochondrial membrane, carnitine reacts with acyl CoA in the presence of **carnitine-palmitoyl transferase I** to form acylcarnitine and CoA. Acylcarnitine moves to the inner surface of the inner mitochondrial membrane. It reacts with CoA present in the matrix in the presence of **carnitine-palmitoyl transferase II** to release acyl CoA into the mitochondrial matrix. Carnitine set free in this reaction moves back to the outer surface of the membrane (Fig. 11.1). The transport

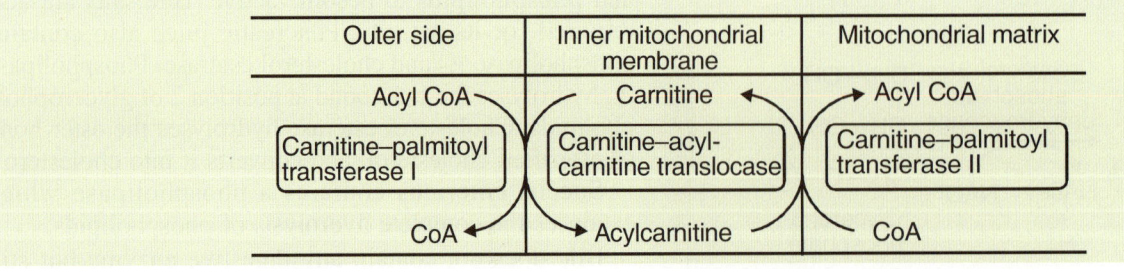

Fig. 11.1: Transport of long- and medium-chain fatty acids into mitochondria

of carnitine and acylcarnitine through the inner mitochondrial membrane is catalysed by **carnitine-acylcarnitine translocase**.

β-Oxidation Pathway

This pathway was elucidated by Franz Knoop. He labelled the methyl end of the fatty acids with a phenyl group and fed them to animals. The end products of oxidation were recovered from urine and identified. It was seen that when fatty acids having an even number of carbon atoms were fed, phenylacetic acid was recovered from urine. When fatty acids having an odd number of carbon atoms were fed, benzoic acid was recovered from urine. From these observations, Knoop concluded that oxidation of fatty acids involved removal of the last two carbon atoms from the carboxyl end in one cycle. In case of fatty acids having an even number of carbon atoms, the last two carbon atoms on the methyl end remain tagged with the label as phenylacetic acid. In case of fatty acids having an odd number of carbon atoms, the last carbon atom remains tagged with the label in the form of benzoic acid (Fig. 11.2).

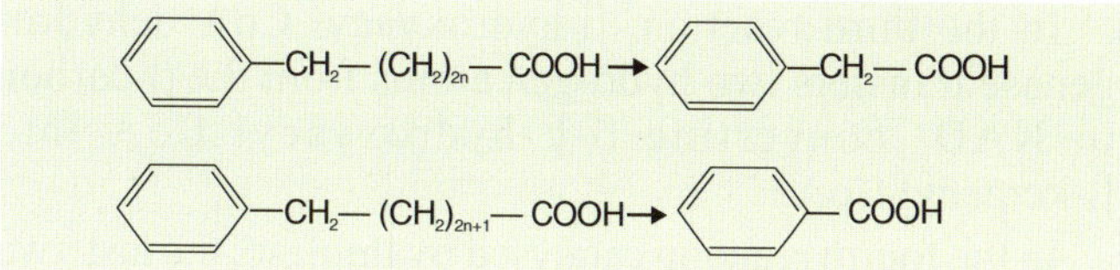

Fig. 11.2: Oxidation of labelled fatty acids having even and odd number of carbon atoms

This was termed as β-oxidation because after each cycle, the **β-carbon atom** (C_3) gets oxidised to a carboxyl group.

In the first reaction of the β-oxidation pathway, catalysed by acyl CoA dehydrogenase, one hydrogen atom from α-carbon and another from β-carbon of acyl CoA are transferred to FAD which is a prosthetic group of the enzyme. A double bond is formed between the α- and β-carbon atoms converting acyl CoA into α, β-unsaturated acyl CoA (Fig. 11.3).

In the second reaction, crotonase splits a molecule of water, and adds a hydrogen atom to α-carbon and a hydroxyl group to β-carbon converting α, β-unsaturated acyl CoA into β-L-hydroxyacyl CoA.

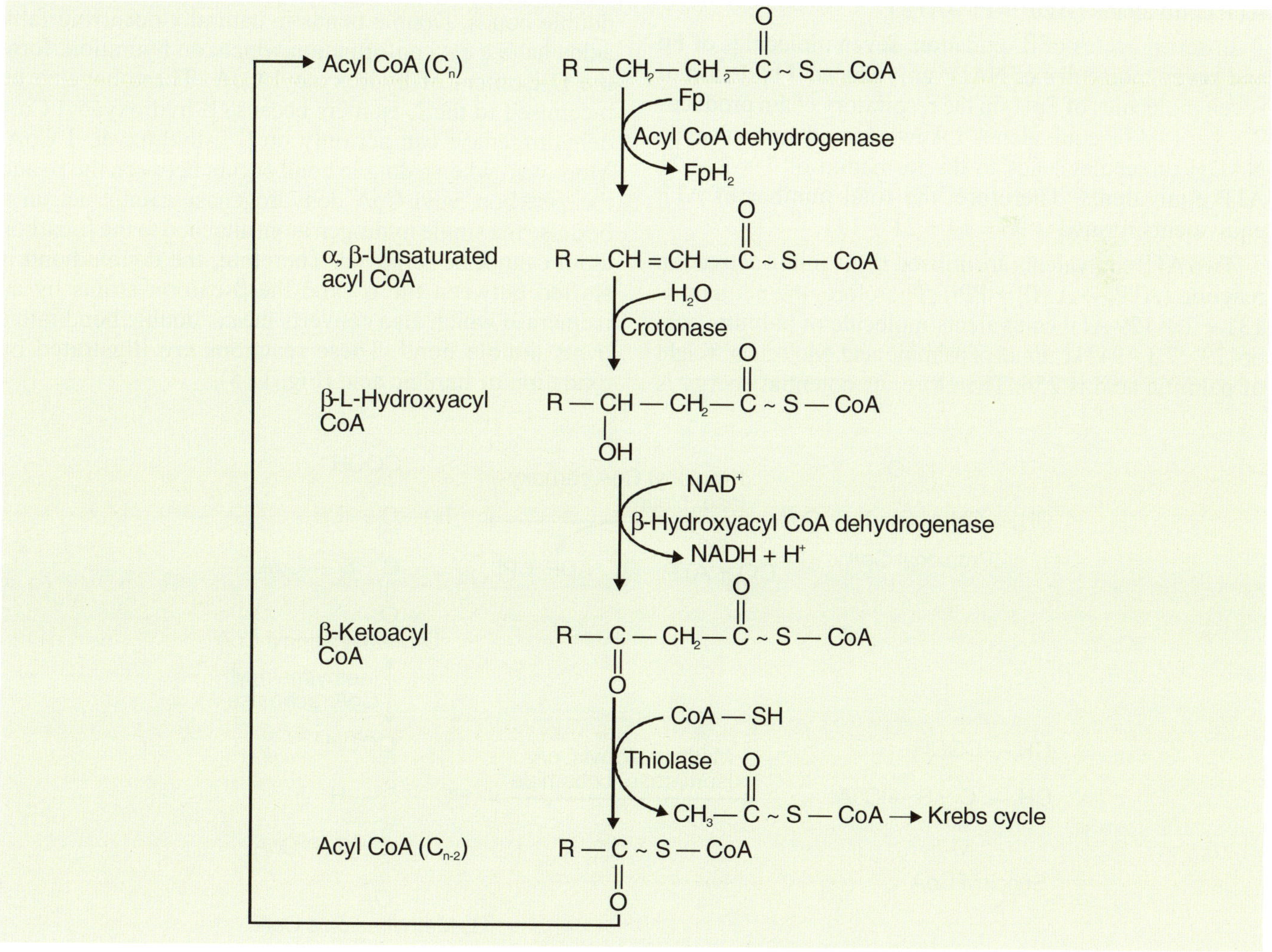

Fig. 11.3: β-Oxidation of fatty acids

In the third reaction, β-hydroxyacyl CoA dehydrogenase transfers two hydrogen atoms from the β-carbon to NAD⁺ converting β-L-hydroxyacyl CoA into β-ketoacyl CoA.

In the fourth reaction catalysed by thiolase, the last two carbon atoms along with CoA are released as acetyl CoA, and a new CoA molecule is added to the acyl chain forming an acyl CoA shorter by two carbon atoms than the initial acyl CoA. This acyl CoA goes through the cycle again, and two more carbon atoms are removed in the form of acetyl CoA. This process continues until only a two-carbon compound (acetyl CoA) is left as the final acyl CoA.

Energetics

If the fatty acid being oxidised is palmitic acid having 16 carbon atoms (C_{16}), seven cycles of β-oxidation will remove 14 carbon atoms in the form of seven molecules of acetyl CoA, and a two-carbon acyl CoA (acetyl CoA) will be left at the end of the seventh cycle. Thus, eight molecules of acetyl CoA will be formed. When these are oxidised in the citric acid cycle, they will form $8 \times 12 = 96$ ATP equivalents (ADP + Pi→ATP).

In seven cycles of β-oxidation, seven molecules of Fp and seven molecules of NAD⁺ are reduced. Oxidation of seven molecules of FpH_2 in the respiratory chain produces $7 \times 2 = 14$ ATP equivalents. Likewise, oxidation of seven NADH molecules leads to the formation of $7 \times 3 = 21$ ATP equivalents. Therefore, the total number of ATP equivalents formed is $96 + 14 + 21 = 131$.

Two ATP equivalents are utilised in the initial activation reaction (ATP → AMP + PPi). Therefore, the net gain is $131 - 2 = 129$ ATP equivalents/molecule of palmitic acid or $129 \times 7.3 = 942$ kcal/mol of palmitic acid. Molecular weight of palmitic acid is 256. Therefore, its potential energy is

$256 \times 9.1 = 2,330$ kcal/mol. Thus, the efficiency of β-oxidation is $942/2,330 \times 100$ or nearly 40 per cent.

Oxidation of stearic acid (C_{18}) requires eight cycles of β-oxidation and results in the formation of nine molecules of acetyl CoA, eight molecules of FpH_2 and eight molecules of NADH. Therefore, the total number of ATP equivalents formed is $(9 \times 12) + (8 \times 2) + (8 \times 3) = 108 + 16 + 24 = 148$. After subtracting the two ATP equivalents utilised in the initial activation reaction, the net gain is 146. This equals $146 \times 7.3 = 1,066$ kcal/mol of stearic acid. Molecular weight of stearic acid is 284. Therefore, its potential energy is $284 \times 9.1 = 2,584$ kcal/mol. Efficiency of its oxidation is $1,066/2,584 \times 100$ or nearly 41 per cent.

When fatty acids having an odd number of carbon atoms are oxidised, the final cycle of β-oxidation leaves behind a 3-carbon acyl CoA which is propionyl CoA. This is converted by a series of reactions into succinyl CoA. Succinyl CoA can enter the citric acid cycle (Fig. 11.4).

Oxidation of Unsaturated Fatty Acids

Unsaturated fatty acids are also oxidised by β-oxidation but two additional enzymes are needed to deal with the double bonds. Double bonds in naturally occurring fatty acids have a *cis* conformation which, on hydration, form the D-isomers of hydroxyacyl CoA. These have to be racemised to the L-isomers because β-hydroxyacyl CoA dehydrogenase can act only on β-L-hydroxyacyl CoA. Moreover, when a double bond occurs between the β- and the γ-carbon, acyl CoA dehydrogenase cannot act on it because the single hydrogen atom attached to the β-carbon atom cannot be removed. Therefore, the double bond is shifted between the α- and the β-carbon atoms by an isomerase which also converts the *cis* double bond into a *trans* double bond. These reactions are illustrated by oxidation of linoleic acid (Fig. 11.5).

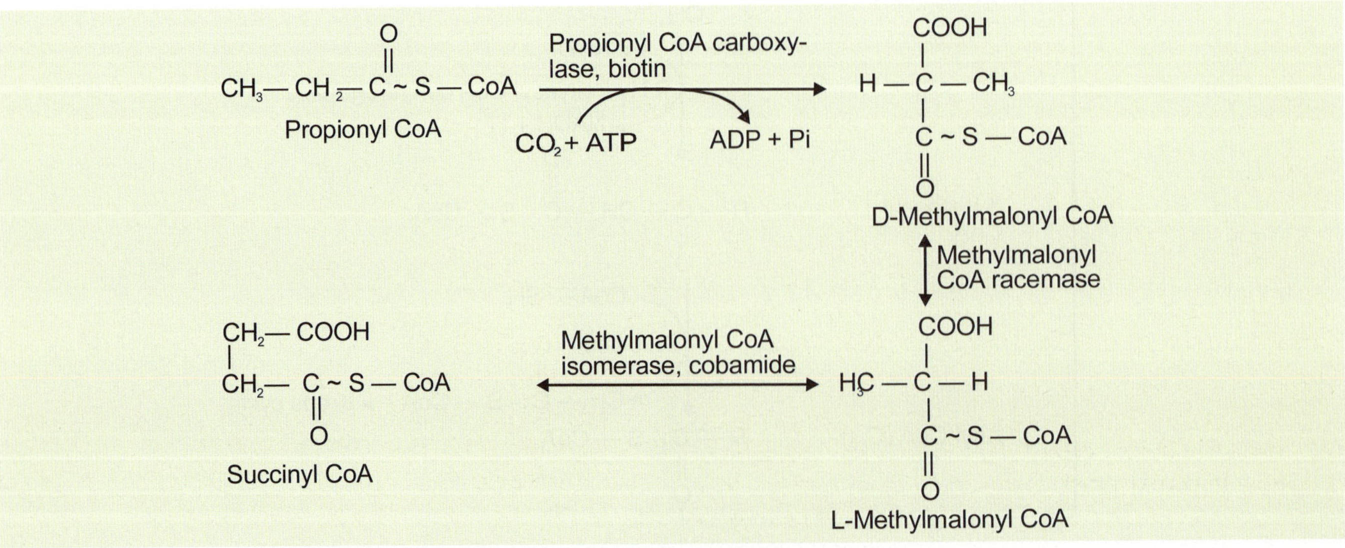

Fig. 11.4: Utilisation of propionyl CoA

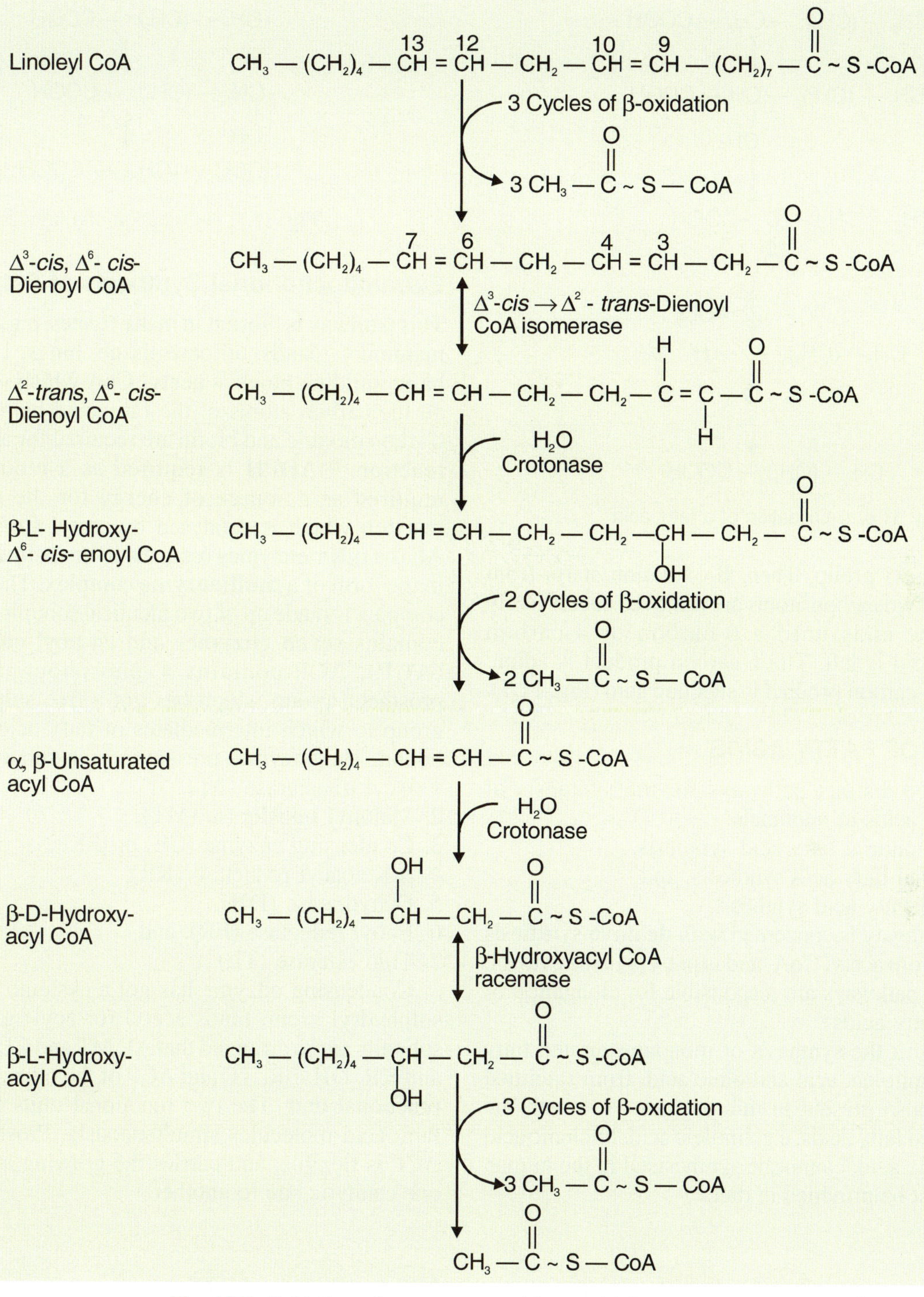

Fig. 11.5: Oxidation of an unsaturated fatty acid (linoleic acid)

Other Pathways for Oxidation of Fatty Acids

There are two other pathways for oxidation of fatty acids which are quantitatively insignificant. Their physiological importance is not very clear. Of these, α-oxidation pathway is present in peroxisomes. One carbon atom is removed at a time from the carboxyl end in the form of carbon dioxide (Fig. 11.6). This pathway is concerned mainly with the oxidation of phytanic acid which is formed from phytol, present in plants. Phytanic acid cannot be oxidised by the β-oxidation pathway because of the presence of methyl group at the β-carbon.

An inherited defect in this pathway blocks the oxidation of phytanic acid. This produces **Refsum's disease** in which large amounts of phytanic acid accumulate in the body leading to neurological abnormalities.

Another minor oxidative pathway is ω-oxidation in which the ω-carbon, i.e. the methyl group is first oxidised to a hydroxymethyl group, then an aldehyde group and

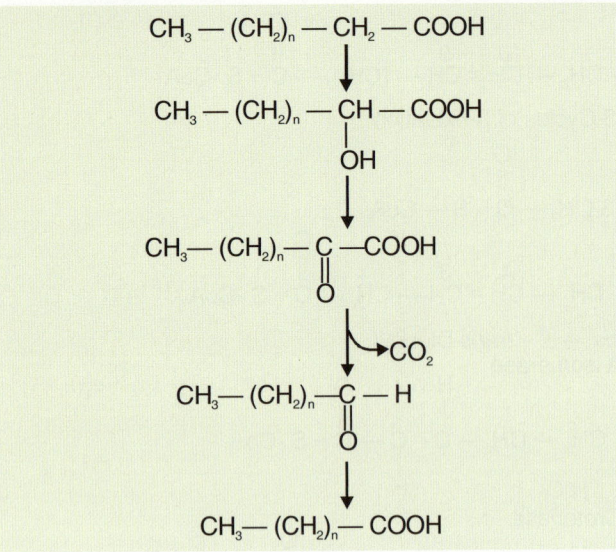

Fig. 11.6: α-Oxidation of a fatty acid

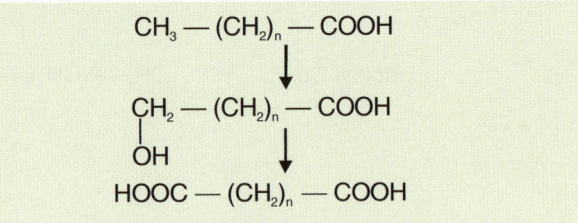

Fig. 11.7: ω-Oxidation of a fatty acid

finally a carboxyl group. Then, β-oxidation starts from both the ends. Two carbon atoms are removed successively from both the ends until a 6-carbon or 4-carbon dicarboxylic acid is left. The 6-carbon product is adipic acid, and the 4-carbon product is succinic acid (Fig. 11.7).

SYNTHESIS OF FATTY ACIDS

There are three distinct pathways for the synthesis of saturated fatty acids in mammals:
1. Extramitochondrial fatty acid synthesis,
2. Mitochondrial fatty acid synthesis, and
3. Microsomal fatty acid synthesis.

The first pathway is concerned with **de novo synthesis** of fatty acids from acetyl CoA, and is present in the cytosol. The other two pathways are responsible for elongation of pre-existing fatty acids.

A pathway for the synthesis of monounsaturated fatty acids, e.g. palmitoleic acid and oleic acid, from saturated fatty acids is also present in microsomes. However, the polyunsaturated fatty acids, e.g. linoleic acid, linolenic acid and arachidonic acid, cannot be synthesised in the human body, and must be provided in diet.

Extramitochondrial Synthesis of Fatty Acids

This pathway is present in many tissues, e.g. liver, kidneys, mammary glands, adipose tissue, lungs, brain, etc. The basic building block is **acetyl CoA** which is the source of all the carbon atoms of the fatty acid being synthesised. Carbon dioxide and biotin are required for a carboxylation reaction. NADPH is required as a reductant. ATP is required as a source of energy for the carboxylation reaction which is catalysed by acetyl CoA carboxylase. All the other enzymes required in the pathway are present in the form of a **multienzyme complex**. The multienzyme complex is made up of two identical subunits. Each subunit contains **seven enzymes** and an **acyl carrier protein (ACP)**. ACP contains 4'-phosphopantetheine as a prosthetic group which has got a free sulphydryl (–SH) group to which intermediates of fatty acid synthesis are bound. The enzymes present in each subunit are:
1. Acyl transferase (AT),
2. Malonyl transferase (MT),
3. Condensing enzyme (CE) or β-Ketoacyl synthetase,
4. β-Ketoacyl reductase (KR),
5. Dehydratase (DH),
6. Enoyl reductase (ER), and
7. Thio esterase (TE)

Condensing enzyme has got a cysteine residue whose sulphydryl group binds acetyl (or acyl) group. The two subunits are so arranged that AT, MT and CE of one subunit and KR, DH, ER, TE and ACP of the other subunit form a functional unit. The two functional units synthesise two fatty acid molecules simultaneously. Prosthetic group of ACP is flexible, and carries the growing acyl chain from one catalytic site to another.

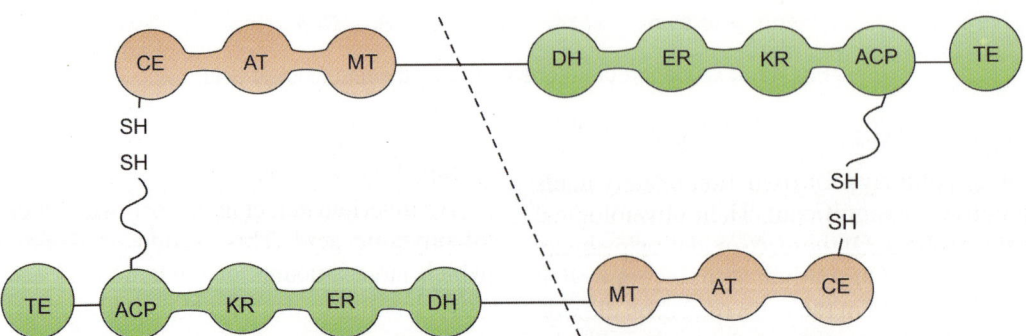

Fig. 11.8: Multienzyme complex having two functional units divided by discontinuous line

The initial reaction is carboxylation of acetyl CoA to form malonyl CoA. ATP provides energy for formation of the covalent bond.

$$CH_3 - \overset{\overset{\displaystyle O}{\|}}{C} \sim S - CoA$$
Acetyl CoA

$CO_2 + ATP$ ⟍ Acetyl CoA carboxylase
$ADP + Pi$ ↙

$$\overset{\overset{\displaystyle COOH}{|}}{CH_2} - \overset{\overset{\displaystyle O}{\|}}{C} \sim S - CoA$$
Malonyl CoA

The malonyl group is transferred to ACP, and an acetyl group from acetyl CoA is transferred to CE of one functional unit of multienzyme complex on which the subsequent reactions leading to the synthesis of palmitate occur.

Malonyl group is decarboxylated and condensed with the acetyl group by CE to form a β-ketoacyl group which is bound to the –SH group of ACP. The –SH group of CE becomes free. The β-ketoacyl group is reduced to a β-hydroxyacyl group by KR. The reducing equivalents are provided by NADPH. The –OH group attached to the β-carbon atom and a hydrogen atom from the α-carbon atom are removed as water by DH. The β-hydroxyacyl group is converted into an α, β-unsaturated acyl (enoyl) group. The double bond between the α- and the β-carbon atoms is reduced by transfer of reducing equivalents from NADPH by ER. A butyryl group is, thus, formed which is subsequently transferred to the –SH group of CE. This completes one cycle of reactions in which the 2-carbon acetyl group is converted into a 4-carbon butyryl group.

Another cycle begins with the binding of another malonyl group to ACP. Two carbon atoms are added to the butyryl group by the end of the cycle. These cycles are repeated until the growing acyl group is converted into a palmityl group. The enzyme system is incapable of increasing the length of the acyl chain beyond 16 carbon atoms. Palmitate is hydrolytically split off the multienzyme complex by thio esterase (Fig. 11.9).

The acetyl CoA molecules required for fatty acid synthesis are obtained from pyruvate. Pyruvate, formed mainly from glucose, enters the mitochondria, and is converted into acetyl CoA. When the energy content of the cells is high, acetyl CoA is diverted to fatty acid synthesis. As the mitochondrial membrane is not permeable to acetyl CoA, it combines with oxaloacetate to form citrate. Citrate comes out of the mitochondria and is cleaved into oxaloacetate and acetyl CoA by ATP-citrate lyase.

NADPH required for fatty acid synthesis comes mainly from hexose monophosphate shunt. Two other minor sources are:

i. Extramitochondrial oxidation of isocitrate by isocitrate dehydrogenase which uses $NADP^+$ as a coenzyme.
ii. Oxidative decarboxylation of malate in cytosol in which $NADP^+$ is used as a coenzyme.

Mitochondrial Synthesis of Fatty Acids

This is a minor pathway for elongation of medium-chain fatty acids. It is just a reversal of β-oxidation pathway with the difference that α, β-unsaturated acyl CoA is reduced by a different enzyme, α, β-unsaturated acyl CoA reductase which uses NADPH as a coenzyme instead of NAD.

α, β-Unsaturated acyl CoA
$$R-CH = CH-\overset{\overset{\displaystyle O}{\|}}{C}\sim S-CoA$$
⟍ $NADPH + H^+$
α, β-Unsaturated acyl CoA reductase
↙ $NADP^+$

Acyl CoA
$$R-CH_2-CH_2-\overset{\overset{\displaystyle O}{\|}}{C}\sim S-CoA$$

Microsomal Synthesis of Fatty Acids

This is the major pathway for elongation of medium-chain fatty acids into long-chain fatty acids. The pathway is present in endoplasmic reticulum. Two carbon atoms are added to the carboxyl end of a pre-existing fatty acid in one cycle. The source of these carbon atoms is malonyl CoA. NADPH is required as a reductant (Fig.11.10). Two molecules of NADPH are used in each cycle.

Thus, the chain length increases by two carbon atoms after every cycle of elongation. These cyclic reactions continue until the medium-chain fatty acid has been converted into a long-chain fatty acid. This pathway also elongates the long-chain fatty acids into very long-chain fatty acids in brain required for the synthesis of sphingolipids.

SYNTHESIS OF UNSATURATED FATTY ACIDS

Unsaturated fatty acids, e.g. oleic acid, linoleic acid, linolenic acid and arachidonic acid are necessary in human nutrition. Of these, linoleic acid, linolenic acid and arachidonic acid are polyunsaturated fatty acids (PUFAs) which cannot be synthesised by human beings. Therefore, these are known as essential fatty acids, and must be supplied in diet. Their deficiency causes dermatitis, hypercholesterolaemia and impairment of lipid transport. Presence of PUFAs in membrane lipids increases the fluidity of membranes.

PUFAs are present in most of the plant lipids. Safflower oil, sunflower oil, cottonseed oil and soya bean oil are very rich in PUFAs.

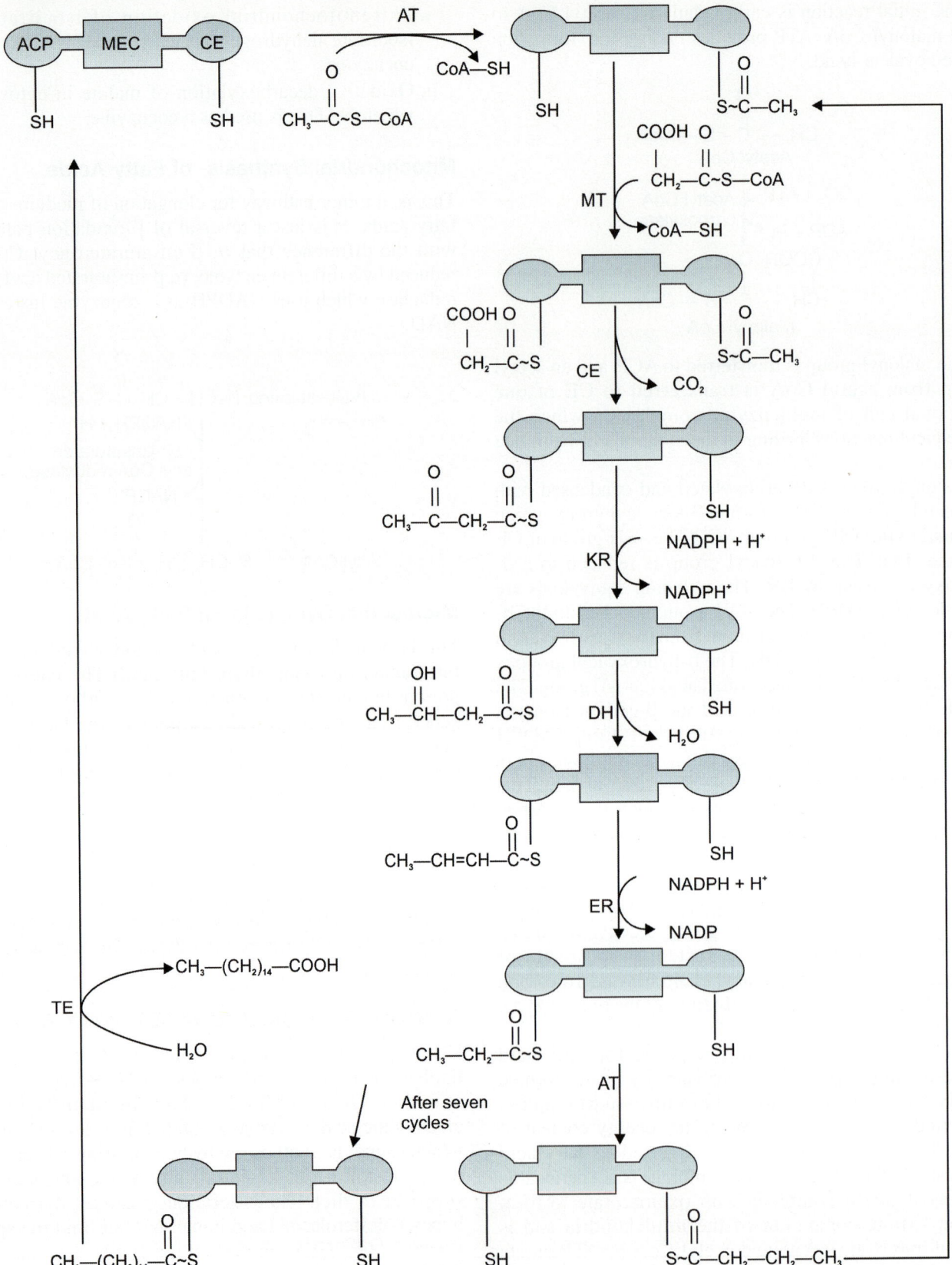

Fig. 11.9: De novo synthesis of a fatty acid (palmitate) on one functional unit of multienzyme complex (MEC). (AT-acyl transferase; MT-malonyl transferase; CE-condensing enzyme; KR-β-ketoacyl reductase; DH-dehydratase; ER-enoyl reductase; TE-thio esterase; ACP-acyl carrier protein)

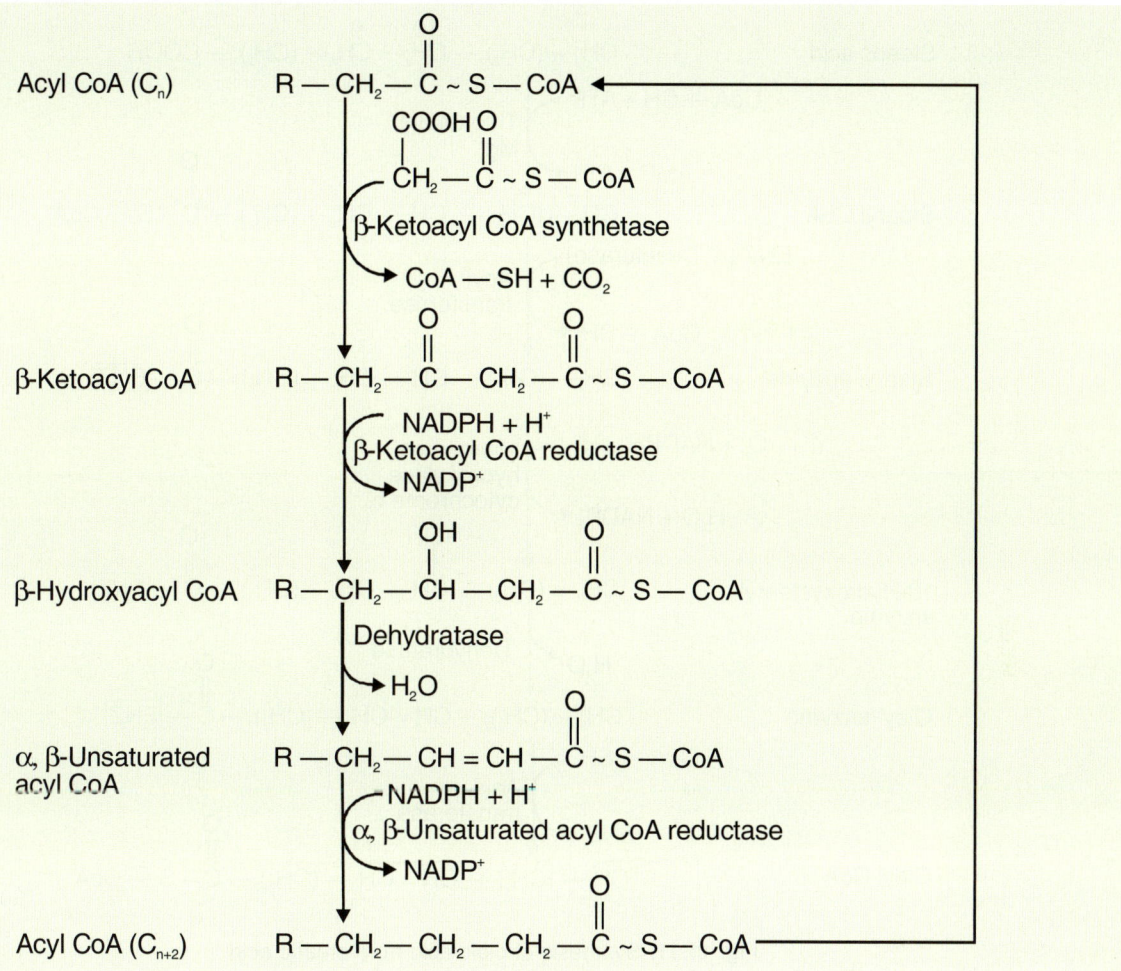

Fig. 11.10: Microsomal elongation of a fatty acid

Monounsaturated fatty acids, e.g. oleic acid and palmitoleic acid, can be synthesised in the human body from saturated fatty acids.

The synthesis occurs in microsomes of liver cells. Microsomal hydroxylase system introduces a hydroxyl group in the fatty acids. NADPH is required as a source of hydrogen atoms. The complete system is known as the **desaturase** system. Oleic acid is synthesised by this system from stearic acid, and palmitoleic acid from palmitic acid (Fig. 11.11).

The desaturase system is incapable of introducing a double bond beyond C_9. Hence, linoleic acid and α-linolenic acid cannot be synthesised by this system.

Synthesis of Arachidonic Acid

Arachidonic acid (20:4;5,8,11,14) is an important PUFAs as several prostaglandins, thromboxanes and leukotrienes are synthesised from it. Human beings can synthesise it from linoleic acid (Fig.11.12). The synthesis begins with the introduction of a double bond between C_6 and C_7 by Δ^6 desaturase to convert linoleyl CoA into γ-linolenyl CoA (18:3;6,9,12). One cycle of chain elongation follows,

adding two carbon atoms at the carboxyl end, so that a 20-carbon acyl CoA is formed (20:3; 8,11,14). Then, a double bond is introduced between C_5 and C_6 by Δ^5 desaturase forming arachidonyl CoA (20:4;5,8,11,14).

Thus, arachidonic acid and γ-linolenic acid both of which are ω-6 PUFAs, can be synthesised by human beings from linoleic acid. Linoleic acid (ω-6) and α-linolenic acid (ω-3) cannot be synthesised by human beings. The dietary requirements of ω-6 and ω-3 PUFAs are roughly in the ratio of 10:1.

REGULATION OF FATTY ACID METABOLISM

Metabolism of fatty acids is regulated in such a way that when there is abundance of energy, synthesis of fatty acids in increased and oxidation of fatty acids is decreased. The reverse occurs when energy is scarce. The rate of oxidation of fatty acids depends mainly on the availability of substrates, i.e. fatty acids. Fatty acids are released from fat depots by lipolysis. When energy is scarce, secretion of **glucagon** and **epinephrine** is increased which activate the adipocyte lipase through cAMP. Lipolysis is increased and fatty acids are released from stored triglycerides.

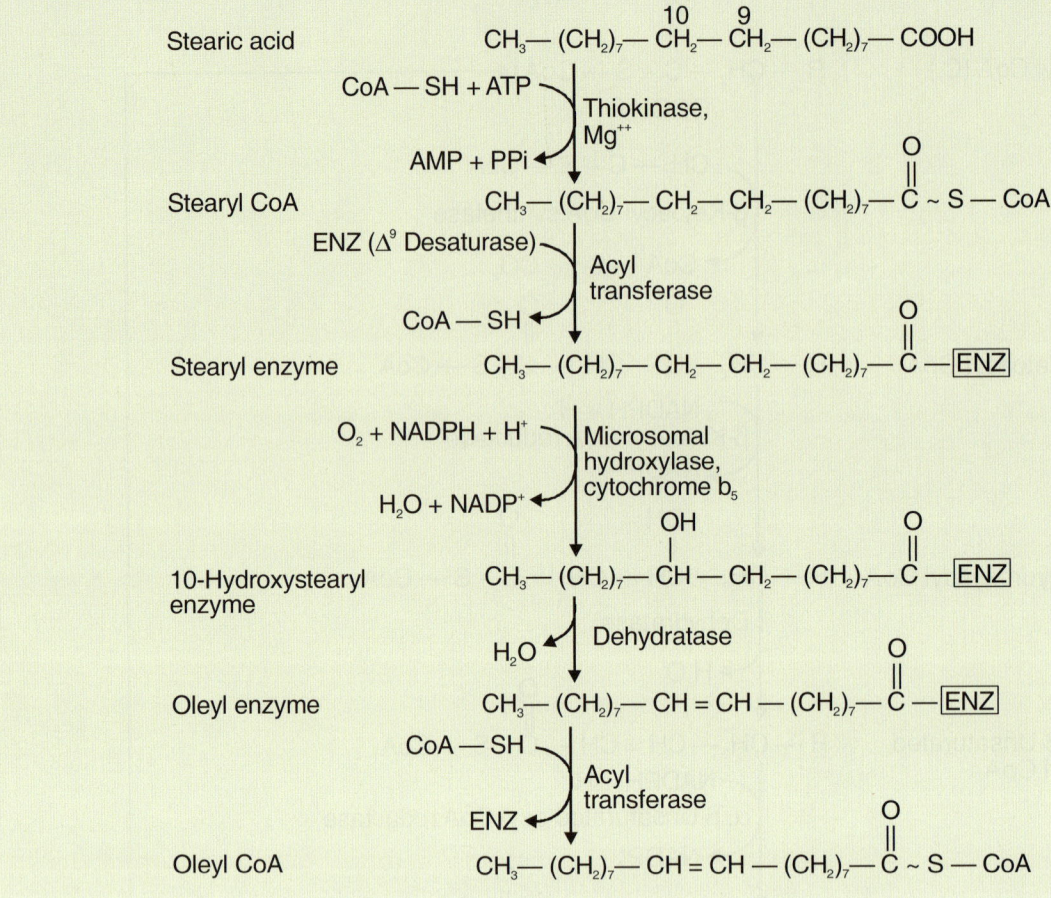

Fig. 11.11: Synthesis of oleic acid from stearic acid

Increased availability of fatty acids increases the rate of their oxidation.

When energy is abundant, **insulin** secretion is high which inhibits lipolysis. In times of plenty, the concentrations of **acetyl CoA, malonyl CoA** and **NADH** are also high. Malonyl CoA inhibits carnitine-palmitoyl transferase I, NADH inhibits β-hydroxyacyl CoA dehydrogenase, and acetyl CoA inhibits thiolase. Thus, both mitochondrial uptake and oxidation of fatty acids are decreased.

When energy is abundant, fatty acid synthesis is increased. Concentration of citrate is high in times of plenty. **Citrate** activates **acetyl CoA carboxylase** and increases the synthesis of malonyl CoA which, in turn, increases fatty acid synthesis. When enough fatty acids have been synthesised, concentration of **palmityl CoA** increases which inhibits acetyl CoA carboxylase. Palmityl CoA also inhibits glucose-6-phosphate dehydrogenase which provides NADPH for fatty acid synthesis.

Acetyl CoA carboxylase is also regulated by **covalent modification**. Phosphorylated form of this enzyme is inactive, and the dephosphorylated form is active. When energy is scarce, glucagon secretion rises. It increases the

concentration of cAMP in liver cells. Protein kinase A is activated, and acetyl CoA carboxylase is phosphorylated. The enzyme becomes inactive, and fatty acid synthesis decreases. The reverse occurs in times of plenty when insulin secretion is high. cAMP level decreases and more of the enzyme is present in the dephosphorylated, active form. Insulin also **induces** the synthesis of acetyl CoA carboxylase.

SYNTHESIS OF TRIGLYCERIDES

Triglycerides are synthesised in many tissues e.g. liver, kidneys, lactating mammary glands, intestinal mucosa, adipose tissue, muscles, etc. The building blocks are glycerol and fatty acids both of which have to be activated before they can be used for triglyceride synthesis. The fatty acids are activated to acyl CoA by thiokinase:

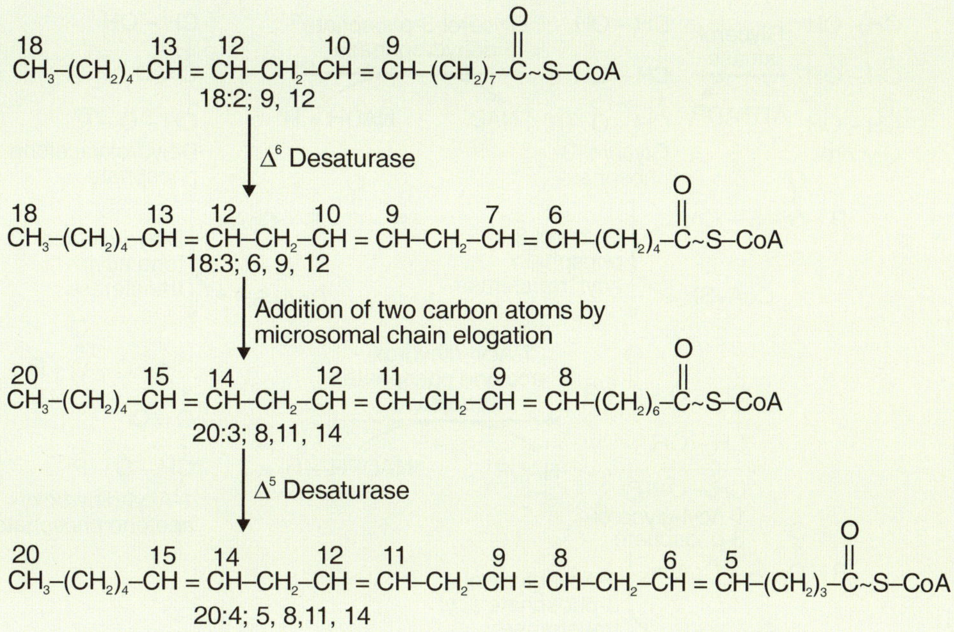

Fig. 11.12: Synthesis of arachidonyl CoA from linoleyl CoA

Glycerol is activated to glycerol-3-phosphate by glycerol kinase:

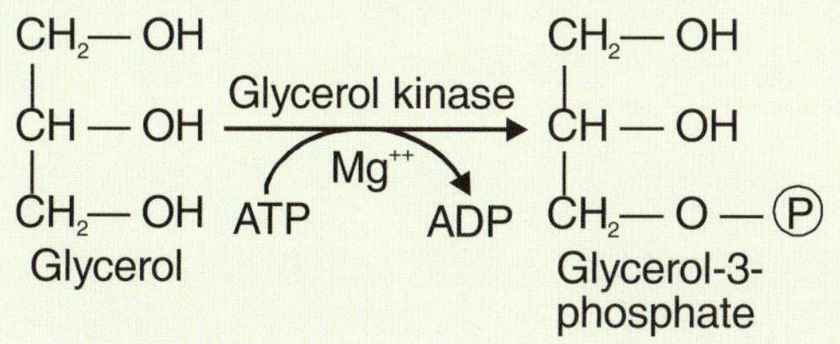

Glycerol kinase is not present in **adipose tissue** and **muscles**. These tissues can use dihydroxyacetone phosphate (formed in glycolytic pathway) to synthesise glycerol-3-phosphate with the help of glycerol-3-phosphate dehydrogenase. In intestinal mucosal cells, 2-mono-acylglycerol formed by partial hydrolysis of dietary triglycerides, can enter the synthetic pathway at an intermediate stage (Fig. 11.13).

CATABOLISM OF TRIGLYCERIDES

Triglycerides can be hydrolysed in tissues as well as plasma. Triglycerides are sequentially broken down into diglycerides, monoglycerides and glycerol and free fatty acids. The hydrolysis is catalysed by a hormone-sensitive lipase in tissues, and by lipoprotein lipase in plasma.

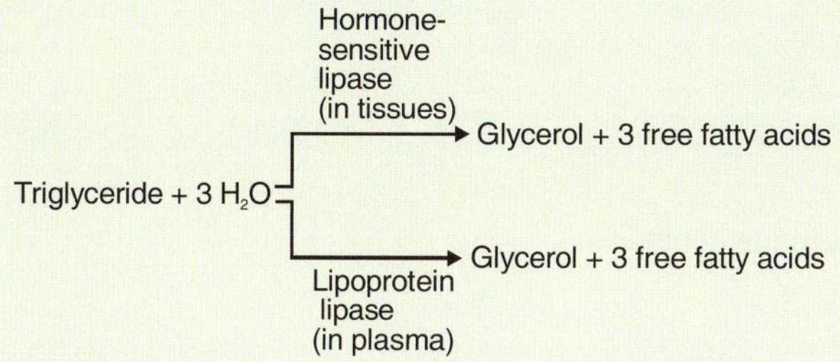

Hormone-sensitive lipase can exist in an active (phosphorylated) form and an inactive (dephosphorylated) form. Protein kinase A converts the inactive form into the active form. Protein kinase A is activated by cAMP. Therefore, hormones that raise the concentration of cAMP, e.g. epinephrine, glucagon, etc. stimulate lipolysis. Insulin has an opposite effect.

Hydrolysis of triglycerides is catalysed in plasma by lipoprotein lipase. The substrates are chylomicrons and VLDL which are rich in triglycerides. Lipoprotein lipase is normally present in an inactive form attached to the surface of the endothelial cells of capillaries. It can be activated by apo C-II and phospholipids. When blood containing chylomicrons and VLDL circulates through tissues, lipoprotein lipase is activated by apo C-II and phospholipids present in chylomicrons and VLDL. The triglycerides present in these lipoproteins are hydrolysed by the active enzyme. The free fatty acids released are taken up by the tissues. Most of the glycerol goes via circulation to liver where it can be converted into glucose.

SYNTHESIS OF PHOSPHOLIPIDS

Phospholipids include glycerophospholipids, e.g. phosphatidyl choline (lecithin), phosphatidyl ethanolamine (cephalin), phosphatidyl inositol, phosphatidyl serine, diphosphatidyl glycerol (cardiolipin) and plasmalogens, and sphingophospholipids, e.g. sphingomyelin.

Synthesis of Lecithin and Cephalin

Synthetic pathways for lecithin and cephalin are similar. Choline and ethanolamine are converted into CDP-choline

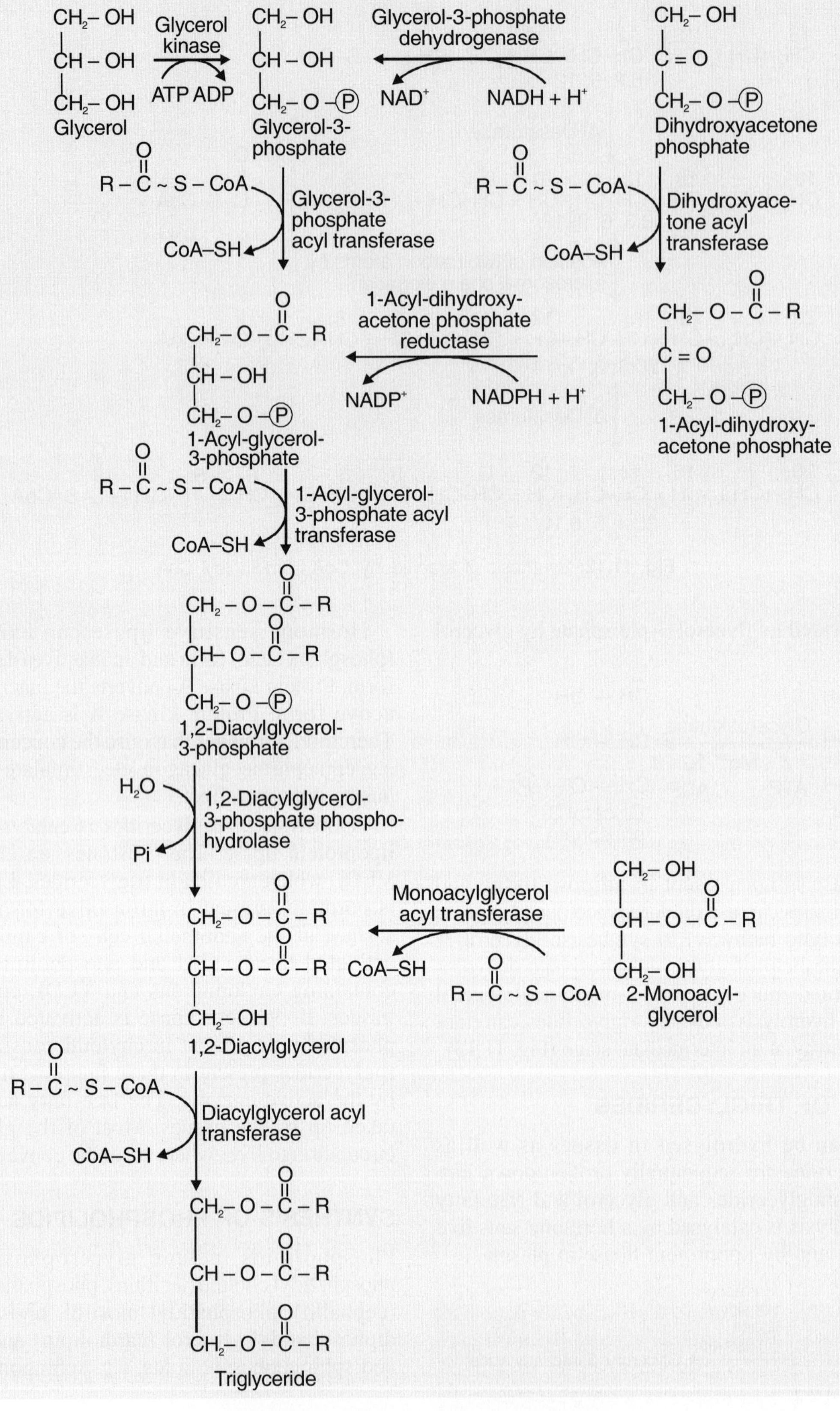

Fig. 11.13: Pathway of triglyceride synthesis

and CDP-ethanolamine respectively which react with 1,2-diacylglycerol forming lecithin and cephalin respectively (Fig. 11.14).

Synthesis of Phosphatidyl Inositol and Phosphatidyl Serine

Synthetic pathways for phosphatidyl inositol and phosphatidyl serine are similar. 1, 2-Diacylglycerol is converted into CDP-diacylglycerol which reacts with inositol to form phosphatidyl inositol, and with serine to form phosphatidyl serine (Fig.11.14).

Synthesis of Plasmalogens

Plasmalogens are synthesised from dihydroxyacetone phosphate, acyl CoA, a long-chain alcohol and CDP-ethanolamine (Fig.11.15). If an acetate group is esterified with C_2 of plasmalogen, it is known as **platelet activating factor** which causes aggregation of platelets and vasodilatation.

Synthesis of Cardiolipin

Cardiolipin is diphosphatidyl glycerol. It is synthesised from two molecules of CDP-diacylglycerol and one molecule of glycerol-3-phosphate (Fig.11.16).

Synthesis of Sphingomyelin

Sphingomyelin is synthesised from sphingosine, acyl CoA and CDP-choline. Sphingosine is a complex amino alcohol which is synthesised from palmityl CoA and serine (Fig. 11.17).

CATABOLISM OF PHOSPHOLIPIDS

Glycerophospholipids are hydrolysed by enzymes known as phospholipases. There are several different phospholipases which act on different bonds present in glycerophospholipids.

Phospholipase A_1 hydrolyses the ester bond at position 1 of the phospholipid molecule. Phospholipase A_2 hydrolyses the ester bond at position 2 converting the phospholipid into lysophospholipid, e.g. lecithin into lysolecithin. The fatty acid at position 2 is usually a polyunsaturated fatty acid. Phospholipase B removes the fatty acid from position 1 of the lysophospholipid. Phospholipase C hydrolyses the ester bond at position 3 between phosphate and glycerol. Phospholipase D hydrolyses the bond between phosphate and the nitrogenous base (Fig. 11.18). The partially hydrolysed products can be reutilised for the synthesis of new phospholipid molecules.

Sphingomyelin is hydrolysed into phosphocholine and ceramide (acylsphingosine) by sphingomyelinase. Ceramide can be hydrolysed into sphingosine and fatty acid by ceramidase.

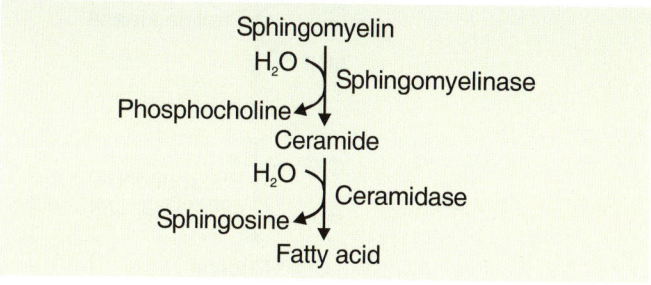

SYNTHESIS OF GLYCOLIPIDS

Glycolipids include cerebrosides, sulphatides and gangliosides. These are present mainly in nervous tissue. Glycolipids and sphingomyelin are known collectively as **sphingolipids** as the alcohol present in all these is **sphingosine**.

Synthesis of Cerebrosides

Cerebrosides are synthesised from ceramide and UDP-galactose (Fig. 11.19). Galactose forms a glycosidic bond with the primary alcohol group of sphingosine and UDP is released.

The fatty acids present in cerebrosides are very long-chain (24-carbon) fatty acids, e.g. cerebronic acid in cerebron, nervonic acid in nervon, oxynervonic acid in oxynervon and lignoceric acid in kerasin.

Synthesis of Sulphatides

Sulphatides (sulpholipids) are formed from cerebrosides and phosphoadenosine phosphosulphate (PAPS; active sulphate). The sulphate group is transferred from PAPS to C_3 of galactose.

$$Cerebroside + PAPS \longrightarrow Sulphatide + PAP$$

Synthesis of Gangliosides

Gangliosides are synthesised from ceramide and a number of activated hexoses and hexosamines, and N-acetyl neuraminic acid (NANA). The sugar residues are added to ceramide one by one by specific glycosyl transferases by different types of glycosidic bonds. Various gangliosides, e.g. G_{M3}, G_{M2} and G_{M1}, are formed at different stages (Fig. 11.20).

The glycosidic bonds in gangliosides are:

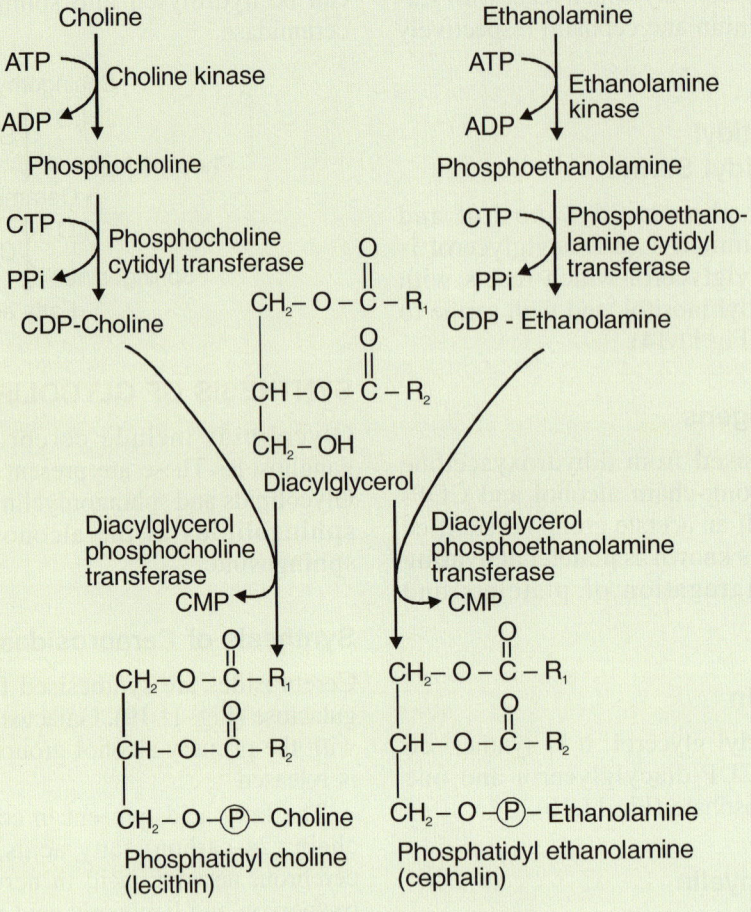

Synthesis of lecithin and cephalin

Synthesis of phosphatidyl inositol and phosphatidyl serine

Fig. 11.14: Synthesis of lecithin, cephalin, phosphatidyl inositol and phosphatidyl serine

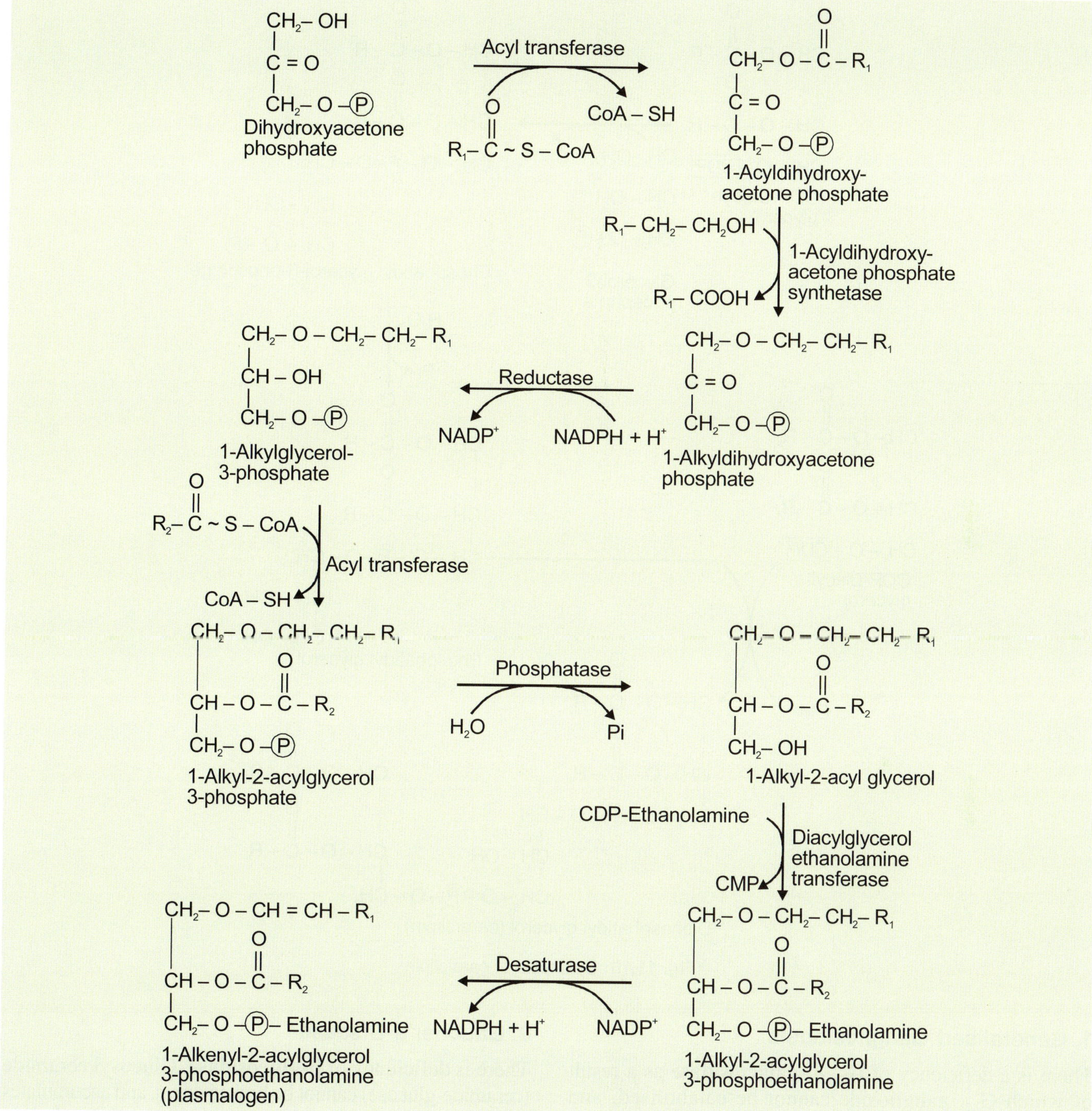

Fig. 11.15: Synthesis of plasmalogen

Catabolism of Glycolipids

Glycolipids are catabolised by removal of carbohydrate residues. The sugar residues are split off one by one by specific lysosomal glycosidases. Finally, ceramide is hydrolysed into sphingosine and fatty acid (Fig. 11.21).

SPHINGOLIPIDOSES

Sphingolipidoses are a group of inborn errors of sphingolipid metabolism. Synthesis of sphingolipids occurs normally in the affected persons but the breakdown of sphingolipids is impaired due to deficiency of some catabolic enzyme. Since sphingolipids occur in large amounts in nervous tissue, it is the nervous system which bears the brunt of the disease though there is abnormal accumulation of sphingolipids in all the tissues. Antenatal diagnosis of these disorders is possible by detection of abnormal sphingolipids in foetal cells recovered from amniotic fluid. The following are the major sphingolipidoses:

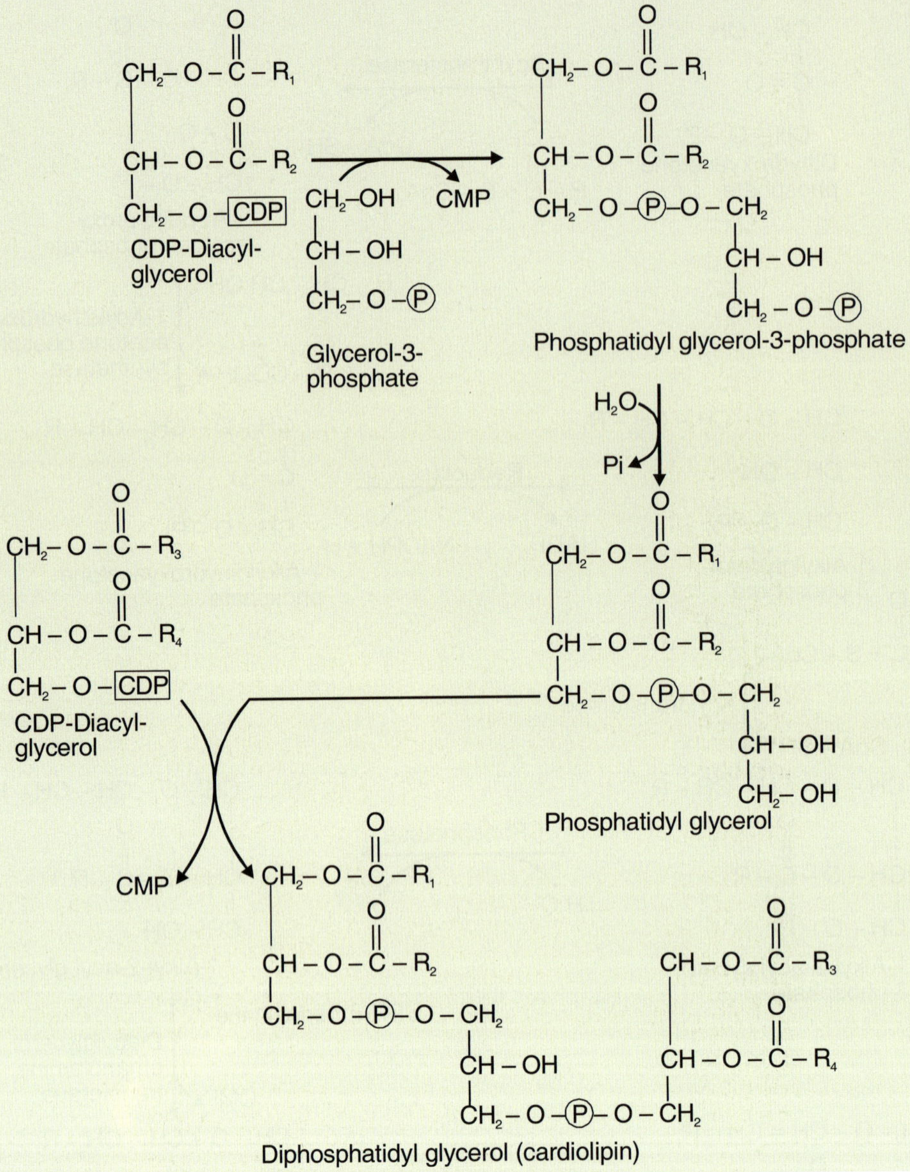

Fig. 11.16: Synthesis of cardiolipin

1. Generalised Gangliosidosis

There is a deficiency of G_{M1}-β-galactosidase as a result of which G_{M1} ganglioside cannot be catabolised, and accumulates in the tissues. The disease is characterised by mental retardation, hepatomegaly and skeletal deformities.

2. Tay-Sachs Disease

Hexosaminidase A is deficient which leads to accumulation of G_{M2} ganglioside. The clinical features include mental retardation, blindness, hypotonia and paralysis. Death occurs by 3 to 4 years of age.

3. Gaucher's Disease

There is deficiency of β-glucosidase. Glucosyl ceramide (ceramide-glucose) cannot be broken down, and accumulates in tissues. The clinical features are mental retardation, hepatosplenomegaly, hypersplenism and erosion of bones.

4. Krabbe's Disease

There is deficiency of β-Galactosidase which leads to accumulation of galactosyl ceramide (cerebrosides). The clinical features include mental retardation, blindness, deafness, hypertonia, hyperirritability.

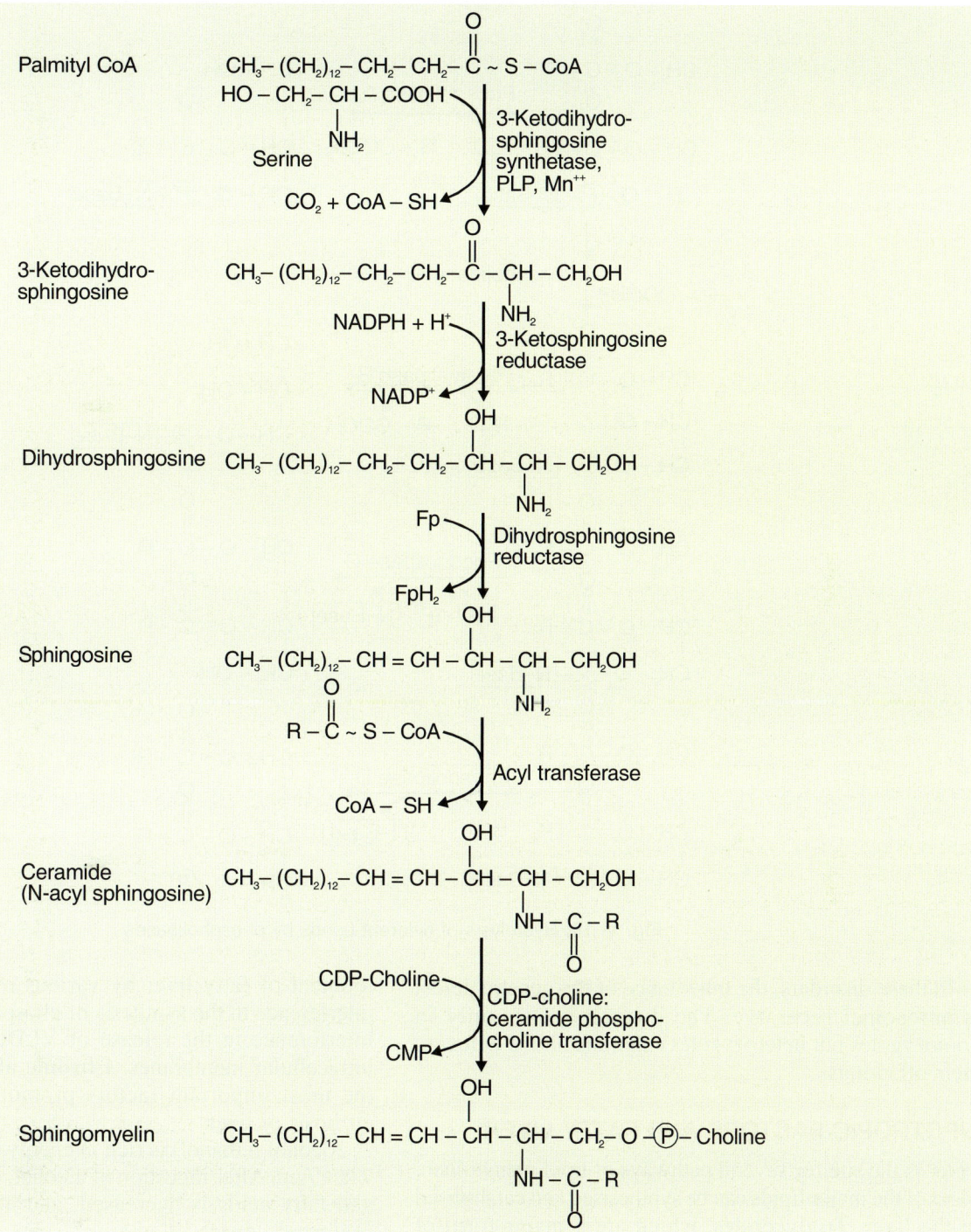

Fig. 11.17: Synthesis of sphingomyelin

5. Metachromatic Leukodystrophy

There is deficiency of **arylsulphatase A**. Sulphatides accumulate in the tissues. The clinical features are dementia and progressive paralysis. Death occurs by 3–10 years of age.

6. Niemann-Pick Disease

There is deficiency of **Sphingomyelinase** which leads to accumulation of sphingomyelin. The clinical features include mental retardation, motor disturbances, growth failure and hepatosplenomegaly. Death occurs by four years of age.

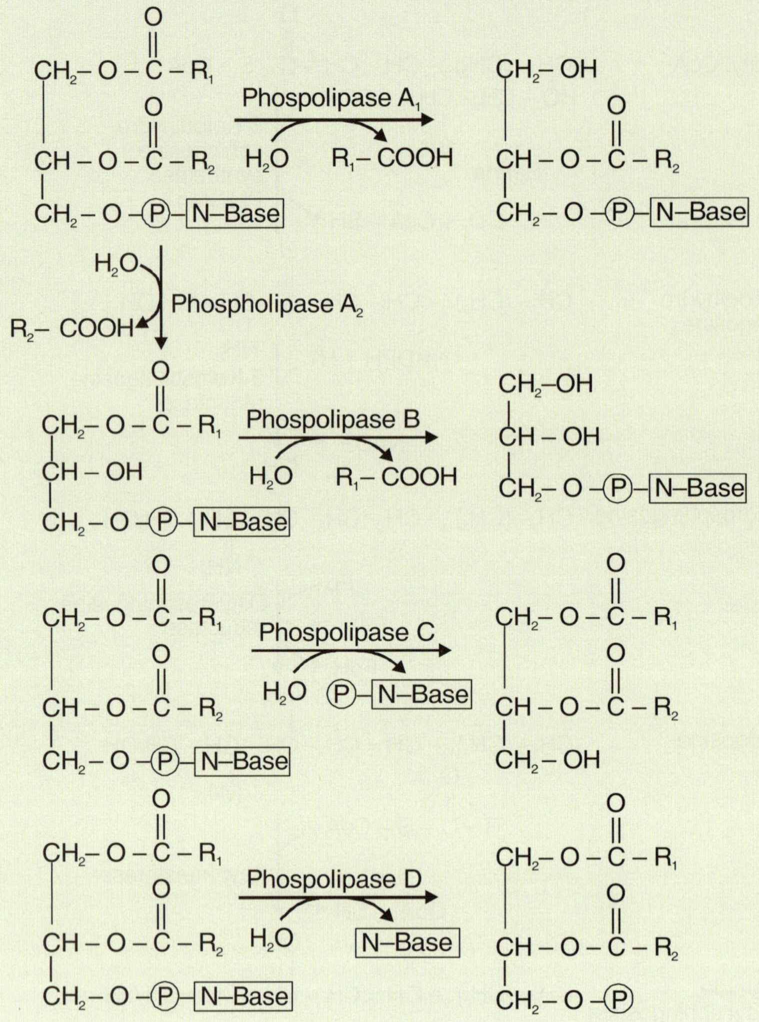

Fig. 11.18: Hydrolysis of different bonds by phospholipases

In these disorders, the inheritance of the genetic defect is autosomal recessive. The disease occurs only in homozygotes but heterozygotes can transmit the defect to their offsprings.

LIPOTROPIC FACTORS AND FATTY LIVER

Liver is the site for several pathways of lipid metabolism. Most of the major lipids can be synthesised and catabolised in the liver. Triglycerides, which are a major form of reserve energy, are synthesised in liver, and are transported out in the form of VLDL. Certain compounds, known as lipotropic factors, are essential for the transport of lipids out of liver. These include **choline, methionine** and **betaine**. Their deficiency causes abnormal accumulation of lipids, particularly triglycerides, in liver leading to a condition known as fatty liver. This can ultimately result in the destruction of liver cells and their replacement by fibrous tissue, a condition known as **cirrhosis of liver**.

Certain agents, e.g. alcohol, carbon tetrachloride, ethionine, puromycin, orotic acid, etc. promote the deve-

lopment of fatty liver by various mechanisms such as interference in the synthesis of phospholipids and VLDL, interference in the release of VLDL and disruption of intracellular membranes. **Chronic alcoholism** is one of the most important factors promoting fatty liver and cirrhosis of liver.

Alcohol (ethanol) is rich in energy. Its calorific value is 7 kcal/gm. After ingestion of alcohol, oxidation of glucose and fatty acids is decreased, and alcohol becomes the preferred source of energy. Since fatty acids are not oxidised, they are esterified with glycerol to form triglycerides. Increased synthesis of triglycerides in liver over a period of time leads to their accumulation in liver cells causing fatty liver.

Choline acts as a lipotropic factor as it is required to form **lecithin**, a phospholipid which is a component of **lipoproteins** that help in the transport of lipids from liver. Phospholipids are also required for the formation of **membranes** such as those of endoplasmic reticulum on which the apoprotein components of lipoproteins are synthesised. Betaine and methionine act as lipotropic

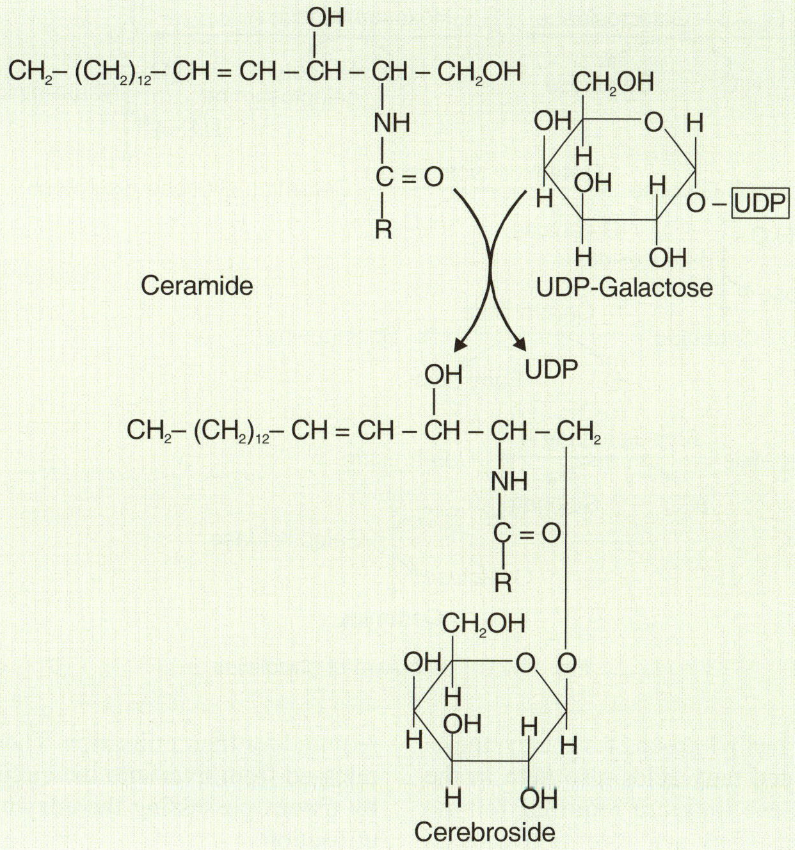

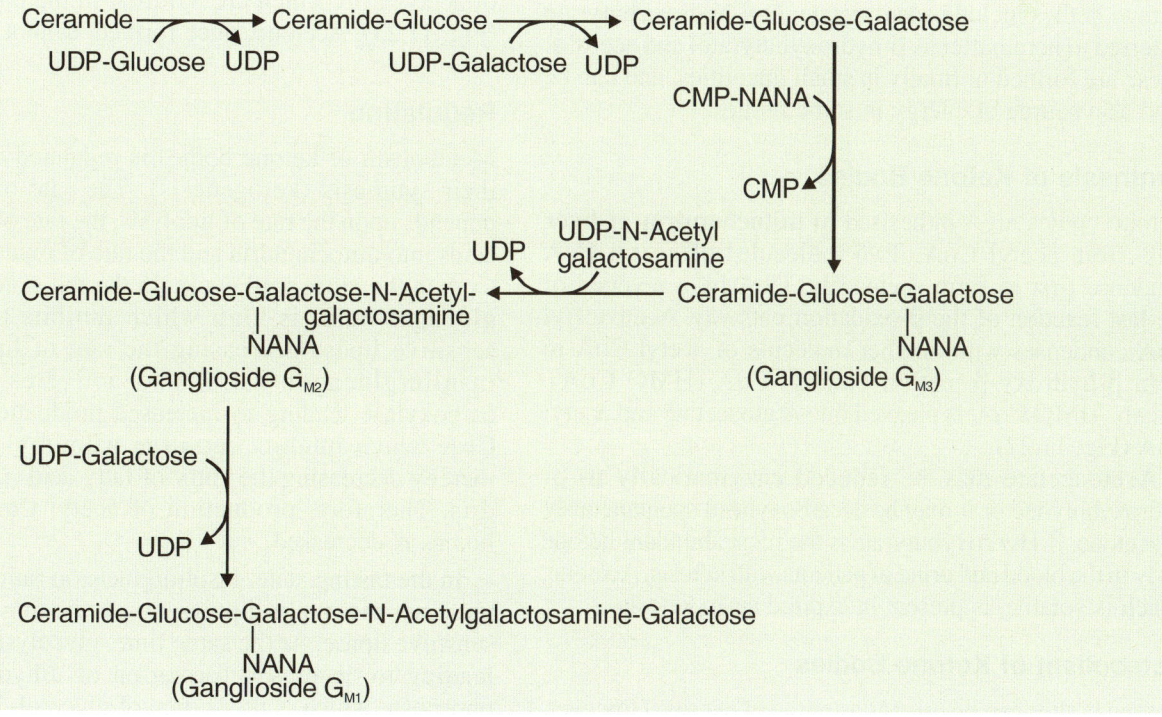

Fig. 11.19: Synthesis of cerebrosides

Fig. 11.20: Synthesis of gangliosides

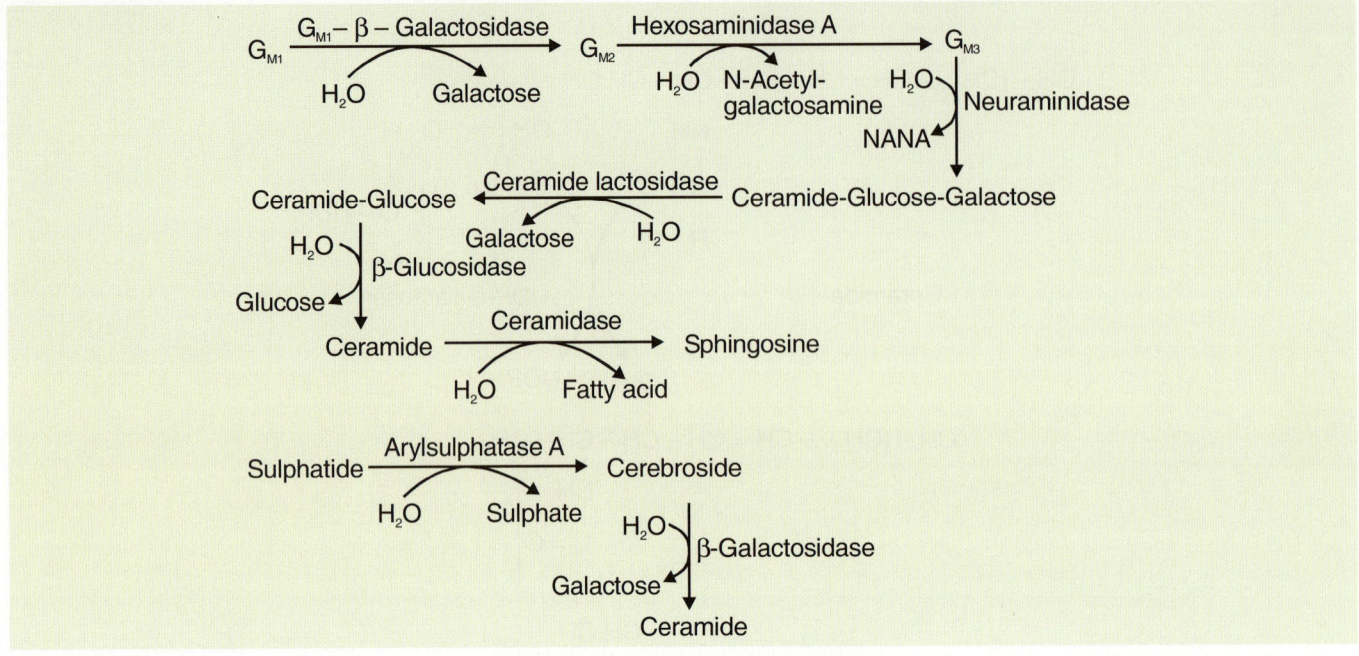

Fig. 11.21: Catabolism of glycolipids

factors by providing the methyl groups for the synthesis of choline. Polyunsaturated fatty acids also help in the transport of lipids because they are required for the synthesis of phospholipids (fatty acid esterified with C_2 of glycerophospholipids is usually a polyunsaturated fatty acid).

METABOLISM OF KETONE BODIES

Ketone bodies include acetoacetate, D-β-hydroxybutyrate (referred to hereinafter as β-hydroxybutyrate) and acetone. These are formed normally in small quantities, and can be used as a source of energy in some tissues.

Synthesis of Ketone Bodies

Ketone bodies are synthesised in **mitochondria** of **liver cells** from acetyl CoA. Two molecules of acetyl CoA condense first to form acetoacetyl CoA by a reversal of the last reaction of the β-oxidation pathway. Acetoacetyl CoA condenses with another molecule of acetyl CoA to form β-hydroxy-β-methyl glutaryl CoA (HMG CoA). Finally, HMG CoA is cleaved into acetoacetate and acetyl CoA (Fig. 11.22).

Acetoacetate may be reduced enzymatically to β-hydroxybutyrate or it may be decarboxylated spontaneously to acetone. β-Hydroxybutyrate is the most abundant ketone body in the blood and urine of patients with ketosis. Acetone, which is volatile, is present in expired air in ketosis.

Catabolism of Ketone Bodies

Ketone bodies can be used as a source of energy. However, liver which produces the ketone bodies lacks the enzymes required for their utilisation. Therefore, ketone bodies are released from liver into the circulation, and are taken up by tissues possessing the enzymatic machinery for their utilisation.

The first step is their activation to acetoacetyl CoA. β-Hydroxybutyrate is oxidised to acetoacetate. Acetoacetate reacts with succinyl CoA to form succinate and acetoacetyl CoA. Acetoacetyl CoA is converted into two molecules of acetyl CoA which are oxidised in the citric acid cycle (Fig. 11.23). Acetone, once formed, cannot be oxidised.

Regulation

Metabolism of ketone bodies is regulated at the level of their synthesis (ketogenesis). The rate of ketogenesis depends upon the rate of lipolysis, the rate of entry of fatty acids into mitochondria and the rate of oxidation of acetyl CoA in the citric acid cycle. In the fed state, the **insulin/ glucagon** ratio is high which inhibits the hormone-sensitive lipase decreasing the rate of lipolysis. High insulin/glucagon ratio also activates acetyl CoA carboxylase leading to increased production of malonyl CoA which inhibits carnitine palmitoyl transferase I thereby decreasing the entry of fatty acids into mitochondria. Therefore, production of acetyl CoA and ketone bodies is decreased.

In the fasting state, insulin/glucagon ratio is low which increases the rate of lipolysis by activating the hormone-sensitive lipase. At the same time, glycolysis is decreased leading to decreased formation of dihydroxy-acetone phosphate which is the source of glycerol-3-phosphate in adipose tissue and muscles. Therefore, esterification of

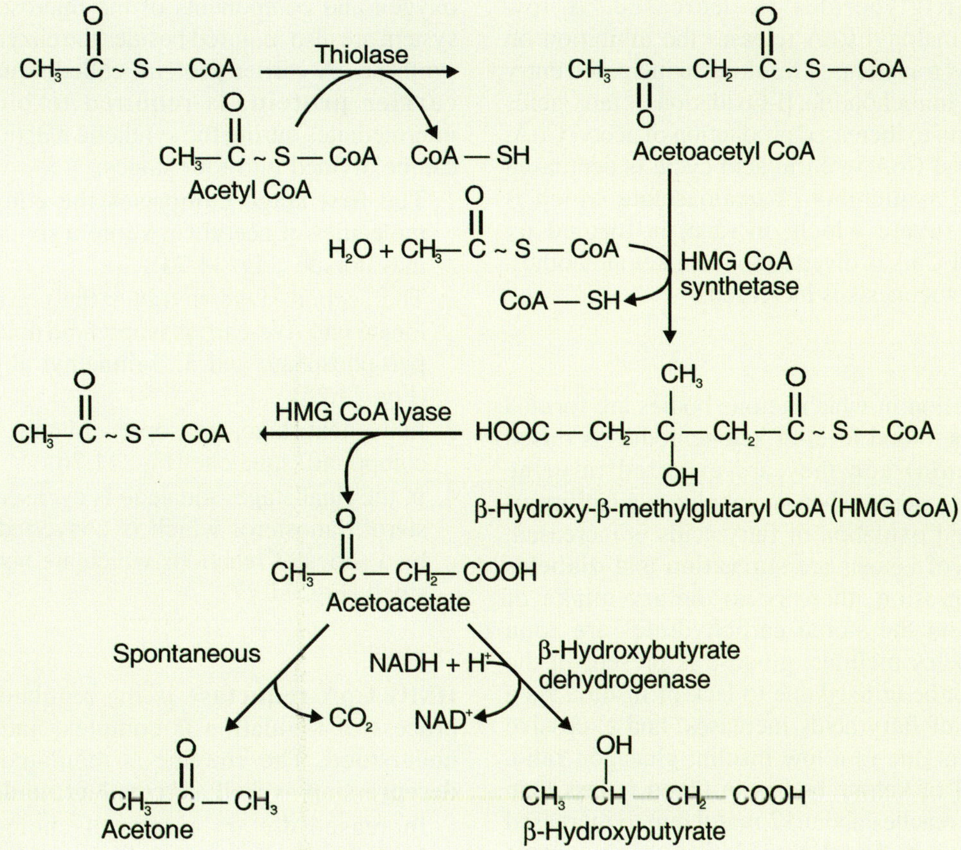

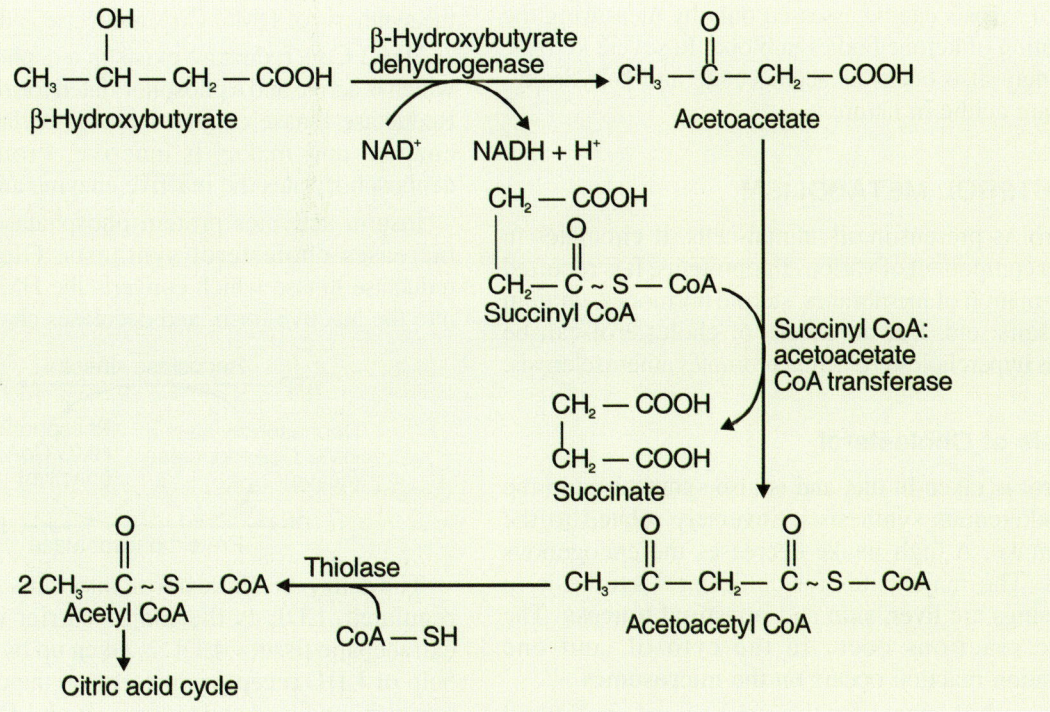

Fig. 11.22: Synthesis of ketone bodies

Fig. 11.23: Oxidation of ketone bodies

fatty acids to triglycerides is decreased. A low concentration of malonyl CoA releases the inhibition on carnitine palmitoyl transferase I resulting in increased entry of fatty acids into mitochondria. β-Oxidation of fatty acids is increased leading to increased production of acetyl CoA. Oxidation of acetyl CoA in citric acid cycle is decreased due to decreased availability of oxaloacetate which is formed from pyruvate which, in turn, is formed by glycolysis. Acetyl CoA is diverted to form ketone bodies, and the rate of ketogenesis is increased.

Ketosis

Ketosis is a condition in which ketone bodies are formed in large quantities, blood level of ketone bodies is raised (**hyperketonaemia**) and they are excreted in urine (**ketonuria**). This occurs when metabolic availability of glucose is low and oxidation of fatty acids is increased. The main causes of ketosis are **starvation** and **diabetes mellitus**. In starvation, there is no dietary intake of carbohydrates, and the stored carbohydrates are soon depleted. In diabetes mellitus, glucose is present in the body but it cannot be utilised due to lack of insulin. As a result, oxidation of fatty acids increases, and excessive ketogenesis occurs due to a low insulin: glucagon ratio. The normal level of ketone bodies in blood is less than 2 mg/dl. When it reaches about 12 mg/dl due to increased ketogenesis, the extrahepatic oxidative machinery is saturated, and ketone bodies accumulate in blood and are excreted in urine. Acetone is lost in expired air. Therefore, ketosis can be detected from the smell of acetone in breath, and the presence of ketone bodies in urine. However, the severity of ketosis can be assessed only by measuring the concentration of ketone bodies in blood. In severe ketosis, acidosis may also occur as acetoacetate and β-hydroxybutyrate are acidic in nature.

CHOLESTEROL METABOLISM

Cholesterol is present in all animal cells. It circulates in blood as a component of various lipoproteins. It is required for the formation of membranes, steroid hormones, vitamin D_3, bile salts, etc. But an excess of cholesterol can be harmful as hypercholesterolaemia promotes atherosclerosis.

Synthesis of Cholesterol

Cholesterol is taken in diet and is also synthesised in the body. Endogenous synthesis is inversely related to the dietary intake. A high intake decreases the endogenous synthesis. The major sites for cholesterol synthesis in human beings are **liver, skin** and **intestinal mucosa**. The synthetic reactions occur in the cytosol, and one hydroxylation reaction occurs on the **microsomes**.

All the carbon atoms for the synthesis of cholesterol are provided by **acetyl CoA**. ATP, NADPH, molecular oxygen and components of the microsomal hydroxylase system are also required besides the enzymes of cholesterol synthesis. A carrier protein, called **squalene and sterol carrier protein**, is required to bind some of the intermediates during the synthetic reactions. The reactions can be divided into four stages:

1. The first stage comprises the conversion of three molecules of acetyl CoA into a six-carbon compound, mevalonate (Fig. 11.24).
2. The second stage involves the conversion of mevalonate into five-carbon isoprenoid units, i.e. isopentenyl pyrophosphate and 3, 3-dimethyl allyl pyrophosphate (Fig. 11.25).
3. In the next stage, six isoprenoid units form a 30-carbon compound, squalene (Fig. 11.26).
4. In the final stage, squalene is cyclised to form the first sterol, lanosterol which is converted into cholesterol by a series of reactions which are not perfectly understood (Fig. 11.27).

Regulation

HMG CoA reductase is the regulatory enzyme. The process of regulation is complex, and is not perfectly understood. The enzyme is regulated by **repression-derepression** as well as **covalent modification**.

Increased dietary intake of cholesterol decreases endogenous synthesis of cholesterol. It has been proposed that cholesterol or some metabolite of cholesterol, when present in excess, represses the synthesis of HMG CoA reductase. This decreases the rate of cholesterol synthesis. When the intracellular concentration of cholesterol decreases, the synthesis of HMG CoA reductase is derepressed.

HMG CoA reductase exists in a dephosphorylated form which is active and a phosphorylated form which is inactive. Reductase kinase catalyses phosphorylation of the active enzyme and makes it inactive. Protein phosphatase dephosphorylates the inactive enzyme and makes it active.

Insulin activates protein phosphatase which converts increases cholesterol synthesis. Glucagon activates reductase kinase which converts the HMG CoA reductase into the inactive form, and decreases cholesterol synthesis.

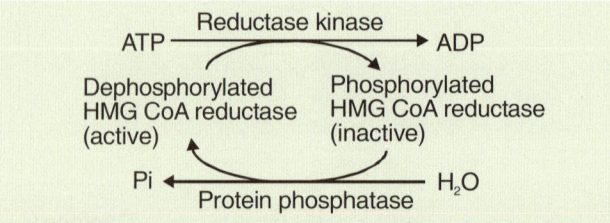

The entry of cholesterol into cells is also precisely regulated. LDL is the major carrier of cholesterol to extrahepatic tissues. LDL is taken up by the cells with the help of **LDL receptors** present on the cell membrane by receptor-mediated endocytosis. Both LDL and its receptor enter the cell. As more and more LDL enters the cell, the

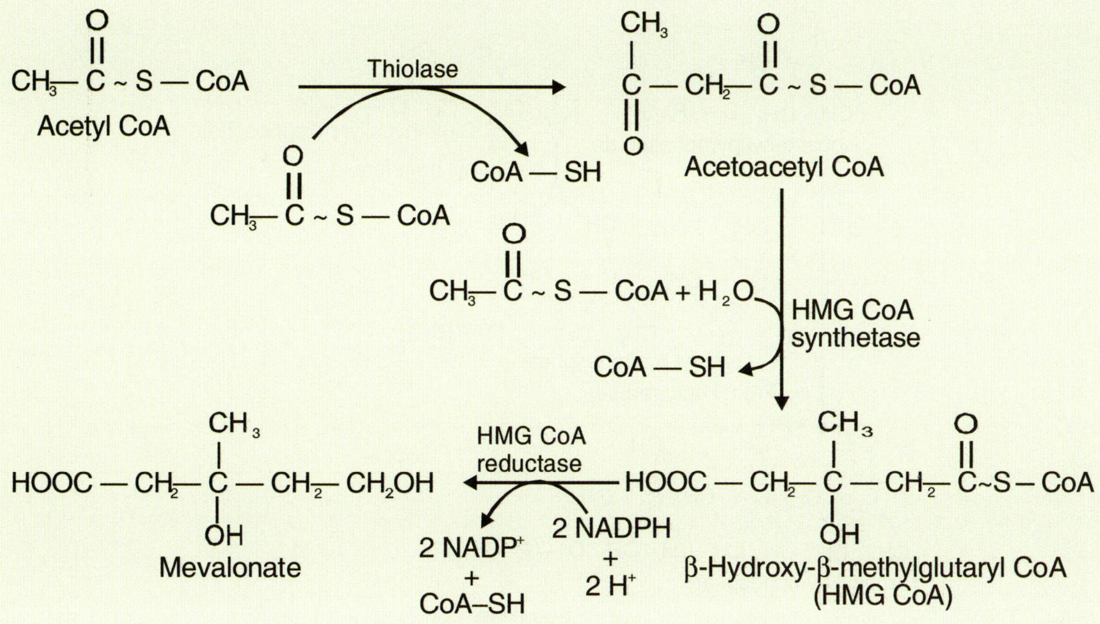

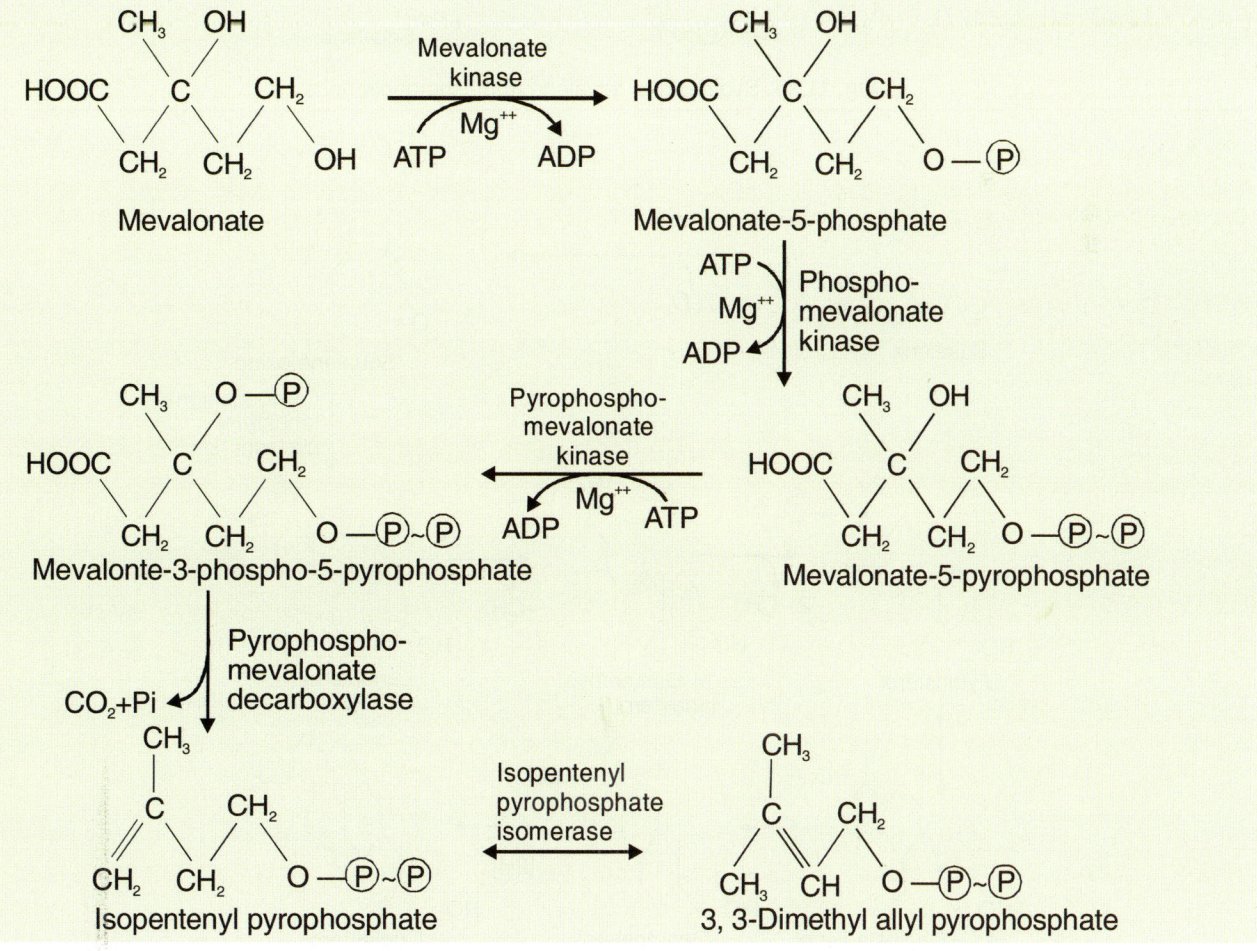

Fig. 11.24: Synthesis of mevalonate from acetyl CoA

Fig. 11.25: Conversion of mevalonate into isoprenoid units

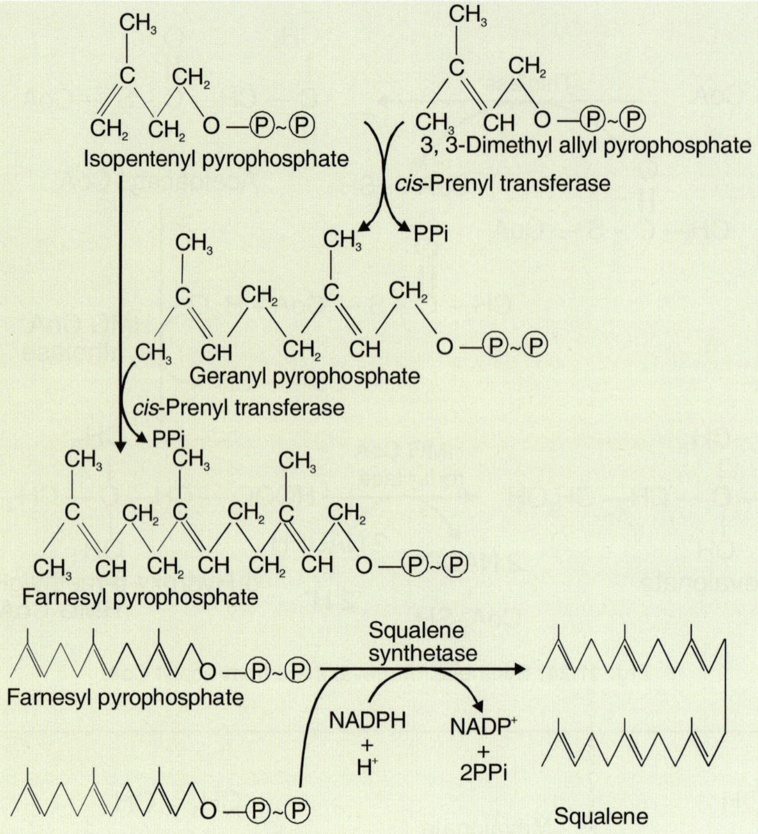

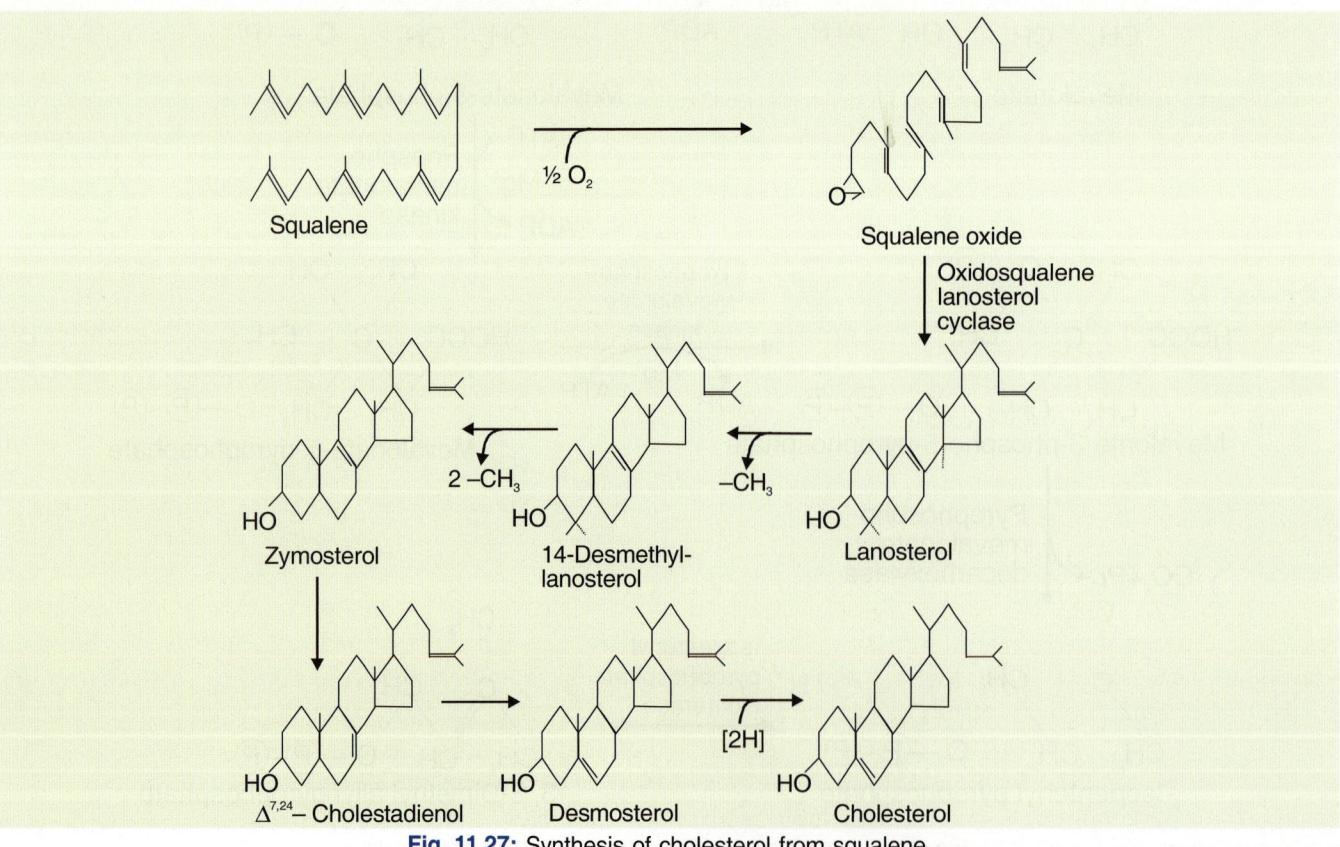

Fig. 11.26: Synthesis of squalene from isoprenoid units

Fig. 11.27: Synthesis of cholesterol from squalene

where they are utilised. Glycerol is transported to liver via circulation. After loss of triglycerides, apoproteins A and C are transferred from chylomicrons to HDL, and chylomicrons are converted into small '**chylomicron remnants**'.The chylomicron remnants are taken up by the liver cells with the help of a receptor specifc for apoprotein E. Chylomicron remnants are catabolised in liver (Fig. 11.30).

Metabolism of VLDL

Synthesis of VLDL is very similar to that of chylomicrons with the difference that the site of synthesis is liver. Nascent VLDL contains only apoprotein **B-100**. It acquires apoproteins **C** and **E** in circulation from HDL, and is converted into VLDL. Catabolism of VLDL is also similar to that of chylomicrons. After hydrolysis of a major portion of triglycerides, apoprotein C is transferred to HDL, and VLDL are converted into VLDL remnants or IDL (intermediate density lipoproteins). Nearly half of the

VLDL remnants are taken up by liver cells with the help of an **apoprotein E-specific receptor**, and are catabolised. The rest are converted into LDL (Fig. 11.31).

Metabolism of LDL

LDL is synthesised from IDL in plasma. It is rich in cholesterol. The only apoprotein present in LDL is B-100. Apoprotein B-100 is made up of a single long polypeptide chain which is wrapped around the LDL particle. Only one molecule of apoprotein B-100 is present in one LDL particle.

Catabolism of LDL occurs mainly in extrahepatic tissues. LDL is taken up by the cells with the help of LDL receptors which are specific for apoprotein B-100. The receptors bind LDL, and the receptor-LDL complex enters the cell by endocytosis. Apoprotein B-100 and cholesteryl esters are hydrolysed by lysosomal enzymes. The free receptors can return to the cell membrane.

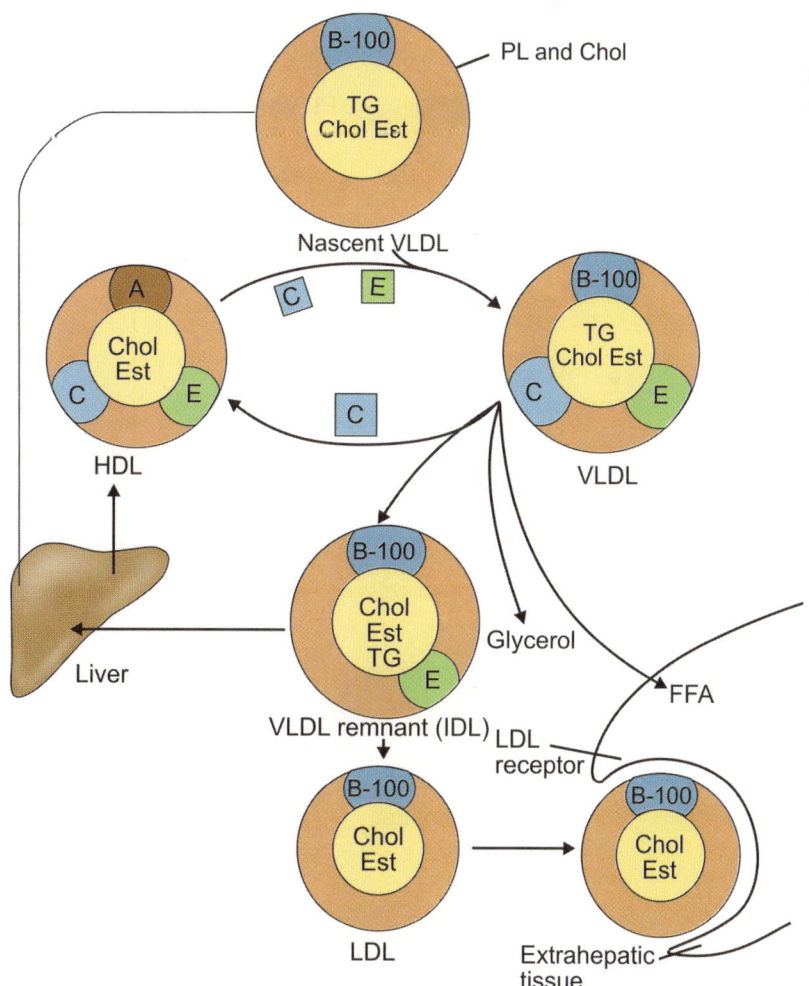

Fig. 11.31: Metabolism of VLDL and LDL (VLDL-very low density lipoprotein; LDL-low density lipoprotein; HDL-high density lipoprotein; IDL-intermediate density lipoprotein; A-apoprotein A; B-100, apoprotein B-100; C-apoprotein C; E-apoprotein E; TG-triglyceride; PL-phospholipid; Chol- free cholesterol; Chol Est-cholesteryl ester; FFA-free fatty acid)

Metabolism of HDL

HDL is synthesised in **liver** and **intestine**. The newly synthesised HDL is known as 'nascent HDL'. Nascent HDL formed in liver contains apoproteins A-I, C-I, C-II, C-III and E. Nascent HDL formed in the intestine contains apoprotein A-I and acquires apoproteins C and E after entering the circulation. Nascent HDL is disc-shaped, and consists of a phospholipid bilayer, free cholesterol and apoproteins. An enzyme, **lecithin cholesterol acyl transferase (LCAT)** is also present on the surface of HDL.

After entering the circulation, LCAT is activated by **apoprotein A-I** of nascent HDL. LCAT transfers a fatty acid from lecithin to cholesterol converting them into lysolecithin and cholesteryl ester, respectively. Lysolecithin is released into circulation. Cholesteryl esters accumulate in the interior and push the phospholipids outwards converting the disc-shaped particle into spherical and mature HDL_3. HDL_3 takes up cholesterol from extra-hepatic tissues and from the circulating chylomicrons and VLDL, and is converted into HDL_2. HDL_2 transfers cholesterol to liver, and is reconverted into HDL_3. Thus, the **HDL_2-HDL_3 cycle** serves to transport cholesterol from the extrahepatic tissues to liver (Fig. 11.32).

Cholesteroyl ester transfer protein (CETP), also known as plasma lipid transfer protein, is a protein present in plasma which transfers lipids between different lipoproteins, e.g. exchange of triglycerides present in LDL and VLDL with cholesteroyl esters present in HDL. It can also exchange triglycerides with triglycerides or cholesteroyl esters with cholesteroyl ester.

INHERITED DISORDERS OF LIPOPROTEIN METABOLISM

Inherited disorders of lipoprotein metabolism (dyslipoproteinaemias) may be divided into hypolipoproteinaemia and hyperlipoproteinaemia.

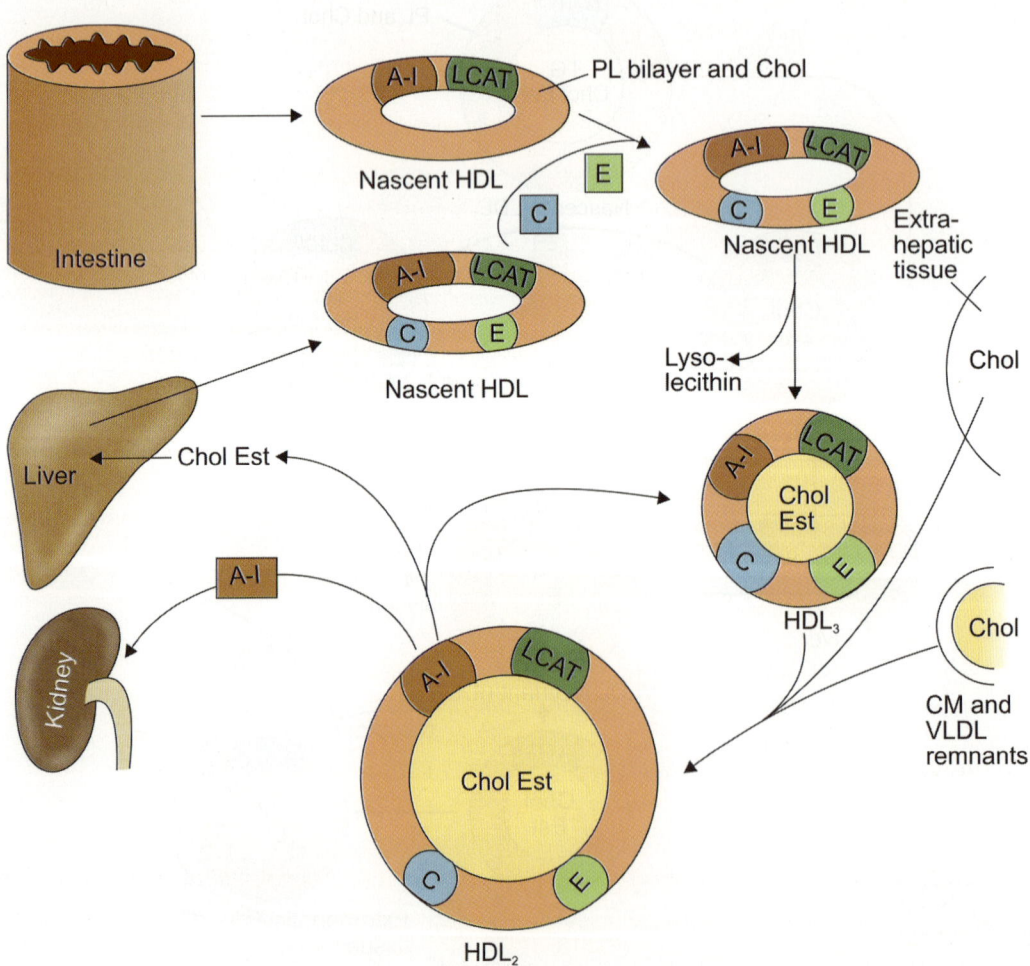

Fig. 11.32: Metabolism of HDL (HDL-high density lipoprotein; CM-chylomicron; VLDL-very low density lipoprotein; A-I-apoprotein A-I; C-apoprotein C; E-apoprotein E; PL-phospholipid; Chol-cholesterol; Chol Est-cholesteryl ester; LCAT-lecithin cholesterol acyl transferase)

Hypolipoproteinaemia

This group includes disorders in which the concentration of one or more lipoproteins in plasma is decreased. The disorders are:

Abetalipoproteinaemia

This is a rare autosomal recessive disorder. There is a defect in the **incorporation of lipids** in the lipoproteins containing **apoprotein B,** i.e. chylomicrons, VLDL and LDL. These lipoproteins are absent or greatly decreased in plasma. Serum cholesterol and triglycerides are very low. Transport of dietary lipids (and fat-soluble vitamins) from the intestine to various tissues is impaired. Availability of fatty acids is decreased. Synthesis of cholesterol, glycolipids and sphingomyelin is decreased. Many patients die in childhood. Those who survive develop steatorrhoea, intestinal malabsorption, neurological abnormalities and retinitis pigmentosa.

Hypobetalipoproteinaemia

This is an autosomal dominant disorder. The defect is decreased synthesis of apoprotein B. Plasma LDL and cholesterol are low. Clinical abnormalities are mild and compatible with life.

Hypoalphalipoproteinaemia

This is an autosomal recessive disorder of α-lipoprotein (HDL) metabolism. It is also known as Tangier disease as it was first discovered on the **Tangier island**. Synthesis of apoprotein A is decreased resulting in a decreased level of HDL in plasma and impaired transport of cholesterol. Cholesterol is deposited in liver, spleen, tonsils, lymph nodes and other reticuloendothelial tissues. Risk of atherosclerotic diseases is increased. Mild neurological abnormalities are also common.

Hyperlipoproteinaemia

A classification of hyperlipoproteinaemias of genetic origin was proposed by Frederickson and his associates in 1967. It was slightly modified by WHO in 1970. In the WHO classification, hyperlipoproteinaemia is divided into six types on the basis of plasma levels of lipids and lipoproteins after a 14-hour fast and the appearance of serum after standing it for 48 hours (serum storage test). Characteristic features of these hyperlipoproteinaemias are summarised in Table 11.1. All of these, except type I, are associated with an increased risk of atherosclerotic diseases.

A hyperlipoproteinaemia, termed as hyperalphalipoproteinaemia, has also been identified in which plasma HDL (α-lipoprotein) is congenitally raised. This is a beneficial condition because a high level of HDL protects against atherosclerotic diseases.

SERUM LIPIDS, LIPOPROTEINS AND ATHEROSCLEROSIS

Atherosclerosis is a condition in which cholesterol and some other substances are deposited in the walls of blood vessels leading to a narrowing of the lumen of the affected

Table 11.1: Classification of hyperlipoproteinaemia (WHO, 1970)

	Type I	Type IIa	Type IIb	Type III	Type IV	Type V
CM	Present	Absent	Absent	Absent	Absent	Present
VLDL	Normal or mildly ↑	Normal	↑	↑	↑	↑
LDL	Normal or mildly ↑	↑	↑	↑ (Broad β-band)	Normal	Normal
HDL	Normal	Normal	Normal	Normal	Normal	Normal
Serum cholesterol	Normal or mildly ↑	↑	↑	↑	Normal or mildly ↑	↑
Serum triglycerides	↑	Normal	↑	↑	↑	↑
Appearance (serum storage test)	Creamy top over clear infranatant	Clear	Turbid	Turbid	Turbid	Creamy top over turbid infranatant
Genetic defect	Lipoprotein lipase deficient	LDL receptors deficient	Variant of type IIa	Abnormal apo E, CM and VLDL remnants not removed	Not known, associated with diabetes and obesity	Not known

vessels. This impedes the blood flow and decreases the supply of blood to the affected organs. Coronary arteries are affected most commonly leading to **ischaemic heart disease** (IHD) or **coronary artery disease** (CAD). Involvement of cerebral arteries causes **cerebral thrombosis**. The arteries supplying blood to lower limbs may also be affected resulting in **peripheral vascular disease**.

The risk of atherosclerotic IHD is increased by many factors. The association between serum lipids and IHD has been proved in many epidemiological and clinical studies. There is a positive correlation between hyper-cholesterolaemia and the incidence of IHD. Cholesterol is present in plasma mainly in LDL and HDL. LDL-Cholesterol increases the risk of IHD while HDL-cholesterol has a protective effect. Recent studies have shown that measurements of apoproteins A-I and B in plasma are more informative than HDL and LDL. A rise in apoprotein B level indicates an increased risk of IHD while a rise in apoprotein A-I indicates a decreased risk.

Lp (a) is another risk factor for IHD. Lp (a) migrates with pre-β-liproprotein on electrophoresis. It is similar to LDL in lipid composition, contains apo B-100 and another apolipoprotein, apo (a). Apo (a) has a close resemblance with plasminogen in amino acid sequence. Apo (a) competes with plasminogen for binding to fibrin, and interferes with fibrinolysis. Some people have an elevated level of plasma Lp (a). Levels above 30 mg/dl increase the risk of premature IHD.

When serum cholesterol (or LDL or apoprotein B) is elevated, dietary or pharmacological measures are required to decrease the risk of IHD. The dietary measures include a reduction in total fat intake, a reduction in cholesterol intake and a reduction in the intake of saturated fatty acids while increasing the intake of PUFA. Hypocholes-terolaemic drugs which decrease serum cholesterol (and/or triglycerides) may be needed in more severe cases.

Hypocholesterolaemic Drugs

Three classes of drugs are commonly used as hypocho-lesterolaemic drugs – **bile acid-binding resins, nicotinic acid** and **inhibitors of HMG CoA reductase**. A fourth class, **fibric acid derivatives** is more effective in reducing serum triglycerides.

Bile acid-binding resins include **colestipol** and **cholestyramine**. They bind bile acids in the intestine preventing their reabsorption. Enterohepatic circulation of bile acids is interrupted. Decreased reabsorption necessitates increased synthesis of bile acids from cholesterol in the liver. Thus, more cholesterol is diverted to bile acid synthesis resulting in a decrease in serum cholesterol level.

Nicotinic acid (**niacin**) in large doses decreases the level of serum cholesterol. Mechanism of action of nicotinic

acid is not known. It decreases the secretion of lipoproteins containing apo B-100 from liver.

Statin family of drugs inhibit HMG CoA reductase and, thereby, decrease the synthesis of cholesterol. They are the most effective hypocholesterolaemic drugs with the least side effects. They also cause a modest decrease in serum triglycerides. **Lovastatin** and **mevastatin** are the oldest members of this family. The newer members include atorvastatin, fluvastatin, simvastatin, etc.

Fibric acid derivatives include **clofibrate, fenfibrate, gemfibrozil,** etc. They activate lipoprotein lipase and increase the hydrolysis of triglycerides present in the lipoproteins. VLDL concentration is decreased. Serum triglycerides are consequently decreased. They cause a modest decrease in serum cholesterol also.

EICOSANOIDS

Eicosanoids are **20-carbon** hormone-like compounds which are synthesised from polyunsaturated fatty acids, e.g. arachidonic acid. Eicosanoids include prostaglandins (PG), thromboxanes (TX) and leukotrienes (LT). Prostaglandins structurally resemble prostanoic acid, a 20-carbon fatty acid having a five-carbon ring and two side chains attached to the ring (Fig. 11.33).

The important prostaglandins are PGE_1, PGE_2, PGE_3, $PGF_{1\alpha}$, $PGF_{2\alpha}$ and $PGF_{3\alpha}$. Thromboxanes are similar in structure to prostaglandins with the difference that they have a six-membered oxane ring. The important thrombanes are TXA_1, TXA_2 and TXA_3. Leukotrienes are 20-carbon polyenoic fatty acids having a number of substituents. The most important leukotrienes are LTB_4, LTC_4, LTD_4 and LTE_4. Structures of eicosanoids were described in Chapter 4.

Synthesis of Eicosanoids

Prostaglandins E_1 and $F_{1\alpha}$, thromboxane A_1, and leuko-trienes A_3, C_3 and D_3 are synthesised from 8,11,14-eicosatrienoic acid (20:3;8,11,14) which, in turn, is synthesised from linoleic acid. Linoleic acid (18:2;9,12) is first converted into g-linolenic acid (18:3;6,9,12) by δ^6-desaturase. Then, chain elongation occurs by addition of two carbon atoms at the carboxyl end of γ-linolenic acid to convert it into 8,11,14-eicosatrienoic acid.

Prostaglandins E_2 and $F_{2\alpha}$, thromboxane A_2, and leukotrienes A_4, B_4, C_4, D_4 and E_4 are synthesised from arachidonic acid (20:4;5,8,11,14).

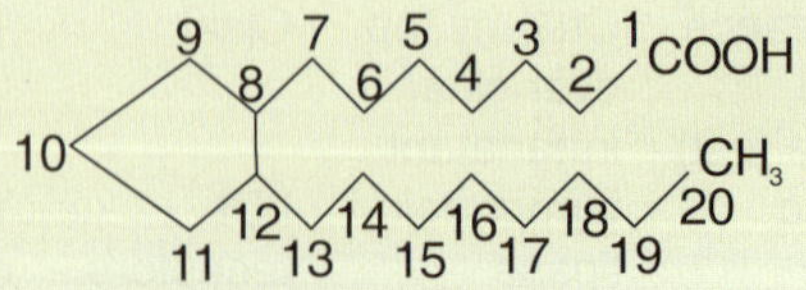

Fig. 11.33: Prostanoic acid

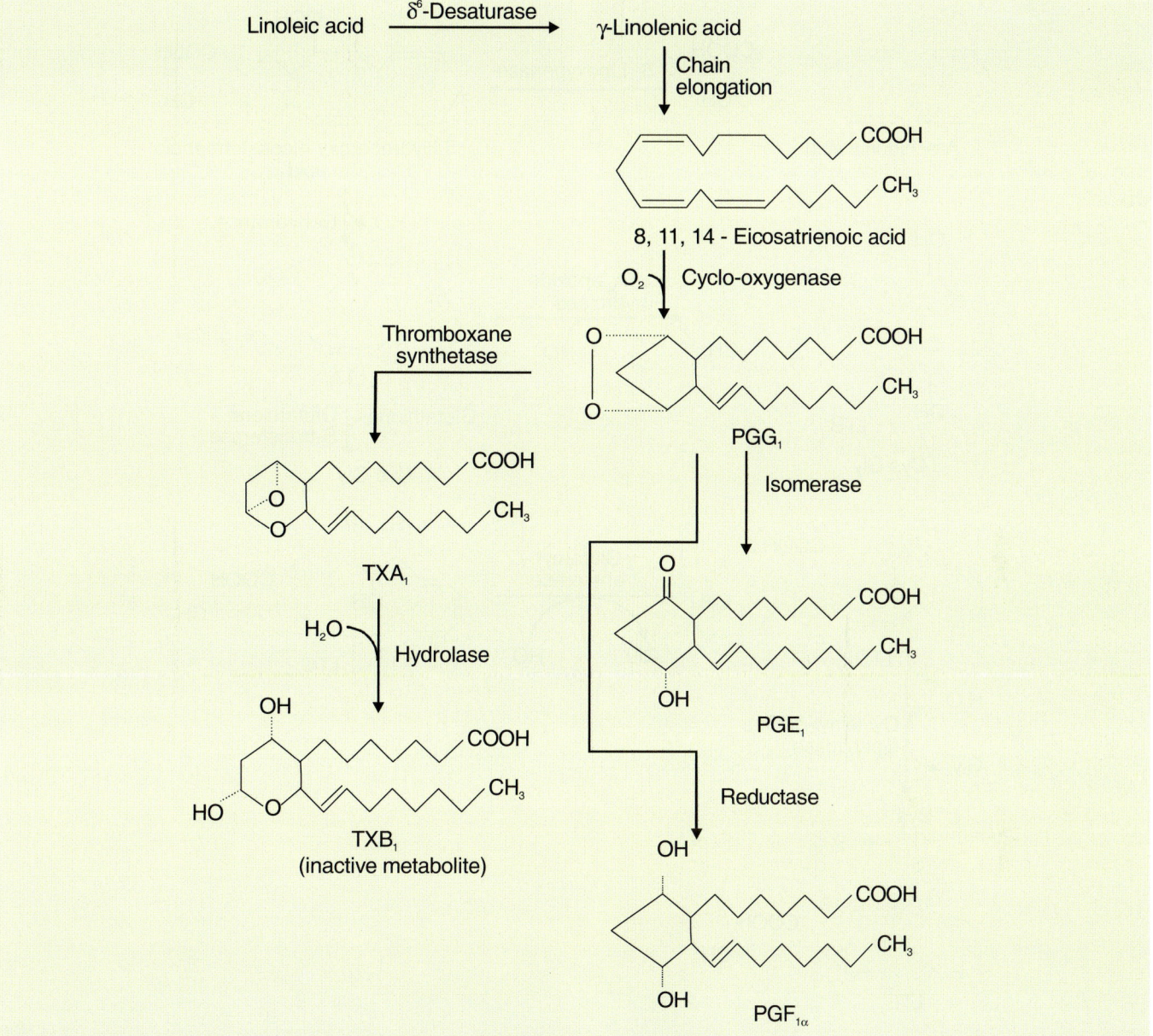

Fig. 11.34: Synthesis of prostaglandins and thromboxanes of series 1. Prostaglandins and thromboxanes of series 2 and 3 are synthesised similarly from arachidonic acid and eicosapentaenoic acid respectively

Prostaglandins E_3 and $F_{3\alpha}$, thromboxanes A_3 and leukotrienes A_5, B_5 and C_5 are synthesised from 5,8,11,14,17-eicosapentaenoic acid (20:5;5,8,11,14,17) which, in turn, is synthesised from α-linolenic acid.

α-Linolenic acid (18:3;9,12,15) is converted, by δ⁶-desaturase, into octadecatetraenoic acid (18:4;6,9, 12,15). Two carbon atoms are added at the carboxyl end by the chain elongation system to form eicosatetraenoic acid (20:4;8,11,14,17).

Finally, a double bond is introduced between carbon atoms 5 and 6 by δ⁵-desaturase to form eicosapentaenoic acid (20:5;5,8, 11,14,17).

Catabolism of Eicosanoids

Eicosanoids are very short-lived compounds. They produce their effects locally, and are quickly inactivated. Prostaglandins are inactivated by 15-hydroxyprostaglandin dehydrogenase. Thromboxanes of type A are catabolised by hydration to type B which are inactive. Inactivation of leukotrienes is not very clear.

Functions of Eicosanoids

Eicosanoids are physiologically very potent. Some of them are being used as pharmacological agents and some others are being evaluated as possible pharmacological agents.

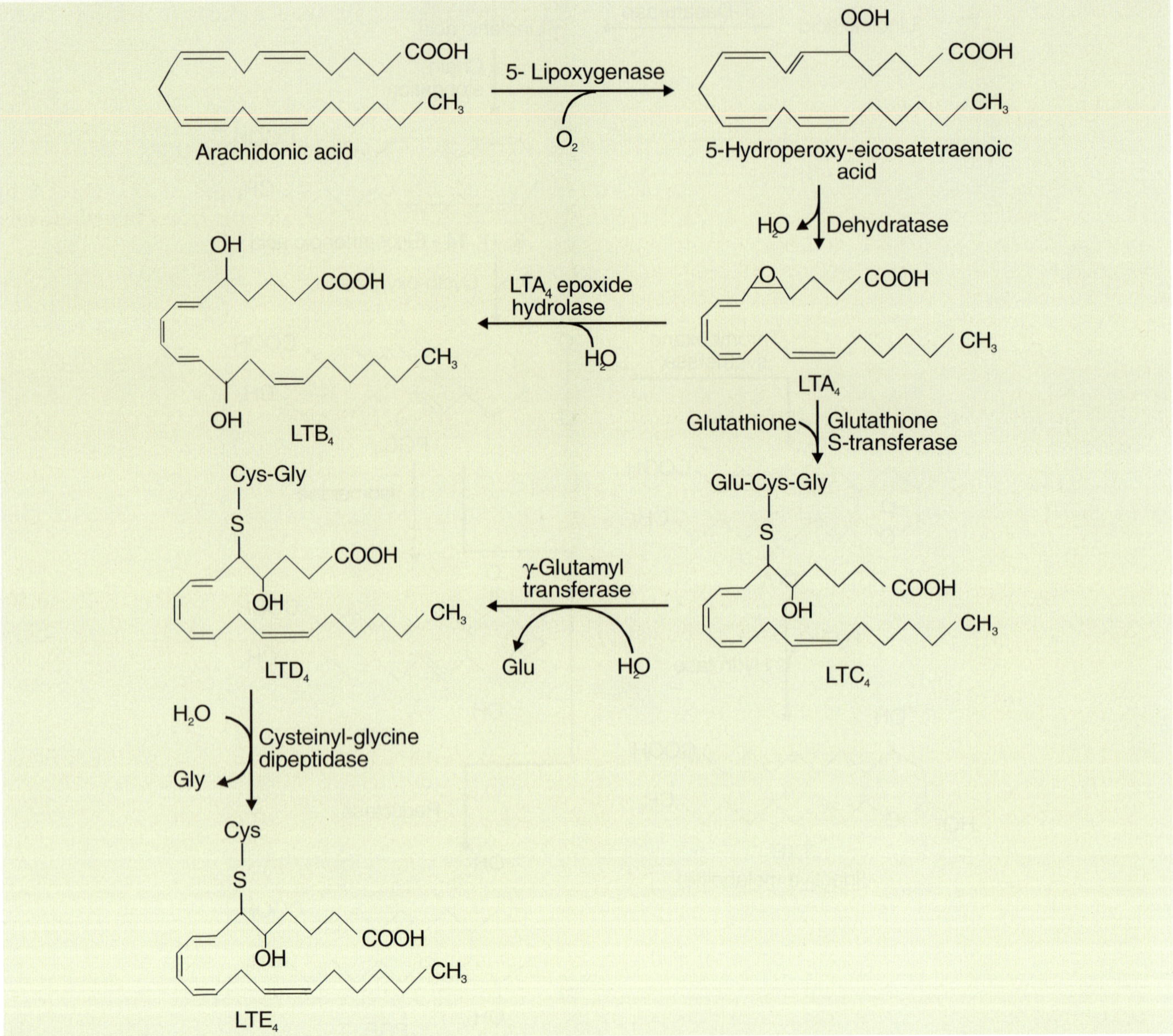

Fig. 11.35: Synthesis of leukotrienes of series 4. Series 3 and 5 are synthesised similarly from eicosatrienoic acid and eicosapentaenoic acid respectively

The effects of eicosanoids vary in different tissues, e.g. prostaglandins increase the concentration of cAMP in some tissues but decrease it in other tissues.

Actions of Prostaglandins

1. Prostaglandins inhibit lipolysis in adipose tissue.
2. They increase the contractility of uterine muscle, and induce labour.
3. They are bronchodilators and, hence, may be of pharmacological use in bronchial asthma.
4. They decrease gastric hydrochloric acid secretion.
5. They cause vasodilatation, and decrease blood pressure.

6. They increase the permeability of capillaries.
7. They inhibit aggregation of platelets.
8. They stimulate intestinal peristalsis.
9. They increase the tubular reabsorption of water and sodium.
10. They are required for spermatogenesis, maturation and transport of sperms.

Actions of Thromboxanes

1. They stimulate aggregation of platelets.
2. They cause vasoconstriction, and increase blood pressure.

Actions of Leukotrienes

1. They are powerful bronchoconstrictors. The slow reacting substance of anaphylaxis (SRS-A), which is responsible for constriction of bronchioles in bronchial asthma is, in fact, a mixture of LTC_4, LTD_4 and LTE_4.
2. They increase capillary permeability.
3. They are chemotactic agents, and attract leukocytes to the site of inflammation.

Several drugs produce their effects by inhibiting the synthesis of eicosanoids. Production of eicosanoids begins with the release of a polyunsaturated fatty acid from carbon atom 2 of glycerophospholipids present in the cell membrane.

This reaction is catalysed by phospholipase A_2. **Corticosteroids** decrease the production of all the eicosanoids by inhibiting phospholipase A_2.

Aspirin decreases the synthesis of PG and TX by irreversible inhibition of cyclo-oxygenase. **Phenylbutazone** and **indomethacin** decrease PG and TX synthesis by reversibly inhibiting cyclo-oxygenase.

EXERCISE

1. Describe β-oxidation of a 16-carbon saturated fatty acid and its energetics. What is the role of carnitine in the oxidation of fatty acids?

2. Describe de novo synthesis of palmitic acid and its regulation.

3. Describe the synthesis and oxidation of ketone bodies. Discuss the regulation of ketogenesis.

4. Describe the synthesis of cholesterol and its regulation.

5. Discuss the role of cholesterol in atherosclerosis. Describe the mechanism of action of hypocholesterolaemic drugs.

6. Describe the synthesis and catabolism of VLDL and LDL. Discuss the role of various lipoproteins in coronary artery disease.

7. Write short notes on:
   a. Ketosis
   b. Fatty liver
   c. HDL
   d. Abetalipoproteinaemia
   e. HMG CoA reductase
   f. Prostaglandins
   g. Sphingolipidoses
   h. Bile salts

8. Write 'true' or 'false':
   a. Glycerol kinase is not present in adipose tissue.
   b. Long chain fatty acids are activated in mitochondria.
   c. β-Oxidation of fatty acids occurs in mitochondria.
   d. Propionyl CoA is formed on β-oxidation of fatty acids having an odd number of carbon atoms.
   e. Unsaturated fatty acids cannot undergo β-oxidation.
   f. α-Oxidation of fatty acids is defective in Refsum's disease.
   g. De novo synthesis of fatty acids occurs in cytosol.
   h. Acetyl CoA synthetase is activated by citrate, and is inhibited by palmityl CoA.
   i. Monounsaturated fatty acids can be synthesised in human beings.
   j. Arachidonic acid can be synthesised from linoleic acid.
   k. Hormone-sensitive lipase is activated by insulin.
   l. Sphingosine is synthesised from palmityl CoA and methionine.
   m. Sphingomyelinase is deficient in Gaucher's disease.
   n. Chronic alcoholism can cause fatty liver.
   o. Ketosis can occur in starvation and uncontrolled diabetes mellitus.
   p. Vitamin C is required for synthesis of cholesterol.
   q. Lecithin cholesterol acyl transferase is activated by apoprotein C-II.
   r. HDL decreases the risk of coronary artery disease.
   s. Lovastatin and mevastatin inhibit HMG CoA reductase.
   t. Aspirin decreases the synthesis of eicosanoids by inhibiting phospholipase A_2.

9. Fill in the blanks:
   a. Pancreatic lipase is activated by .... and ....
   b. ATP is converted into .... during activation of fatty acids.
   c. Carnitine is required for entry of fatty acids into ....
   d. End product of β-oxidation of fatty acids having an even number of carbon atoms is ....
   e. α-Oxidation of fatty acids occurs mainly in ....
   f. Multienzyme complex for de novo synthesis of fatty acids consists of ....and seven enzymes.
   g. The end product of de novo synthesis of fatty acids is ....
   h. HMP shunt is the major source of .... for the synthesis of fatty acids.
   i. Synthesis of acetyl CoA carboxylase is induced by ....
   j. Deficiency of .... causes generalised gangliosidosis.
   k. .... is deficient in Niemann-Pick disease.
   l. Lipotropic factors are required for the transport of lipids out of ....
   m. Ketone bodies are synthesised in ....and are utilised in ....
   n. HMG CoA is regulated by .... as well as ....
   o. Ascorbic acid is required for the conversion of .... into bile acids.
   p. Chylomicrons transport .... from the intestine to peripheral tissues.
   q. .... transports cholesterol from peripheral tissues to liver.
   r. LDL receptors are specific for ....
   s. Apo B-100 is the only apoprotein present in ....
   t. Corticosteroids decrease the production of eicosanoids by inhibiting ....

ANSWERS TO SHORT QUESTIONS

8. a. True
   c. True
   e. False
   g. True
   i. True
   k. False
   m. False
   o. True
   q. False
   s. True

   b. False
   d. True
   f. True
   h. True
   j. True
   l. False
   n. True
   p. False
   r. True
   t. False

9. a. Co-lipase, phospholipids
   c. Mitochondria
   e. Brain
   g. Palmitic acid
   i. Insulin
   k. Sphingomyelinase
   m. Liver, extrahepatic tissues
   o. Cholesterol
   q. HDL
   s. LDL

   b. AMP
   d. Acetyl CoA
   f. Acyl carrier protein
   h. NADPH
   j. G_{M1}-gangliosidase
   l. Liver
   n. Covalent modification, repression-derepression
   p. Triglycerides
   r. Apo B-100
   t. Phospholipase A_2

12

Metabolism of Amino Acids

Carbohydrates, lipids and proteins are known as the proximate principles of diet as they can provide energy. While monosaccharides and fatty acids are metabolised mainly to provide energy, provision of energy is not the primary purpose of amino acid metabolism. Amino acids are used mainly to form various structural and functional proteins and, to some extent, some specialised non-protein products. If the availability of carbohydrates and lipids is low or if the availability of amino acids is very high, the amino acids can be used as a source of energy.

Amino acids are obtained from:
1. Digestion of dietary proteins,
2. Breakdown of body proteins, and
3. Endogenous synthesis.

The amino acids are used for:
1. Synthesis of body proteins,
2. Synthesis of non-protein specialised products, and
3. Provision of energy.

In plasma as well as in tissues, there is an amino acid pool to which amino acids are continuously added and from which amino acids are continuously removed.

Nitrogen Balance

Proteins are the main nitrogenous constitutent of our diet. Proteins are broken down into amino acids. Catabolism of amino acids results in the release of their amino groups in the form of ammonia. In human beings and other mammals, ammonia is converted into urea which is excreted in urine. Urea is the main nitrogenous compound excreted from the body. Thus, nitrogen is mostly taken in as proteins and excreted mainly as urea. The relative intake and excretion of nitrogen is known as the nitrogen balance.

In healthy adults, nitrogen excretion equals nitrogen intake, and the person is said to be in **nitrogen equilibrium**. In growing age, amino acids are used to form tissue proteins. Therefore, nitrogen excretion is less than the intake, and the individual is said to be in a **positive nitrogen balance**. In starvation and wasting diseases, there is excessive breakdown of body proteins. Nitrogen excretion exceeds the intake, and the individual is said to be in **negative nitrogen balance**.

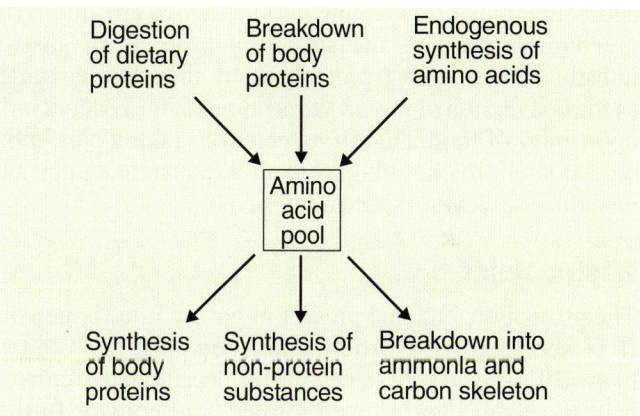

Fig. 12.1: Addition to and removal from amino acid pool

ESSENTIAL AND NON-ESSENTIAL AMINO ACIDS

Proteins are synthesised from twenty L-amino acids (standard amino acids). All these amino acids are equally important for protein synthesis is. However, the presence of all these amino acids in diet is not imperative as some of these can be synthesised in human beings. Those amino acids which cannot be synthesised by human beings are said to be nutritionally essential or indispensable, and their presence in diet is imperative. These include valine, leucine, isoleucine, threonine, methionine, lysine, phenylalanine and tryptophan. Two amino acids, arginine and histidine, are said to be semi-essential as their endogenous synthesis is not sufficient to meet the requirements of protein synthesis in growing age. The remaining amino acids can be synthesised in the body in adequate amounts, and are considered to be nutritionally non-essential or dispensable.

Our study of amino acid metabolism will include:
1. Digestion of proteins and absorption of amino acids,
2. Synthesis of non- and semi-essential amino acids,
3. Catabolism of amino acids (disposal of amino groups and catabolism of carbon skeletons of amino acids),
4. Synthesis of non-protein specialised products from amino acids, and
5. Inborn errors of amino acid metabolism.

DIGESTION AND ABSORPTION

Proteins are macromolecules. Dietary proteins have to be hydrolysed into amino acids in the alimentary tract as only amino acids can be absorbed by the intestinal mucosa. A large variety of proteins are present in the diet but the number of proteolytic enzymes in digestive secretions is small. These enzymes are specific for peptide bonds and not for the actual substrate. Some are **endopeptidases** and some are **exopeptidases**. The proteolytic enzymes are generally secreted in the form of inactive **precursors (proenzymes)** in which the catalytic site is concealed by a portion of the polypeptide chain of the enzyme itself. Removal of the covering peptide reveals the catalytic site, and converts the proenzyme into the active enzyme. This mechanism protects the structural proteins of gastro-intestinal tract against proteolysis by digestive enzymes as the conversion of proenzymes into enzymes occurs only upon entry of food. Digestive secretions taking part in the digestion of proteins are gastric juice, pancreatic juice and intestinal secretion (succus entericus).

Gastric Juice

The proteolytic enzyme present in gastric juice is **pepsin**. It is secreted as a proenzyme, pepsinogen. Gastric hydrochloric acid splits a peptide off pepsinogen to convert it into pepsin. Pepsin, once formed, can convert further molecules of pepsinogen into pepsin. Pepsin is an endopeptidase which hydrolyses internal peptide bonds of proteins to convert them into polypeptides. It acts preferentially on peptide bonds formed by aromatic and dicarboxylic amino acids.

Another enzyme, **rennin** is present in the gastric juice of infants which acts on casein of milk, and converts it into calcium paracaseinate. The latter is hydrolysed by pepsin into polypeptides.

Pancreatic Juice

The proteolytic enzymes present in pancreatic juice are **trypsin, chymotrypsin, elastase** and **carboxypeptidase**.

These are initially secreted as trypsinogen, chymotrypsinogen, proelastase and procarboxypeptidase respectively which are proenzymes. Trypsinogen is converted into trypsin by enterokinase. Trypsin can convert further molecules of trypsinogen into trypsin. Trypsin also converts chymotrypsinogen into chymotrypsin, proelastase into elastase, and procarboxypeptidase into carboxypeptidase.

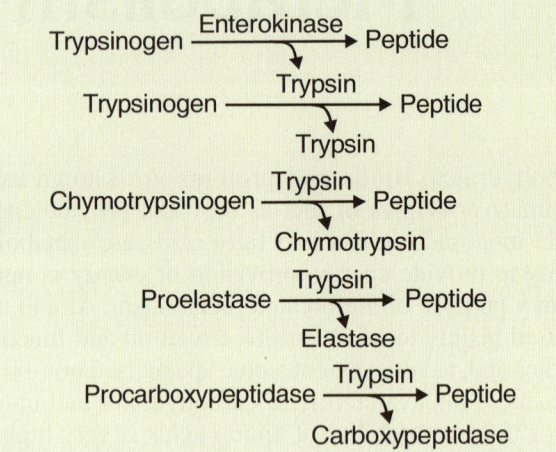

Trypsin, chymotrypsin and elastase are endopeptidases which hydrolyse proteins and polypeptides into small peptides. Trypsin acts preferentially on peptide bonds formed by basic amino acids. Chymotrypsin acts preferentially on peptide bonds in which the carboxyl group is contributed by aromatic amino acids. Elastase acts preferentially on peptide bonds in which the carboxyl group is contributed by glycine, alanine or serine.

Carboxypeptidase is an exopeptidase which removes amino acids one by one from the carboxyl end of proteins and peptides.

Intestinal Secretion

Intestinal secretion contains an **aminopeptidase** and several **dipeptidases**. Aminopeptidase is an exopeptidase which removes amino acids one by one from the amino end. Dipeptidases hydrolyse dipeptides into amino acids.

The final products of digestion of proteins are L-amino acids which are absorbed by the mucosal cells of the small intestine. The absorption is active and energy-requiring. Several active transport systems are present for absorption of different groups of amino acids. Some of these transport systems are linked with sodium pump in the same way as the active transport system for glucose (SGLT 1).

SYNTHESIS OF NON- AND SEMI-ESSENTIAL AMINO ACIDS

These amino acids can be synthesised in human beings from amphibolic intermediates (intermediates common to catabolism and anabolism) or from some other amino acids.

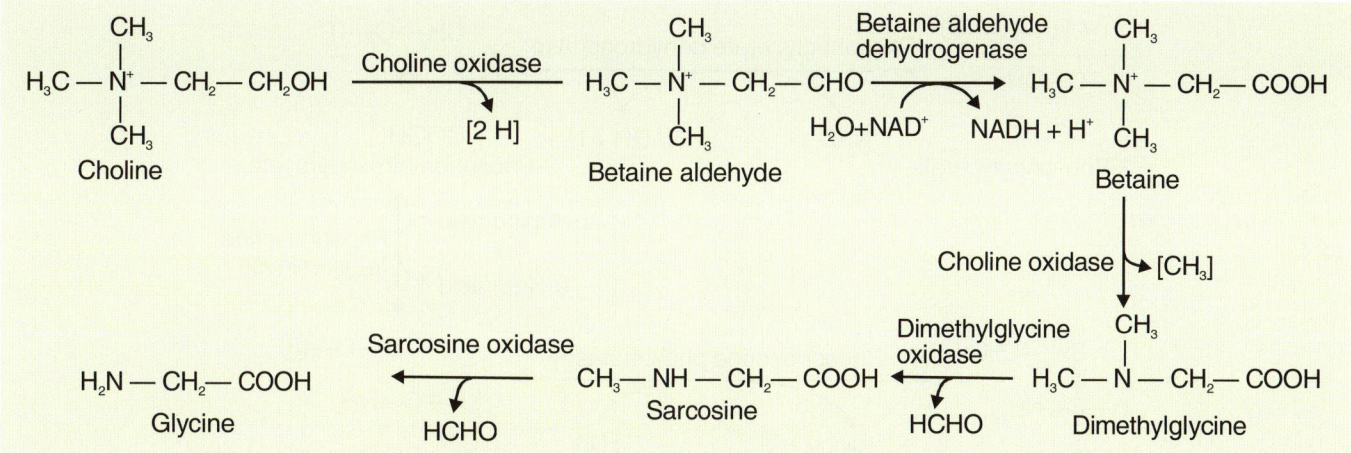

Fig. 12.2: Synthesis of glycine from choline

From Amphibolic Intermediates

Glycine, alanine, serine, aspartate and glutamate can be synthesised from amphibolic intermediates.

Glycine

Glycine can be synthesised from choline (Fig. 12.2). The hydroxymethyl group of choline is oxidised to a carboxyl group and three methyl groups are removed.

Alanine

Alanine can be synthesised from pyruvate by the transamination reaction catalysed by glutamate pyruvate transaminase (GPT) in the presence of pyridoxal phosphate.The amino group of glutamate is transferred to pyruvate. and the keto group of pyruvate is transferred to glutamate (Fig.12.3).

Aspartate

Aspartate can be synthesised from oxaloacetate by transamination. The reaction is catalysed by glutamate oxaloacetate transaminase (GOT) in the presence of pyridoxal phosphate (FIg.12.3).

Glutamate

Glutamate can be synthesised from α-ketoglutarate, an intermediate in citric acid cycle, in an NADPH-dependent reaction catalysed by glutamate dehydrogenase. There is an NAD-dependent glutamate dehydrogenase also which probably catalyses the reverse reaction (Fig.12.3).

Serine

Serine can be synthesised from 3-phosphoglycerate, an intermediate of glycolysis (Fig. 12.4).

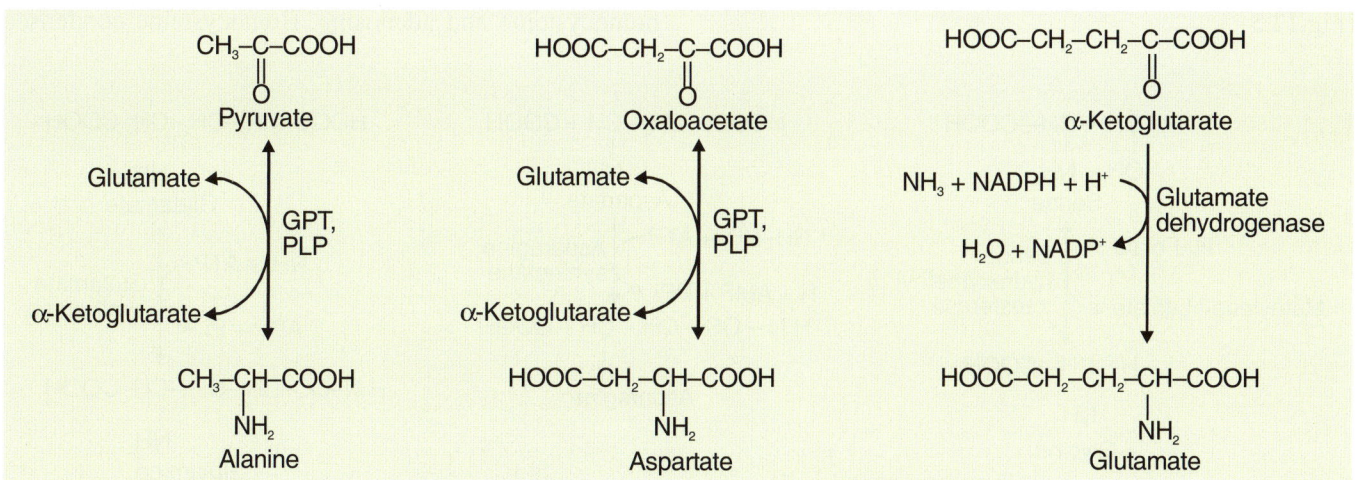

Fig. 12.3: Synthesis of alanine, aspartate and glutamate

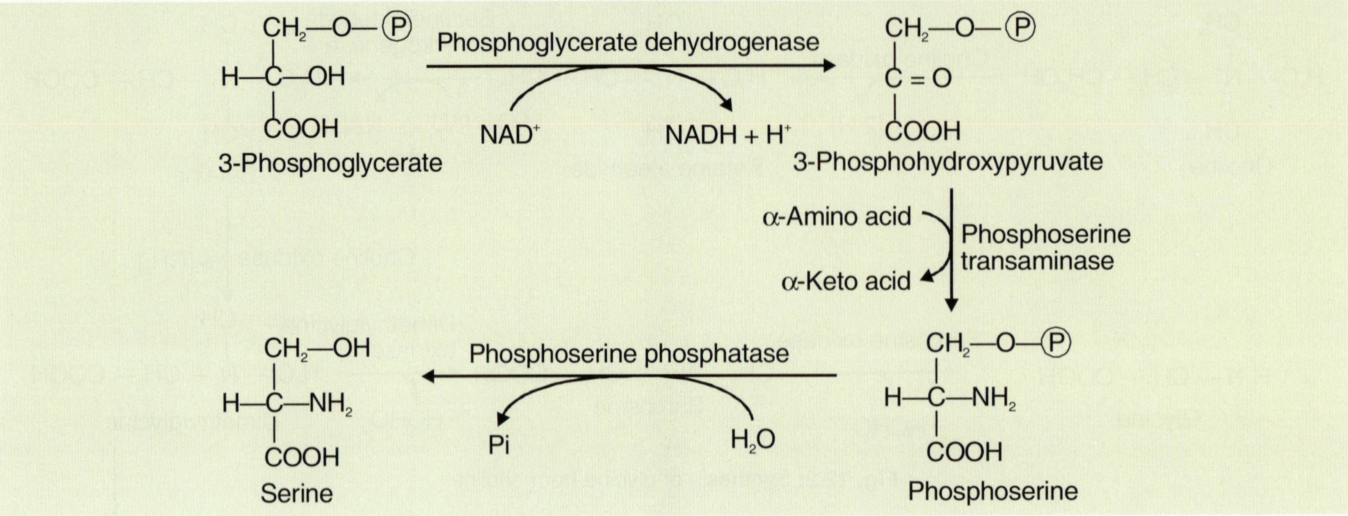

Fig. 12.4: Synthesis of serine from 3-phosphoglycerate

From other Amino Acids

Several amino acids can be synthesised from other essential or non-essential amino acids.

Glycine

Glycine can be synthesised from serine (Fig. 12.5).

Serine

Serine can be synthesised from glycine as the reaction catalysed by serine hydroxymethyl transferase is reversible.

Asparagine

Asparagine can be synthesised from aspartate and a donor of amino group ($RH–NH_2$) which is generally glutamine. The energy for the formation of the covalent bond is provided by hydrolysis of ATP into AMP and PPi (Fig.12.5).

Glutamine

Glutamine is synthesised from glutamate and free ammonia. Energy is provided by hydrolysis of ATP into ADP and Pi (Fig.12.5).

Cysteine

Cysteine can be synthesised from methionine and serine which are converted into homoserine and cysteine respectively. In the first reaction, methionine reacts with ATP to form S-Adenosyl methionine (SAM; active methionine). ATP is converted into adenosine in this reaction. This is the only reaction in which all the phosphate groups of ATP are removed, two in the form of inorganic pyrophosphate and one as inorganic phosphate (Fig.12.6). S-Adenosyl methionine acts as a donor of labile methyl groups in a number of methylation reactions. Specfic methyl transferases transfer the methyl group from SAM to different acceptors converting SAM into S-adenosyl homocysteine. The latter is hydrolysed into homocysteine and adenosine. Homocysteine condenses

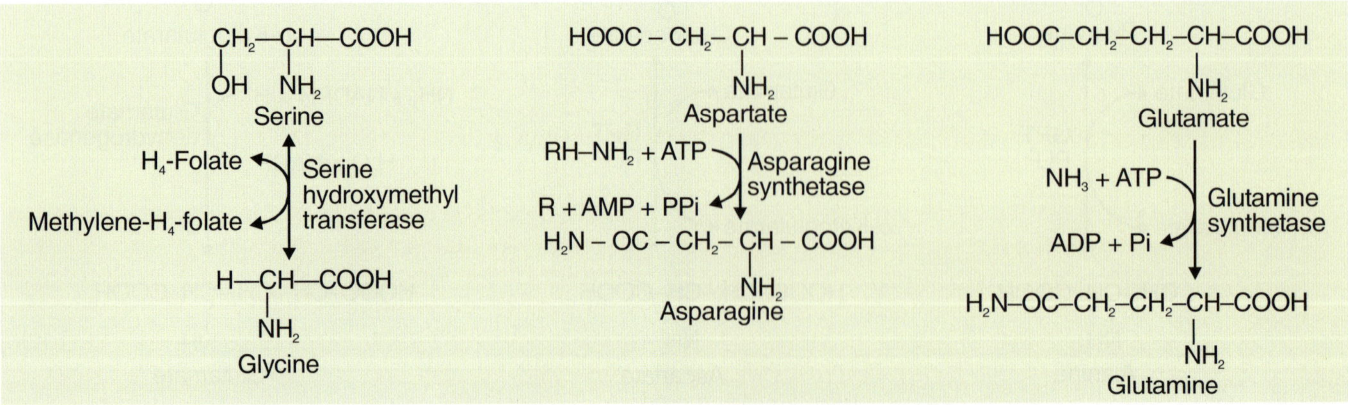

Fig. 12.5: Synthesis of glycine, asparagine and glutamine

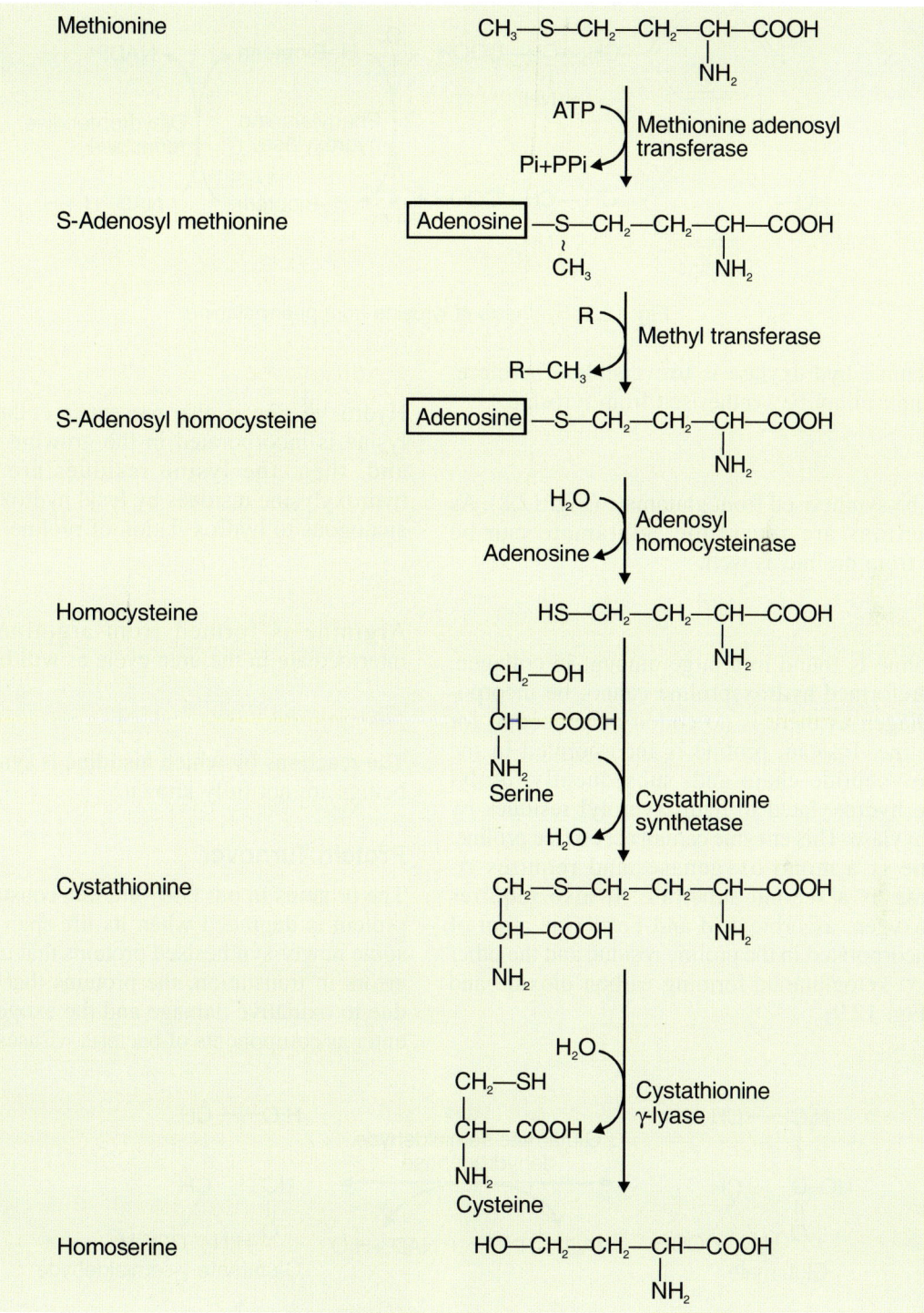

Fig. 12.6: Synthesis of cysteine

with serine to form cystathionine which splitts into cysteine and homoserine.

Tyrosine

Tyrosine can be synthesised by hydroxylation of phenylalanine. The reaction is catalysed by phenylalanine hydroxylase which is a mono-oxygenase. One atom of

molecular oxygen is incorporated in phenylalanine and the other is reduced to water. The two hydrogen atoms for formation of water are provided by tetrahydrobiopterin (H_4-biopterin) which is oxidised to dihydrobiopterin (H_2-biopterin). H_4-Biopterin is regenerated from H_2-biopterin by transfer of two hydrgen atoms from NADPH. Dihydropteridine reductase catalyses the reduction of H_2-biopterin to H_4-biopterin (Fig. 12.7). The reaction catlysed

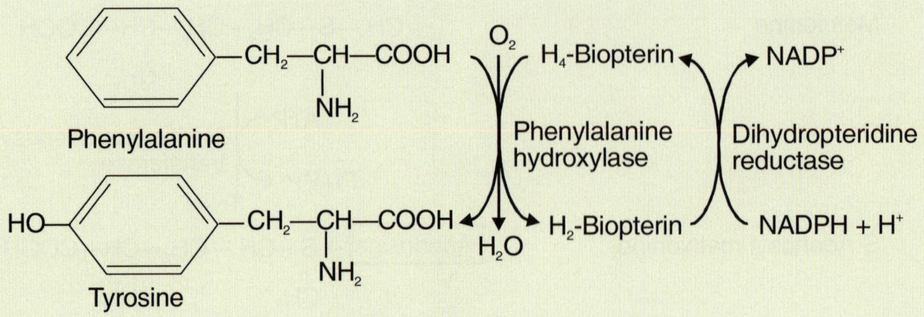

Fig. 12.7: Synthesis of tyrosine from phenylalanine

by phenylalanine hydroxylase is irreversible. Therefore, phenylalanine can not be synthesised from tyrosine.

Proline

Proline can be synthesised from glutamate (Fig. 12.8). As all the reactions are reversible, glutamate can be synthesised from proline as well.

Hydroxyproline

Hydroxyproline is found in a large amount in collagen. However, preformed hydroxyproline cannot be incorporated in collagen as there is no codon or anticodon for hydroxyproline. Instead, proline is incorporated in the growing polypeptide chain and, subsequently, prolyl residues are hydroxylated to hydroxyprolyl residues by prolyl hydroxylase. This enzyme cannot act on free proline. The enzyme is a mono-oxygenase, and requires α-ketoglutarate as a second substrate. It also requires molecular oxygen, ascorbic acid and Fe++. One atom of oxygen is incorporated in the proline residue and the other reacts with α-ketoglutarate forming carbon dioxide and succinate (Fig. 12.9).

Hydroxylysine

Hydroxylysine is also present in collagen. Like proline, lysine is incorporated in the growing polypeptide chain and, then, the lysine residues are hydroxylated to hydroxylysine residues by lysyl hydroxylase in a reaction analogous to hydroxylation of proline residues.

Arginine

Arginine is formed from argininosuccinate as an intermediate in the urea cycle as will be seen later.

Histidine

The reactions by which histidine is synthesised in human beings are not fully known.

Protein Turnover

The proteins in our body are in a constant state of flux. A protein is degraded when its life-span is over. However, some newly-synthesised proteins that are defective due to errors in translation, the proteins that become defective due to oxidative damage and the exogenous proteins that enter as components of bacteria, viruses, etc. are promptly

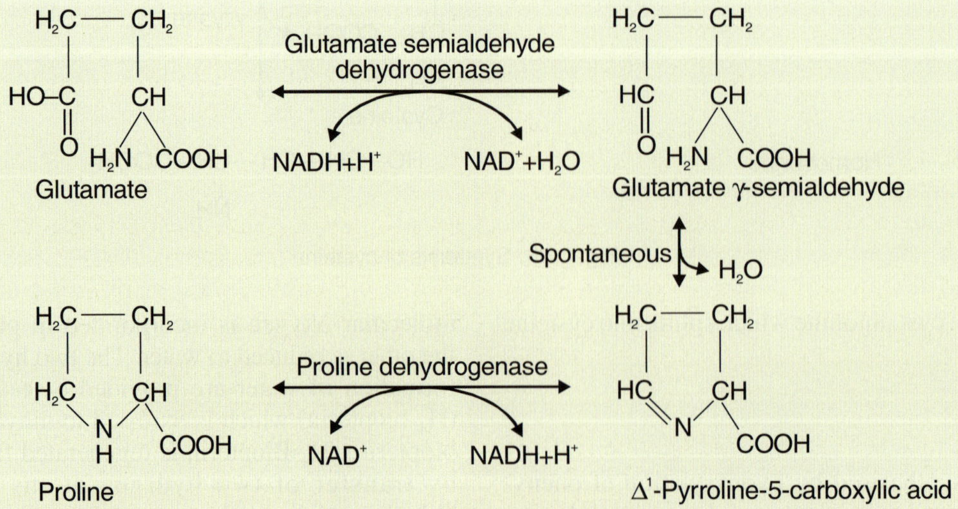

Fig. 12.8: Synthesis of proline

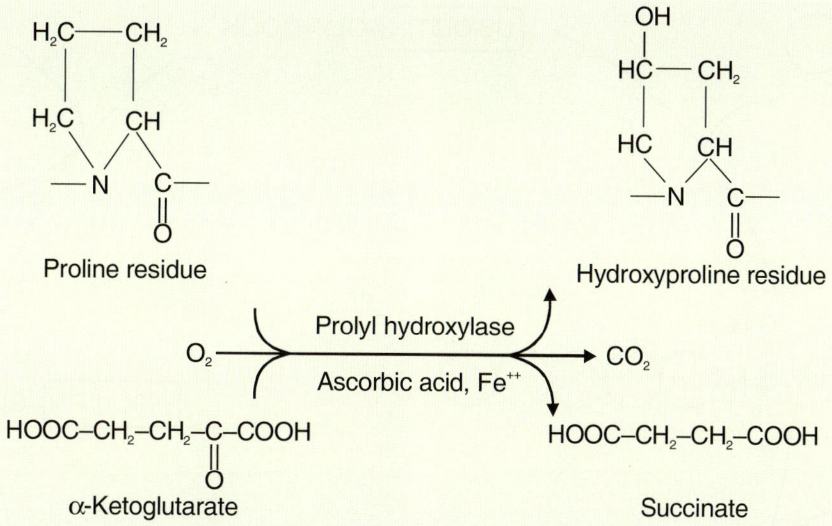

Fig. 12.9: Hydroxylation of a proline residue

degraded. There are two different pathways for degradation of proteins–lysosomal degradation and cytosolic degradation.

Lysosomal Degradation

Lysosomal proteolytic enzymes (cathepsins) hydrolyse proteins having long half-lives, circulating proteins, membrane proteins and the exogenous microbial proteins residing in endosomes. No energy is required for lysosomal hydrolysis of proteins. Loss of sialic acid from the prosthetic group of circulating glycoproteins destines them for destruction. These proteins are taken up by hepatocytes with the help of **asialoglycoprotein receptors**.

Cytosolic Degradation

Proteins having short half-lives, defective proteins, and exogenous proteins of most viruses and some bacteria are degraded in the cytosol. The degradation is ATP-dependent, and requires **26 S protease complex** (proteasome), three other enzymes (ENZ_1, ENZ_2 and ENZ_3) and **ubiquitin** (Fig. 12.10). Ubiquitin is a ubiquitous protein found in all organisms. It is made up of 76 amino acids, and has a molecular weight of 8,500. There is very little difference in the primary structure of ubiquitin in different species. Its C-terminal residue is glycine which forms a peptide bond with the epsilon-amino group of a lysine residue of the target protein to be degraded. If there are more than one lysine residues in the target protein, several ubiquitin molecules may be attached to it. First, the C-terminal glycine residue of ubiquitin forms a thioester bond with the –SH group of ENZ_1 in a reaction driven by hydrolysis of ATP into AMP and PPi. In the second reaction, ENZ_1 is replaced by ENZ_2. In the presence of ENZ_3, ENZ_2 is replaced by the target protein. Once the

target protein is tagged with ubiquitin, it is destined for destruction. The 26 S protease complex hydrolyses the target protein. Ubiquitin is not hydrolysed and is recycled

Half-lives of Proteins

Half-lives of proteins vary over a wide range. Regulatory enzymes usually have half-lives of minutes, circulating proteins have half-lives of days to months while structural proteins have half-lives of years. Half-life of a protein depends upon its N-terminal amino acid. Proteins having methionine, valine, glycine, threonine or serine at their N-terminus have long half-lives. Proteins having arginine, histidine, lysine, phenylalanine or aspartate at their N-terminus have short half-lives. A protein is degraded when its life-span is over. ENZ_3 recognises the N-terminal amino acid of the protein and targets it for degradation.

In adult human beings, the protein turnover is 1–2%, i.e. 1–2% of the body proteins are degraded and replaced by newly-synthesised proteins everyday. Three-fourths of the amino acids released from breakdown of proteins are reutilised and the rest are catabolised.

CATABOLISM OF AMINO ACIDS

Catabolism of amino acids includes catabolism of their amino groups and catabolism of their carbon skeletons. While carbon skeletons of different amino acids have different fates, the fate of their amino groups is the same. The amino groups are removed as **ammonia**. Since ammonia is very toxic, it has to be converted into a non-toxic metabolite. In **ureotelic** organisms, e.g. mammals, ammonia is converted into urea which is excreted in urine. In **uricotelic** organisms, e.g. birds and reptiles, ammonia is converted into uric acid. In **ammonotelic** organisms, e.g. bony fish, ammonia is excreted as such.

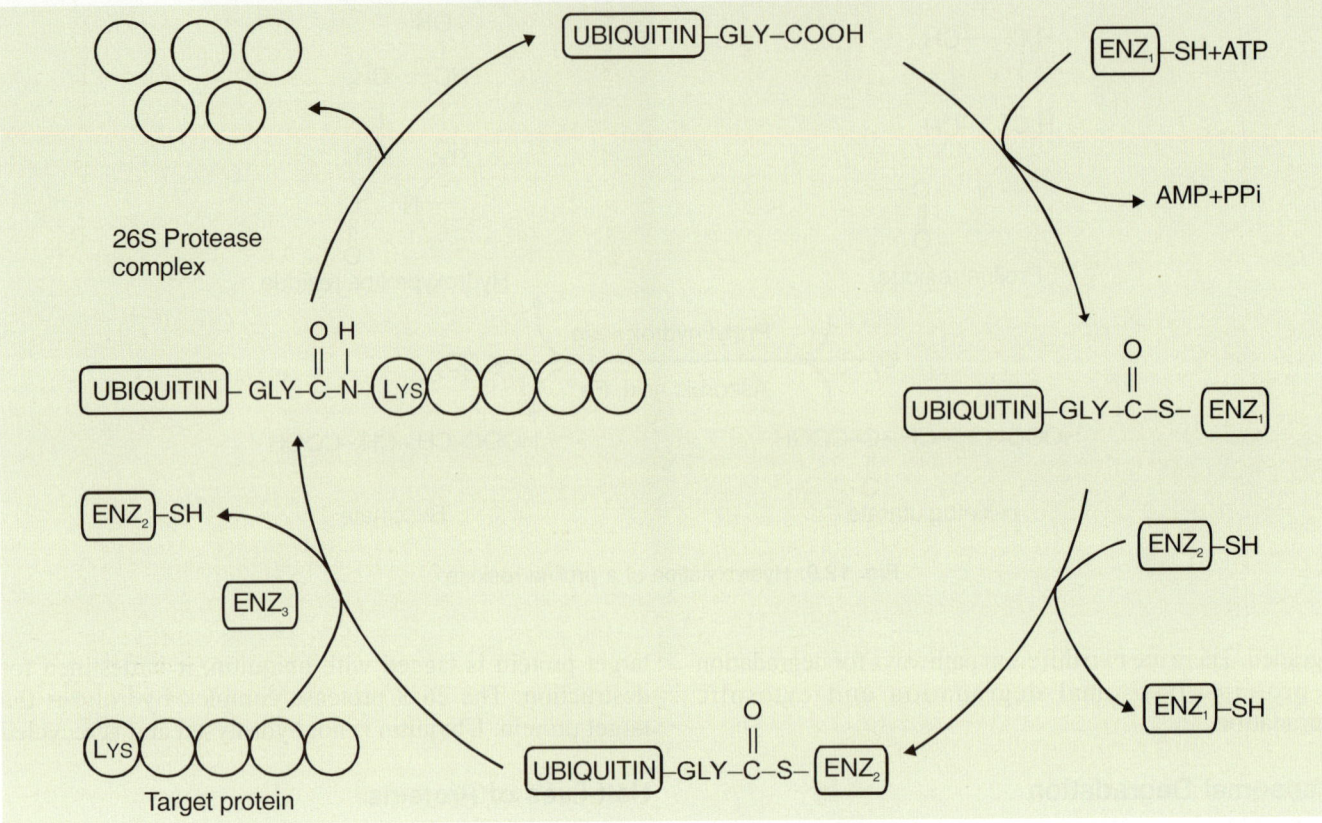

Fig. 12.10: Cytosolic degradation of proteins

REMOVAL AND DISPOSAL OF AMINO GROUPS

In human beings, disposal of amino groups of amino acids involves four steps:

1. Transfer of amino groups of different amino acids to α-ketoglutarate to form glutamate,
2. Oxidative deamination of glutamate and release of ammonia,
3. Transport of ammonia to liver and
4. Synthesis of urea in liver.

The carbon atom of urea ($H_2N–CO–NH_2$) is provided by carbon dioxide, one of the nitrogen atoms comes from ammonia and the other from aspartate (Fig. 12.11).

Transfer of Amino Groups to α-Ketoglutarate

For disposal of amino groups, the amino groups of amino acids have to be removed. This is done by deamination.

However, there is only one amino acid, i.e. glutamate which can undergo deamination at a significant rate. Therefore, amino groups of all the amino acids have to be transferred to α-ketoglutarate. This usually occurs by transamination. Amino groups of some amino acids, e.g. threonine, lysine, proline and hydroxyproline, are transferred to α-ketoglutarate by other mechanisms.

Transamination reactions are readily reversible. No energy is spent or released during these reactions. These reactions are important not only for catabolism of amino acids but also for their interconversion. Transamination reactions are catalysed by transaminases (amino-transferases). Pyridoxal phosphate (PLP) is required as a coenzyme by all transaminases, and it forms an integral part of the enzyme molecule. There are several transa-minases, each transferring the a-amino group of a particular amino acid to an α-keto acid. The α-keto acid is generally

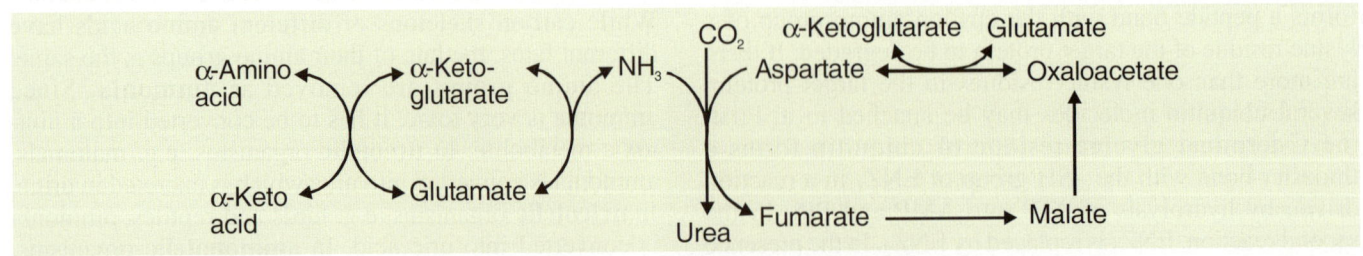

Fig. 12.11: Disposal of amino groups – An outline

α-ketoglutarate which is converted into glutamate. The enzyme is named after the amino acid donating the amino group, e.g. alanine aminotransferase (glutamate pyruvate transaminase) and aspartate aminotransferase (glutamate oxaloacetate transaminase).

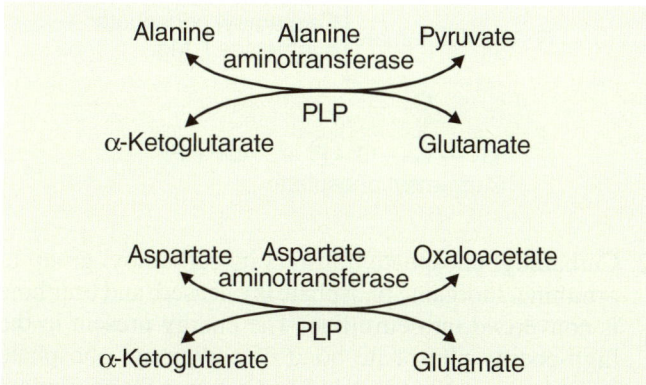

Thus, the amino groups are concentrated in glutamate, which is the only amino acid that can undergo oxidative deamination at a significant rate.

Oxidative Deamination of Glutamate

Oxidative deamination of glutamate is catalysed by glutamate dehydrogenase.

$$HOOC - CH_2 - CH_2 - CH - COOH$$
$$| \atop NH_2$$
Glutamate

$$NAD(P)^+ + H_2O$$

Glutamate dehydrogenase

$$NAD(P)H + H^+ + NH_3$$

$$HOOC - CH_2 - CH_2 - C - COOH$$
$$\| \atop O$$
α-Ketoglutarate

Glutamate dehydrogenase can use NAD⁺ as well and NADP⁺ as coenzyme. NADP⁺ is probably used for synthesis of glutamate from α-ketoglutarate and NAD⁺ for oxidative deamination of glutamate.

Apart from the ammonia liberated by oxidative deamination of glutamate, some ammonia can be liberated from amino acids by the actions of L-amino acid oxidase and D-amino acid oxidase. L-Amino acid oxidase acts on L-amino acids using FMN as a coenzyme. D-Amino acid oxidase acts similarly on D-amino acids with the difference that it uses FAD as a coenzyme. However, the contribution of L-amino acid oxidase and D-amino acid oxidase to the overall oxidative deamination of amino acids is very small as L-amino acid oxidase is very low in activity and D-amino acids do not occur in significant quantities in human beings.

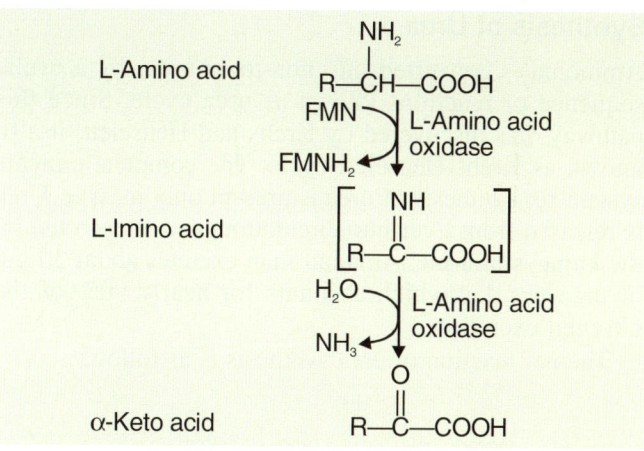

Transport of Ammonia

The complete enzyme system for the synthesis of urea is present only in liver though some enzymes are present in other tissues also. Though liver is the major site for catabolism of amino acids as well, some ammonia is produced in other tissues also which must be transported to liver without causing ammonia intoxication. Normal concentration of ammonia in blood is 10 to 80 µg/dl. Even a small rise in blood ammonia level, which may occur if hepatic function is impaired or if a portocaval shunt is formed, may damage nervous tissue.

Since brain tissue is extremely sensitive to ammonia, it possesses a mechanism for immediate detoxification of ammonia. Ammonia is combined with glutamate to form glutamine by glutamine synthetase. A constant supply of glutamate is required for this reaction, which is formed mainly from α-ketoglutarate, an intermediate of citric acid cycle.

Glutamine released into circulation can be taken up by liver and kidneys wherein glutaminase converts it into glutamate and ammonia. Thus, ammonia can be transported from brain in the form of non-toxic glutamine.

Glutamate, which is formed by transamination of α-ketoglutarate in many tissues, transports the amino groups of various amino acids to liver in a non-toxic form.

In muscles, amino groups of many amino acids are transferred to pyruvate forming alanine. Alanine is transported to liver where pyruvate is reformed, and the amino group of alanine is transferred to α-ketoglutarate. Thus, glucose-alanine cycle not only transports pyruvate from muscles to liver for gluconeogenesis but also transports the amino groups of amino acids from muscles to liver.

Significant quantities of ammonia are formed in the intestine by the action of bacterial enzymes on amino acids and urea. Catabolism of dietary purines and pyrimidines in the intestine also releases their amino groups in the form of ammonia. All this ammonia is released into portal blood. Liver extracts all the ammonia when portal blood passes through it.

Synthesis of Urea

Ammonia is converted into non-toxic urea by a cyclic sequence of reactions known as urea cycle. Since this pathway was discovered by Krebs and Henseleit, it also known as Krebs-Henseleit cycle. The complete enzyme system for synthesis of urea is present only in liver. Urea is released from liver into circulation, and is excreted by the kidneys in urine. An adult man excretes about 30 gm of urea per day which accounts for nearly 90% of the nitrogen excretion.

The net reaction of urea synthesis is as follows:

$$CO_2 + NH_3 + HOOC-CH_2-\overset{\overset{\displaystyle NH_2}{|}}{CH}-COOH + 3\,ATP + 2\,H_2O$$

$$\downarrow$$

$$H_2N-\overset{\overset{\displaystyle O}{\|}}{C}-NH_2 + HOOC-\overset{\overset{\displaystyle H}{|}}{C}=\overset{\overset{\displaystyle }{\underset{\underset{\displaystyle H}{|}}{C}}}-COOH + 2\,ADP + 2\,Pi + AMP + PPi$$

Thus, the $>C=O$ group of urea is provided by carbon dioxide, one $-NH_2$ group is provided by ammonia and the other $-NH_2$ group is provided by aspartate. Four high-energy phosphate bonds of ATP are utilised in the process as two ATP molecules are converted into ADP and one into AMP.

After losing its amino group, aspartate is converted into fumarate. For continuation of the cycle, aspartate has to be regenerated. For this, fumarate enters the citric acid cycle to form oxaloacetate which is, then, transaminated to aspartate. Thus, urea cycle is linked with citric acid cycle.

Synthesis of urea occurs partly in mitochondria and partly in cytosol. The first two reactions of urea cycle, i.e. synthesis of carbamoyl phosphate and synthesis of citrulline occur in mitochondria while the rest of the reactions occur in cytosol. Conversion of fumarate into oxaloacetate and aspartate also occurs in mitochondria.

Reactions of the urea cycle are as follows:

1. Carbamoyl phosphate synthetase I (CPS I) catalyses the synthesis of carbamoyl phosphate from ammonia, carbon dioxide and ATP. Two molecules of ATP are converted into ADP, one inorganic phosphate is released and the other phosphate is incorporated in carbamoyl phosphate.

   N-acetylglutamate is an activator of carbamoyl phosphate synthetase I. It is synthesised from acetyl

CoA and glutamate. Binding of N-acetylglutamate to carbamoyl phosphate synthetase I converts the inactive enzyme into its active form.

$$CO_2 + NH_3 + 2\,ATP$$

N-Acetylglutamate $\left|\begin{array}{l}\text{Carbamoyl phosphate}\\ \text{synthetase I, }Mg^{++}\end{array}\right.$

$$\downarrow$$

$$H_2N-\overset{\overset{\displaystyle O}{\|}}{C}-O\!-\!\textcircled{P} + 2\,ADP + Pi$$
Carbamoyl phosphate

2. Carbamoyl phosphate transfers its carbamoyl group to ornithine. Inorganic phosphate is released, and ornithine is convertwd into citrulline. The energy present in the high-energy phosphate bond of carbamoyl phosphate is used to form the covalent bond between the carbamoyl group and the δ-amino group of ornithine. The reaction is catalysed by ornithine transcarbamoylase (ornithine carbamoyl transferase).

Ornithine enters the mitochondria from cytosol for this reaction and citrulline leaves the mitochondria for the next reaction which occurs in cytosol. Ornithine-citrulline antiport is required for this transport.

3. Citrulline combines with aspartate to form argininosuccinate. A covalent bond is formed between the amino group of aspartate and the keto group of citrulline. The energy for the formation of this bond is provided by hydrolysis of ATP into AMP and inorganic pyrophosphate. The reaction is catalysed by argininosuccinic acid synthetase.

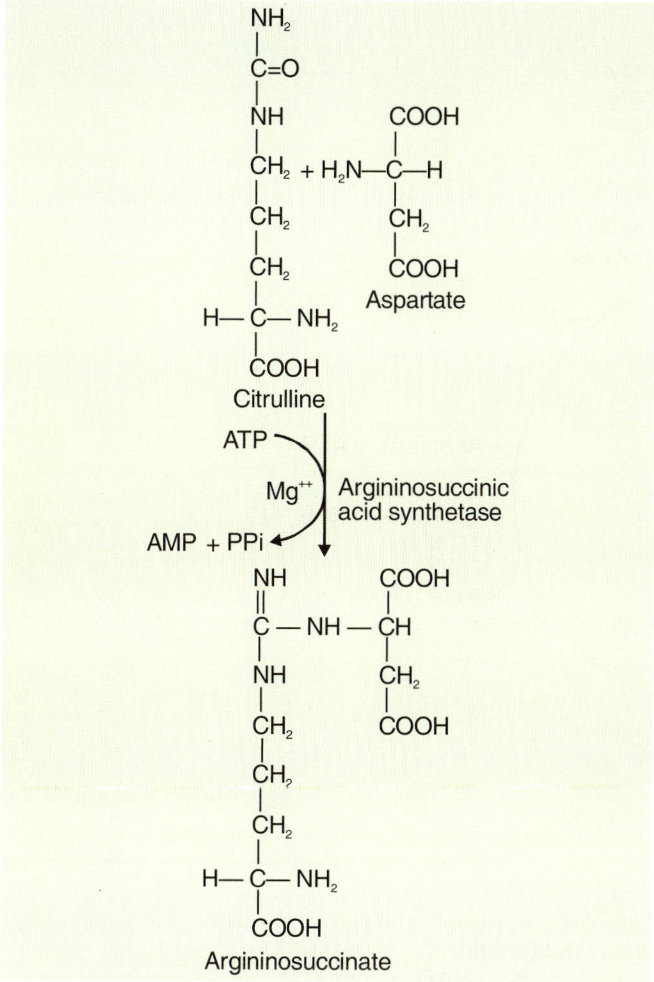

The structures shown (left column, top):

Citrulline + Aspartate → (ATP, Mg^{++}, Argininosuccinic acid synthetase, AMP + PPi) → Argininosuccinate

4. Argininosuccinate is cleaved into arginine and fumarate. The reaction is catalysed by argininosuccinase. The net effect of this and the preceding reaction is that aspartate loses its amino group and is converted into fumarate. This is also the reaction by which human beings can synthesise arginine, a semi-essential amino acid. However, arginine synthesised in liver is not released into circulation, and is used only for the synthesis of urea. The most likely site for endogenous synthesis of arginine for use within the body is the renal cortex.

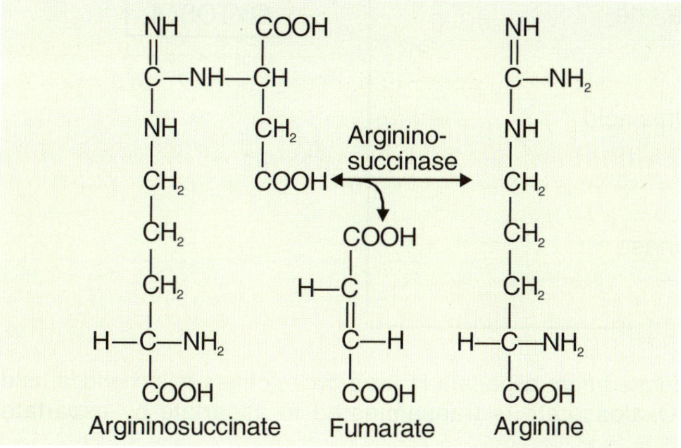

Argininosuccinate ⇌ (Arginino-succinase) Fumarate + Arginine

5. The last reaction of the cycle is hydrolytic cleavage of arginine into urea and ornithine which is catalysed by arginase. Ornithine goes back to begin another cycle by reacting with yet another molecule of carbamoyl phosphate.

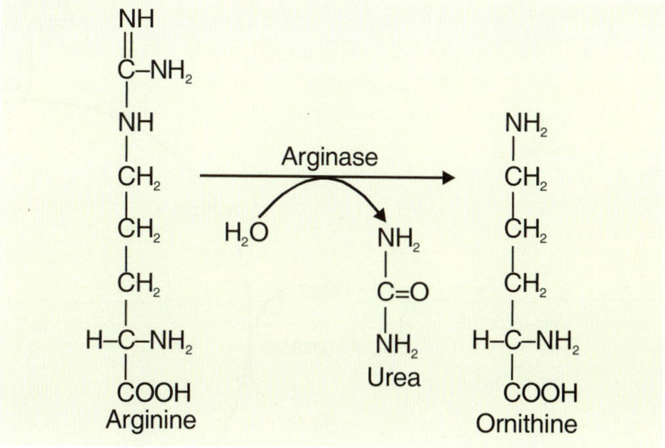

Arginine + H_2O → (Arginase) → Urea + Ornithine

Regulation of Urea Synthesis

Glutamate dehydrogenase, which provides ammonia for urea synthesis, is an allosteric enzyme. ATP and GTP are its allosteric inhibitors, and ADP and GDP are its allosteric activators. Thus, a decrease in energy status increases the catabolism of amino acids and synthesis of urea. Mitochondrial carbamoyl phosphate synthetase is also a regulatory enzyme. It is activated by N-acetyl glutamate which is formed by transfer of the acetyl group from acetyl CoA to glutamate.

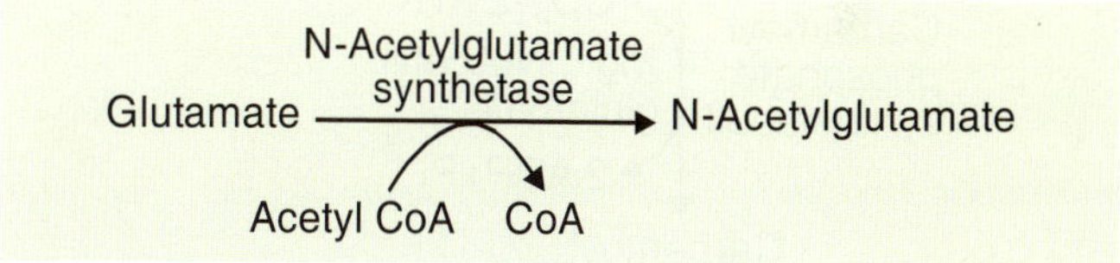

Glutamate → (N-Acetylglutamate synthetase, Acetyl CoA → CoA) → N-Acetylglutamate

Hepatic Encephalopathy

Life-threatening neurological abnormalities can occur in severe liver diseases, e.g. cirrhosis of liver. Disturbed hepatic architecture can lead to the formation of porto-caval shunt. Portal blood which is rich in ammonia mixes with systemic blood. Decrease in the number of functioning liver cells impairs the ability of liver to convert ammonia into urea. All this can result in severe hyperammonaemia. Hyperammonaemia causes encephalo-pathy manifesting as **blurring of vision, slurring of speech, flapping tremors, hepatic coma** and **death**.

As mentioned earlier, brain possesses a mechanism for immediate detoxification of ammonia viz. synthesis of glutamine from glutamate and ammonia. Glutamate required for this reaction is formed from α-ketoglutarate, an intermediate of citric acid cycle. Excessive removal of α-ketoglutarate can result in impairment of citric acid cycle limiting the production of ATP. Apart from energy deficit,

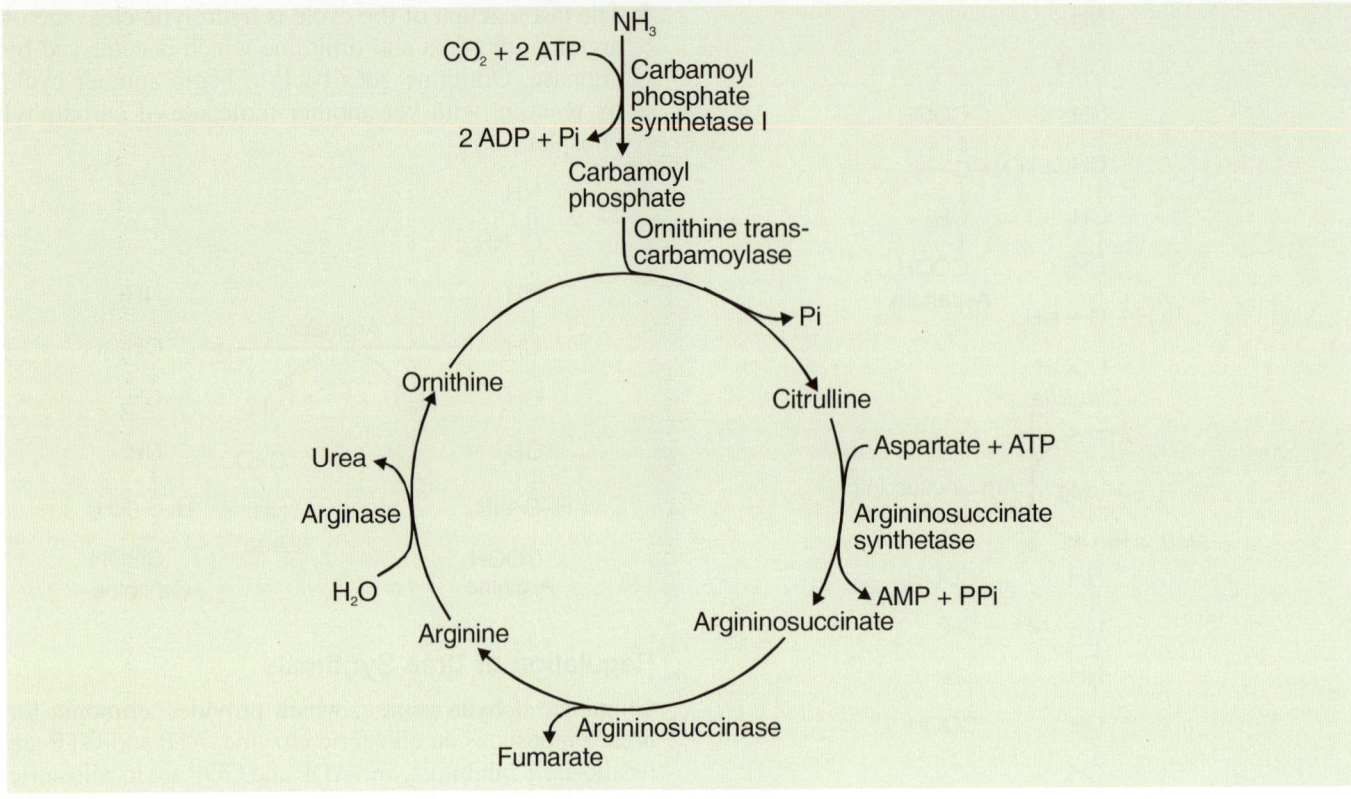

Fig. 12.12: Urea cycle

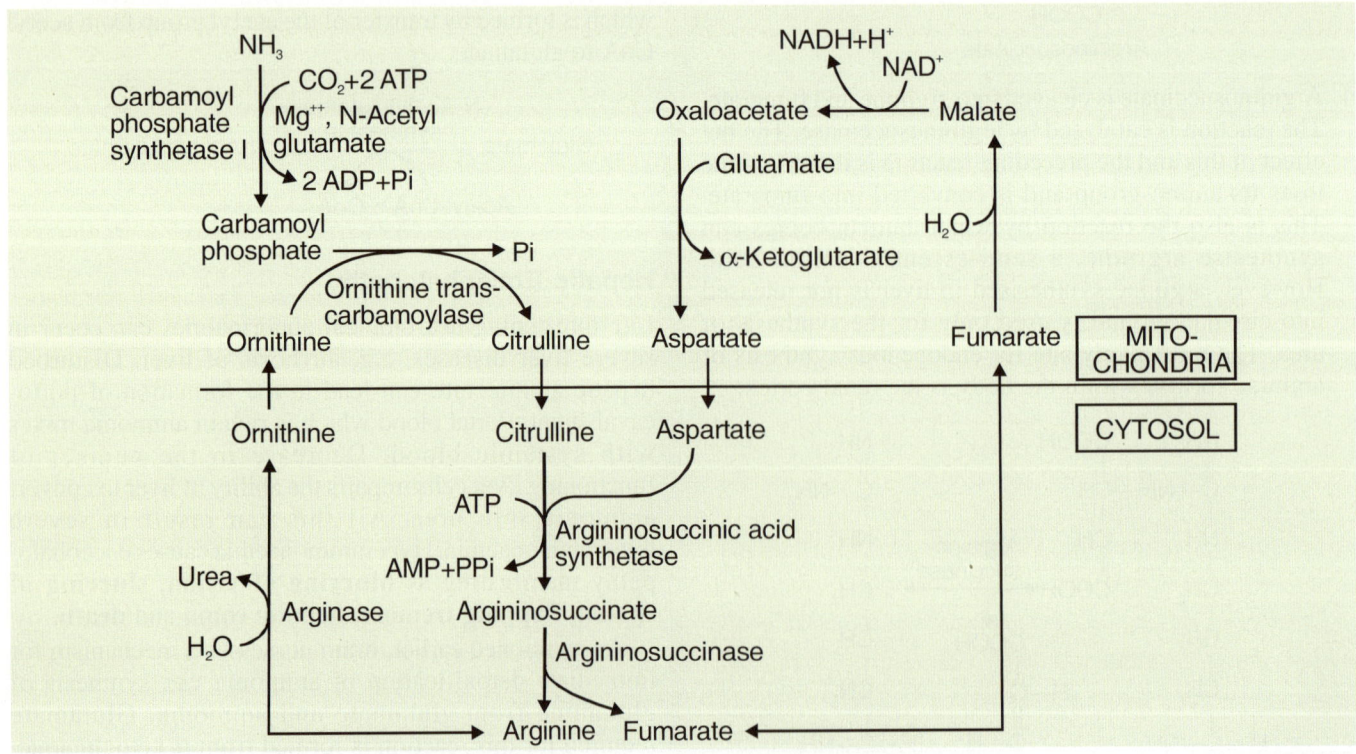

Fig. 12.13: Linkage of urea cycle with citric acid cycle. Fumarate, formed from aspartate in urea cycle, enters mitochondria, and is converted into oxaloacetate by citric acid cycle enzymes. Oxaloacetate is transaminated to aspartate by aspartate aminotransferase

increased synthesis of gamma-aminobutyric acid from glutamate and inhibition of uptake of some amino acids by brain cells due to increased level of glutamine have been proposed to cause encephalopathy.

Low protein diet and sterilisation of gut by antibiotics are useful in decreasing the production of ammonia.

Inborn Errors of Urea Cycle

Each of the five enzymes involved in urea synthesis may be congenitally absent or deficient. This leads to decreased urea synthesis and accumulation of ammonia. Varying degrees of **ammonia intoxication** occur. Clinical abnormalities are more severe when the defect occurs at an early stage in the pathway. The disorders (name of the enzyme in parenthesis) are:

1. Hyperammonaemia, type I (carbamoyl phosphate synthetase),
2. Hyperammonaemia, type II (ornithine transcarbamoylase),
3. Citrullinaemia (argininosuccinic acid synthetase),
4. Argininosuccinic aciduria (argininosuccinase) and
5. Hyperargininaemia (arginase).

These disorders are very rare. Clinical features, which are common to all though varying in severity, are vomiting, distaste for protein-rich foods, lethargy, irritability, ataxia and mental retardation. Small and frequent meals, low in protein, help in preventing sudden and excessive rise in blood ammonia and lead to improvement.

FATE OF CARBON SKELETONS

The carbon skeletons of amino acids are converted into pyruvate, acetyl CoA or intermediates of citric acid cycle viz. α-ketoglutarate, succinyl CoA, fumarate and oxaloacetate. Conversion of carbon skeletons into acetyl CoA may occur directly or via acetoacetyl CoA.

Pyruvate and all the intermediates of citric acid cycle can be converted into glucose (and glycogen) by gluconeogenesis. Therefore, the amino acids which are catabolised to pyruvate or intermediates of citric acid cycle are known as **glycogenic amino acids**. These include glycine, alanine, valine, serine, threonine, cysteine, methionine, aspartate, asparagine, glutamate, glutamine, arginine, histidine, proline and hydroxyproline.

Those amino acids which give acetyl CoA on catabolism are known as **ketogenic amino acids** as acetyl CoA can be converted into fatty acids. Leucine is the only amino acid in this group.

Those amino acids whose carbon skeletons form acetyl CoA as well as pyruvate or citric acid cycle intermediates are known as **glyco- and ketogenic amino acids** as their carbon skeletons can form glucose as well as fatty acids. The amino acids in this group are isoleucine, lysine, phenylalanine, tyrosine and tryptophan.

Amino Acids Forming Pyruvate

Carbon skeletons of threonine, glycine, serine, alanine, cysteine (and cystine) and hydroxyproline are converted into pyruvate. Some of these amino acids may have additional fates also. For example, glycine, besides forming pyruvate, may also be cleaved into ammonia, carbon dioxide and a methylene group which is taken up by tetrahydrofolate. Thus, glycine can act as a donor of single-carbon moieties.

$$\text{Glycine} + H_4 - \text{Folate} + NAD^+ \underset{\text{Glycine synthetase}}{\rightleftharpoons} \text{Methylene} - H_4 - \text{folate} + NH_3 + CO_2 + NADH + H^+$$

Conversion of **alanine** into pyruvate occurs by a simple transamination reaction catalysed by glutamate pyruvate transaminase (GPT):

$$\text{Alanine} + \alpha\text{-Ketoglutarate} \underset{\text{GPT}}{\rightleftharpoons} \text{Pyruvate} + \text{Glutamate}$$

Cysteine is catabolised to pyruvate. The catabolism may occur via mercaptopyruvate or cysteine sulphinate and β-sulphinylpyruvate. In the former case, the sulphur atom is released as hydrogen sulphide. In the latter case, it is released as sulphur dioxide (Fig. 12.14).

Threonine, glycine and **serine** are catabolised to pyruvate by a common pathway. In fact, glycine and serine are formed as intermediates during the conversion of threonine into pyruvate, and free glycine and serine can enter the pathway at intermediate stages (Fig. 12.15).

Threonine is cleaved into acetaldehyde and glycine. Glycine is converted into serine by serine hydroxymethyl transferase. Serine is converted into pyruvate by serine dehydratase, a pyridoxal phosphate-dependent enzyme.

Hydroxyproline is catabolised to pyruvate and glyoxylate (Fig. 12.16). Glyoxylate can be transaminated to glycine or it can be oxidised to formate.

Amino Acid Forming Oxaloacetate

Asparagine and **aspartate** are catabolised to oxaloacetate. Asparagine is first converted into aspartate by asparaginase in a reaction analogous to the conversion of glutamine into glutamate.

Aspartate is transaminated by glutamate oxaloacetate transaminase (GOT) to oxaloacetate which is a citric acid cycle intermediate:

$$\text{Asparagine} \xrightarrow[\substack{H_2O \quad NH_3}]{\text{Asparaginase}} \text{Aspartate} \xrightarrow[\substack{\alpha\text{-KG} \quad GLU}]{\text{GOT,PLP}} \text{Oxaloacetate}$$

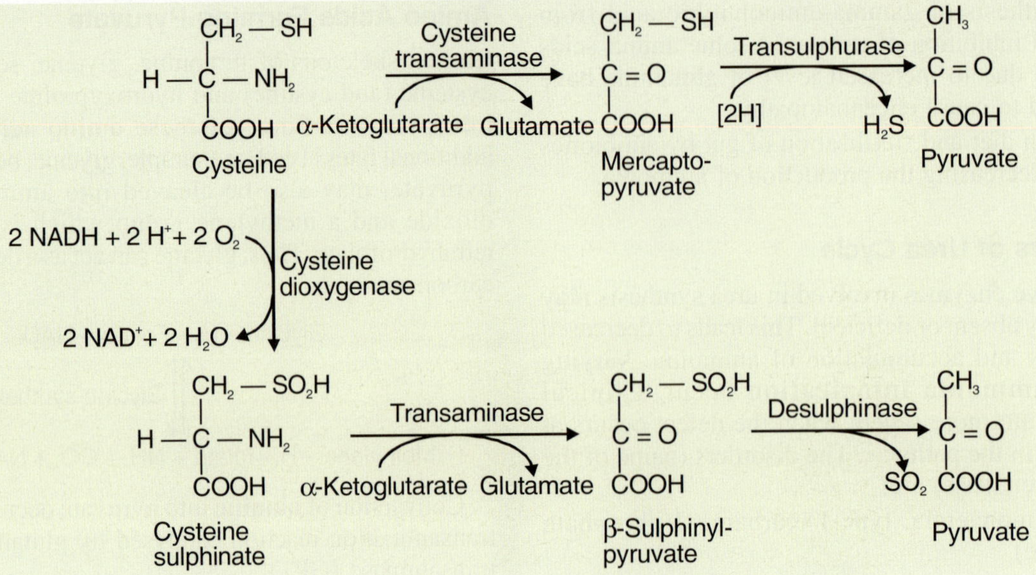

Fig. 12.14: Catabolism of cysteine to pyruvate

Amino Acids Forming α-Ketoglutarate

Histidine, proline, arginine, glutamine and glutamate are converted into α-ketoglutarate which is an intermediate of citric acid cycle. Histidine, proline, arginine and glutamine are converted into glutamate which is transaminated to α-ketoglutarate.

Histidine is converted, via urocanic acid and 4-imidazolone-5-propionic acid, into **N-formiminoglutamic acid** (FIGLU). The latter transfers its formimino group to H_4-folate, and is converted into glutamic acid. Thus, histidine can also act as a donor of single-carbon moieties. If tetrahydrofolate is not available, FIGLU will not be converted into glutamic acid and urinary FIGLU excretion will be increased. Therefore, measurement of urinary excretion of FIGLU after a test dose of histidine is an important test for diagnosis of folic acid deficiency (Fig. 12.17).

Proline is converted into glutamate by a reversal of the pathway for the synthesis of proline (Fig. 12.18).

Arginine is hydrolysed into urea and ornithine by arginase which is present in several tissues. Ornithine is transaminated at the δ-carbon to glutamate γ-semialdehyde which is oxidised to glutamate. The latter is converted into α-ketoglutarate by transamination (Fig. 12.19).

Glutamine is converted into glutamate by glutaminase as described earlier.

$$\text{Glutamine} + H_2O \xrightarrow{\text{Glutaminase}} \text{Glutamate} + NH_3$$

Glutamate is converted into the citric acid cycle intermediate, α-ketoglutarate by transamination as described earlier.

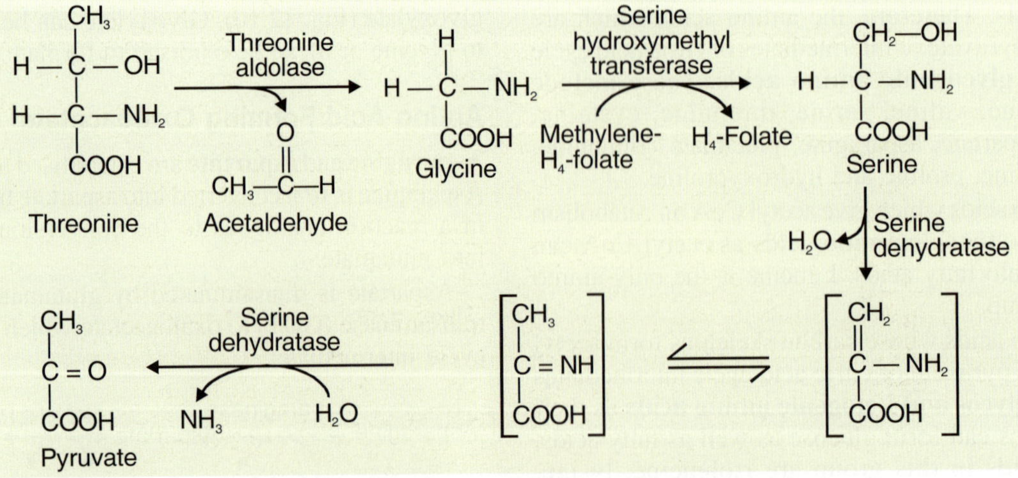

Fig. 12.15: Catabolism of threonine, glycine and serine

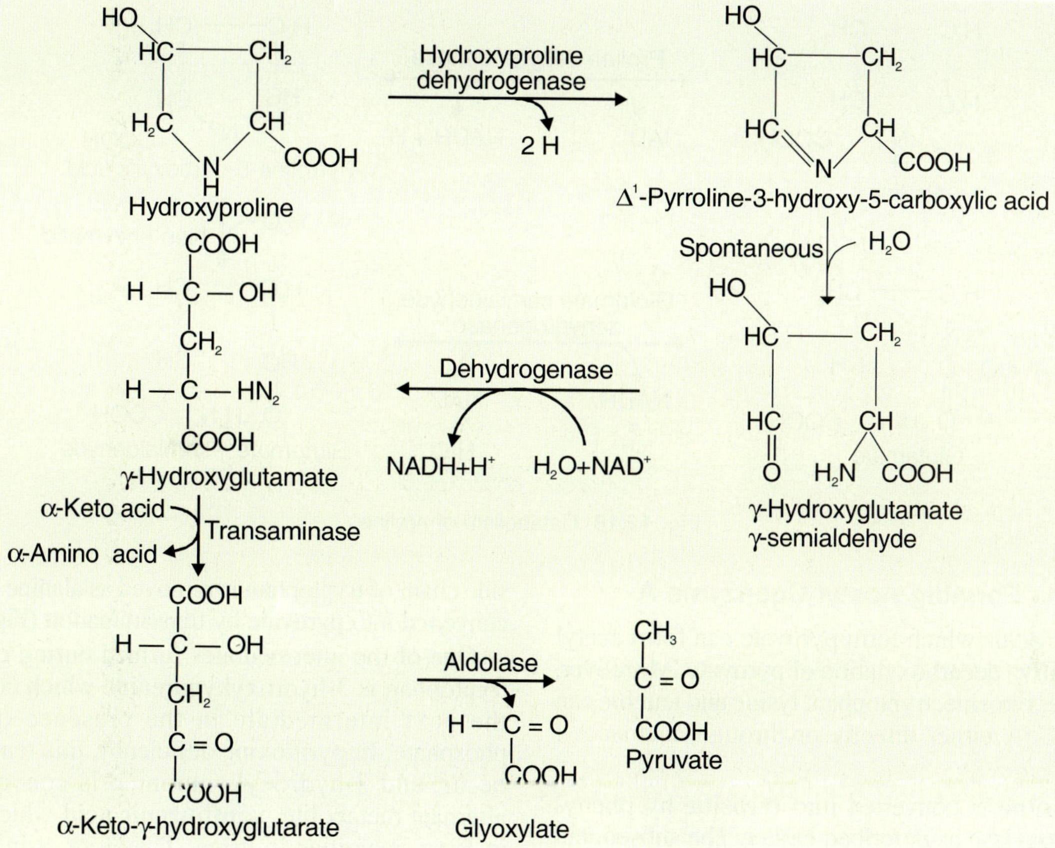

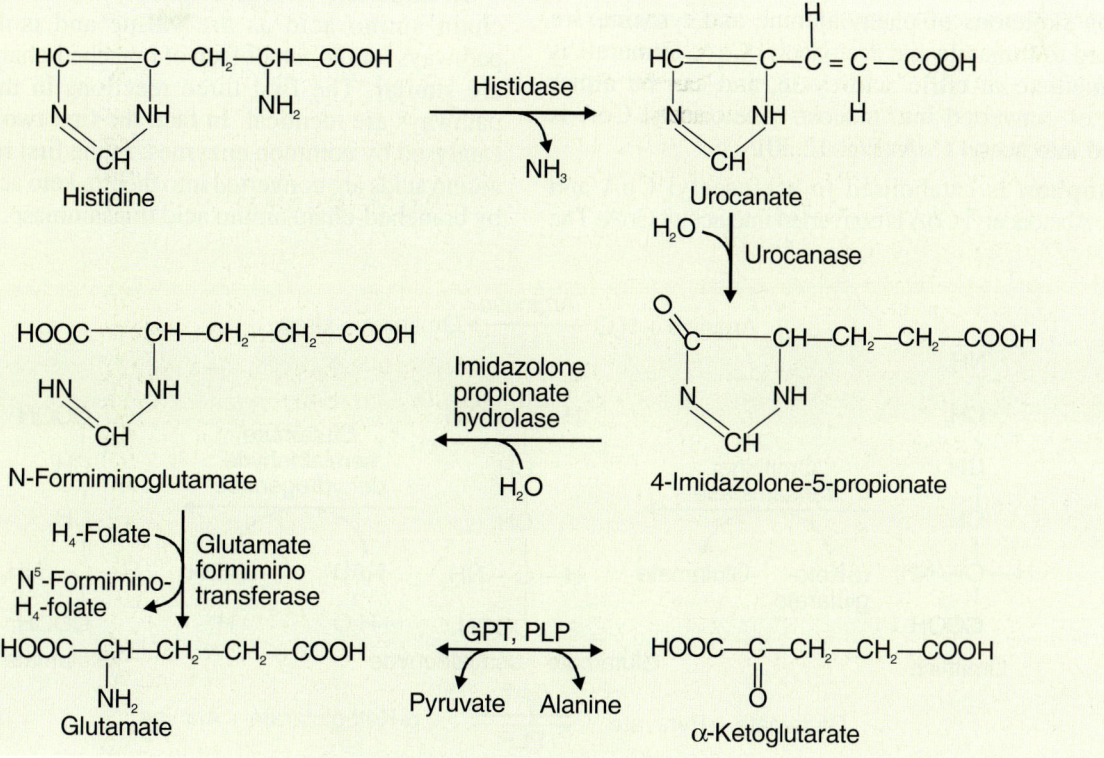

Fig. 12.16: Catabolism of hydroxyproline

Fig. 12.17: Catabolism of histidine

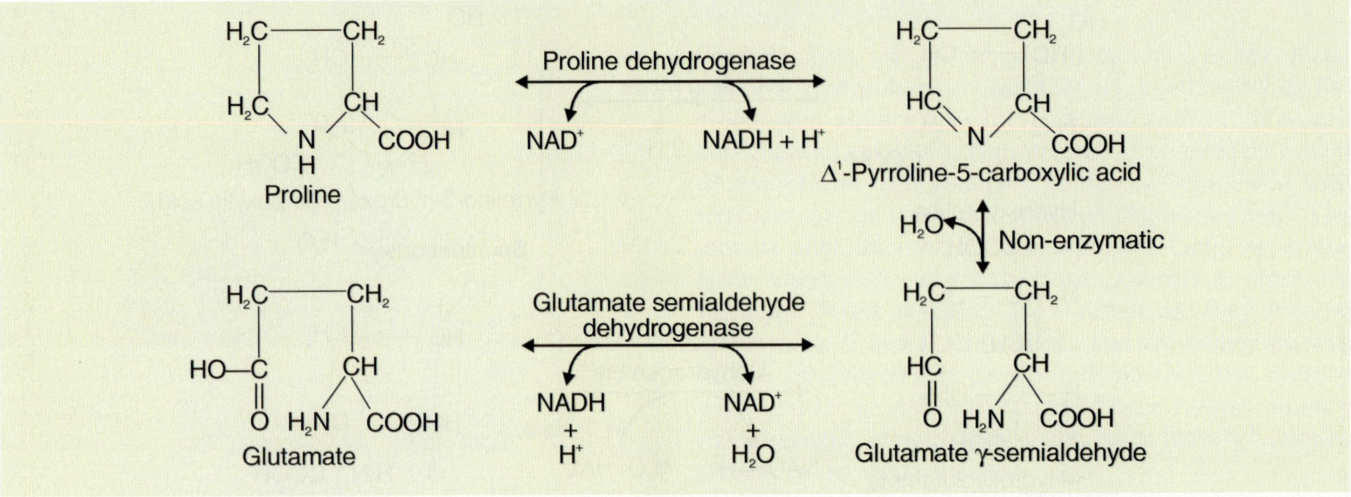

Fig. 12.18: Catabolism of proline

Amino Acids Forming Acetyl Coenzyme A

All the amino acids which form pyruvate can form acetyl CoA by oxidative decarboxylation of pyruvate. Moreover, phenylalanine, tyrosine, tryptophan, lysine and leucine can form acetyl CoA either directly or through acetoacetyl CoA.

Phenylalanine is converted into **tyrosine** by phenylalanine hydroxylase as described earlier. The subsequent pathway for catabolism of these amino acids is common. Apart from other coenzymes, ascorbic acid is required for their catabolism.

Carbon skeletons of phenylalanine and tyrosine are catabolised to fumarate and acetoacetyl CoA. Fumarate is an intermediate of citric acid cycle, and can be either oxidised or converted into glucose. Acetoacetyl CoA is converted into acetyl CoA (Fig. 12.20).

Tryptophan is catabolised to acetoacetyl CoA and pyruvate. Acetoacetyl CoA is converted into acetyl CoA. The side chain of tryptophan is removed as alanine which can be converted into pyruvate by transamination (Fig. 12.21).

One of the intermediates formed during catabolism of tryptophan is 3-hydroxykynurenine which converted into the next intermediate in the presence of pyridoxal phosphate. In pyridoxine deficiency, this reaction doesn't occur, and 3-hydroxykynurenine is converted into an alternate metabolite, **xanthurenic acid** which is excreted in large quantities in urine. Therefore, urinary excretion of xanthurenic acid after a test dose of tryptophan is a useful test for diagnosis of pyridoxine deficiency.

Leucine is a ketogenic amino acid. It is a branched-chain amino acid as are valine and isoleucine. The pathways for the catabolism of branched-chain amino acids are similar. The first three reactions in their catabolic pathways are identical. In fact, the first two reactions are catalysed by common enzymes. In the first reaction, these amino acids are converted into their α-keto acid derivatives by branched-chain amino acid transaminase. In the second

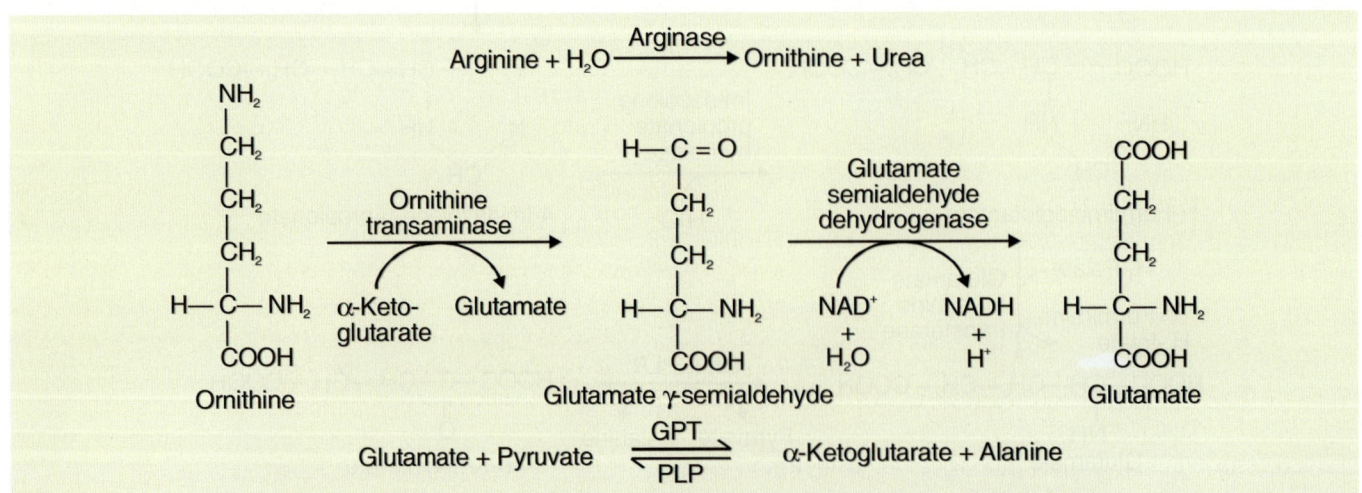

Fig. 12.19: Arginine is converted into α-ketoglutarate via ornithine and glutamate

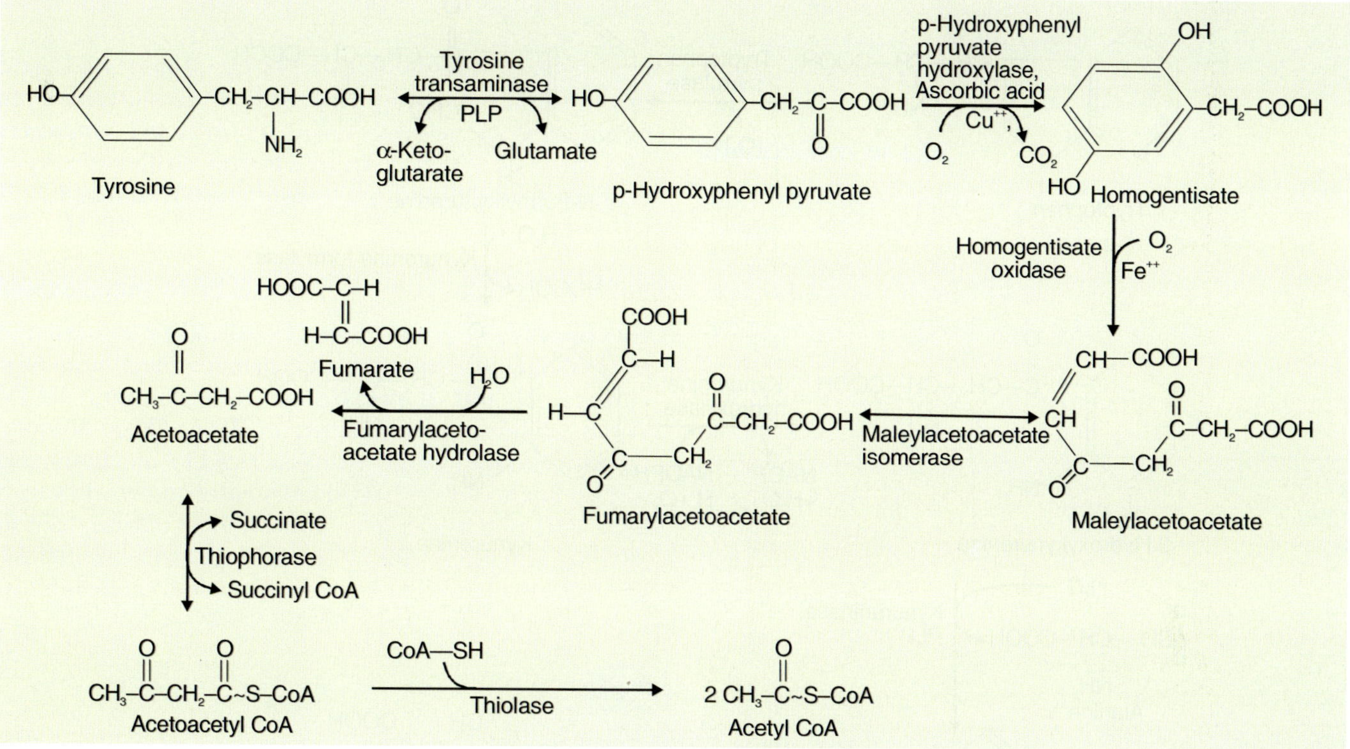

Fig. 12.20: Catabolism of tyrosine

reaction, the α-keto acids are oxidatively decarboxylated by α-ketoisovalerate dehydrogenase to their CoA derivatives with one carbon atom less. In the third reaction, the CoA derivatives are oxidised by specific dehydrogenases by removal of two hydrogen atoms. From this reaction onwards, the pathways differ.

Leucine has six carbon atoms which are converted into three molecules of acetyl CoA (Fig. 12.22).

Lysine is catabolised to acetylCoA via α-ketoadipic acid (Fig. 12.23).

Amino Acids Forming Succinyl Coenzyme A

Valine, isoleucine and methionine are catabolised to form succinyl CoA, another intermediate of citric acid cycle.

Valine is a glycogenic amino acid. Valine is converted into methylmalonyl CoA (Fig. 12.24) which is, subsequently, converted into succinyl CoA by methymalonyl CoA isomerase as described earlier.

Isoleucine is a glyco- and keto-genic amino acid. Carbon skeleton of isoleucine is converted into one molecule of propionyl CoA which is glycogenic and one molecule of acetyl CoA which is ketogenic (Fig. 12.25). Propionyl CoA, as described earlier, can be converted into succinyl CoA via methylmalonic acid. Acetyl CoA can form fatty acids and other lipids.

Methionine is converted into S-adenosyl methionine which acts as a donor of labile methyl groups for various methylation reactions. Its conversion into homoserine has been described earlier (Fig.12.5). Homoserine is deaminated to α-ketobutyrate by homoserine deaminase. The reaction involves the formation of a number of unstable intermediates. α-Ketobutyrate is converted into propionyl CoA by oxidative decarboxylation analogous to that of pyruvate and α-ketoglutarate (Fig. 12.26). Propionyl CoA is then converted into succinyl CoA as described in Chapter 11.

Amino Acids Forming Fumarate

A part of the carbon skeletons of phenylalanine and tyrosine is converted into fumarate. The major portion of the carbon skeletons is converted into acetyl CoA. The reactions leading to the formation of fumarate and acetyl CoA from phenylalanine and tyrosine have been described earlier.

SYNTHESIS OF NON-PROTEIN SPECIALISED PRODUCTS FROM AMINO ACIDS

Amino acids are used mainly as building blocks for protein synthesis but some amino acids or their carbon skeletons are used for the synthesis of some specialised products, e.g. hormones, porphyrins, purines, etc. The amino acids which form specialised products are the following:

Glycine

Glycine acts as a **neurotransmitter** in brain. It is used for the formation of many specialised products. The entire

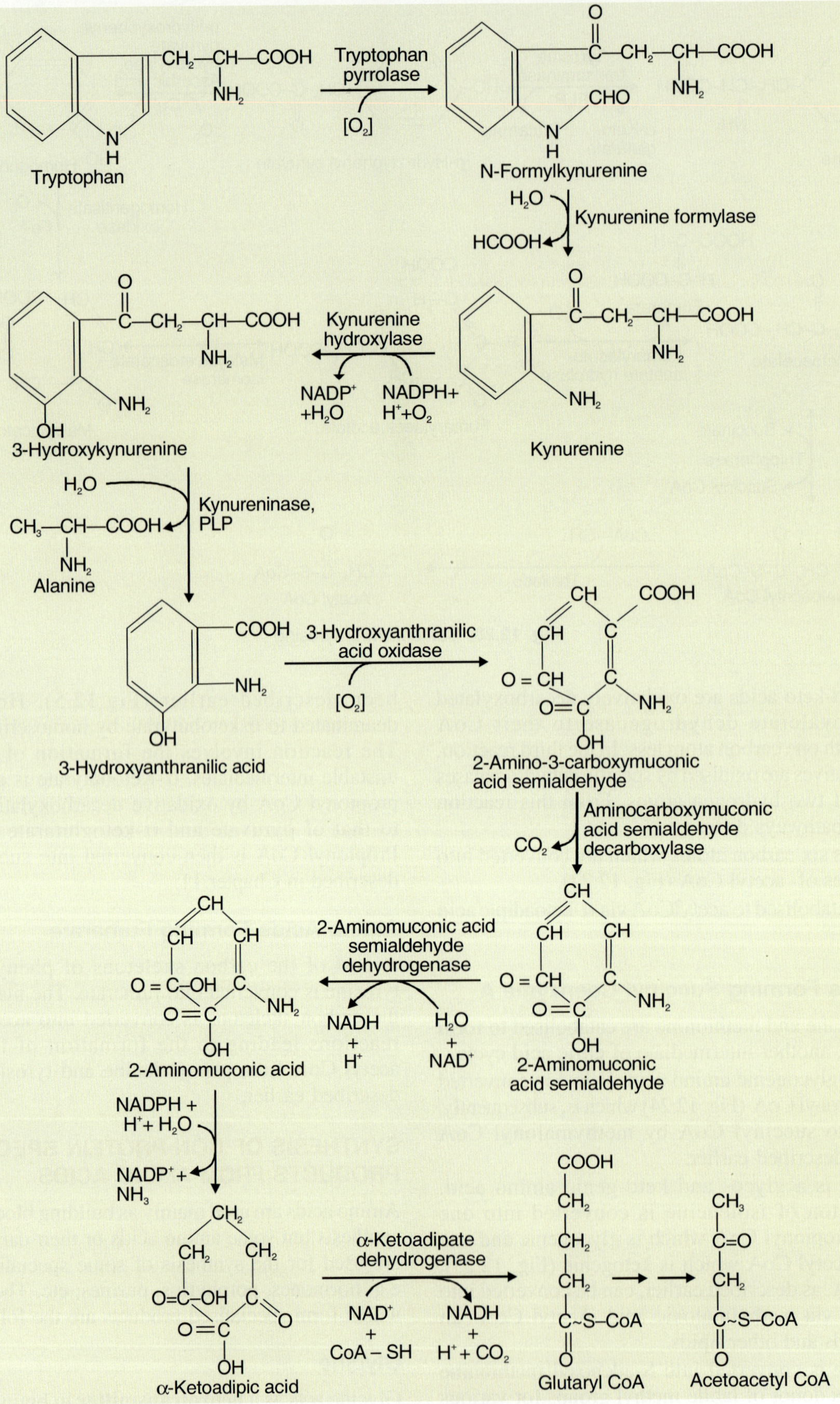

Fig. 12.21: Catabolism of tryptophan

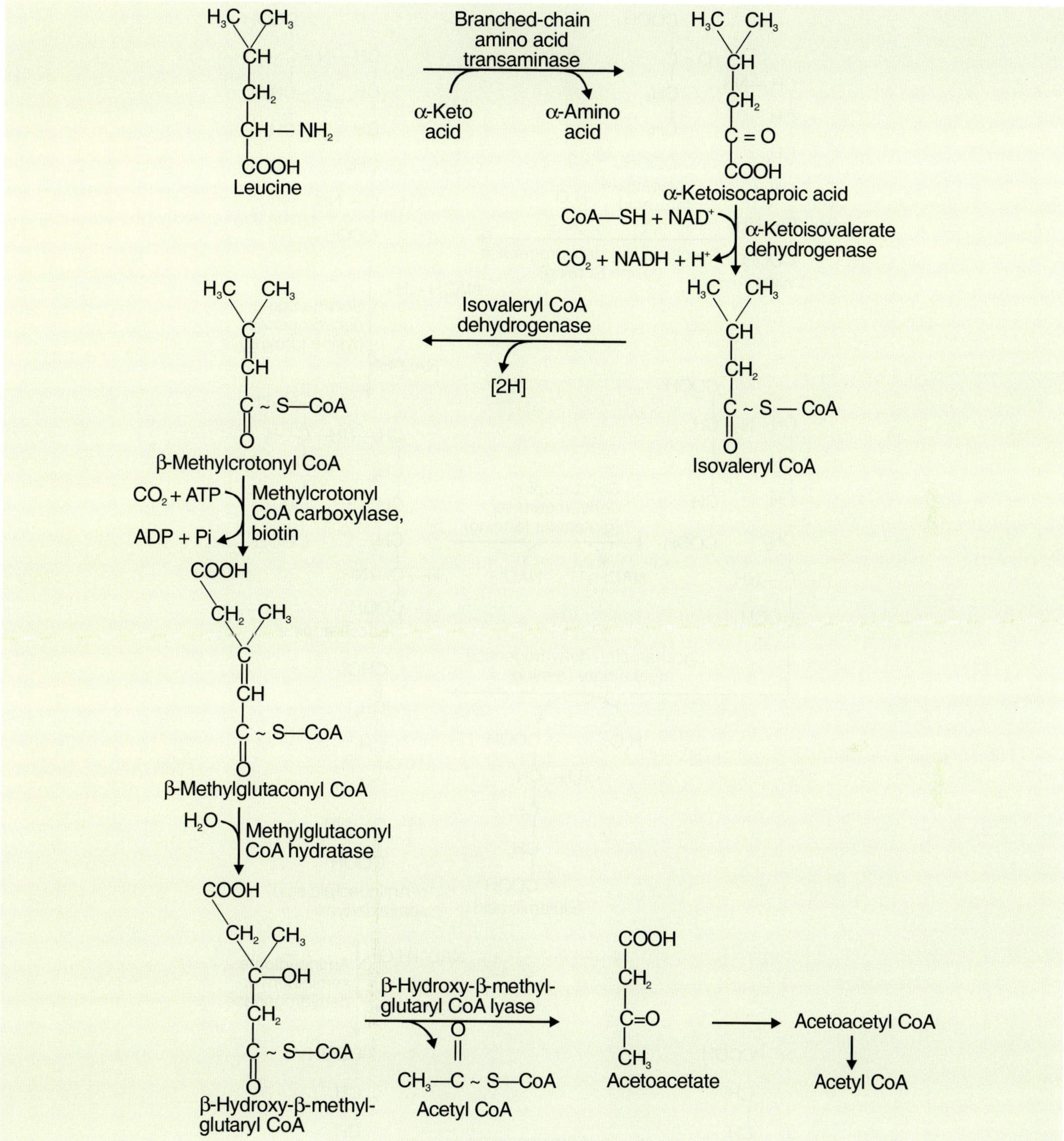

Fig. 12.22: Catabolism of leucine

glycine molecule is incorporated in the **purine nucleus**. The carbon atoms at positions 4 and 5, and the nitrogen atom at position 7 of the purines are provided by glycine (see Chapter 13). Glycine also forms a part of the **porphyrin nucleus**. Porphyrin synthesis begins with condensation of glycine with succinyl CoA (see Chapter 20). The bile acid, **glycocholic acid** is formed by conjugation of glycine with cholic acid. Glycine is one of

the amino acids present in the biologically important tripeptide, **glutathione** (γ-glutamyl-cysteinyl-glycine). Glycine can provide a one-carbon unit to tetrahydrofolate. It can be converted into serine. It can combine with benzoyl CoA to form hippuric acid. Glycine also forms part of the **creatine** molecule.

Creatine is present in significant quantities in muscles, mainly as creatine phosphate(a high-energy

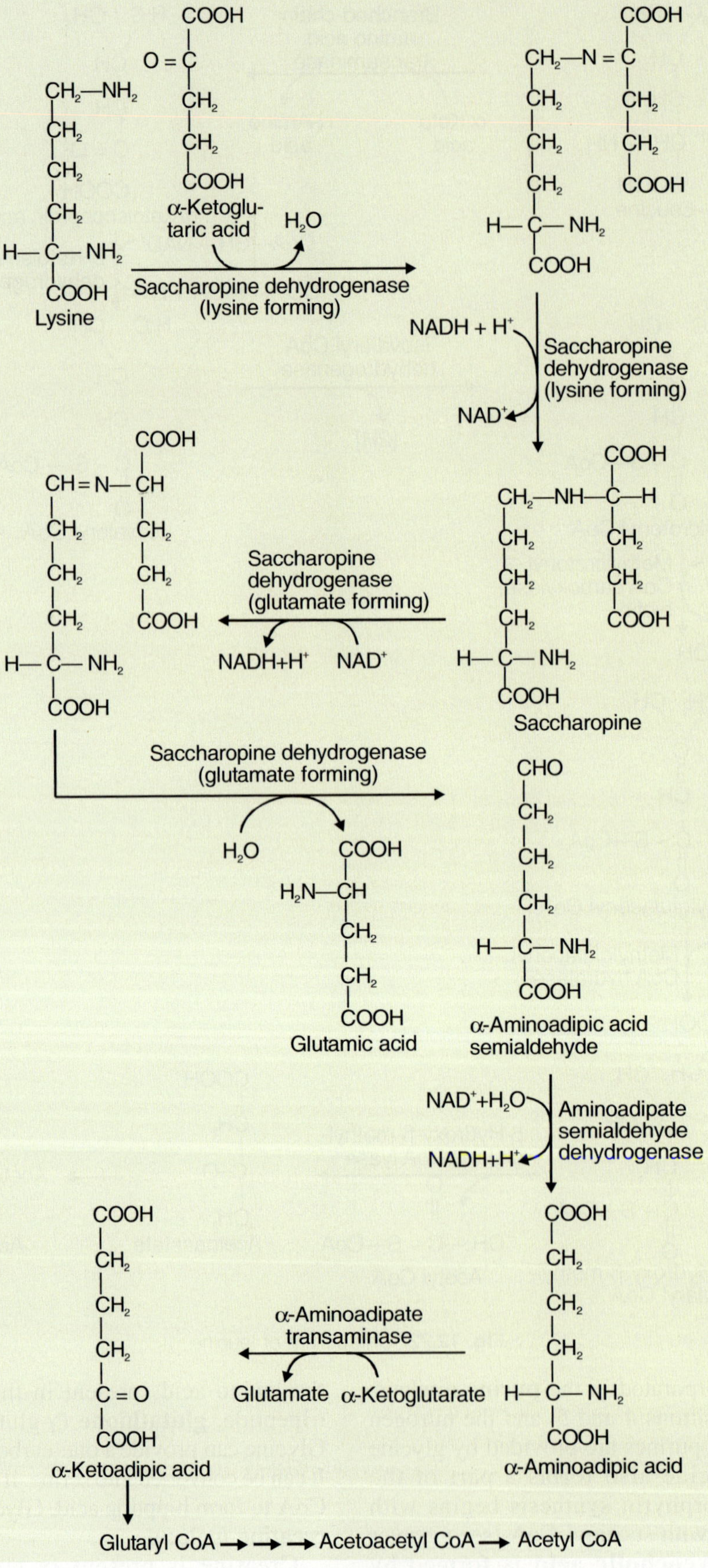

Fig. 12.23: Catabolism of lysine

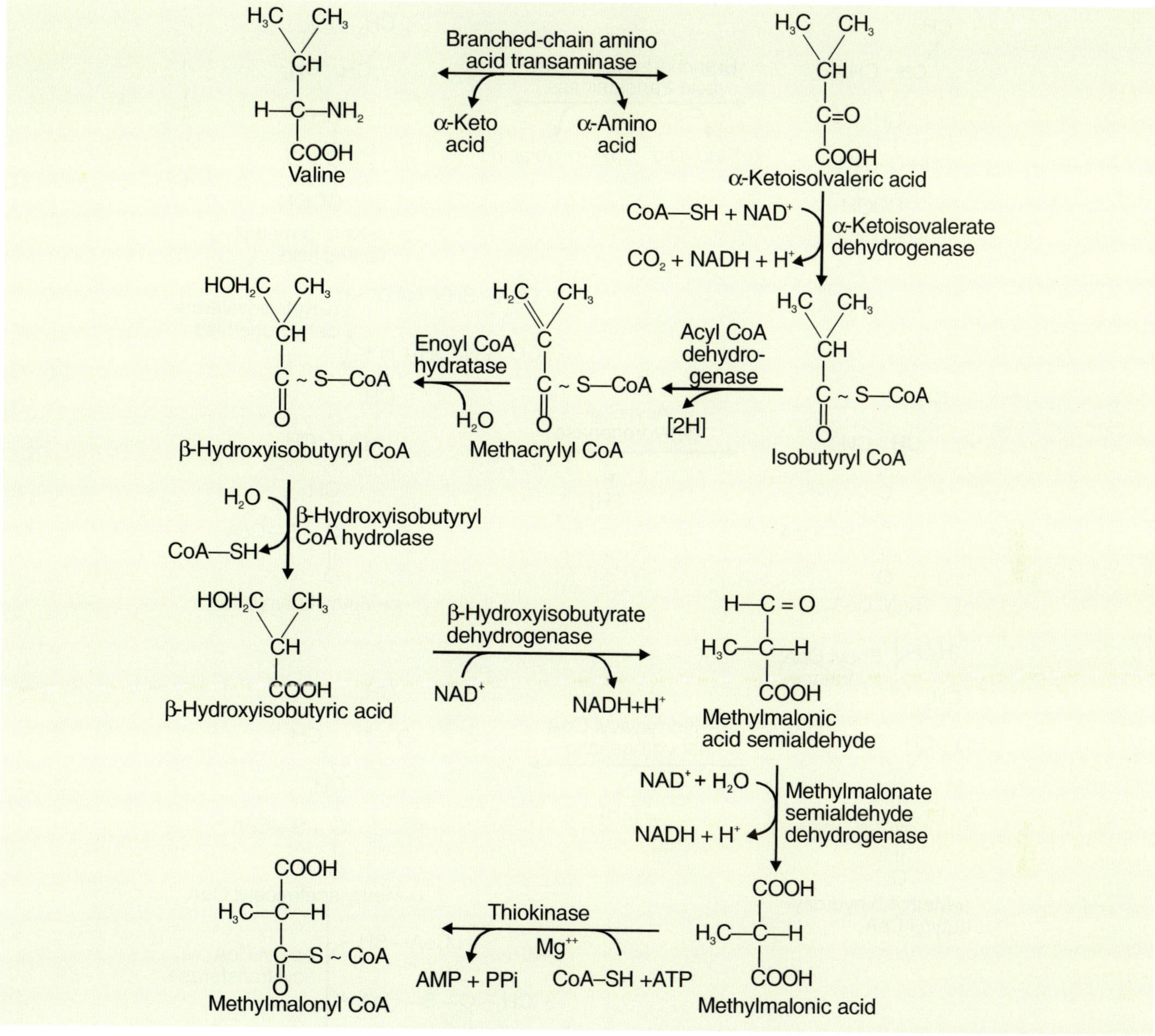

Fig. 12.24: Catabolism of valine

phosphate). It plays an important role in energy-transfer reactions in muscles. For muscle contraction, energy is provided by hydrolysis of ATP to ADP. During sustained muscle activity, ATP may be depleted. However, ATP is rapidly regenerated by transfer of a high-energy phosphate group from creatine phosphate to ADP. Thus, a continuous supply of energy is ensured during muscle contraction. When muscles are relaxing, creatine phosphate is regenerated by transfer of a high-energy phosphate group from ATP to creatine. This is a reversible reaction catalysed by creatine kinase (CK), also known in the past as creatine phosphokinase (CPK).

$$\text{Creatine phosphate + ADP} \underset{}{\overset{\text{CK}}{\rightleftharpoons}} \text{Creatine + ATP}$$

Glycine is one of the amino acids, besides arginine and methionine, required to synthesise creatine (Fig. 12.27).

Creatine is catabolised to creatinine which is released into circulation, and is excreted in urine. Urinary creatinine excretion, over a 24-hour period, is fairly constant in an individual, and depends upon his muscle mass. Creatinine clearance is used as one of the kidney function tests as the urinary excretion of creatinine is decreased in kidney diseases.

Methionine

The biologically important compound formed from methionine is **S-adenosyl methionine** which acts as a donor of labile methyl groups for various methylation reactions (Fig. 12.5). It supplements the action of

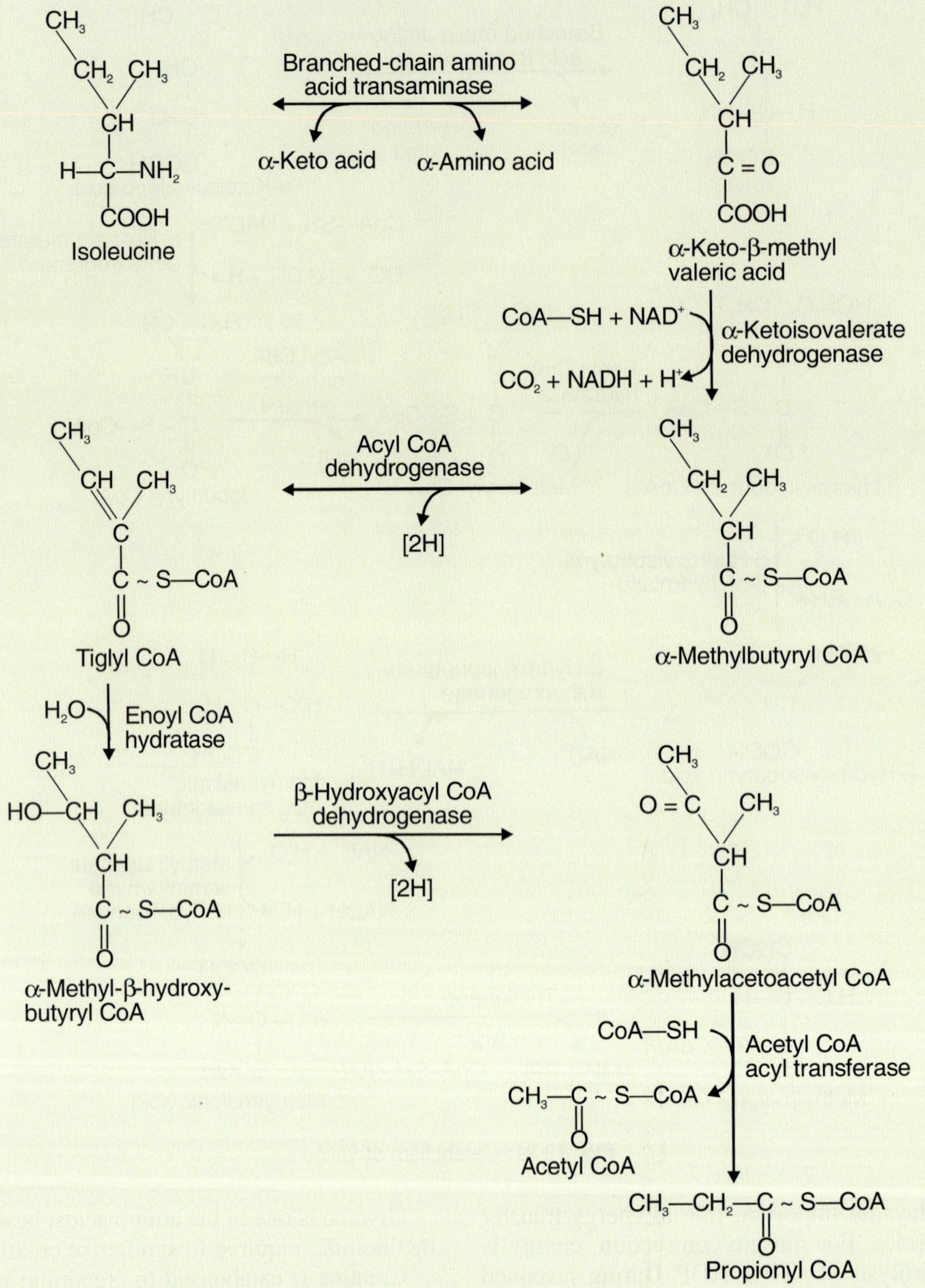

Fig. 12.25: Catabolism of isoleucine

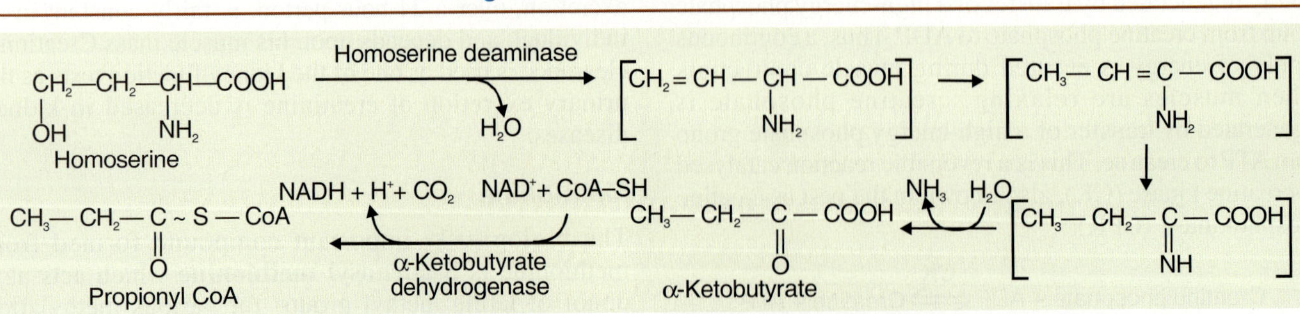

Fig. 12.26: Conversion of homoserine into propionyl CoA

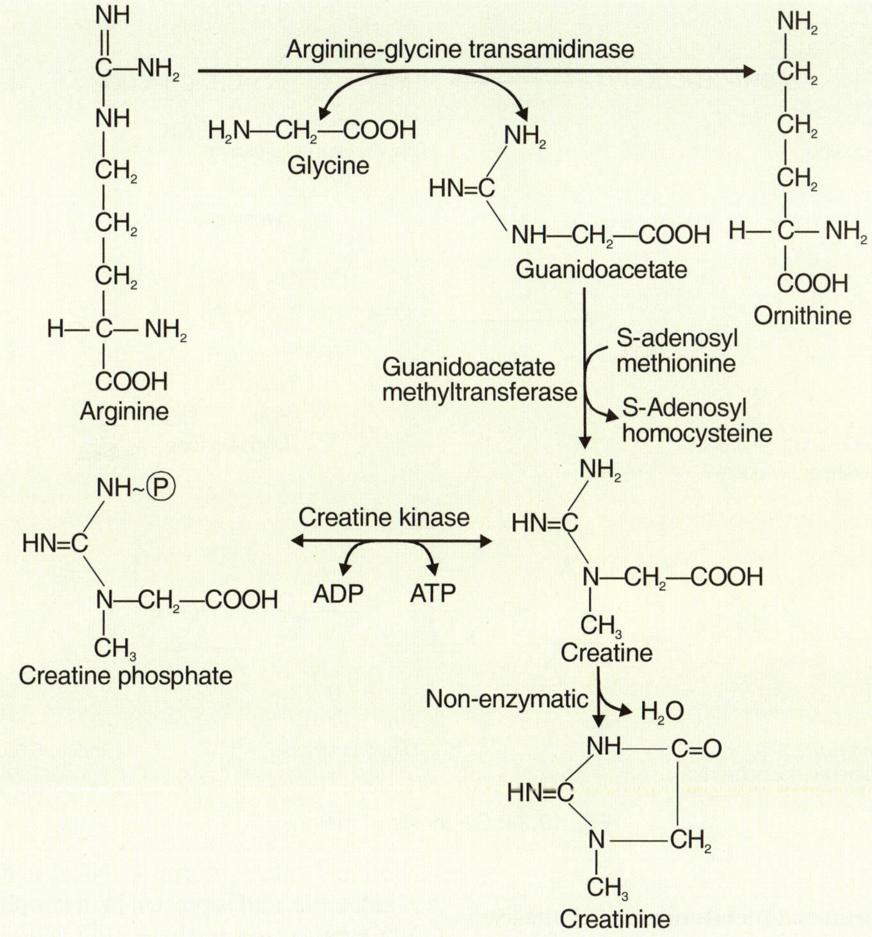

Fig. 12.27: Synthesis and catabolism of creatine

methyltetrahydrofolate which has a limited methyl transfer potential.

Cysteine

Cysteine forms **taurine** which acts as a **neurotransmitter** in brain. Taurine also conjugates with cholic acid to form **taurocholic acid**, a bile acid. Cysteine is also used in the synthesis of **coenzyme A** from pantothenic acid. The mercaptoethanolamine portion of coenzyme A is derived from cysteine. Cysteine is also a constituent of **glutathione**.

Glutamate

Gamma-aminobutyric acid (GABA) is formed by decarboxylation of the α-carboxyl group of glutamate.

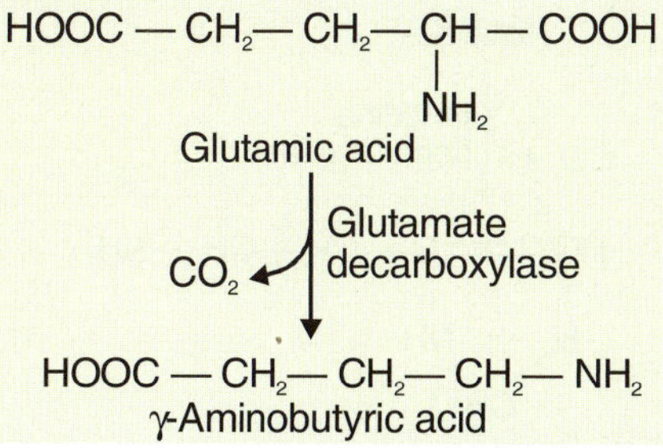

$$HOOC - CH_2 - CH_2 - CH - COOH$$
$$|$$
$$NH_2$$
Glutamic acid

Glutamate
decarboxylase
CO_2

$$HOOC - CH_2 - CH_2 - CH_2 - NH_2$$
γ-Aminobutyric acid

Gamma-aminobutyric acid acts as a **neurotransmitter** in brain. Glutamate itself is also a neurotransmitter. Glutamate is also a constituent of **glutathione**.

Tyrosine

A number of specialised compounds are formed from tyrosine (or phenylalanine after its hydroxylation to tyrosine). Formation of **epinephrine, norepinephrine, triiodo-thyronine** and **thyroxine** from tyrosine or phenylalanine will be discussed later (see Chapter 17).

Melanin, the black pigment present in skin, hair and iris, is also formed from tyrosine. The exact structure of melanin is not known but it is believed to be a polymer of 5,6-dihydroxyindole and indole-5,6-quinone which are formed from tyrosine (Fig. 12.28).

The first two reactions in the synthetic pathway are catalysed by tyrosinase which is a copper-dependent enzyme but the identity of the enzymes catalysing the subsequent reactions is not clearly established. According to one view, all the reactions are catalysed by tyrosinase. According to another view, the reactions after the formation of dopaquinone occur spontaneously.

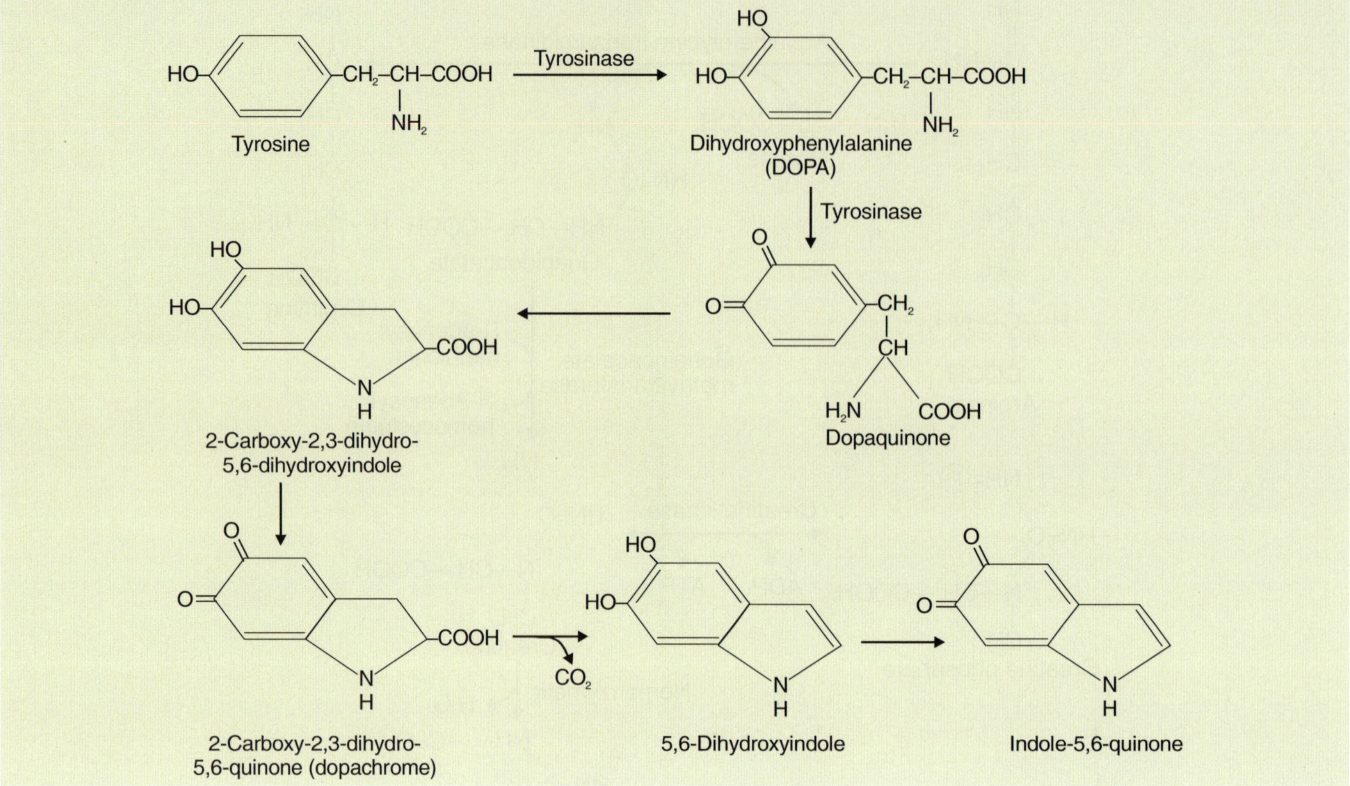

Fig. 12.28: Synthesis of melanin

Tryptophan

Two hormones, **serotonin** and **melatonin**, are synthesised from tryptophan (see Chapter 17). Tryptophan can also be converted into **nicotinic acid (niacin)** in the body.It has been estimated that one mg of niacin is synthesised from 60 mg of tryptophan.

During the catabolism of tryptophan, 3-hydroxyanthranilic acid is formed as an intermediate. This can be converted into nicotinic acid (Fig. 12.29).

Arginine

Besides forming creatine, arginine is used to synthesise some polyamines, e.g. spermine and putrescine. **Nitric oxide** is also synthesised from arginine by nitric oxide synthase (NOS). The reaction occurs in stages.

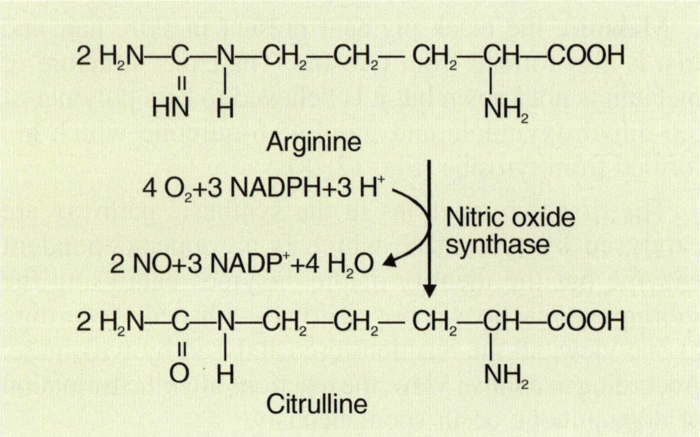

NOS has three isoforms – iNOS, nNOS and eNOS. iNOS is inducible, and is present in macrophages and neutrophils. NO synthesised in these cells aids in the destruction of phagocytosed cells, e.g. bacteria. nNOS is present in neurons. NO synthesised in neurons acts as a neurotransmitter. eNOS is present in endothelial cells. NO formed in endothelial cells diffuses into adjacent smooth muscles, and causes vasodilatation by relaxing the smooth muscles (coronary vasodilatation caused by nitroglycerin is due to release of nitric oxide during its breakdown). Nitric oxide synthesised in the endothelial cells acts as a local hormone.

Histidine

The local hormone, **histamine** is formed by decarboxylation of histidine (*see* Chapter 17 for more details).

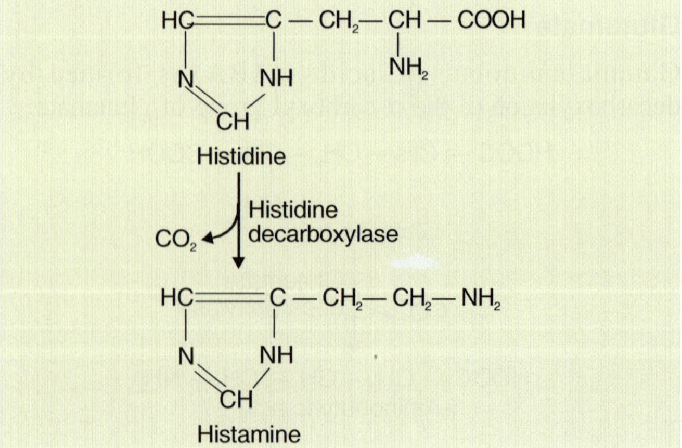

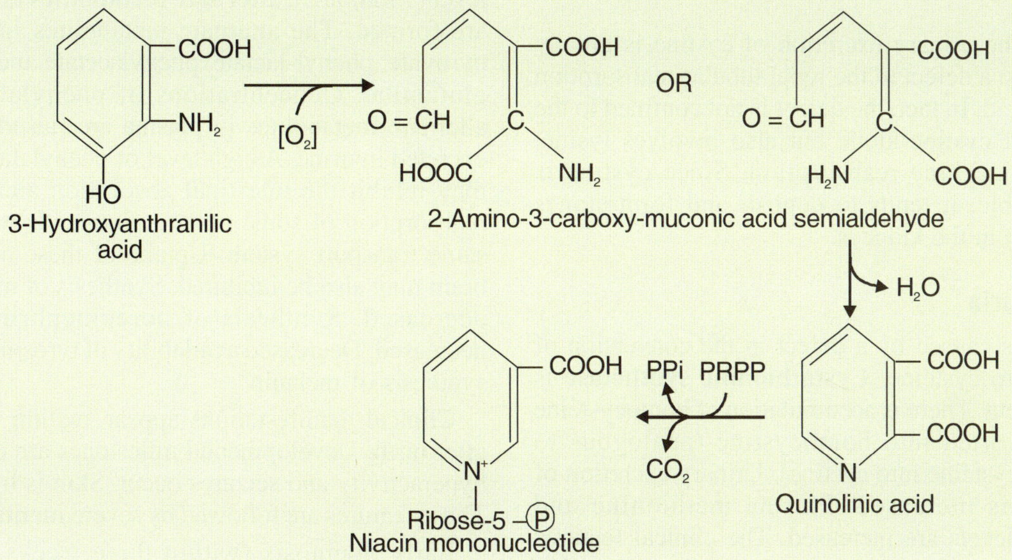

Fig. 12.29: Endogenous synthesis of niacin

Another compound formed from histidine is **ergothioneine** in red blood cells which plays a role in oxidation-reduction reactions.

INBORN ERRORS OF AMINO ACID METABOLISM

Mutations in genes encoding enzymes concerned with the metabolism of amino acids can lead to the synthesis of defective enzymes which may be devoid of catalytic activity or may have decreased catalytic activity. When catalytic activity is absent or deficient, the metabolism of the concerned amino acid is impaired resulting in an inborn error of metabolism. Over 50 inborn errors of metabolism of amino acids have been discovered. Clinical abnormalities occur because of decreased synthesis of products or accumulation of intermediates or formation of alternate metabolites. Many of the disorders of amino acid metabolism are very rare. Some of these are fatal in infancy or early childhood. Many result in mental retardation and other neurological abnormalities. Early diagnosis of these disorders is important so that treatment can be started early and neurological abnormalities may be prevented. In most of these disorders, the treatment consists of **restricted intake** or **exclusion** of the affected amino acid from the diet. Some relatively common inborn errors of amino acid metabolism are the following:

Primary Hyperoxaluria

Urinary excretion of oxalate is increased in primary hyperoxaluria. This is really a disorder of **glyoxylate** metabolism but glyoxylate is formed from amino acids viz. glycine and hydroxyproline. Normally, glyoxylate is transaminated to glycine or is oxidised to formate. A deficiency of glycine transaminase together with a disturbance in the oxidation of glyoxylate into formate results in the formation of oxalate from glyoxylate. This leads to hyperoxaluria and recurrent formation of **oxalate stones** in the urinary tract.

Maple Syrup Urine Disease (MSUD)

This disorder involves the branched-chain amino acids, **valine, leucine** and **isoleucine**. As described earlier, the enzymes catalysing the first two reactions in the catabolism of these amino acids (transamination and oxidative decarboxylation) are common to all the three amino acids. Absence or decreased activity of **α-ketoisovalerate dehydrogenase (α-keto acid decarboxylase)**, which catalyses oxidative decarboxylation of the α-keto acid derivatives of branched-chain amino acids, leads to accumulation of valine, leucine, isoleucine and their respective α-keto acid derivatives in blood and their excessive excretion in urine. This imparts a typical odour to urine resembling that of maple syrup or burnt sugar.

The clinical signs and symptoms appear within one week of birth. Lethargy, vomiting and aversion to food are early signs followed later by severe brain damage and ultimately death. The treatment consists of exclusion of branched-chain amino acids from diet until their plasma levels fall to normal and, then, restricted intake to maintain the plasma levels.

A milder variant of maple syrup urine disease, known as **intermittent branched-chain ketonuria**, has also been recognised. In this, the decrease in enzyme activity is only moderate. The signs and symptoms are milder and appear much later. The excretion of branched-chain α-keto acids is intermittently increased.

Cystinuria

In cystinuria, the urinary excretion of cystine is greatly increased due to a defect in the renal tubular reabsorption of this amino acid. In fact, the defect is not confined to the reabsorption of cystine alone but also involves lysine, arginine and ornithine reabsorption. Since cystine is sparingly soluble, it tends to deposit and form stones (cystine stones) in the kidneys.

Homocystinuria

This disorder is caused by a defect in the conversion of **methionine** into cysteine. **Cystathionine synthetase** is severely deficient. There is accumulation of homocysteine which is converted into homocystine (analogous to conversion of cysteine into cystine). Urinary excretion of homocystine is increased. Plasma methionine and homocysteine levels are increased. The clinical features include thrombotic phenomena, osteoporosis, dislocation of lenses in the eyes, mental retardation and ischaemic vascular disease.

Accumulation of homocysteine produces several abnormalities. It impairs the normal cross-linking of collagen. It produces abnormalities in the ground substance of walls of blood vessels. It increases platelet adhesiveness. Dislocation of ocular lenses and osteoporosis occur due to abnormal collagen. Thrombotic phenomena occur because of abnormalities in the walls of blood vessels. Increased platelet adhesiveness and abnormal vessel walls cause **ischaemic heart disease, cerebral thrombosis** and **peripheral vascular disease**. Ischaemic vascular diseases occur at a young age. Homocysteine has been described as the **'new cholesterol'** because of its propensity to cause ischaemic vascular diseases.

Early diagnosis and a **low-methionine, high-cysteine** diet prevents most of the clinical abnormalities. **Pyridoxine** supplements may be given to activate the residual cystathionine synthetase.

Hyperhomocysteinaemia may also occur due to deficiency of folic acid and vitamin B_{12}. In such cases, vitamin supplements correct the abnormality.

Phenylketonuria (PKU)

This is the commonest inborn error of amino acid metabolism. Its incidence is about 1 in 10,000 livebirths. It was the first inborn error of amino acid metabolism treated successfully by diet manipulation. The biochemical abnormality is a block in the conversion of **phenylalanine** into tyrosine (Fig.12.30). Two-thirds of the patients suffer from phenylketonuria, type I in which **phenylalanine hydroxylase** is deficient. Several mutations can cause this abnormality. The degree of enzyme deficiency is variable but it is severe in majority of the patients.

Plasma phenylalanine concentration rises after ingestion of phenylalanine. When the concentration exceeds a certain level (1 mmol/L), **alternate metabolites** of phenylalanine are formed. The alternate metabolites include phenyl-pyruvate, phenyl-lactate, phenylacetate and phenylacetyl-glutamine. Concentrations of phenylalanine and its alternate metabolites in plasma are raised, and they are excreted in urine. A high level of phenylalanine in plasma may inhibit the intestinal absorption and renal tubular reabsorption of some other amino acids which share the same transport system. Uptake of these amino acids by brain may also be inhibited. Synthesis of myelin sheath is decreased. Synthesis of norepinephrine in brain is decreased. Decreased availability of tyrosine decreases the synthesis of melanin.

Clinical manifestations appear within days or weeks after birth. Developmental milestones are delayed. Motor hyperactivity and seizures occur. Skin is hypopigmented. These features are followed by severe **mental retardation**.

Early diagnosis (within three weeks of birth) and treatment prevent the clinical abnormalities. Since phenylalanine is an essential amino acid, it can not be excluded from the diet. A **low-phenylalanine diet** is given to keep the plasma phenylalanine level below 6 mg/dl. As tyrosine can not be synthesised in the body due to severe deficiency of phenylalanine hydroxylase, tyrosine becomes an essential amino acid for patients with phenylketonuria. Therefore, the diet needs **tyrosine supplements**.

In phenylketonuria, type II, **dihydropteridine reductase** is deficient. In phenylketonuria, type III, there is a block in the **synthesis of tetrahydrobiopterin** from GTP. The end result is decreased conversion of phenylalanine into tyrosine. Moreover, synthesis of dopamine, norepinephrine and epinephrine from tyrosine and synthesis of serotonin and melatonin from tryptophan are also affected as tetrahydrobiopterin is required for **hydroxylation of tyrosine and tryptophan** also. Therefore, the clinical abnormalities in phenylketonuria, types II and III are more severe, appear early and do not improve despite diet manipulation.

Alkaptonuria

Alkaptonuria is an inborn error of **tyrosine** metabolism. Homogentisate, an intermediate in the catabolism of tyrosine, can not be metabolised further due to absence of **homogentisate oxidase**. Homogentisate is excreted in urine. Characteristically, freshly voided urine is normal in colour but becomes dark on exposure to atmosphere due to oxidation of homogentisate by oxygen.

Homogentisate and its oxidation product form polymers that bind to **collagen**. This leads to generalised pigmentation of connective tissues (**ochronosis**). Chemical irritation of collagen and/or defective cross-linking of collagen lead to degenerative changes in connective tissue. Damage to joint cartilages produces arthritis (**ochronotic arthritis**). Arthritis usually occurs in hip joints, knee joints, shoulder

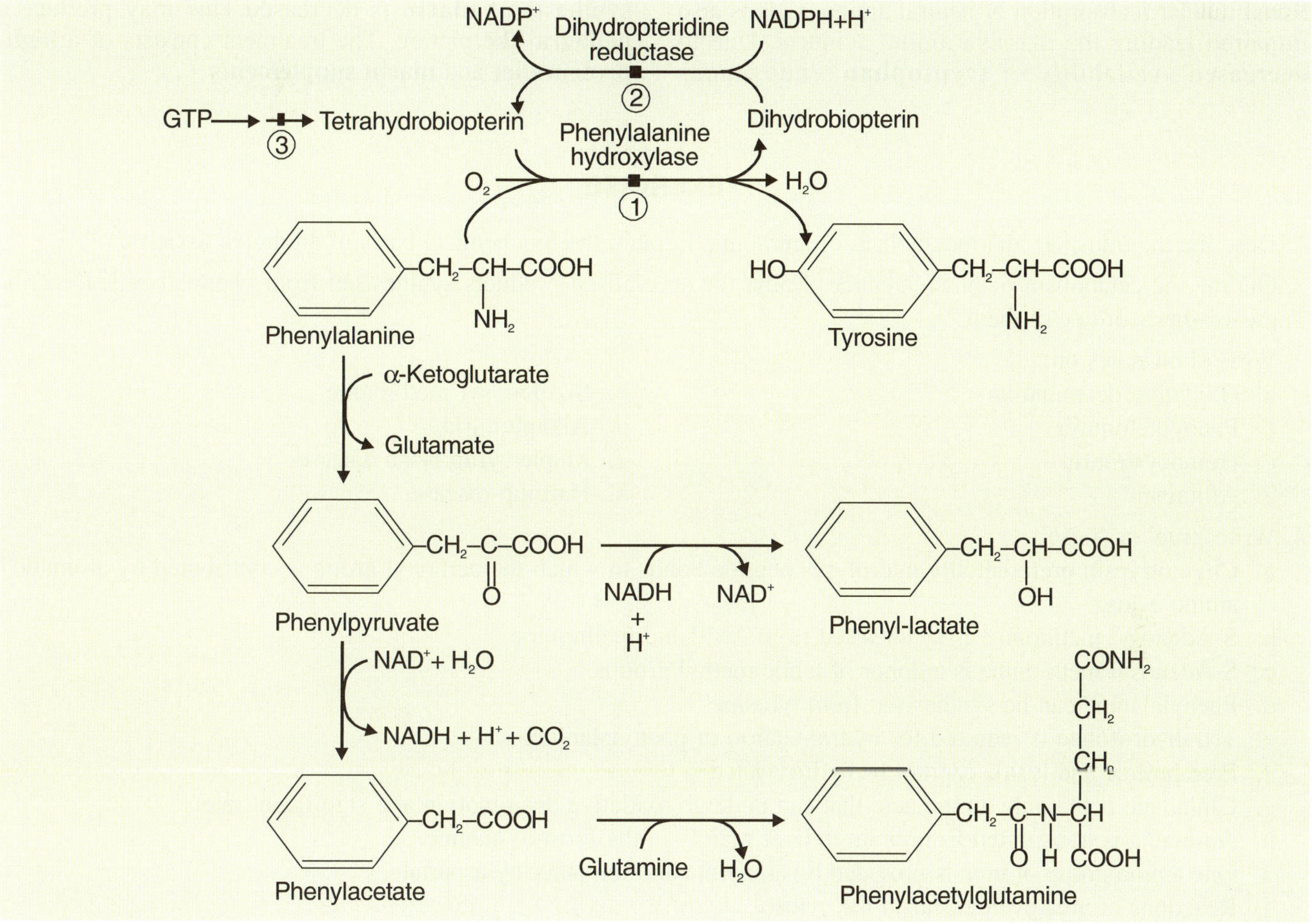

Fig. 12.30: Blocks in phenylketouria. ① Block in type I; ② Block in type II; ③ Block in type III. Alternate metabolites are formed due to the block

joints and the vertebral column. Pigmented spots may be seen on **sclera** and **ears**.

Treatment is symptomatic. Ascorbic acid supplements have been tried but without much success.

Tyrosinaemia

This is another inborn error of **tyrosine** metabolism in which plasma tyrosine level is increased. Tyrosine and its metabolites are excreted in urine. Two distinct genetic defects are known. Tyrosinaemia, **type I** is due to a deficiency of **fumarylacetoacetate hydrolase**, and is characterised by neurological abnormalities, liver damage and renal tubular dysfunction. Tyrosinaemia, **type II** is due to a deficiency of **tyrosine transaminase**, and affects eyes and skin.

Albinism

This is another inborn error of **tyrosine** metabolism. **Tyrosinase** is absent from **melanocytes**. Melanin can not be synthesised due to absence of tyrosinase, and skin, hair and iris become white. Such patients are called albinos.

Photophobia and skin hypersensitivity are the common clinical problems. The incidence of skin cancer is also high as sunlight cannot be blocked due to absence of melanin.

Histidinaemia

This is an inborn error of **histidine** metabolism in which **histidase** is deficient. Histidine can not be converted into urocanic acid. Concentration of histidine in plasma is increased. Histidine is converted into some alternate metabolites, viz imidazole pyruvate, imidazole lactate and imidazole acetate, which are excreted in urine. Development of **speech** is retarded in histidinaemia.

Hartnup Disease

This was believed to be a disorder of **tryptophan** metabolism at first but later evidence showed a **transport defect** involving all **neutral amino acids** including tryptophan. Intestinal absorption of neutral amino acids is impaired. Tryptophan stagnating in the intestinal lumen is converted by the intestinal bacteria into indole and indoxyl derivatives which are absorbed and are excreted in urine.

Renal tubular reabsorption of neutral amino acids is also impaired leading the massive amino aciduria. Due to decreased availability of **tryptophan**, endogenous synthesis of **niacin** is decreased. This may produce a **pellagra-like** picture. The treatment consists of a **high-protein diet** and **niacin supplements**.

EXERCISE

1. Describe the transport and metabolism of ammonia. Explain the biochemical basis of ammonia toxicity.

2. Outline the catabolism of phenylalanine. Name the specialised products synthesised from phenylalanine. Describe the synthesis of one of them.

3. Write short notes on:
   a. Oxidative deamination
   b. S-Adenosyl methionine
   c. Phenylketonuria
   d. Alkaptonuria
   e. Homocystinuria
   f. Maple syrup urine disease
   g. Albinism
   h. Hartnup disease

4. Write 'true' or 'false':
   a. Chymotrypsin preferentially hydrolyses peptide bonds in which the carboxyl group is contributed by aromatic amino acids.
   b. S-Adenosyl methionine is synthesised from AMP and methionine.
   c. S-Adenosyl methionine is a donor of labile methyl groups.
   d. Phenylalanine can be synthesised from tyrosine.
   e. Tetrahydrofolate is required for hydroxylation of phenylalanine.
   f. Free proline and lysine can not be hydroxylated.
   g. Glutamate is the only amino acid that can undergo oxidative deamination at a significant rate.
   h. Ammonia is transported from brain to liver mainly in the form of alanine.
   i. One amino group of urea is provided by ammonia and the other by aspartate.
   j. Reactions of urea cycle occur in the cytosol.
   k. N-Acetylglutamate is an activator of carbamoyl phosphate synthetase II.
   l. Arginine is an intermediate of urea cycle.
   m. Urea cycle is linked with citric acid cycle.
   n. Four ATP equivalents are utilised for the synthesis of one molecule of urea.
   o. Leucine is a glycogenic amino acid.
   p. N-Formiminoglutamate (FIGLU) is a metabolite of histidine.
   q. In pyridoxine deficiency, tyrosine is converted into xanthurenic acid.
   r. Creatine is synthesised from glycine, arginine and S-adenosyl methionine.
   s. Risk of ischaemic vascular diseases is increased in homocystinuria.
   t. Tetrahydrobiopterin deficiency causes a more severe type of phenylketonuria than phenylalanine hydroxylase deficiency.

5. Fill in the blanks:
   a. S-Adenosyl methionine is an intermediate in the catabolism of........................ .
   b. Tyrosine can be synthesised from ....
   c. Vitamin .... is required for hydroxylation of proline and lysine residues.
   d. Ammonia is transported from muscles to liver mainly in the form of ....
   e. Reactions of urea cycle in which energy is spent are synthesis of .... and ....
   f. .... is an activator of carbamoyl phosphate synthetase I.
   g. Glutamine can be synthesised from .... and ....
   h. An inorganic cofactor for prolyl hydroxylase is ....
   i. .... catalyses oxidative deamination of glutamate.
   j. .... is the organ most susceptible to ammonia toxicity.
   k. Nitric oxide is formed from ....

l. Melanin is synthesised from ....

m. .... is an inborn error of metabolism of branched-chain amino acids.

n. Deficiency of .... causes homocystinuria.

o. A low-methionine, high-cysteine diet is recommended for the treatment of ....

p. A low-phenylalanine, high-tyrosine diet is recommended for the treatment of ....

q. Tetrahydrobiopterin can be synthesised from ....

r. Absence of .... causes alkaptonuria.

s. Ochronosis occurs in ....

t. Albinism occurs due to absence of ....

ANSWERS TO SHORT QUESTIONS

4. a. True
   b. False
   c. True
   d. False
   e. False
   f. True
   g. True
   h. False
   i. True
   j. False
   k. False
   l. True
   m. True
   n. True
   o. False
   p. True
   q. False
   r. True
   s. True
   t. True

5. a. Methionine
   b. Phenylalanine
   c. C
   d. Alanine
   e. Carbamoyl phosphate, argininosuccinate
   f. N-Acetylglutamate
   g. Glutamate, ammonia
   h. Fe^{++}
   i. Glutamate dehydrogenase
   j. Brain
   k. Arginine
   l. Tyrosine
   m. Maple syrup urine disease
   n. Cytathionine synthetase
   o. Homocystinuria
   p. Phenylketonuria
   q. GTP
   r. Homogentisate oxidase
   s. Alkaptonuria
   t. Tyrosinase

Metabolism of Nucleotides

Nucleotides are small intracellular nitrogenous compounds essential for life. They are made up of a nitrogenous base, a pentose sugar and phosphate. The nitrogenous base may be a purine base or a pyrimidine base. The most important purine bases are adenine and guanine. The most important pyrimidine bases are cytosine, uracil and thymine. The sugar may be ribose or deoxyribose.

The nucleotides are required for the synthesis of the information molecules, deoxyribonucleic acid (DNA) and ribonucleic acid (RNA). The bases present in DNA are adenine, guanine, cytosine and thymine. The sugar present in DNA is deoxyribose.The bases present in RNA are adenine, guanine, cytosine and uracil. The sugar present in RNA is ribose. In addition to synthesis of DNA and RNA, many nucleotides, e.g. ATP, GTP, CTP, UTP, cAMP, cGMP, etc. perform other important functions as well.

Nucleotides are present in our diet and are also synthesised in the body. However, dietary nucleotides are not used for any purpose in our body. For our requirement of nucleotides, we are dependent solely on endogenous synthesis.

DIGESTION

In food, nucleotides are present mainly in the form of nucleoproteins. The protein portion is digested by the proteolytic enzymes present in the gastrointestinal tract. The nucleic acids are hydrolysed by nucleases. DNA is hydrolysed by deoxyribonuclease and RNA by ribonuclease into small polynucleotides. Polynucleotidases hydrolyse the small polynucleotides into mononucleotides. The nucleotides are hydrolysed into nucleosides and phosphate by nucleotidases and phosphatases. The nucleosides are absorbed by intestinal mucosal cells where they are broken down to their final metabolic end products. The end products are released into circulation, and are excreted in urine.Thus, the only fate of dietary nucleotides is digestion, absorption and excretion.

SYNTHESIS OF NUCLEOTIDES

Synthesis of purine and pyrimidine nucleotides is important because only the endogenously synthesised nucleotides are used for various purposes in our body. There are two pathways for the synthesis of nucleotides. In one pathway, known as **de novo synthesis**, the nucleotides are synthesised afresh from various amphibolic intermediates. Both purine and pyrimidine nucleotides can be synthesised by de novo pathway. In the second pathway, known as the **salvage pathway,** the bases or the nucleosides released during the catabolism of pre-existing nucleic acids and nucleotides are reutilised for the synthesis of new nucleotides. Salvage pathways exist for both purine nucleotides and pyrimidine nucleotides.Since the salvage pathway is energy-efficient and prevents wastage of raw materials, it is the preferred pathway for the synthesis of nucleotides. However, some tissues, for example **brain**, do not possess the salvage pathway and are dependent exclusively on de novo pathway for their requirement of nucleotides.

De novo Synthesis of Purine Nucleotides

Liver is the major site for de novo synthesis of purine nucleotides though synthesis can occur in several other tissues. The intracellular location of the pathway is the cytosol. The different carbon and nitrogen atoms for the synthesis of the purine nucleus are provided by glycine, glutamine, aspartate, carbon dioxide and the single-carbon moiety carried by tetrahydrofolate. The nitrogen at position 1 is provided by **aspartate**. Carbon 2 is contributed by the formyl group present in N^{10}- **formyl tetrahydrofolate**. Nitrogen 3 and nitrogen 9 are contributed by the amide group of **glutamine**. Carbon atoms 4 and 5, and the nitrogen atom at position 7 are provided by **glycine**. Carbon 6 comes from CO_2, and carbon 8 from N^5, N^{10}-**methenyl tetrahydrofolate** (Fig. 13.1).

The synthesis begins with the formation of **5-phosphoribosyl-1-pyrophosphate (PRPP).** PRPP is synthesised from ribose-5-phosphate and ATP. A pyrophosphate group is transferred from ATP to carbon 1 of ribose-5-phosphate by PRPP synthetase. PRPP is also required for the synthesis of pyrimidine nucleotides. Purine nucleus is formed atom by atom on carbon 1 of ribose.

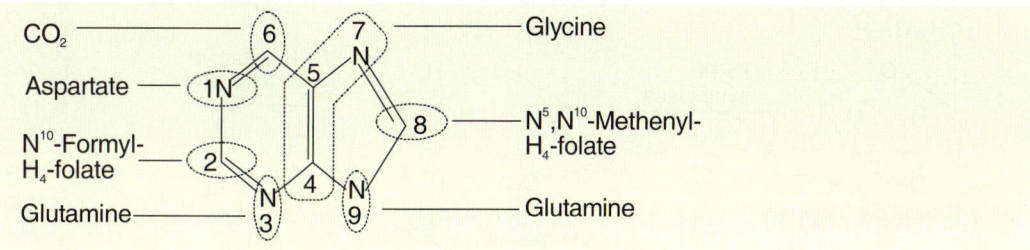

Fig. 13.1: Sources of various carbon and nitrogen atoms for the purine nucleus

In the second reaction, an amide group from glutamine replaces the pyrophosphate group on carbon 1 of ribose forming 5-phospho-β-D-ribosylamine. This reaction is the committed step of the pathway.

In the third reaction, the entire glycine molecule condenses with the amino group of 5-phospho-β-D-ribosylamine forming glycinamide ribosyl-5-phosphate. In the next reaction, a formyl group is transferred to the terminal amino group from N^5, N^{10}-methenyl tetrahydrofolate forming formylglycinamide ribosyl-5-phosphate. In the next reaction, an amide group from glutamine replaces the keto group forming formylglycinamidine ribosyl-5-phosphate. This is followed by ring closure. The product is aminoimidazole ribosyl-5-phosphate. By this stage, the imidazole portion of the purine nucleus has been formed.

In the next reaction, aminoimidazole ribosyl-5-phosphate is carboxylated to aminoimidazole carboxylate ribosyl-5-phosphate. The latter condenses with the entire molecule of aspartate forming aminoimidazole succinyl carboxamide ribosyl-5-phosphate. The condensation occurs between the amino group of aspartate and the carboxyl group of aminoimidazole carboxylate ribosyl-5-phosphate. From the latter, fumarate is split off leaving behind aminoimidazole carboxamide ribosyl-5-phosphate.

A formyl group is now transferred from N^{10}-formyl-tetrahydrofolate to aminoimidazole carboxamide ribosyl-5-phosphate forming formimidoimidazole carboxamide ribosyl-5-phosphate. In the next reaction, ring closure occurs between the formyl group and the amino group. The product of the reaction is inosine monophosphate (IMP). Inosine monophosphate is the first purine nucleotide to be formed in the pathway in which the base, hypoxanthine is attached to ribose and phosphate (Fig.13.2).

Hypoxanthine can be converted into adenine as well as guanine by a series of reactions. In this way both AMP and GMP can be formed from inosine monophosphate (Fig. 13.3).

In eukaryotes, some of the enzymes are present in the form of **multienzyme complexes**. One such complex consists of phosphoribosyl glycinamide synthetase and phosphoribosyl aminoimidazole synthetase. A second complex consists of phosphoribosyl aminoimidazole carboxylase and phosphoribosyl aminoimidazole succinyl carboxamide synthetase. A third complex consists of formyl transferase and IMP synthetase.

Formation of ATP and GTP

AMP and GMP are converted into ADP and GDP respectively by nucleoside monophosphate kinase. ADP and GDP are converted into ATP and GTP respectively by nucleoside diphosphate kinase.

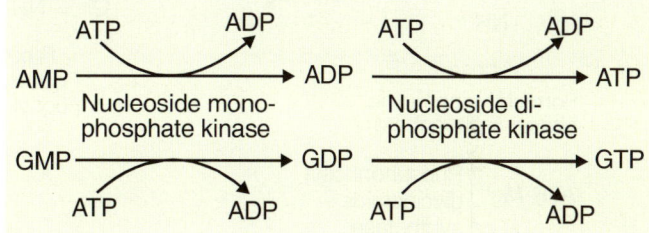

Regulation of de novo Synthesis

PRPP synthetase is an allosteric enzyme. It is inhibited by **AMP, ADP, GMP** and **GDP**. However, this enzyme is not unique to purine nucleotide synthesis as PRPP is required for the synthesis of pyrimidine nucleotides as well. **PRPP glutamyl amidotransferase** catalyses the first reaction unique to purine nucleotide synthesis. This enzyme is allosterically inhibited by **GMP**.

Moreover, the synthesis of adenine and guanine nucleotides is cross-regulated in such a way that the production of these two groups of nucleotides is always balanced. Conversion of IMP into AMP requires GTP, and conversion of IMP into GMP requires ATP. This ensures a balanced production of AMP and GMP.

Conversion of IMP into AMP and GMP is also regulated by allosteric mechanism. **AMP** is an allosteric inhibitor of **adenylosuccinate synthetase**. Similarly, **GMP** is an allosteric inhibitor of **IMP dehydrogenase**.

Synthesis of Purine Nucleotides by Salvage Pathway

Pre-existing purine bases and purine nucleosides may be salvaged to form new purine nucleotides. Conversion of purine bases into nucleotides is catalysed by two enzymes– **adenine phosphoribosyl transferase (APRT)** and **hypoxanthine-guanine phosphoribosyl transferase (HGPRT)**. The former acts on adenine while the latter acts on hypoxanthine as well as guanine. A phosphoribosyl moiety is transferred from PRPP to the base (Fig. 13.4).

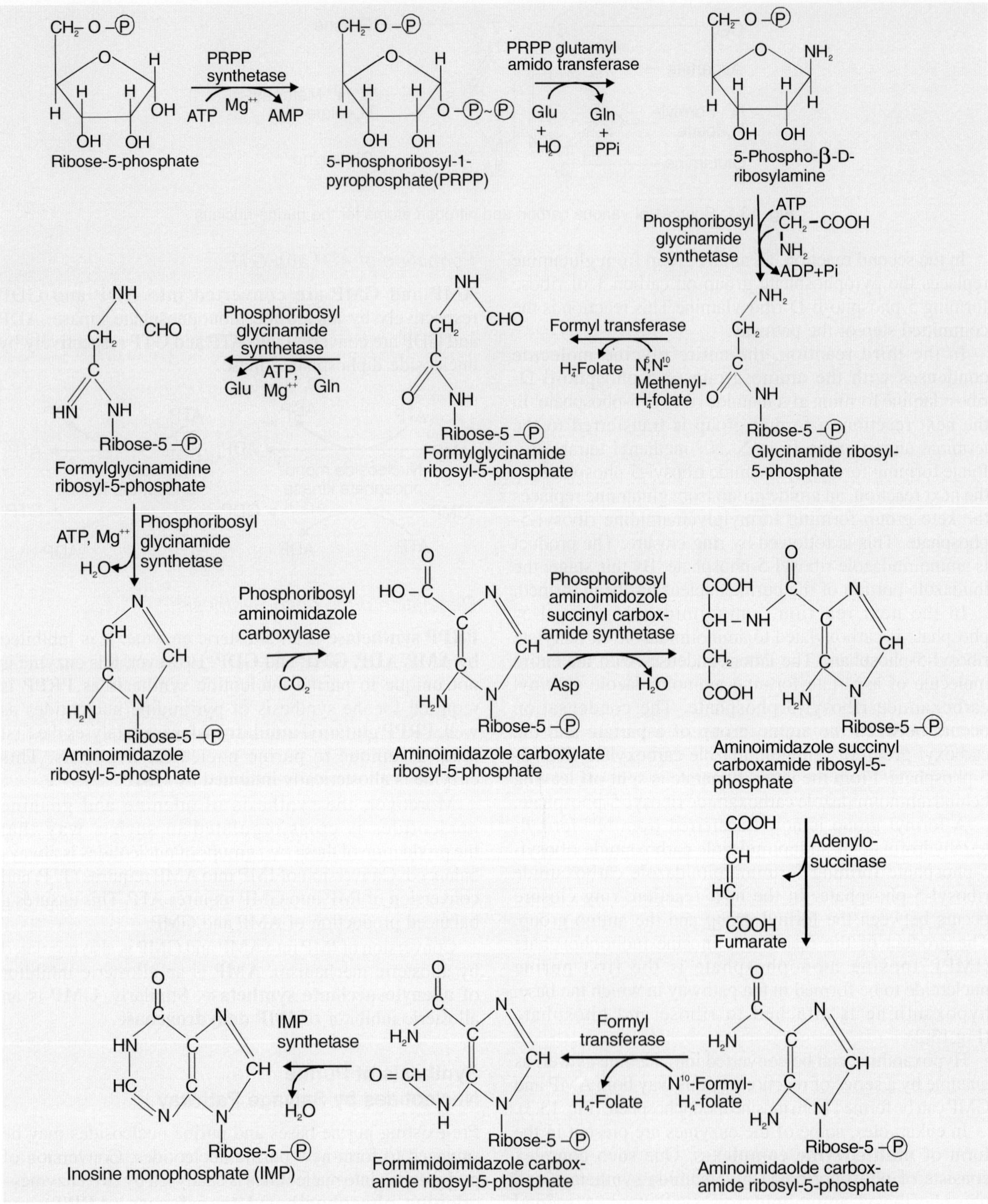

Fig. 13.2: De novo synthesis of purine nucleotides

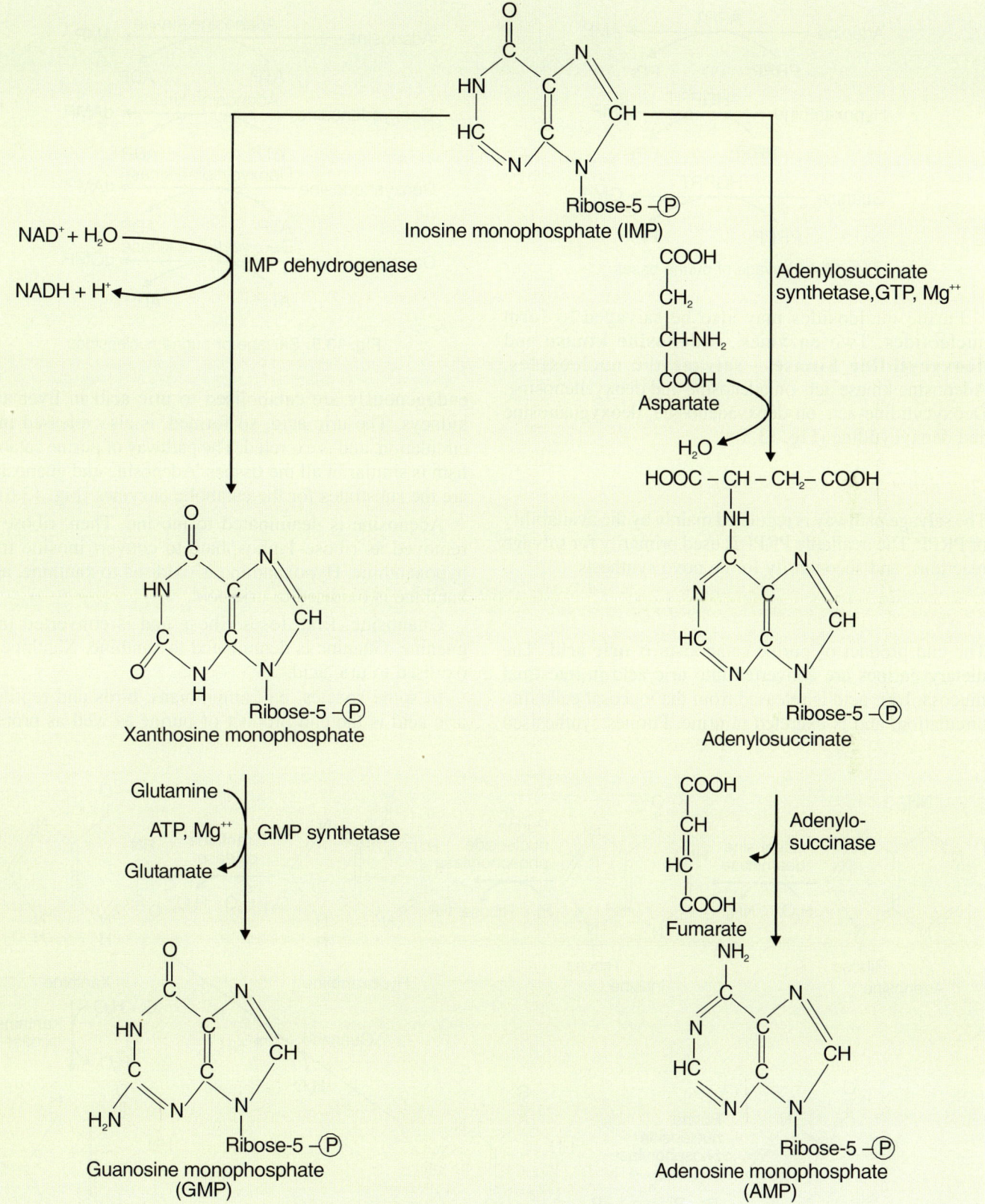

Fig. 13.3: Synthesis of GMP and AMP from IMP

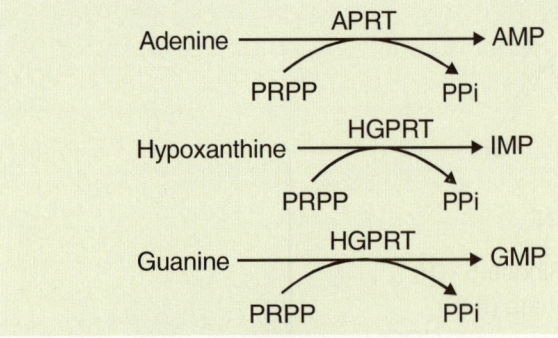

Fig. 13.4: Salvage of purine bases

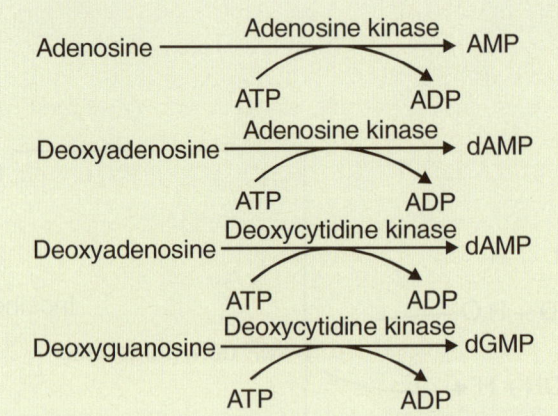

Fig. 13.5: Salvage of purine nucleosides

Purine nucleosides may also be salvaged to form nucleotides. Two enzymes – **adenosine kinase** and **deoxycytidine kinase** – salvage the nucleosides. Adenosine kinase acts on adenosine and deoxyadenosine. Deoxycytidine acts on deoxyadenosine, deoxyguanosine and deoxycytidine (Fig. 13.5).

Regulation of Salvage Pathway

The salvage pathway is regulated mainly by the availability of PRPP. The available PRPP is used primarily for salvage reactions, and secondarily for de novo synthesis.

Catabolism of Purines

The end product of purine catabolism is **uric acid**. The dietary purines are converted into uric acid in intestinal mucosa. Uric acid is released from the mucosal cells into circulation, and is excreted in urine. Purines synthesised endogenously are catabolised to uric acid in liver and kidneys. The uric acid, so formed, is also released into circulation, and is excreted. The pathway of purine catabolism is similar in all the tissues. Adenosine and guanosine are the substrates for the catabolic enzymes (Fig. 13.6).

Adenosine is deaminated to inosine. Then, ribose is removed as ribose-1-phosphate to convert inosine into hypoxanthine. Hypoxanthine is oxidised to xanthine, and xanthine is oxidised to uric acid.

Guanosine, first, loses ribose and is converted into guanine. Guanine is deaminated to xanthine. Xanthine is oxidised to uric acid.

In some species, e.g. amphibians, birds and reptiles, uric acid is the end product of purine as well as protein

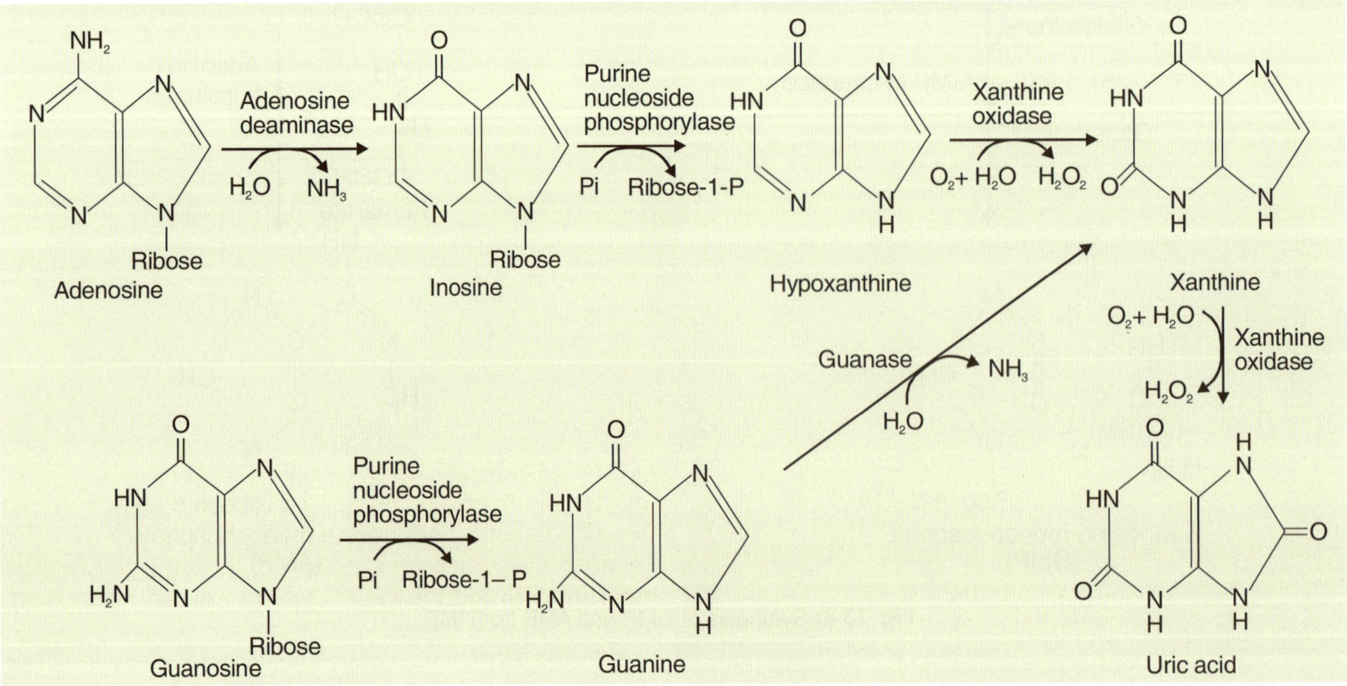

Fig. 13.6: Catabolism of purines

catabolism. In these organisms, uric acid is the main vehicle for excretion of nitrogenous waste. Such organisms are said to be uricotelic. Those organisms, e.g. human beings, in whom urea is the major form of nitrogenous waste are said to be ureotelic. Aquatic animals eliminate ammonia as such in the surrounding water, and are said to be ammonotelic.

De novo Synthesis of Pyrimidine Nucleotides

The first reaction in de novo synthesis of pyrimidine nucleotides is formation of **carbamoyl phosphate** from glutamine, CO_2 and ATP. Formation of carbamoyl phosphate is also the first reaction in the synthesis of urea. However, this reaction occurs in mitochondria in urea cycle and the amino group of carbamoyl phosphate comes from ammonia.

In contrast, for synthesis of pyrimidine nucleotides, carbamoyl phosphate is synthesised in the cytosol. The amino group is provided by glutamine. The enzyme catalysing this reaction is **carbamoyl phosphate synthetase II (CPS II).**

In the second reaction, the carbamoyl group is transferred from carbamoyl phosphate to aspartate forming carbamoyl aspartate. This reaction is catalysed by aspartatate transcarbamoylase.

The third reaction is a ring closure reaction catalysed by dihydro-orotase. The product of this reaction is dihydro-orotate.

In the next reaction, dihydro-orotate is reduced to orotate by dihydro-orotate dehydrogenase. This is the only reaction of the pathway which occurs in **mitochondria**. All the other reactions occur in **cytosol**.

In the next reaction, a phosphoribosyl group is transferred from PRPP to orotate by orotate phosphoribosyl transferase forming orotidine monophosphate (OMP) or ortidylate. This shows a contrast between de novo synthesis of purines and pyrimidines. The purine ring is assembled on ribose phosphate. During pyrimidine synthesis, ribose phosphate is added after formation of the ring.

OMP is, then, decarboxylated to uridine monophosphate (UMP) by OMP decarboxylase (Fig. 13.7).

UMP is the first pyrimidine nucleotide to be formed in the pathway. Cytidine and thymidine nucleotides are formed from UMP. For the formation of cytidine nucleotides, UMP is converted into UDP, and UDP into UTP. UTP is aminated to CTP. The amino group is provided by the amide group of glutamine (Fig. 13.8).

Thymidine nucleotides occur only in DNA. Therefore, the sugar portion in thymidine nucleotides is deoxyribose. The synthesis occurs from UDP. UMP is first converted into UDP. The ribose residue of UDP is reduced to deoxyribose by ribonucleotide reductase. Deoxyuridine diphosphate (dUDP) is dephosphorylated to dUMP. dUMP is methylated to form dTMP (also termed TMP) by thymidylate (TMP) synthetase. The methyl group is provided by N^5, N^{10}-**methylene-H$_4$-folate** (Fig. 13.9). During this reaction, the methylene group is reduced to a methyl group, and tetrahydrofolate gets oxidised to dihydrofolate. For continued synthesis of TMP, dihydro-folate has to be reduced to tetrahydrofolate, a reaction catalysed by **dihydrofolate reductase.**

Competitive inhibitiors of dihydrofolate reductase, e.g. amethopterin and aminopterin, are used as anti-cancer drugs as they decrease TMP synthesis. This, in turn, retards cell division.

Formation of Deoxyribonucleotides

Deoxyribonucleotides, required for DNA replication, are formed from ribonucleotides. Formation of dUDP from UDP has been shown in Fig. 13.9 but the actual reaction is far more complex. It requires the participation of **ribonucleotide reductase, thioredoxin** (a protein having two sulphydryl groups) and **thioredoxin reductase** (a flavoprotein). First, the oxygen atom attached to carbon 2 of ribose residue reacts with two sulphydryl groups of thioredoxin in the presence of ribonucleotide reductase. Water is formed, and thioredoxin is oxidised. Then, thioredoxin reductase regenerates reduced thioredoxin by transferring reducing equivalents from **NADPH** to oxidised thioredoxin (Fig. 13.10). This enzyme system can act on **ADP, GDP, CDP** and **UDP** to form dADP, dGDP, dCDP and dUDP respectively. Regulation occurs by allosteric mechanism. dADP is an inhibitor while ATP is an activator.

Regulation of de novo Synthesis

Carbamoyl phosphate synthetase and aspartate trans-carbamoylase are the regulatory enzymes. Both are allosteric enzymes. **Carbamoyl phosphate synthetase** is activated by **PRPP**, and is inhibited by **UTP**. **Aspartate transcarbamoylase** is inhibited by **CTP**.

Synthesis of Pyrimidine Nucleotides by Salvage Pathway

Human beings lack enzymes that can salvage free pyrimidine bases. However, pyrimidine nucleosides can be salvaged and used for nucleotide synthesis. Uridine and cytidine can be phosphorylated by a common enzyme, **uridine-cytidine kinase**. Thymidine (deoxythymidine) can be phosphorylated by **thymidine kinase**. Deoxy-cytidine is phosphorylated by **deoxycytidine kinase** which can also phosphorylate deoxyadenosine and deoxy-guanosine (Fig. 13.11).

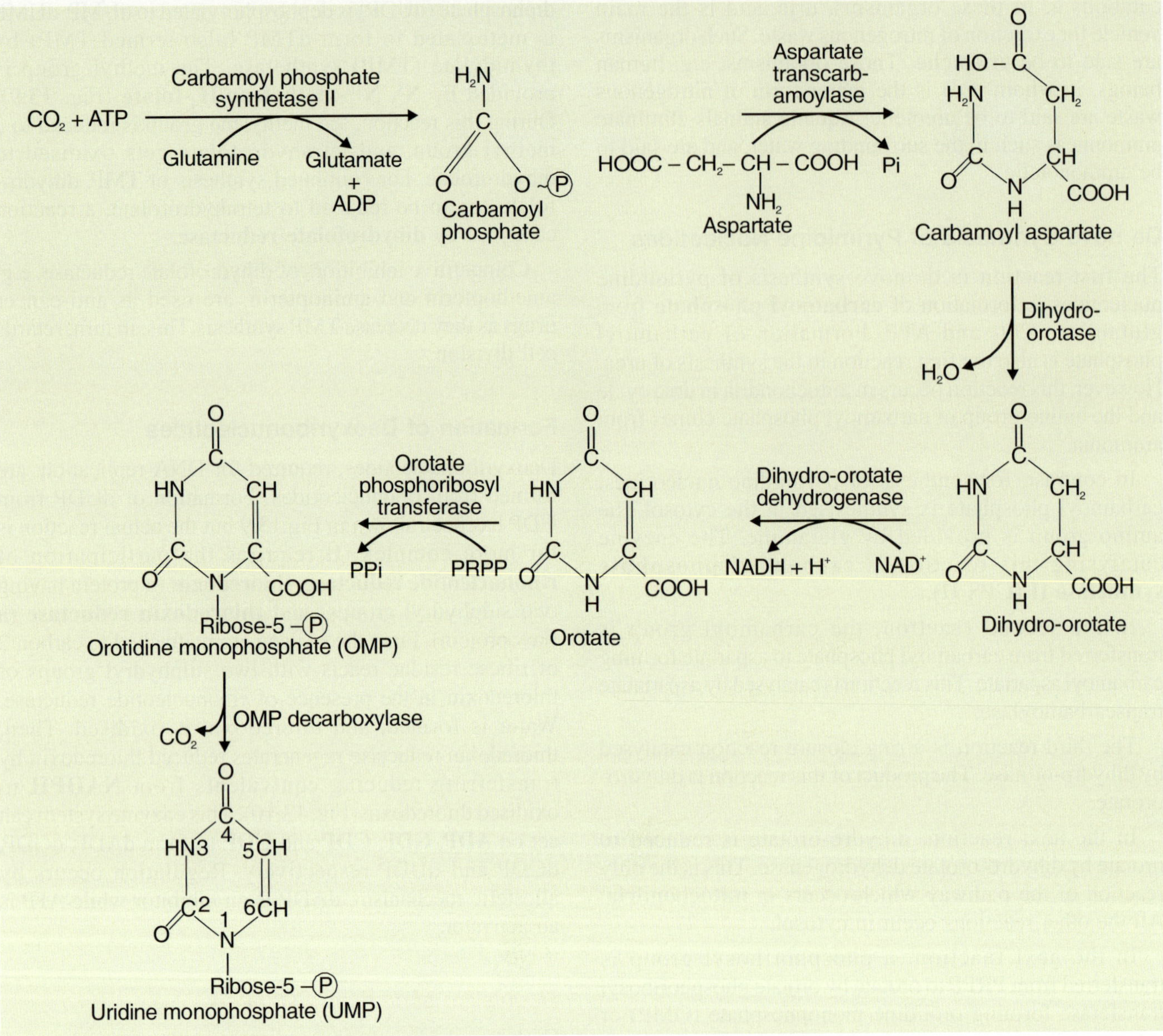

Fig. 13.7: De novo synthesis of uridine monophosphate

Catabolism of Pyrimidines

Cytosine and uracil are catabolised to **β-alanine, carbon dioxide** and **ammonia** (Fig. 13.12). β-Alanine may be utilised in the body or excreted in urine. Thymine is catabolised to **β-aminoisobutyrate**, carbon dioxide and ammonia (Fig. 13.13). Ammonia released from pyrimidines and purines is disposed off in the same way as that released from amino acids.

β-Aminoisobutyrate is excreted in urine. Urinary excretion of β-aminoisobutyrate is a rough indicator of the rate of DNA turnover.

INBORN ERRORS OF NUCLEOTIDE METABOLISM

Disorders of purine and pyrimidine nucleotide metabolism occur due to mutations in genes encoding the enzymes involved in the metabolism of purines and pyrimidines.

The affected enzyme may be absent, deficient or even superactive. Inborn errors of purine metabolism are more common and more severe than those of pyrimidine metabolism.

Some important disorders of purine metabolism are the following:

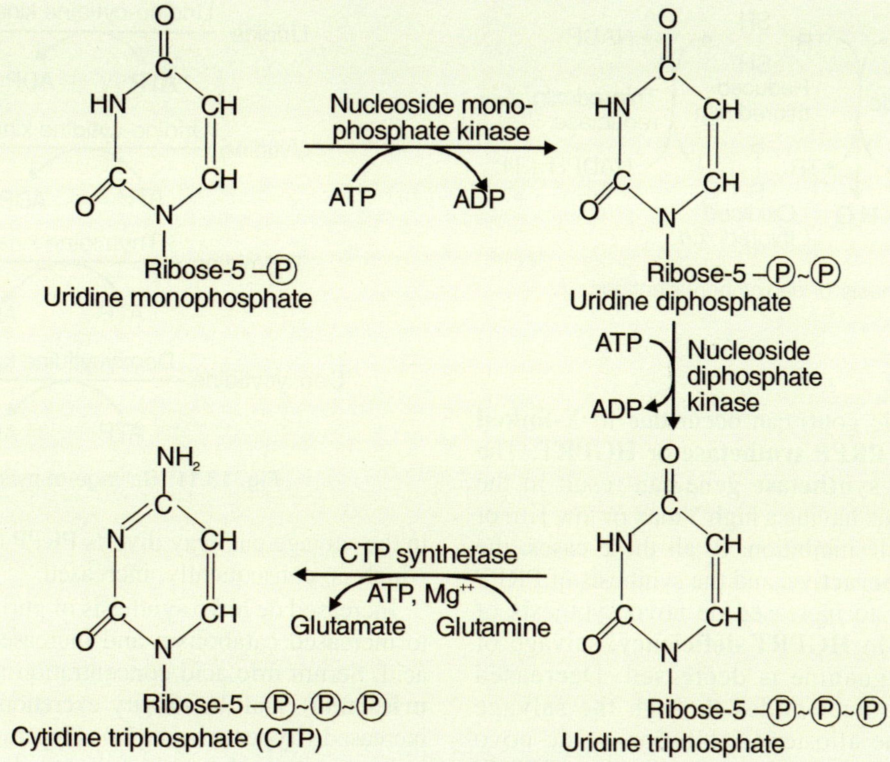

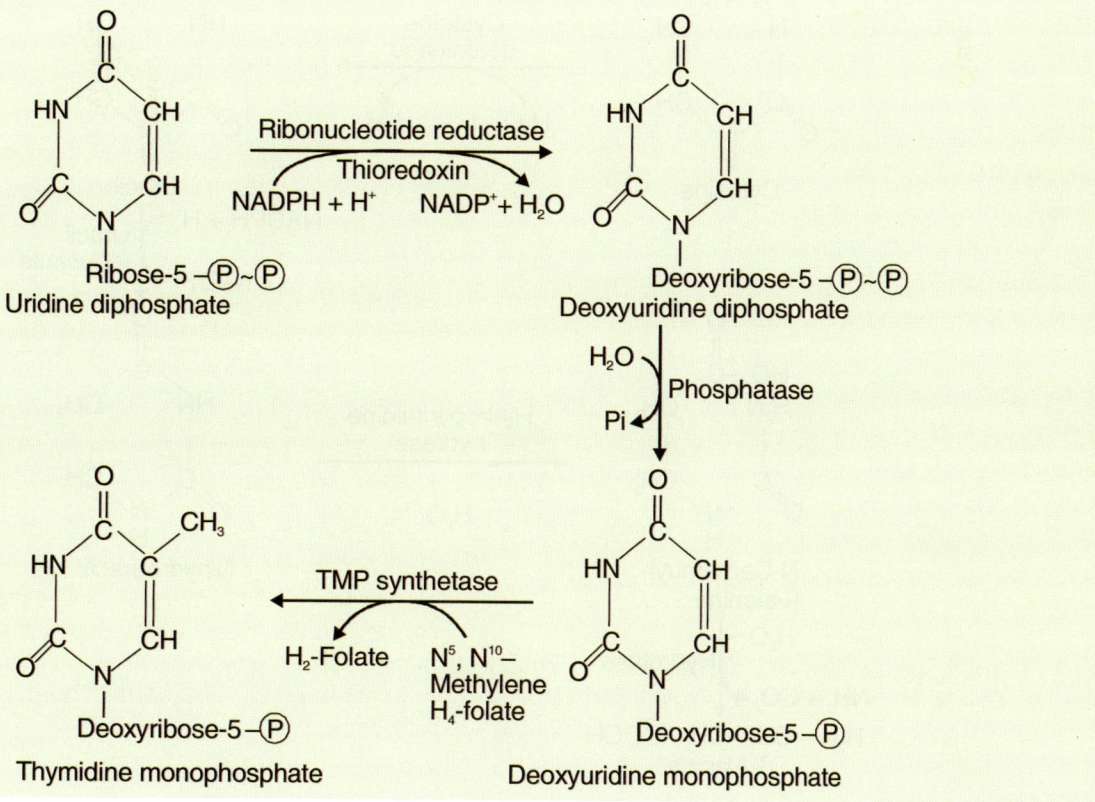

Fig. 13.8: Synthesis of cytidine triphosphate

Fig. 13.9: Synthesis of thymidine monophosphate

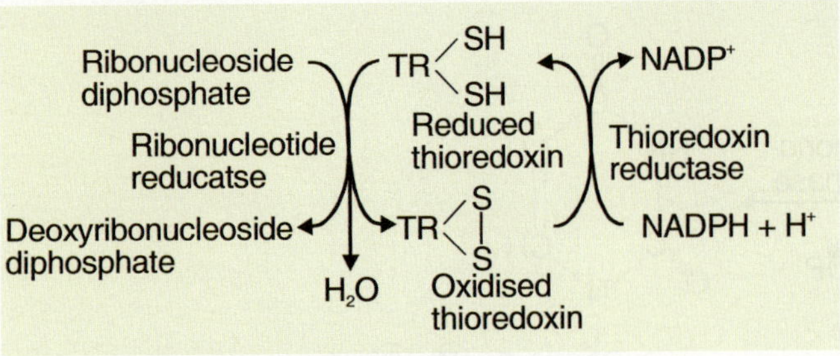

13.10: Synthesis of deoxyribonucleotides

Primary Gout

Primary gout (genetic gout) can occur due to **X-linked recessive** defects in **PRPP synthetase** or **HGPRT**. The mutations in **PRPP synthetase** gene can result in the synthesis of an enzyme having a high Vmax or low Km or resistance to allosteric inhibition. In all these cases, the enzyme becomes **superactive**, and the synthesis of PRPP is increased leading to increased de novo synthesis of purine nucleotides. In **HGPRT deficiency**, salvage of hypoxanthine and guanine is decreased. Decreased synthesis of purine nucleotides through the salvage pathway relieves the allosteric inhibition on de novo synthesis. At the same time, decreased utilisation of PRPP

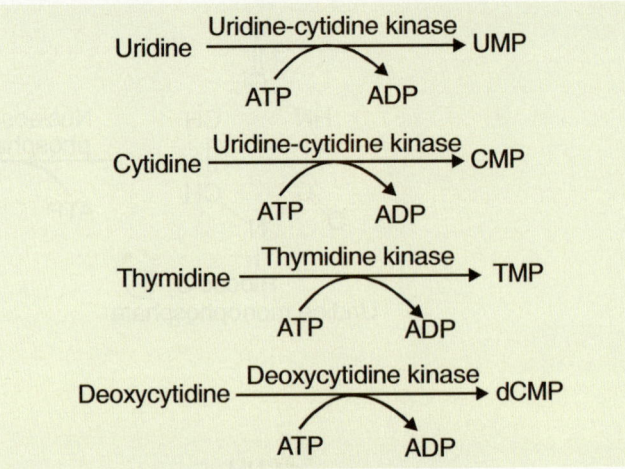

Fig. 13.11: Salvage of pyrimidines

in the salvage pathway diverts PRPP to de novo synthesis which is, consequently, increased.

Increased de novo synthesis of purine nucleotides leads to increased catabolism and increased formation of uric acid. Serum uric acid concentration is increased (**hyperuricaemia**), and the urinary excretion of uric acid is also increased (**hyperuricosuria**). Hyperuricaemia and hyperuricosuria cause the various signs and symptoms of gout.

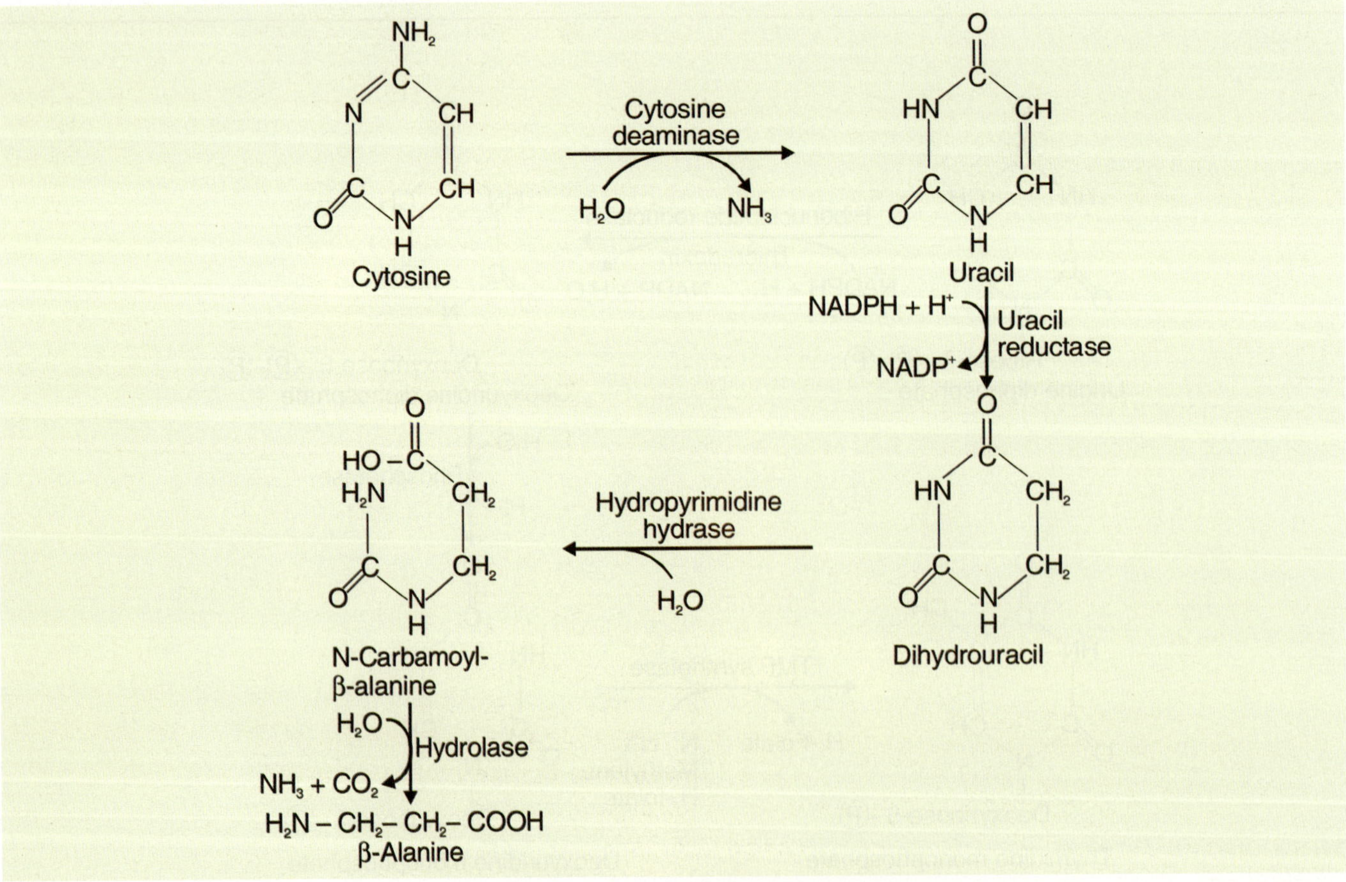

Fig. 13.12: Catabolism of cytosine and uracil

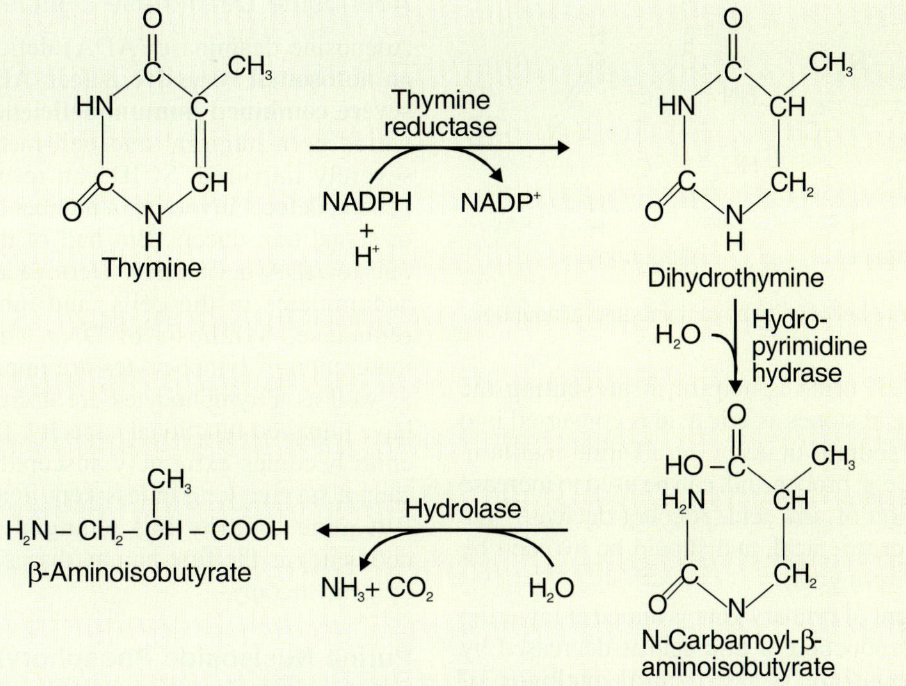

Fig. 13.13: Catabolism of thymine

Uric acid is a weak acid. Its keto and enol forms exist in equilibrium (Fig. 13.14). From the enol form, the first hydrogen ion dissociates at pH 5.8 (pKa$_1$ of uric acid) forming urate (or sodium urate). At pH below 5.8, uric acid is undissociated. At pH above 5.8, it is dissociated to form urate (or sodium urate or monosodium urate). At pH 5.8, uric acid and sodium urate are present in equimolar concentrations. Both uric acid and sodium urate are **poorly soluble** substances but uric acid is even less soluble than sodium urate.

Since the pH of plasma is above 5.8, uric acid is present predominantly in the form of sodium urate in plasma. When its concentration exceeds 7 mg/dl, it begins to get precipitated, mainly in and around joints. Deposits of urate crystals are known as **tophi**. The needle-shaped crystals of sodium urate in synovial fluid first attract neutrophils and later on macrophages which engulf the crystals. The neutrophils release oxygen-derived free radicals, leukotriene B$_4$, chemotactic factors and lysosomal hydrolytic enzymes, e.g. collagenase and protease. The macrophages release PGE$_2$, tumour necrosis factor$_\alpha$ (TNF$_\alpha$), interleukin-1(IL-1) and lysosomal enzymes. The resultant acute inflammatory response produces acute **gouty arthritis** which may later progress to chronic gouty arthritis. Metatarsophalangeal joint of big toe is affected most frequently. Less commonly, other small joints may also be affected. Acute attacks of gouty arthritis are treated with colchicine and anti-inflammatory drugs. **Colchicine** prevents the activation of neutrophils. Anti-inflammatory drugs prevent or suppress inflammatory response.

Increased urinary uric acid can lead to precipitation of uric acid in kidneys which can cause the formation of **uric acid stones**. Such stones are more likely to be formed in the distal convoluted tubules and collecting ducts where urine is acidified. When urinary pH decreases below 5.8, urate is converted into uric acid which is more likely to precipitate due to its low solubility.

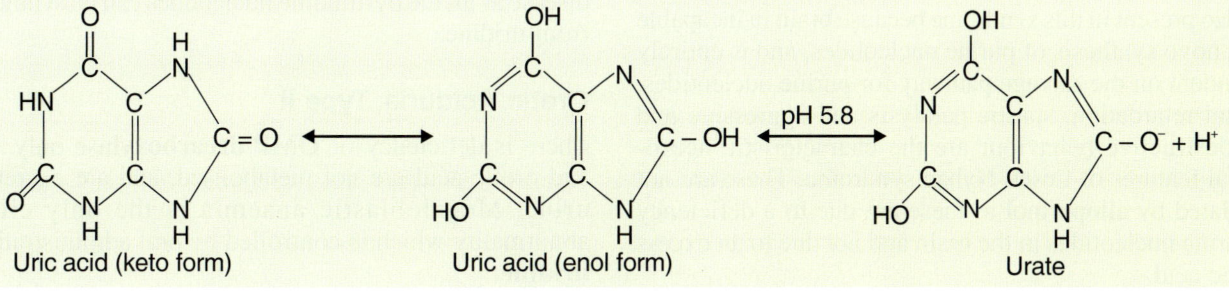

Fig. 13.14: Dissociation of uric acid

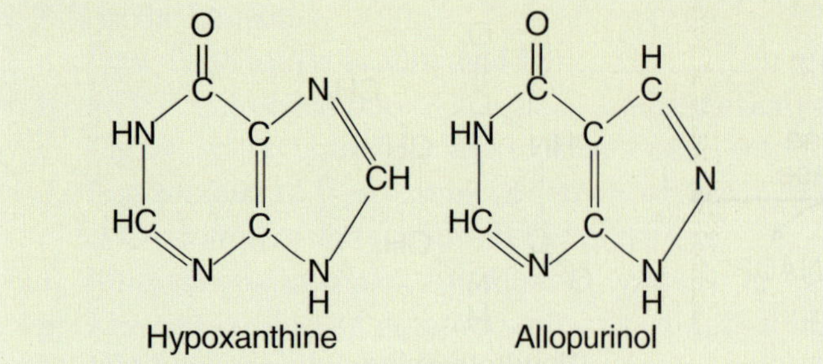

Fig. 13.15: Similarity between hypoxanthine and allopurinol

Alkalinisation of urine is helpful in preventing the formation of uric acid stones as uric acid is converted into the more soluble sodium urate in an alkaline medium. **Uricosuric drugs**, e.g. probenecid, can be used to increase the urinary excretion of uric acid. Alcohol decreases the urinary excretion of uric acid, and should be avoided by persons suffering from gout.

Specific treatment of primary gout is aimed at lowering serum uric acid. Production of uric acid is decreased by **allopurinol**. Allopurinol is a structural analogue of hypoxanthine, and is, therefore, a competitive inhibitor of xanthine oxidase (Fig. 13.15).

On administration of allopurinol, xanthine oxidase is inhibited, formation of uric acid is greatly decreased, and hypoxanthine and xanthine become the major end products of purine catabolism. Since hypoxanthine and xanthine are highly soluble, they are easily excreted in urine, and chances of stone formation are decreased. **Febuxostat** is a newer drug which is a non-competitive inhibitor of xanthine oxidase. It is used in patients who can not tolerate allopurinol.

Sometimes, gout may occur due to raised serum uric acid concentration resulting from excessive breakdown of cells, e.g. in leukaemia, polycythaemia, pernicious anaemia, haemolytic anaemia, etc. or in renal disorders in which urinary excretion of uric acid is decreased. This type of gout is known as secondary gout.

Lesch-Nyhan Syndrome

This is a rare **X-linked recessive** disorder in which HGPRT is completely absent. Besides gouty arthritis and uric acid stones in the kidneys, severe **neurological abnormalities** are also present in this syndrome because brain in incapable of de novo synthesis of purine nucleotides, and is entirely dependent on the salvage pathway for purine nucleotides. Mental retardation, spastic paralysis and aggressive and self-destructive behaviour are the characteristic neurological features of Lesch-Nyhan syndrome. These are not alleviated by allopurinol as these are due to a deficiency of purine nucleotides in the brain and not due to an excess of uric acid.

Adenosine Deaminase Deficiency

Adenosine deaminase (ADA) deficiency is inherited as an **autosomal recessive** defect. ADA deficiency causes **severe combined immunodeficiency disease (SCID)** in which both humoral and cell-mediated immunity are severely impaired. SCID can result from a variety of genetic defects involving a number of enzymes, receptors or signal transducers. But half of the cases of SCID are due to ADA deficiency. Deoxyadenosine triphosphate accumulates in the cells, and inhibits ribonucleotide reductase. Synthesis of DNA and formation and/or maturation of lymphocytes are impaired. B lymphocytes as well as T lymphocytes are decreased in number, and have impaired functional capacity. Therefore, the affected child becomes extremely susceptible to infections and cannot survive long unless kept in a sterile environment. But gene therapy has changed the scenario. ADA deficiency is the first human disease successfully treated by gene therapy.

Purine Nucleoside Phosphorylase Deficiency

Purine nucleoside phosphorylase deficiency is inherited as an **autosomal recessive** defect. It results in selective deficiency of **T lymphocytes** which impairs **cell-mediated immunity**. Increased levels of deoxygua-nosine may be responsible for failure of T lymphocyte differentiation.

Disorders of pyrimidine metabolism are not only rare but are also less severe as compared to disorders of purine metabolism. Overproduction of pyrimidines is harmless as their catabolites are easily excreted. A deficient production of pyrimidines may cause clinical abnormalities which can be easily controlled. The following are the important disorders of pyrimidine metabolism:

Orotic Aciduria, Type I

Orotate phosphoribosyl transferase and **OMP decarboxylase** are deficient. The inheritance is **autosomal recessive**. De novo synthesis of pyrimidines is decreased. There is accumulation of orotic acid which is excreted in urine. The clinical features include retardation of growth, impairment of immune system and megaloblastic anaemia. Megaloblastic anaemia is unresponsive to folic acid and vitamin B_{12}. Oral administration of uridine controls the disease as all the pyrimidine nucleotides can be synthesised from uridine.

Orotic Aciduria, Type II

There is deficiency of **OMP decarboxylase** only. OMP and orotic acid are not metabolised, and are excreted in urine. Megaloblastic anaemia is the only clinical abnormality which is controlled by oral administration of **uridine**.

EXERCISE

1. Describe the salvage of purines and pyrimidines. Describe an inherited disorder resulting from absence of one of the salvage enzymes.

2. Describe the enzyme defect(s) and biochemical abnormalities in primary gout. Explain the biochemical basis of clinical abnormalities in and treatment of primary gout.

3. Write short notes on:
   a. Synthesis of deoxyribonucleotides
   b. Lesch-Nyhan syndrome
   c. Adenosine deaminase deficiency
   d. Orotic aciduria

4. Write 'true' or 'false':
   a. Dietary purines can be utilised in the body.
   b. PRPP is required for de novo synthesis of purine as well as pyrimidine nucleotides.
   c. Uric acid is the end product of pyrimidine metabolism.
   d. PRPP glutamyl amidotransferase catalyses the first reaction unique to purine nucleotide synthesis.
   e. Adenylosuccinate synthetase is activated by AMP.
   f. Carbamoyl phosphate synthetase II is present in mitochondria.
   g. Dihydro-orotate dehydrogenase is present in mitochondria.
   h. Inhibitors of dihydrofolate reductase decrease the synthesis of UTP and CTP.
   i. Thioredoxin is required for the synthesis of deoxyribonucleotides.
   j. Aspartate transcarbamoylase in allosterically inhibited by UTP.

5. Fill in the blanks:
   a. Dietary purines are catabolised in ....
   b. Carbamoyl phosphate synthetase II is inhibited by ....
   c. PRPP synthetase is superactive in ....
   d. Uric acid is present predominantly in the form of .... in plasma.
   e. Deposits of uric acid are known as ....
   f. .... is a competitive inhibitor of xanthine oxidase.
   g. .... is absent in Lesch-Nyhan syndrome.
   h. Adenosine deaminase deficiency causes ....
   i. Purine nucleoside phosphorylase deficiency impairs ....
   j. Orotic aciduria can be controlled by administration of ....

ANSWERS TO SHORT QUESTIONS

4. a. False
   b. True
   c. False
   d. True
   e. False
   f. False
   g. True
   h. False
   i. True
   j. False

5. a. Intestinal mucosa
   b. UTP
   c. Primary gout
   d. Sodium urate
   e. Tophi
   f. Allopurinol
   g. HGPRT
   h. Severe combined immunodeficiency disease
   i. Cell-mediated immunity
   j. Uridine

14

Metabolism of Nucleic Acids

Nucleic acids include deoxyribonucleic acid (DNA) and ribonucleic acid (RNA). DNA **stores genetic information**. Information about the amino acid sequence of all the proteins is present in the form of **genes** in DNA. The entire genetic material present in the DNA of an organism is known as its **genome**. The information is present in the form of a specific base sequence. The human genome has been sequenced. It consists of 3.2 billion base pairs. About 5% of human DNA contains coded information in the form of 35,000 genes. The remaining non-coding DNA may be involved in regulation of expression of genes, i.e. synthesis of proteins. Different types of RNA are required for the synthesis of proteins. According to the **central dogma** of molecular biology, information flows from DNA to RNA to proteins. The flow of information from DNA to RNA is known as **transcription**, and the use of this information to synthesise proteins is known as **translation.**

$$DNA \xrightarrow{\text{Transcription}} RNA \xrightarrow{\text{Translation}} \text{Proteins}$$

Another function of DNA is to transmit the genetic information from parent cell to the daughter cells when a cell divides. This is ensured by **replication** of DNA, i.e. the newly-synthesised DNA transmitted to the daughter cells is an exact replica of the DNA of the parent cell.

DNA is a double helix made up of two long strands which are anti-parallel and twisted around each other. It can exist in the form of A-DNA, B-DNA and Z-DNA, but B-DNA is the predominant form of DNA. DNA is supercoiled around histone octamers to form nucleosomes. The histone octamer is made up of two molecules each of histones H2A, H2B, H3 and H4. Another histone, H1 is present in between two nucleosomes. Some non-histone proteins are also associated with DNA.

During replication, each strand of parent cell DNA acts as a **template** on which a new **complementary** strand is synthesised. The DNA has to be uncoiled and the two strands have to be separated so that each can act as a template. Separation of the two strands is known as **denaturation** or **melting** of DNA, and requires breaking of hydrogen bonds between the base pairs, i.e. A and T,

and G and C. There are two hydrogen bonds between A and T, and three between G and C. Therefore, melting of DNA is easier in those regions where A and T pairs are more in number than G and C pairs. DNA can be melted *in vitro* by raising the temperature. As DNA melts, its optical density increases. The temperature at which half of the DNA is denatured is known as **Tm (midpoint or melting temperature)** of DNA which depends upon the relative contents of A⋯T and G⋯C pairs. A⋯T pairs decrease the Tm.

CELL CYCLE

Life cycle of a eukaryotic cell can be divided into four phases:
a. Mitotic or **M phase**,
b. Gap$_1$ or **G$_1$ phase**,
c. Synthetic or **S phase** and
d. Gap$_2$ or **G$_2$ phase**.

DNA is synthesised only once in the cell cycle in the S phase. When the cell divides in the M phase, one copy (molecule) of DNA is received by each daughter cell. Progression of the cell cycle from one phase to the next is regulated by some proteins and enzymes. The proteins are **cyclins** and the enzymes are cyclin-dependent protein kinases or **cyclin-dependent kinases (CDKs)**. Cyclin levels keep on changing during the cell cycle. At a certain time in the cell cycle, a particular cyclin increases and activates a CDK. The CDK phosphorylates some proteins which push the cell from one phase to the next. Some of the mammalian cyclins and CDKs have been identified (Fig. 14.1).

REPLICATION OF DNA

Replication of DNA has been studied extensively in prokaryotes, and much of the information available has been obtained in *E.coli*. Eukaryotic replication is somewhat different but the basic processes are similar in prokaryotes and eukaryotes. During replication, the two strands of DNA separate, and each serves as a template for the synthesis of a new strand which is complementary to the template strand in base sequence. The template strand and the

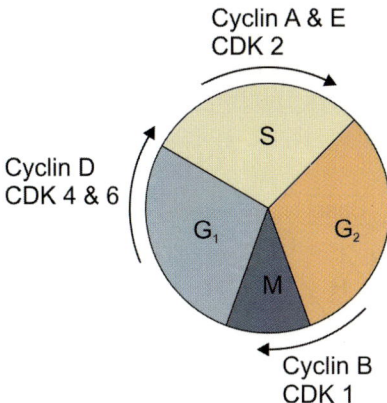

Fig. 14.1: Cell cycle and the periods when the level of various cyclins and cyclin-dependent kinases (CDKs) are raised

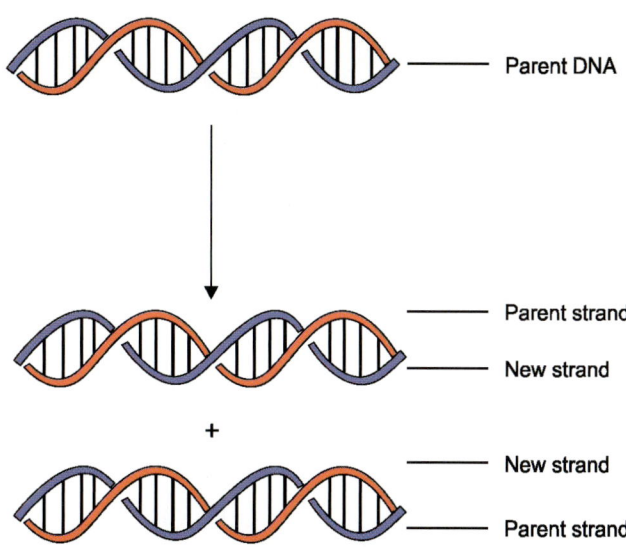

Fig. 14.2: Semi-conservative replication of DNA

newly-synthesised strand wind around each other to form a new double helix. Thus, each new DNA molecule is made up of one strand derived from the parent cell and one newly-synthesised strand (Fig.14.2). Therefore, replication is said to be **semi-conservative**.

Origin of Replication and Replication Fork

Replication of DNA begins at a specific site called origin of replication (Ori). For the two strands of parent DNA to act as templates, they must separate from each other. Origin of replication is a site rich in A=T pairs which makes strand separation easier as the bonding between adenine and thymine is weaker than the bonding between cytosine and guanine. In prokaryotes, there is only one origin of replication. Separation of strands at this site produces a fork-like structure known as replication fork (Fig. 14.3).

Both the strands of DNA are replicated simultaneously. The two strands are anti-parallel, i.e. they are parallel but

run in opposite directions. However, DNA and RNA can be synthesised in one direction only which is from 5´-end to 3´-end. One strand (known as the **leading strand**) is replicated continuously while the other strand (known as the **lagging strand**) is replicated discontinuously.

Primers and Okazaki Fragments (Pieces)

DNA synthesis cannot commence with deoxyribonucleotides because DNA polymerase cannot add a mononucleotide to another mononucleotide. It can add a mononucleotide only to an oligonucleotide. To solve this problem, the synthesis begins with ribonucleotides because a monoribonucleotide can be added to another monoribonucleotide. About ten ribonucleotides are added first to form an oligonucleotide known as **RNA primer** which

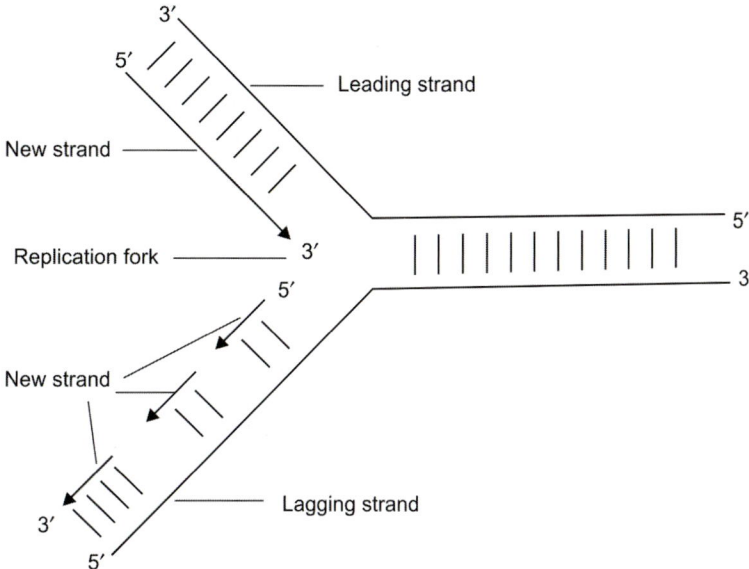

Fig. 14.3: Unwinding of DNA to form a replication fork and synthesis of complementary strands on leading and lagging strands (arrows show the direction of synthesis)

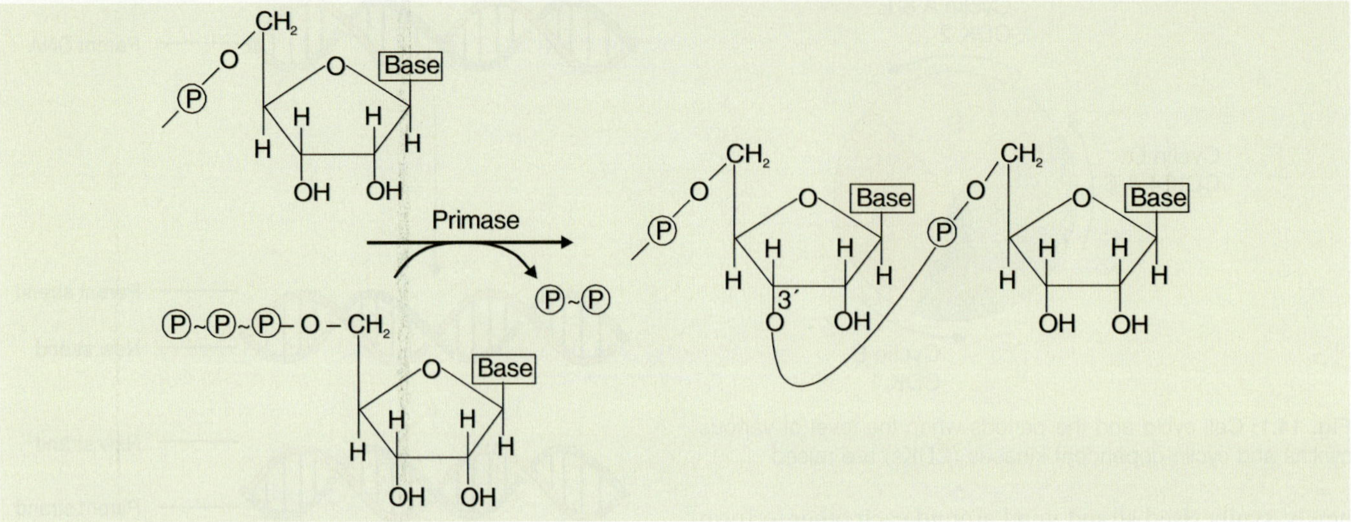

Fig. 14.4: Primase catalyses the formation of a phosphodiester bond between 3′-carbon of the last ribonucleotide and 5′-carbon of the new incoming ribonucleotide

is, then, extended by addition of deoxyribo-nucleotides. Later on, the ribonucleotides of the primer are replaced by deoxyribonucleotides.

The RNA primer is synthesised by **primase**. The ribonucleotide substrates enter in the form of ATP, GTP, CTP and UTP. A new ribonucleotide attaches through its phosphate group to the 3′-hydroxyl group of the previous one with the splitting off of a pyrophosphate. A phosphodiester bond is formed between 3′-carbon of the last nucleotide and 5′-carbon of the new nucleotide (Fig. 14.4).

The selection of nucleotides depends upon the sequence of bases in the template strand according to the **base-pairing rule**. Thus, an adenine nucleotide would enter opposite a thymine nucleotide, a uracil nucleotide opposite an adenine nucleotide, a cytosine nucleotide opposite a guanine nucleotide and a guanine nucleotide opposite a cytosine nucleotide.

After the formation of the RNA primer, deoxyribonucleotides are added one by one in the same manner according to the base-pairing rule. This reaction is catalysed by DNA polymerase. This process continues until about 100 deoxyribonucleotides have been added. The resulting polynucleotide having an RNA primer and several deoxyribonucleotides is known as an Okazaki fragment. Several Okazaki fragments are formed on the template strand (Fig. 14.5).

After the replication of several leading and lagging strands, the ribonucleotides of RNA primers are removed one by one from the 5′-end, and are replaced by appropriate deoxyribonucleotides according to the base-pairing rule. The remaining portions of parent DNA are also replicated. The DNA fragments are, then, sealed together. Each newly-synthesised strand forms a duplex with the template strand of the parent DNA.

Replication Bubbles

Eukaryotic DNA is much bigger than prokaryotic DNA. For example, human genome is 800 times as big as the *E.coli* genome. If replication of human DNA begins at a single site, it will take a long time for the entire DNA to be replicated. For speedy replication, eukaryotic DNA has several sites of origin at which replication begins simultaneously. The template DNA is nicked at a number of places to allow simultaneous unwinding of DNA at several places. The unwound portions form a number of replication bubbles which are replicated simultaneously (Fig. 14.6).

Enzymes and Proteins Involved in Replication

The process of replication requires a number of enzymes and protein factors. In *E.coli*, unwinding of parent DNA is initiated by **dna B** protein. First, **dna A** protein binds to the DNA at the initiation site. Then, it is joined by dna B and **dna C** protein. The dna B protein begins the unwinding. As replication proceeds, the further unwinding is catalysed by **helicase (rep protein)**. Both dna B protein and helicase require ATP as a source of energy for

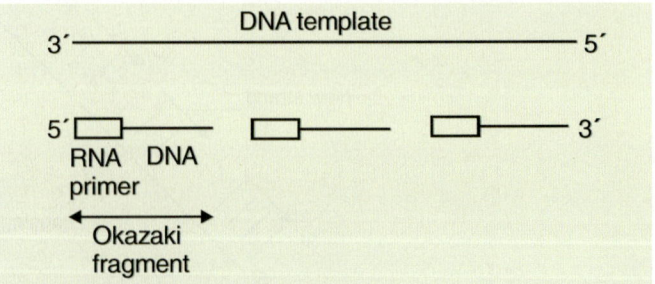

Fig. 14.5: Several Okazaki fragments are synthesised opposite the template strand of DNA

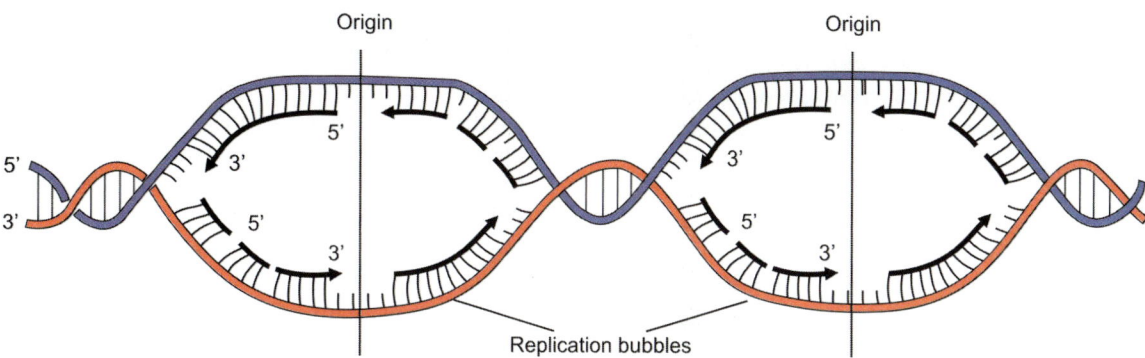

Fig. 14.6: Formation of replication bubbles and simultaneous replication from sites of origin in eukaryotes

unwinding DNA. The unwound strands are held apart by **single strand binding (SSB) protein.** Synthesis of RNA primer is catalysed by **primase.** Deoxyribonucleotides are added to the RNA primer by **DNA polymerase III holoenzyme**. DNA polymerase III possesses two different catalytic activities, i.e. polymerase activity and 3' → 5' exonuclease activity. The latter is required for proof-reading and **error-correction**. The enzyme moves along the template strand, and the polymerase activity adds deoxyribonucleotides one by one. After the addition of each deoxyribonucleotide, the enzyme moves back by one nucleotide distance, and checks the correctness of the base pair. If the pairing is correct, it moves ahead. If a wrong base is detected, the deoxyribonucleotide is split off by the 3' → 5' exonuclease activity of the enzyme. The correct nucleotide is, then, added by the polymerase activity. This ensures a high **fidelity** in replication.

Ribonucleotides of RNA primer are removed and replaced by deoxyribonucleotides by **DNA polymerase I**. DNA polymerase I possesses three different catalytic activities, i.e. 5'→3' exonuclease activity, polymerase activity and 3'→5' exonuclease activity. The 5'→3' exo-nuclease activity removes ribonucleotides from the 5'-end of the primer, the polymerase activity adds deoxyribo-nucleotides, and the 3'→5' exonuclease activity checks the correctness of base-pairing and removes wrong nucleotides

(a DNA polymerase II has also been found in *E.coli* but its function is unclear).

The DNA fragments are joined together by **DNA ligase**. The template strand and the newly-synthesised strand are rewound by **DNA gyrase**. The winding begins even when the replication is going on (Fig. 14.7)

Some of the enzymes involved in **eukaryotic replica-tion** are different. These include:

1. **DNA polymerase α:** It synthesises the lagging strand, and possesses primase activity, DNA polymerase activity and, in some species, 3'→5' exonuclease activity.
2. **DNA polymerase β:** It is a DNA repair enzyme.
3. **DNA polymerase γ:** It is present in mitochondria, and replicates mitochondrial DNA. In eukaryotes, some DNA is present in mitochondria also which is inherited from the mother, and contains genes for some mitochondrial proteins concerned with oxidative phosphorylation.
4. **DNA polymerase δ:** It synthesises the leading strand, and possesses polymerase activity and 3'→5' exonuclease activity.
5. **DNA polymerase ε:** It possesses 5'→3' exonuclease activity (for removal of ribonucleotides), polymerase activity and 3'→5' exonuclease activity.
6. **DNA topoisomerase II:** It rewinds the template strand and the newly-synthesised strand.

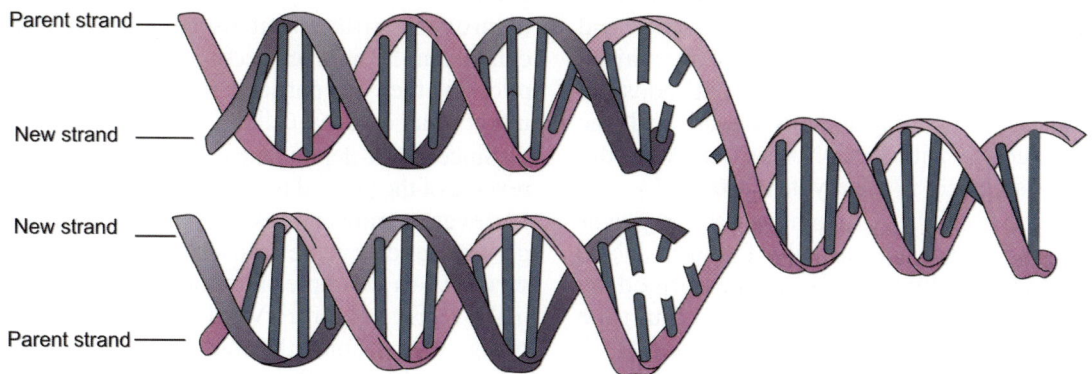

Fig. 14.7: Winding of parent DNA strands and new strands

DNA Repair Mechanisms

Errors in replication of DNA can result in serious consequences. Errors can occur **spontaneously**, and can be brought about by **external agents,** e.g. ultraviolet light, ionising radiation, mutagenic chemicals, chemotherapeutic agents, etc. **Ultraviolet light** can lead to the formation of thymine dimers. **Deaminating agents**, e.g. nitrosamine, can deaminate cytosine to uracil, adenine to hypoxanthine and guanine to xanthine. **Alkylating agents**, e.g. dimethyl sulphate, can methylate the bases. **Acridine** can intercalate between two bases leading to the incorporation of an extra base in the new strand being synthesised. If these errors are not corrected, **mutations** will result. Very efficient repair mechanisms exist to correct the errors.

Proof-reading and error-correcting properties of DNA polymerases have been described earlier which ensure a high fidelity in replication of DNA. Some additional repair systems also exist, both in prokaryotes and eukaryotes, to repair specific defects. All these repair systems comprise elements that:

a. **Detect** the defect,
b. **Remove** the defective portion of DNA,
c. **Add** correct nucleotide(s) in the gap and
d. **Ligate** the newly added nucleotide(s) with pre-existing strand.

The following repair systems correct specific errors in replication:

1. **Mismatch repair system** detects a single mismatched base on the new strand and corrects the mismatch. In *E.coli*, the mismatch repair system comprises three proteins, MutS, MutH and MutL. **Palindromic GATC** sequences are scattered in the DNA in which adenine is methylated. These sequences act as markers for mismatch repair system. GATC sequences on the newly-synthesised strand remain unmethylated for sometime which allows the repair system to recognise the new strand. MutS scans the new strand from one GATC sequence to another. If it finds a mispaired base, it binds to it. MutL binds to MutS. These two activate the **GATC endonuclease** activity of MutH. Active MutH nicks the new strand just upstream of the GATC sequence and goes on removing nucleotides until the mispaired nucleotide is removed. DNA polymerase III adds the correct nucleotides in the gap and DNA ligase seals the new oligonucleotide with the DNA strand. A similar repair system is present in eukaryotes also.

2. **Base excision repair system** removes and replaces modified bases that are not normally found in DNA, e.g. uracil, hypoxanthine and xanthine formed by deamination of cytosine, adenine and guanine respectively. A **DNA glycosylase**, e.g. uracil DNA glycosylase, removes the unusual base. The site lacking the base is nicked by an endonuclease. The gap is filled and sealed by sequential actions of DNA polymerase I and DNA ligase.

3. **Nucleotide excision repair system** corrects errors such as thymine dimerisation or addition of exogenous chemicals to bases. Thymine dimers formed on exposure to ultraviolet light are removed in *E.coli* by **uvr ABC excinuclease** which consists of uvr A, uvr B and uvr C. uvr A and uvr B detect the error and unwind the DNA in the region of the defect. uvr B nicks the strand a few bases downstream of the defect. uvr C nicks it a few bases upstream. Thus, a short oligonucleotide is excised. DNA polymerase I adds the correct nucleotides followed by ligation by DNA ligase. A similar but more elaborate repair system is present in eukaryotes also. An autosomal recessive inherited defect in this repair system causes **xeroderma pigmentosum** in which the damage to DNA caused by ultraviolet light can not be repaired. Skin cells bear the brunt of the disease as they are exposed to sunlight. The disease results in dry and pigmented skin, multiple **skin cancers** and early death. The components of the human nucleotide excision repair system have been named XPA, XPB, XPC, XPD, XPE, XPF and XPG. Mutations in any of these can cause xeroderma pigmentosum.

Reverse Transcriptase

An unusual DNA polymerase, known as **RNA-dependent DNA polymerase**, is present in some RNA viruses. This enzyme can synthesise DNA using RNA as a template. When such a virus infects a cell, the viral RNA-dependent DNA polymerase synthesises a complementary strand of DNA in the infected cell using its own RNA as a template. The DNA strand, then, acts as a template, and a second strand of DNA is synthesised. Thus, a duplex DNA is formed having the genetic information present in the viral genome. This DNA is stably incorporated in the genome of the infected cell by another viral enzyme, integrase.

The infected cell begins to transcribe the viral genes. The mRNA transcript is translated to form the viral proteins. The proteins surround the RNA transcripts of the viral genome to form new virus particles. Thus, a large number of progeny virus particles are formed in the infected cell. When the number becomes too large, the cell ruptures releasing the virus particles. The released viruses can, then, infect other healthy cells.

Since RNA-dependent DNA polymerase catalyses the reverse of the normal transcription process, it is also known as reverse transcriptase. Viruses possessing an RNA genome and reverse transcriptase are known as **retroviruses.** An example is human immunodeficiency virus or HIV (Fig. 14.8). HIV infects helper T cells of human beings and cripples the immune system (*see* Chapter 19 for more details). Reverse transcriptase and retroviruses are being exploited by molecular biologists as useful tools

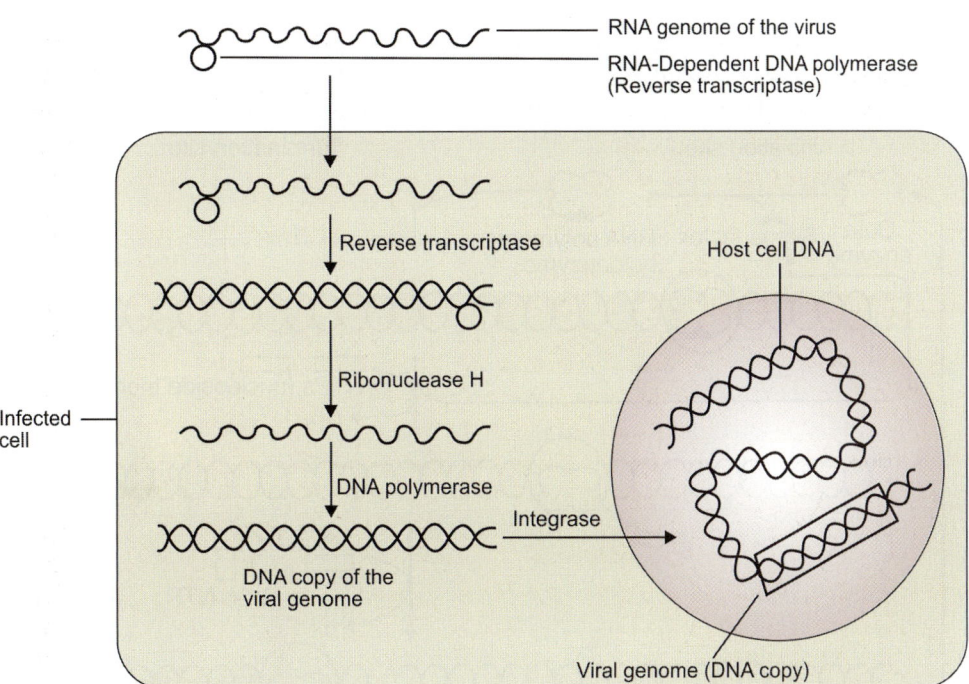

Fig.14.8: A retrovirus, e.g. HIV, injects its RNA genome and reverse transcriptase into a cell. A DNA copy of the viral genome is formed and integrated into the DNA of the infected cell

in recombinant DNA technology (*see* Chapter 16 for more details).

SYNTHESIS OF RNA

Synthesis of RNA is known as **transcription**. One strand of DNA, known as **sense strand** or non-coding strand acts as template for transcription. The other strand of DNA having a complementary base sequence is known as **anti-sense** or coding strand. RNA is synthesised by **RNA polymerase** (DNA-dependent RNA polymerase). The transcription unit is a gene which contains the complete coding for one protein. The genes having coded information for amino acid sequences of proteins are known as **structural genes**. Base sequence is different in different structural genes. However, structural genes are preceded by a **promoter region** or site having some common or consensus sequences which can be recognised by RNA polymerase so that the same enzyme can transcribe different structural genes.

In prokaryotic promoter sites, one common sequence 10 bp (base pairs) upstream of the transcription start site is TATAAT (**Pribnow box**). A second common sequence 35 bp upstream of the transcription start site is TTGACA.

$$—\text{TTGACA}——\text{TATAAT}—\text{GENE}—$$

$$-35 \qquad\qquad -10 \qquad +1$$

In eukaryotic promoters, one consensus sequence 20 to 30 bp upstream of the transcription start site is ATATAA

(**Hogness box or TATA box**). The second consensus sequence 70 to 80 bp upstream of the transcription start site is GGCCAATC (**CAAT box**).

$$—\text{GGCCAATC}——\text{ATATAA}—\text{GENE}—$$

$$-75 \qquad\qquad -25 \qquad +1$$

RNA polymerase of *E.coli* has been studied extensively. It is a tetramer made up of two identical a subunits, one β subunit and one β' subunit. The tetramer is known as the **core enzyme** which is capable of RNA synthesis but can not recognise the promoter site. The core enzyme combines with a protein, **sigma factor** to form **RNA polymerase holoenzyme** which can bind to the promoter site. Thus, sigma factor is necessary for recognition of the promoter site. After attachment of the holoenzyme to the promoter and formation of the first phosphodiester bond, the sigma factor dissociates, and the core enzyme transcribes the gene.

The process of RNA synthesis is similar to primer synthesis. The portion of DNA which is being transcribed is unwound. RNA is synthesised in 5'→3' direction. The substrates are ribonucleoside triphosphates (ATP, GTP, CTP and UTP). Each incoming nucleotide loses an inorganic pyrophosphate, and its α-phosphate group forms an ester bond with 3' –OH group of the last nucleotide. A phosphodiester bond, thus, links the last nucleotide and the new nucleotide. The selection of nucleotides is governed by the base sequence on the template strand of DNA according to the base-pairing rule, i.e. U opposite

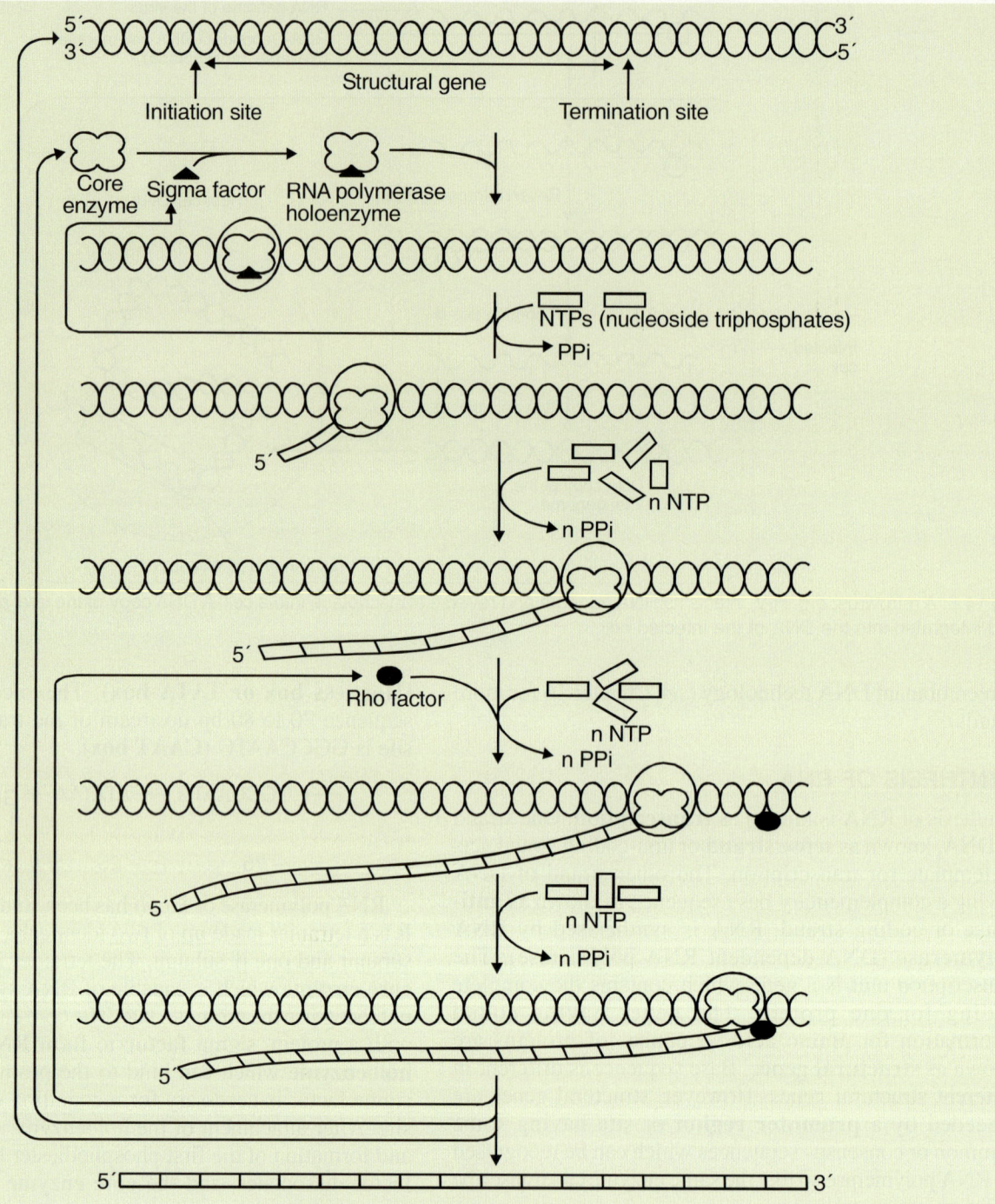

Fig. 14.9: Transcription of a gene

A, A opposite T, C opposite G and G opposite C. The core enzyme moves downstream synthesising RNA. As the transcription nears completion, a protein factor called rho factor binds to the termination site. When the core enzyme reaches the rho factor, the newly transcribed RNA is released and the core enzyme and rho factor are also released (Fig. 14.9). A rho-independent termination has also been described.

EUKARYOTIC TRANSCRIPTION

While the basic process of transcription is similar in pro-karyotes and eukaryotes, the eukaryotic transcription machinery is more complex and more elaborate. Unlike prokaryotes in which a single RNA polymerase can synthesise all types of RNA, eukaryotes have different RNA polymerases to synthesise different types of RNA.

RNA polymerase I synthesises rRNA, **RNA polymerase II** synthesises mRNA and **RNA polymerase III** synthesises tRNA (and also 5S rRNA).

The eukaryotic RNA polymerases are bigger and have more subunits. A wide array of transcription factors are required to form the basal transcription apparatus. Sequences other than promoters also affect the transcription process and its rate.

The eukaryotic genes may be divided into class I, class II and class III genes which are transcribed by RNA polymerase I, RNA polymerase II and RNA polymerase III respectively.

Class I genes are located in the nucleolus. They are transcribed to form 28S rRNA, 18S rRNA and 5.8S rRNA. The rRNAs are not translated. Instead, they combine with some proteins to form ribosomes. Since ribosomes are required in large numbers, multiple copies of class I genes are present in the DNA. The primary transcript is a 45S precursor which is cleaved to form 28S, 18S and 5.8S rRNAs. This ensures a balanced production of rRNAs in the proportion required for the formation of ribosomes.

Class II genes differ from class I and class III genes in the sense that the products of transcription are used for translation. Class II genes are transcribed to form hnRNA in eukaryotes that is processed to form mRNA. mRNA is translated to form a protein. Since the purpose of transcription of class II genes is to form proteins, regulation of transcription is more complex. TATA box is the site for attachment of RNA polymerase II (RNAP II). The first event is the binding of **TATA binding protein (TBP)** to the TATA box. Several other proteins called **TBP-associated factors (TAFs)** bind to TBP. This complex of TBP and TAFs is called **transcription factor IID (TFIID)**. TFIIB joins TFIID. TFIIF brings RNAP II, and both attach to the complex. TFIIF acts like the prokaryotic sigma factor and positions RNAP II at the correct location for initiation of transcription. TFIIA, TFIIE and TFIIH bind to the complex to complete the basal transcription apparatus (analogous to RNA polymerase holoenzyme of prokaryotes). TFIIH possesses kinase activity which is increased by TFIIE. TFIIH phosphorylates some serine and threonine residues present at the carboxyl end of one of the subunits of RNAP II which makes the enzyme active (some other kinases can also activate it). Activated RNAP II transcribes the gene.

CAAT box is another consensus sequence in the eukaryotic promoters which is upstream of the TATA box. A protein, **CAAT-binding transcription factor (CTF)** binds CAAT box. By looping of DNA, CAAT box comes closer to TATA box, and CTF also binds TBP-associated factors which are part of TFIID. This increases the frequency of transcription. Another *cis*-acting element (*cis*-acting elements are sequences within the DNA molecule being transcribed), **GC box** may be present upstream of the CAAT box or between TATA box and CAAT box. A protein, **Sp1** binds to GC box and TBP-associated factors, and increases the frequency of transcription. Several other proteins bind other consensus sequences and increase the rate of transcription.

Enhancer elements are *cis*-acting elements that may be located far away from the gene that they influence. They may be upstream or downstream. Binding of a ***trans*-acting factor** (a molecule other than the DNA molecule being transcribed) to the enhancer element increases the transcription of the gene influenced by the enhancer element. By looping of DNA, enhancer element and the *trans*-acting factor come close to the gene and facilitate the binding of the basal transcription apparatus to the TATA box. Enhancer elements are low in specificity. An example is Burkitt's lymphoma in which myc gene moves from chromosome 8 to chromosome 14 due to reciprocal translocation. Heavy chain immunoglobulin gene is located on chromosome 14. Due to reciprocal translocation, enhancer element of heavy chain gene increases the transcription of myc gene (*see* Chapter 18).

Like enhancer elements, **silencer elements** are located at a distance from the gene they influence, and they may be upstream or downstream. They suppress the transcription of the genes that they influence. Tissue-specific expression of genes may be a function of enhancer elements and silencer elements.

Class III genes are transcribed by RNA polymerase III to form tRNAs and 5S rRNA. These genes are present in multiple copies. The tRNA genes have **intragenic promoters**, i.e. the promoters are located within the gene rather than upstream of the gene. A transcription factor, **TFIIIA** binds to the promoter and positions RNA polymerase III at the correct site to initiate transcription.

The newly-synthesised RNA (**primary transcript**) is not usually the final, functional RNA. Except prokaryotic mRNA, all RNAs undergo extensive post-transcriptional modifications which differ in different types of RNA.

Post-transcriptional Modifications

mRNA

In eukaryotes, the primary transcript is heterogeneous nuclear RNA (**hnRNA**) which is the precursor of mRNA. hnRNA undergoes extensive modifications, two of which are common to all hnRNAs:

a. Addition of 7-methylguanosine triphosphate cap (**7-methyl GTP cap**) at the 5'-end of RNA.
b. Addition of poly-adenylate tail (**poly-A tail**) at the 3'-end of RNA.

The cap at the 5'-end assists in recognition of the proper site on the mRNA where its binding with ribosome has to occur for translation. The tail at the 3'-end probably stabilises mRNA (some mRNAs do not have a poly-A tail, e.g. mRNAs for **histones**).

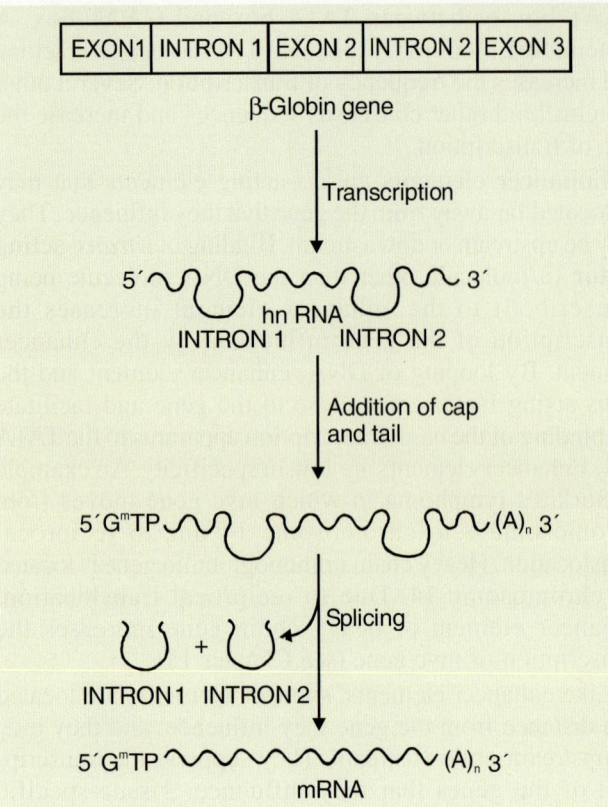

Fig. 14.10: Post-transcriptional modifications in the primary transcript of the β–globin gene

The third modification is deletion of nucleotides which is different in different hnRNAs. Eukaryotic genes contain some coding sequences and some non-coding sequences. The coding sequences, which are expressed, are known as **exons**. The non-coding sequence, which intervene between the coding sequences, are known as **introns**. After transcription and addition of cap and tail, the introns are removed and the exons joined. This process is known as splicing. The number and size of exons and introns are different in different genes. For example, the β-globin gene (the gene for the β polypeptide chain of haemoglobin) has three exons interrupted by two introns (Fig. 14.10).

Splice Sites

Splice sites (splice junctions or intron-exon junctions) in all hnRNAs have some common features. The introns begin with GU and end with AG. In between, there is a branch site having A and a pyrimidine-rich tract of about ten nucleotides (Fig. 14.11).

During splicing, 2'–OH group of adenylate at the branch site forms an ester bond with the phosphate group of G at the 5'-splice site. Exon 1 is released, and its 3'-nucleotide forms an ester bond with the 5'-nucleotide of exon 2. The intron is released in lariat form (Fig. 14.12).

Spliceosome

Spliceosome is an assembly made up of some RNA molecules (< 300 nucleotides) known as small nuclear RNAs (**snRNAs**), some proteins and hnRNA. The snRNAs combine with the proteins to form small nuclear ribonucleoprotein particles (**snRNPs or snurps**). snRNPs are U1, U2, U4, U5 and U6. These combine with hnRNA to form a spliceosome. U1 binds to 5'-splice site, U2 binds to branch site and U5 binds to 3'-splice site of hnRNA. U4 and U6 bind to this complex. The splicing reaction is catalysed by the snRNA components of snRNPs. **Auto-antibodies** against snRNPs are formed in **systemic lupus erythematosus** resulting in wide-spread tissue damage.

In eukaryotes, mRNA is synthesised by RNA polymerase II which binds to the promoter site upstream of the structural gene. Besides promoter site, there are a number of sequences in DNA which control the rate of transcription. Specific protein factors bind to these regulatory sequences, e.g. transcription factors, CTF, Sp1, CREB (cAMP response element binding protein), etc. which facilitate or increase the rate of transcription. Inducers and repressors also bind to regulatory sequences, and increase or decrease the rate of transcription. Mutations in promoter site can decrease the rate of transcription. Two or more different proteins can be synthesised from the same hnRNA by alternative splicing. For example, different types of tropomyosin are present in different tissues which are synthesised from the same gene by **alternative splicing** of hnRNA.

Prokaryotic genes have no introns, and prokaryotic mRNA does not undergo any post-transcriptional modification.

tRNA

In prokaryotes as well as eukaryotes, tRNA is synthesised as a precursor which undergoes post-transcriptional modifications. The modifications include:

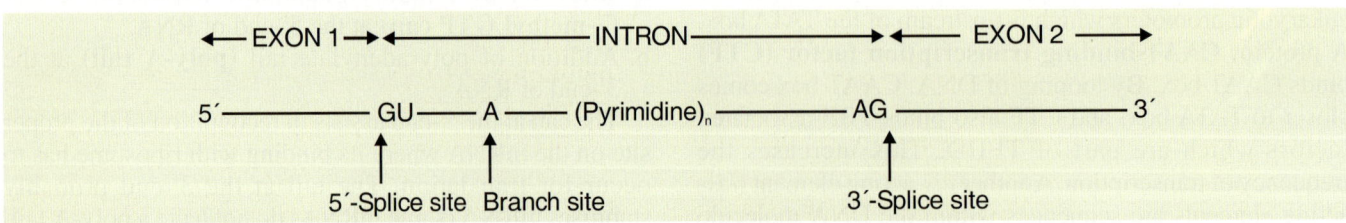

Fig. 14.11: Common features of splice junctions

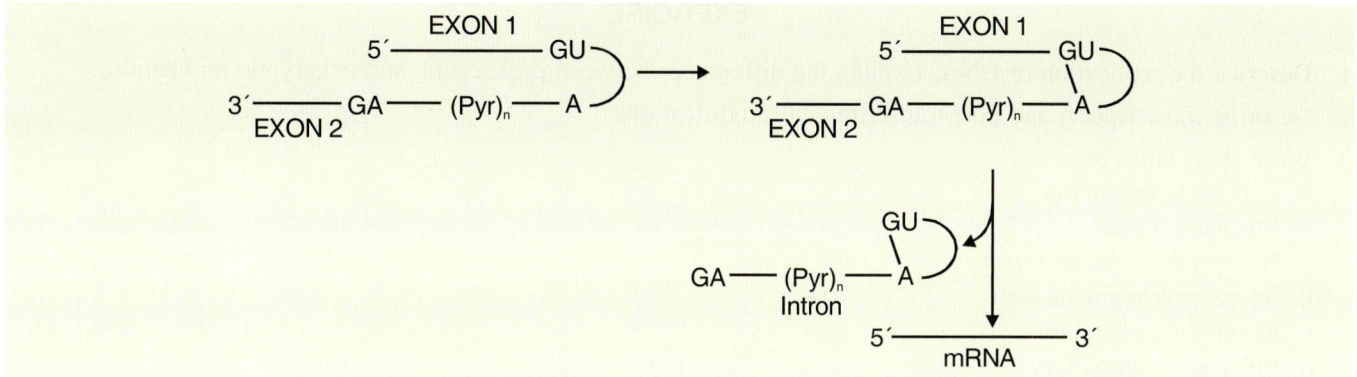

Fig. 14.12: Removal of introns and splicing of exons

a. Removal of some nucleotides,
b. Addition of –CCA terminus at 3'-end,
c. Formation of pseudouridine from uridine and
d. Methylation of several bases (thymine is formed by methylation of a uracil residue).

rRNA

rRNA is a structural constituent of ribosomes. Both eukaryotic and prokaryotic rRNA are synthesised initially as large precursors which are cleaved. Several bases are methylated.

The eukaryotic 80S ribosome is made up of a 40S subunit and a 60S subunit. The 40S subunit is made up of 18S rRNA and about 35 polypeptides. The 60S subunit is made up of 5S rRNA, 5.8S rRNA, 28S rRNA and about 50 polypeptides. 5S rRNA is synthesised as such by RNA

polymerase III. 5.8S rRNA, 18S rRNA and 28S rRNA are synthesised by RNA polymerase I in the form of a 45S precursor. The 45S precursor is cleaved sequentially to yield the final products (Fig. 14.13). The prokaryotic rRNAs are 5S, 16S and 23S. The last two are formed by trimming of a larger precursor.

INHIBITORS OF REPLICATION AND TRANSCRIPTION

Replication of DNA and its transcription are vital for survival. Inhibition of replication prevents cell division. Inhibition of transcription prevents the synthesis of proteins which are essential for every cell. Inhibitors of replication can be used as **anti-cancer drugs** to check the multiplication of cancer cells. Inhibitors of replication or and transcription which act selectively on prokaryotes can be used as **antibiotics** to destroy bacteria without any harmful effects on the human cells. Antibiotics exploit the differences in prokaryotic and eukaryotic replication and transcription. If a compound inhibits a prokaryotic enzyme or protein factor but not the corresponding enzyme or protein factor in eukaryotes, it can be used as an antibiotic.

Some inhibitors of replication and transcription which are used as drugs are:

1. **Cisplatin:** It breaks DNA strands and prevents replication. It is used as an anti-cancer drug.
2. **Mitomycin:** It cross-links adenine and guanine on the DNA strands and prevents unwinding. It is used as an anti-cancer drug.
3. **Daunorubicin:** It intercalates in DNA and prevents access to DNA polymerase. It is used as an anti-cancer drug.
4. **Norfloxacin and ciprofloxacin:** These are used as antibiotics as they prevent prokaryotic replication by inhibiting DNA gyrase. The corresponding human enzyme, DNA topoisomerase II is not inhibited.
5. **Rifampicin:** It prevents transcription by inhibiting the β subunit of RNA polymerase. It is used as an antitubercular drug because it inhibits the bacterial enzyme but not the human RNA polymerase.

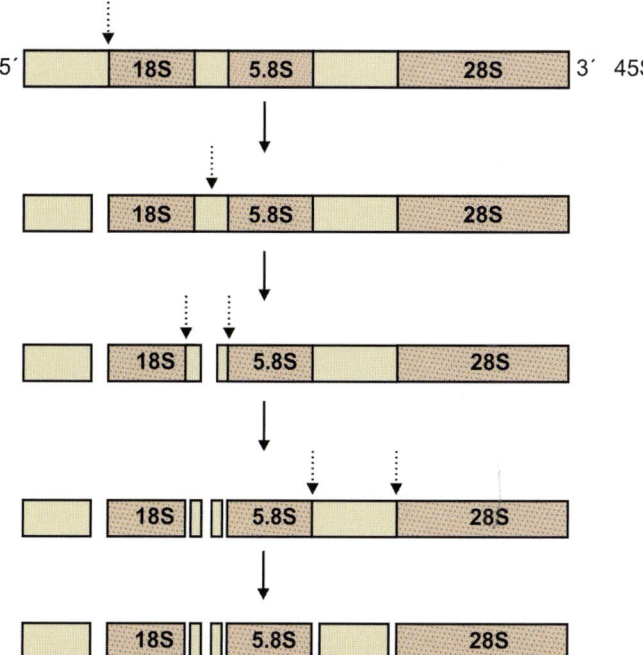

Fig. 14.13: Cleavage of 45S precursor into 5.8S, 18S and 28S rRNAs in eukaryotes. Broken arrows indicate the sites of cleavage

EXERCISE

1. Describe the replication of DNA. Explain the differences between prokaryotic and eukaryotic replication.

2. Describe transcription and post-transcriptional modifications.

3. Write short notes on:
   a. Cell cycle regulation
   b. Mismatch repair
   c. Nucleotide excision repair
   d. Xeroderma pigmentosum
   e. Reverse transcriptase
   f. Eukaryotic promoters
   g. Spliceosome
   h. Inhibitors of replication and transcription

4. Write 'true' or 'false':
   a. Replication of DNA is semi-conservative.
   b. DNA synthesis cannot commence with deoxyribonucleotides.
   c. Direction of DNA synthesis is 3' → 5'.
   d. An Okazaki fragment is made up of about 100 ribonucleotides and 10 deoxyribonucleotides.
   e. The leading strand is synthesised continuously, and the lagging strand discontinuously.
   f. Replication bubbles are formed during eukaryotic replication.
   g. Unwinding of DNA requires energy.
   h. DNA fragments are joined together by DNA ligase.
   i. DNA polymerase III possesses error-correction activity.
   j. DNA polymerase IV removes RNA primer and inserts deoxyribonucletodies.
   k. Deaminating agents can convert thymine into uracil.
   l. GATC endonuclease activity is required for mismatch repair.
   m. Damage to DNA caused by ultraviolet light is corrected by uvr ABC excinuclease.
   n. Xeroderma pigmentosum is an inherited disease in which the damage to DNA caused by ultraviolet light is not repaired.
   o. Reverse transcriptase is present in some bacteria.
   p. Reverse transcriptase is an RNA-dependent DNA polymerase.
   q. Sigma factor recognises the site for termination of transcription.
   r. RNA polymerase II synthesises hnRNA.
   s. rRNA genes have intragenic promoters.
   t. Norfloxacin inhibits prokaryotic DNA gyrase.

5. Fill in the blanks:
   a. Replication of DNA occurs in .... phase of cell cycle.
   b. RNA primer is synthesised in .... direction.
   c. ....is the source of energy for unwinding of DNA.
   d. dna B protein initiates .... of DNA.
   e. DNA polymerase III possesses ....and .... activities.
   f. .... replaces ribonucleotides of RNA primer by deoxyribonucleotides.
   g. Mitochondrial DNA is replicated by ....
   h. .... is the eukaryotic analogue of prokaryotic DNA gyrase.
   i. Palindromic .... sequences act as markers for mismatch repair system.
   j. Viruses possessing reverse transcriptase are known as ....
   k. Reverse transcriptase uses .... as a template.
   l. Prokaryotic RNA polymerase combines with .... to form the RNA polymerase holoenzyme.
   m. .... recognises the site for binding of RNA polymerase.
   n. .... recognises the site for termination of transcription.

o. .... is synthesised by RNA polymerase I in eukaryotes.

p. .... genes have intragenic promoters.

q. .... is the precursor of mRNA in eukaryotes.

r. Poly-A tail is not present in the mRNA for ....

s. Rifampicin inhibits the .... subunit of ....RNA polymerase.

t. Small nuclear RNAs are present in ....

ANSWERS TO SHORT QUESTIONS

4. a. True   b. True

   c. False   d. False

   e. True   f. True

   g. True   h. True

   i. True   j. False

   k. False   l. True

   m. True   n. True

   o. False   p. True

   q. False   r. True

   s. False   t. True

5. a. S   b. $5' \rightarrow 3'$

   c. ATP   d. Unwinding

   e. Polymerase, $3' \rightarrow 5'$ exonuclease   f. RNA polymerase I

   g. DNA polymerase γ h. DNA topoisomerase II

   i. GATC   j. Retroviruses

   k. RNA   l. Sigma factor

   m. Sigma factor   n. Rho factor

   o. rRNA   p. tRNA

   q. hnRNA   r. Histones

   s. β, prokaryotic   t. Spliceosome

15

Genetic Code and Protein Synthesis

Proteins are among the most important biomolecules in all living organisms. Enzymes which are a vital component of the metabolic machinery of living organisms are proteins. In addition, a host of other important functions are performed by proteins in the form of hormones, antibodies, carriers, receptors, signal transducers, coagulation factors, structural constituents, etc. All these myriad proteins are made up of the same twenty amino acids which are assembled in different sequences to give each protein a unique primary structure. Since higher orders of structural organisation depend upon the primary structure, each protein acquires a unique conformation most suited to its function. Even a minor change in the primary structure can change the conformation and the functioning of the protein. Therefore, one of the most important requirements during synthesis of proteins is to ensure a correct sequence of amino acids. A complex and elaborate mechanism has evolved for synthesis of proteins. This mechanism involves the interaction of DNA, various types of RNA, ribosomes, various enzymes and other factors.

AN OVERVIEW OF PROTEIN SYNTHESIS

The information about the amino acid sequence of proteins is present in a coded form in DNA. The coding unit is a **gene**. A gene consists of a specific **sequence of nucleotides** which codes for a specific **sequence of amino acids**. When a protein is to be synthesised, the corresponding gene is transcribed. An mRNA molecule having a base sequence complementary to that of non-coding (sense) strand of the gene is formed.

The code words on mRNA (and the coding or antisense strand of the gene) are known as **codons**. The codons are code words for amino acids. The mRNA goes to cytosol and binds to a ribosome. The tRNA molecules in the cytosol are charged with specific amino acids. Each tRNA possesses an **anticodon** (complementary to a codon) for a particular amino acid. The charged tRNA molecules go to the ribosome and find the complementary codons on mRNA. The amino acids brought by tRNA molecules are

joined to each other in a sequence directed by the codons on mRNA. This process is called **translation**.

GENETIC CODE

The code words for amino acids are made up of purine and pyrimidine bases which are A (adenine), T (thymine), C (cytosine) and G (guanine) in DNA and A, U (uracil), C and G in RNA. How twenty amino acids could be encoded by four bases remained a mystery until 1960. It was surmised that if each base acted as a code word, only four code words would be possible. If a pair of bases formed a code word, $4^2 = 16$ code words could be formed. These are obviously insufficient to encode twenty amino acids. If the code word is made up of a triplet of bases, $4^3 = 64$ combinations are possible.

In the early 1960s, Nirenberg and Matthaei showed that codons are indeed triplets of bases, and they deciphered some of the codons. They prepared synthetic polyribonucleotides containing only one base repeated again and again. The synthetic polyribonucleotides were used in place of mRNA in cell-free protein-synthesising systems. Amino acid sequences of the peptides synthesised were determined, and were compared with the base sequences of the polyribonucleotides.

When a polyribonucleotide containing only uracil (poly-U) was used, the peptide synthesised was poly-phenylalanine. Poly-A resulted in the synthesis of poly-lysine, poly-C in the synthesis of poly-proline and poly-G in the synthesis of poly-glycine. Thus, it was inferred that UUU is a codon for phenylalanine, AAA for lysine, CCC for proline and GGG for glycine (Fig.15.2).

Har Gobind Khorana carried this process further. By chemical and enzymatic methods, he prepared synthetic polyribonucleotides having defined but different base sequences. These were used in place of mRNA in cell-free protein-synthesising system. When two bases were present alternately, a peptide having two amino acids alternately was synthesised. When a polyribonucleotide having three bases repeated again and again was used, a peptide having only one amino acid repeated again and again was synthesised.

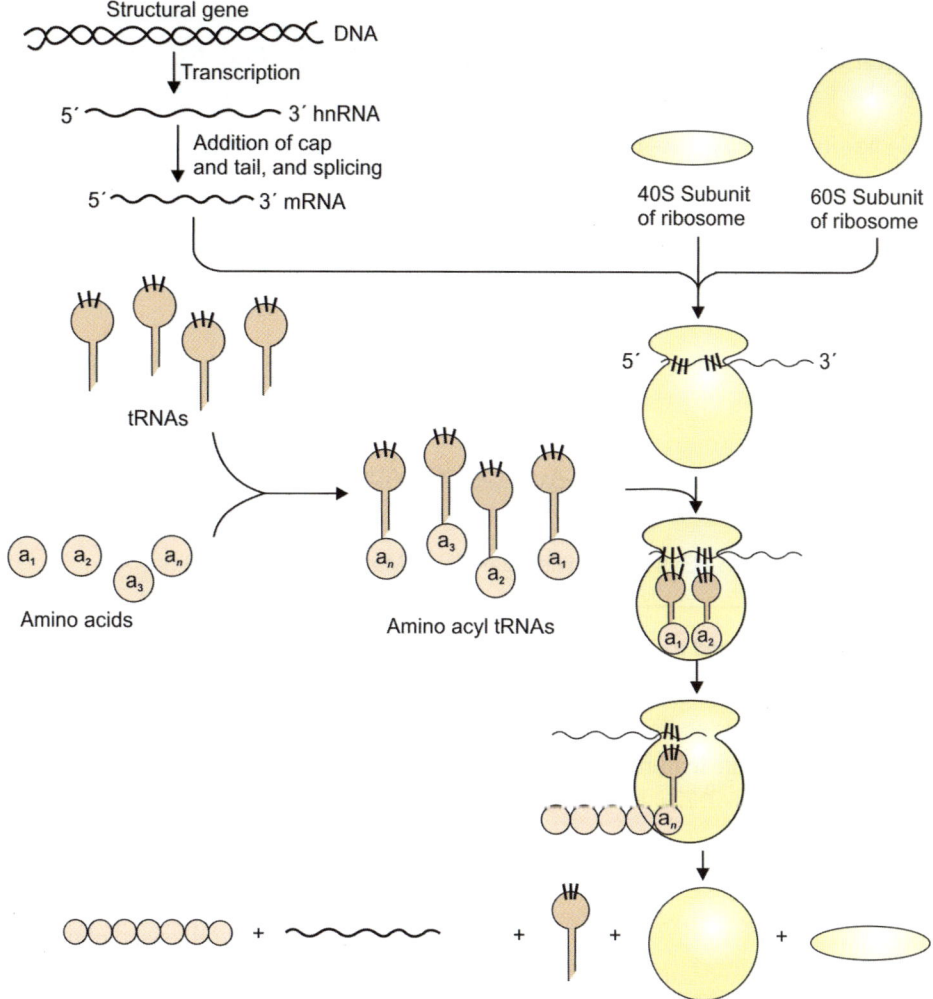

Fig. 15.1: An outline of protein synthesis in eukaryotes

When a polyribonucleotide having four bases repeated again and again was used, the peptide synthesised had four amino acids repeated again and again. These observations revealed the identity of several codons (Fig.15.3).

By using different sequences of bases, Khorana deciphered the entire genetic code by 1966. It was found that all the 64 triplets are code words. There are 61 codons for amino acids. The other three codons do not code for

any amino acid, and are called **nonsense codons**. They act as **chain termination signals (stop signals)**.

SALIENT FEATURES OF GENETIC CODE

Genetic code is the code language for amino acids in all living organisms as proteins are synthesised from the same twenty amino acids in all living beings, and the information is coded by the same four bases.

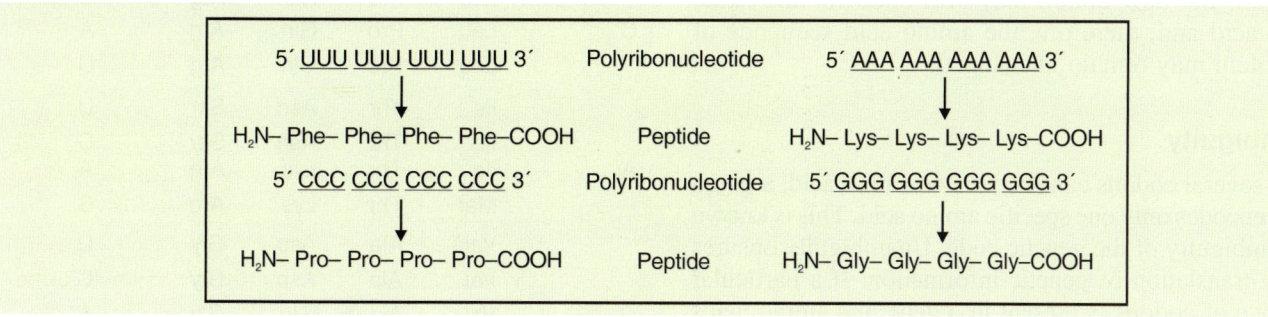

Fig. 15.2: Synthetic polyribonucleotides and peptides synthesised from them showing that UUU is the codon for phenylalanine, AAA for lysine, CCC for proline and GGG for glycine.

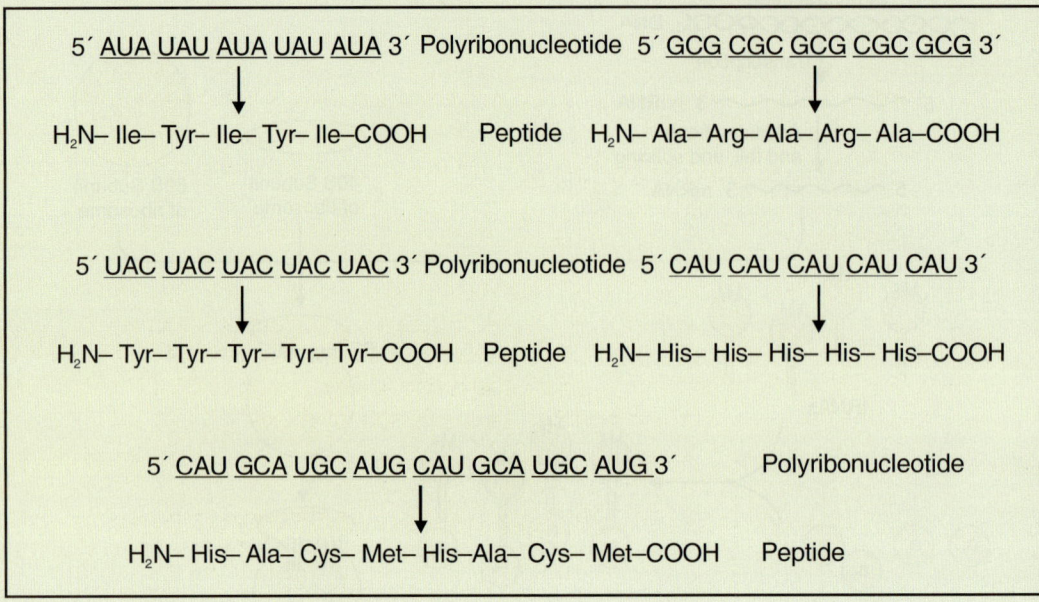

Fig. 15.3: Synthetic polyribonucleotides and peptides synthesised from them showing that AUA is the codon for isoleucine, UAU for tyrosine, GCG for alanine, CGC for argnine, UAC for tyrosine, CAU for histidine, GCA for alanine, UGC for cysteine and AUG for methionine.

The genetic code has some important features:

1. Degeneracy,
2. Unambiguity,
3. Universality, and
4. Absence of punctuations.

Degeneracy

Table 15.1 shows that only tryptophan and methionine have a single codon each. All the other amino acids are encoded by more than one codons. Leucine, serine and arginine have as many as six codons each. **Encoding of one amino acid by more than one codons** is known as degeneracy of the genetic code. Degeneracy resides mainly in the **third base** of the codon. For example, the four codons for alanine are GCU, GCC, GCA and GCG in which the first two bases are identical and only the third base is different. Degeneracy has some advantage too. If the third base of a codon is substituted due to a mutation, the new codon may still code for the same amino acid and, therefore, the amino acid sequence of the protein may remain unchanged.

Unambiguity

While several codons can encode one amino acid, a given codon encodes only one specific amino acid. This is known as unambiguity of the genetic code. Unambiguity ensures correct translation of genetic information. If a particular sequence of codons is present in a gene, the amino acids will be assembled in the correct sequence in the protein as **each codon codes for one specific amino acid**.

Universality

The genetic code consisting of 61 codons for amino acids and three stop codons is **identical in all life forms,** e.g. animals, plants, micro-organisms, etc. However, some variations are found in **mitochondrial DNA**. In eukaryotes, some proteins are synthesised in mitochon-dria also. These proteins are concerned with oxidative phosphorylation. In mitochondrial DNA, AUA is the codon for methionine

Table 15.1: The genetic code (codons on mRNA)

First base at 5'-end	Second base				Third base at 3'-end
	U	**C**	**A**	**G**	
U	Phe	Ser	Tyr	Cys	U
	Phe	Ser	Tyr	Cys	C
	Leu	Ser	Stop	Stop	A
	Leu	Ser	Stop	Trp	G
C	Leu	Pro	His	Arg	U
	Leu	Pro	His	Arg	C
	Leu	Pro	Gln	Arg	A
	Leu	Pro	Gln	Arg	G
A	Ile	Thr	Asn	Ser	U
	Ile	Thr	Asn	Ser	C
	Ile	Thr	Lys	Arg	A
	Met	Thr	Lys	Arg	G
G	Val	Ala	Asp	Gly	U
	Val	Ala	Asp	Gly	C
	Val	Ala	Glu	Gly	A
	Val	Ala	Glu	Gly	G

instead of leucine, UGA is the codon for tryptophan instead of being a stop signal, and AGA and AGG are stop signals instead of being codons for arginine.

Absence of Punctuations

The genetic code is **read continuously** from the start site. There are no punctuations (commas or full stops) to indicate where one codon has ended and another begun. Therefore, insertion or deletion of a base changes the reading frame (Fig. 15.4).

GENE EXPRESSION

Gene expression is the process by which the coded information present in a gene is used to synthesise a protein. The process is broadly similar in prokaryotes and eukaryotes with some small differences. Gene expression in eukaryotes is described below. It comprises:
1. Transcription,
2. Charging of tRNAs,
3. Translation and
4. Post-translational modifications.

Transcription

When a gene is to be expressed, the coded information present in it is transcribed. In eukaryotes, the primary transcript is hnRNA, which is processed to form mRNA. The mRNA leaves the nucleus and goes to ribosomes where proteins are synthesised. The process of transcription has been described earlier (*see* Chapter 14).

Charging of tRNAs

The mRNA binds to a ribosome on which the protein is synthesised. The amino acids are incapable of recognising the codons on the mRNA. Therefore, an **adaptor** molecule is required which can recognise the amino acids as well as the codons present on mRNA. The adaptor molecule is tRNA. Each tRNA has an **anticodon** which is complementary to a codon. The tRNA combines with a specific amino acid according to the anticodon present on it and, then, the anticodon finds the complementary codon on

mRNA. Thus, the amino acids are added to the growing peptide chain in a sequence directed by the sequence of codons on the mRNA. Since 20 amino acids are required for protein synthesis, there must be at least 20 species of tRNA.

The amino acid is bound to the 3'-end of tRNA. The carboxyl group of the amino acid forms an ester bond with the 3'-OH group of the terminal adenylate residue of tRNA. This reaction is catalysed by **amino acyl tRNA synthetase**. ATP is required as a source of energy. The amino acid, ATP and the enzyme form **amino acyl-AMP-enzyme complex**. The complex reacts with tRNA to form **amino acyl tRNA**. The enzyme and AMP are released. Inorganic pyrophosphate released from ATP is hydrolysed (Fig. 15.5). Thus, two ATP equivalents are spent for charging of tRNA.

Binding of amino acid to its tRNA is known as charging of tRNA. The amino acid is attached to tRNA at its 3'-end while the anticodon is present far way. Therefore, the anticodon does not play any role in **recognition of amino acid**. This function is performed by the enzyme, amino acyl tRNA synthetase which is a large molecule, and can recognise the amino acid as well as the corresponding anticodon on the tRNA.

It is obvious that there should be at least 20 different species of amino acyl tRNA synthetase, each capable of charging one particular tRNA with one specific amino acid. Once a tRNA has been charged with its specific amino acid, the anticodon will find the complementary codon on the mRNA. That the amino acid has no role in the recognition process was shown by an experiment in which tRNA for cysteine was charged with cysteine and, then, the cysteine residue was chemically converted into an alanine residue. When this cysteine-specific tRNA carrying alanine was added to cell-free protein-synthesising system, alanine was incorporated in the protein at places where cysteine should have been added (Fig. 15.6).

Wobble

When the anticodon on tRNA pairs with a codon on the mRNA, **recognition of the first two bases** of the codon by the anticodon is **very precise** but the recognition of the

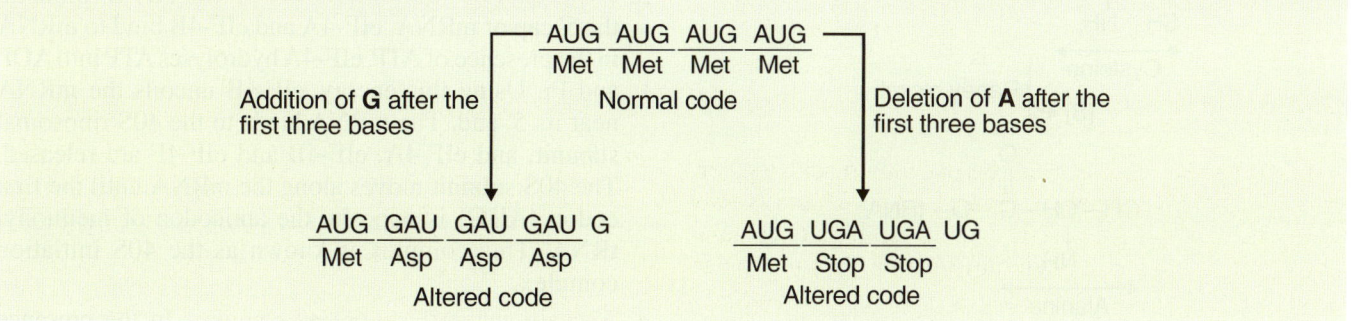

Fig. 15.4: Effect of addition or deletion of a base on the reading of the genetic code

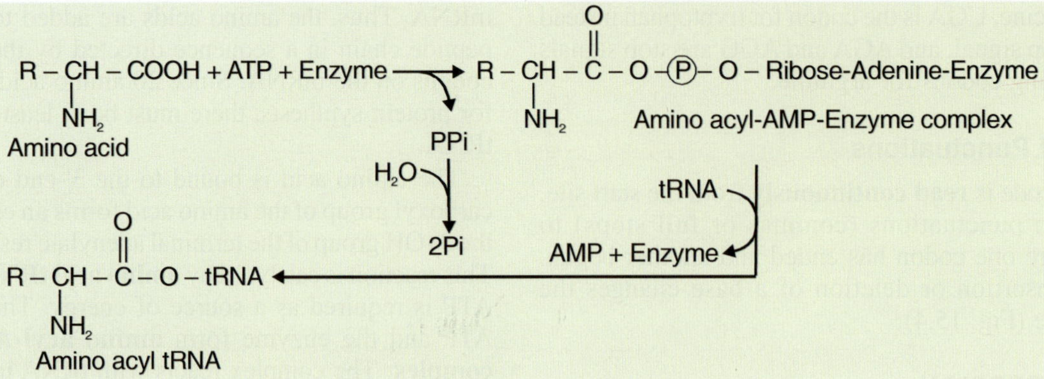

Fig. 15.5: Synthesis of amino acyl tRNA (charging of tRNA)

third base is not so precise. The anticodon can pair with two or three different codons, differing in the third base. This is known as wobble in base pairing. If an amino acid is encoded by more than one codons, the codons usually differ in the third base. These codons will be read by the anticodon as code words for the same amino acid because of wobble, and the correct amino acid will be incorporated in the protein. Thus, wobble is useful in preventing errors in translation which might result from substitution of the third base of a codon due to a mutation in the gene.

Translation

Translation is the actual process of protein synthesis. It occurs on ribosomes. Messenger RNA, which is the transcript of a structural gene, binds to a ribosome. Various tRNA molecules bring amino acids to the ribosome. Anticodons on tRNA molecules pair with the complementary codons on mRNA. Thus, amino acids are assembled according to the sequence of codons on mRNA. Peptide bonds are formed between the amino acids. This process continues until the last codon on mRNA is translated. The newly-synthesised polypeptide and the mRNA are released from the ribosome.

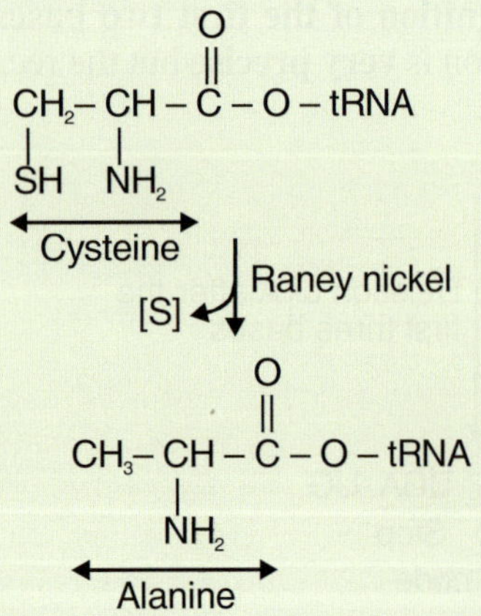

Fig. 15.6: Transformation of amino acid on charged tRNA

The process of translation is complex, and can be divided into three phases:

a. Initiation, i.e. binding of mRNA and the first amino acyl tRNA to the ribosome.

b. Elongation, i.e. addition of subsequent amino acids to the first one.

c. Termination, i.e. conclusion of elongation and release of the polypeptide.

Initiation

Initiation of protein synthesis requires the interaction of ribosome, mRNA, amino acyl tRNA bringing the first amino acid, GTP, ATP and several specific protein factors known as Initiation Factors(IFs).The initiation factors are different in prokaryotes and eukaryotes.In eukaryotes, these are known as eukaryotic initiation factors (eIFs). Eukaryotic translation is being discussed here. The initiation occurs in four steps:

1. *Dissociation of ribosomal subunits:* The 80S ribosome dissociates into 40S and 60S subunits in the presence of eIF-1A and eIF-3 which bind to the 40S subunit, and prevent its re-association with the 60S subunit.

2. *Formation of 40S pre-initiation complex:* In the presence of eIF-2C, eIF-2 and GTP bind to the first amino acyl tRNA which is always methionyl tRNA in eukaryotes. This complex binds to 40S subunit to form the 40S pre-initiation complex.

3. *Formation of 40S initiation complex:* eIF-4F binds to the 5' cap of mRNA. eIF-4A and eIF-4B bind to mRNA in the presence of ATP. eIF-4A hydrolyses ATP into ADP and Pi. Using this energy, eIF-4B uncoils the mRNA near its 5'-end. The mRNA binds to the 40S ribosomal subunit, and eIF-4A, eIF-4B and eIF-4F are released. The 40S subunit moves along the mRNA until the first codon (AUG) is opposite the anticodon of methionyl tRNA. This complex is known as the 40S initiation complex.

4. *Formation of 80S initiation complex:* In the presence of eIF-5, 60 S ribosomal subunit binds to the 40S subunit

to form the 80S initiation complex consisting of 80S ribosome, mRNA and methionyl tRNA. All the eIFs are released, and the GTP attached to eIF-2 is hydrolysed into GDP and Pi. Pi is released. GDP attached to eIF-2 is displaced by GTP in the presence of eIF-2B to a start a new cycle of initiation (Fig. 15.7).

Elongation

The 60S ribosomal subunit has two sites– P(peptidyl) site and A (amino acyl) site. After initiation, the P site is occupied by the first amino acid (methionine) and the A site is vacant. The second amino acid is brought in by the tRNA having anticodon complementary to the second

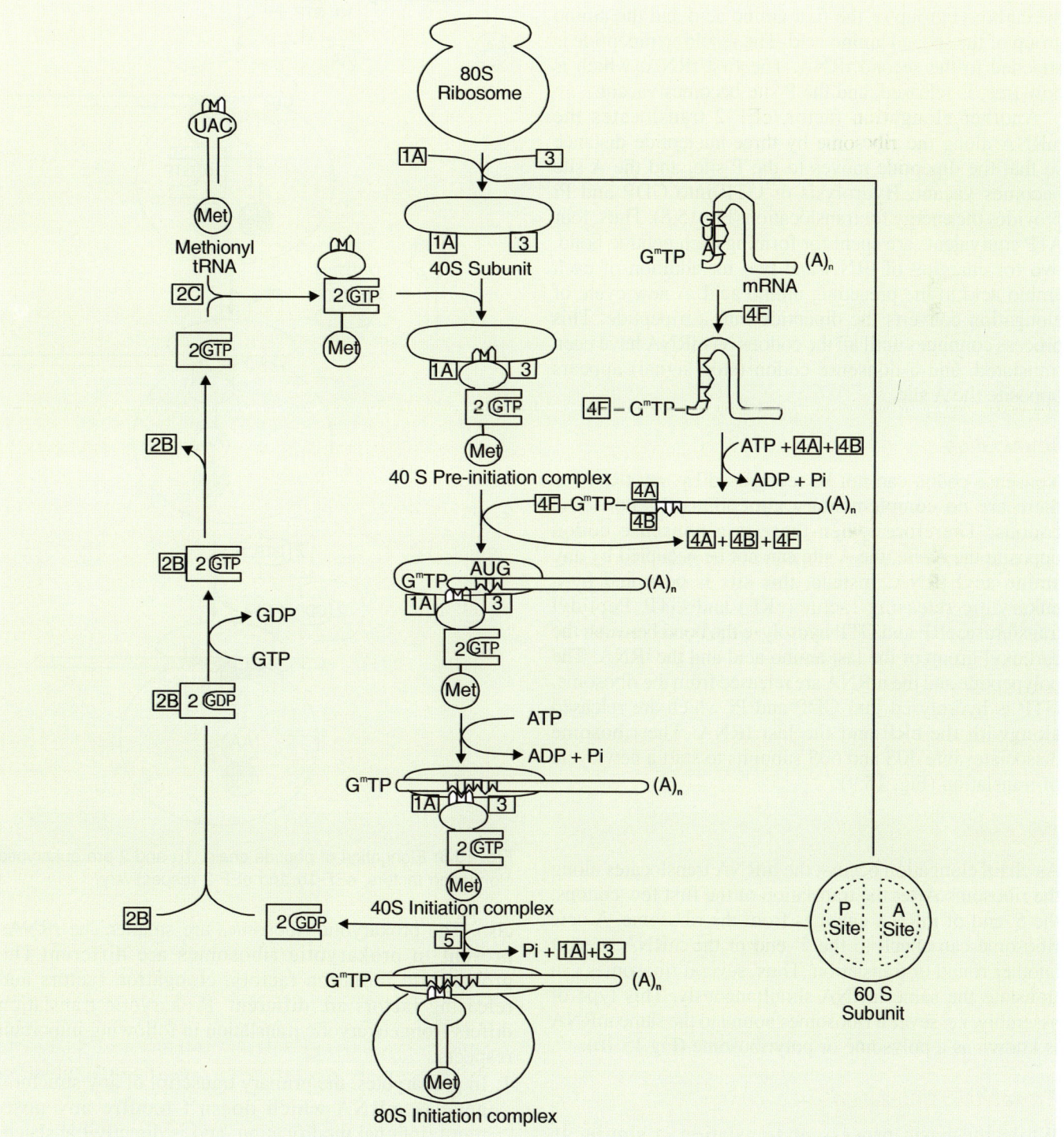

Fig. 15.7: Initiation of translation. Numbers 1A, 2, 2B, 2C, 3, 4A, 4B and 4F are eukaryotic initiation factors

codon on mRNA. Eukaryotic elongation factor 1-α (eEF-1α) and GTP are attached to the amino acyl tRNA before it binds to the ribosome. The second amino acid occupies the A site. After binding of the second amino acyl tRNA, GTP is hydrolysed, and eEF-1a. GDP complex and Pi are released.

The 60S ribosomal subunit possesses peptidyl transferase activity which is present in the 28S rRNA (ribozyme). This enzyme forms a peptide bond between the carboxyl group of the first amino acid and the amino group of the second amino acid. The resulting dipeptide is attached to the second tRNA. The first tRNA, which is now free, is released, and the P site becomes vacant.

Another elongation factor, eEF-2 translocates the mRNA along the ribosome by three-nucleotide distance so that the dipeptide moves to the P site, and the A site becomes vacant. Hydrolysis of GTP into GDP and Pi provides the energy for translocation (Fig.15.8). Thus, four ATP equivalents are spent for forming each peptide bond, two for charging of tRNA and two for addition of each amino acid to the preceding amino acid. A new cycle of elongation converts the dipeptide into a tripeptide. This process continues until all the codons on mRNA have been translated, and a nonsense codon (stop signal) appears opposite the A site.

Termination

Nonsense codon can not be recognised by any tRNA as there are no complementary anticodons for nonsense codons. Therefore, when there is a nonsense codon opposite the A site, the A site can not be occupied by any amino acyl tRNA. Instead, this site is occupied by a eukaryotic releasing factor (eRF) and GTP. Peptidyl transferase, eRF and GTP hydrolyse the bond between the carboxyl group of the last amino acid and the tRNA. The polypeptide and the mRNA are released from the ribosome. GTP is hydrolysed into GDP and Pi which are released alongwith the eRF and the last tRNA. The ribosome dissociates into 40S and 60S subunits to start a new cycle of translation (Fig. 15.9).

Polysome

As chain elongation occurs, the mRNA translocates along the ribosome.After the translation of the first few codons, the 5'-end of mRNA emerges from the ribosome. A new ribosome can attach to the 5'-end of the mRNA to start another round of translation. Thus, several ribosomes can translate the same mRNA simultaneously. This type of assembly, i.e. several ribosomes bound to the same mRNA is known as a polysome or polyribosome (Fig.15.10).

Prokaryotic Translation

While the basic process of translation is similar in eukaryotes and prokaryotes, there are some differences

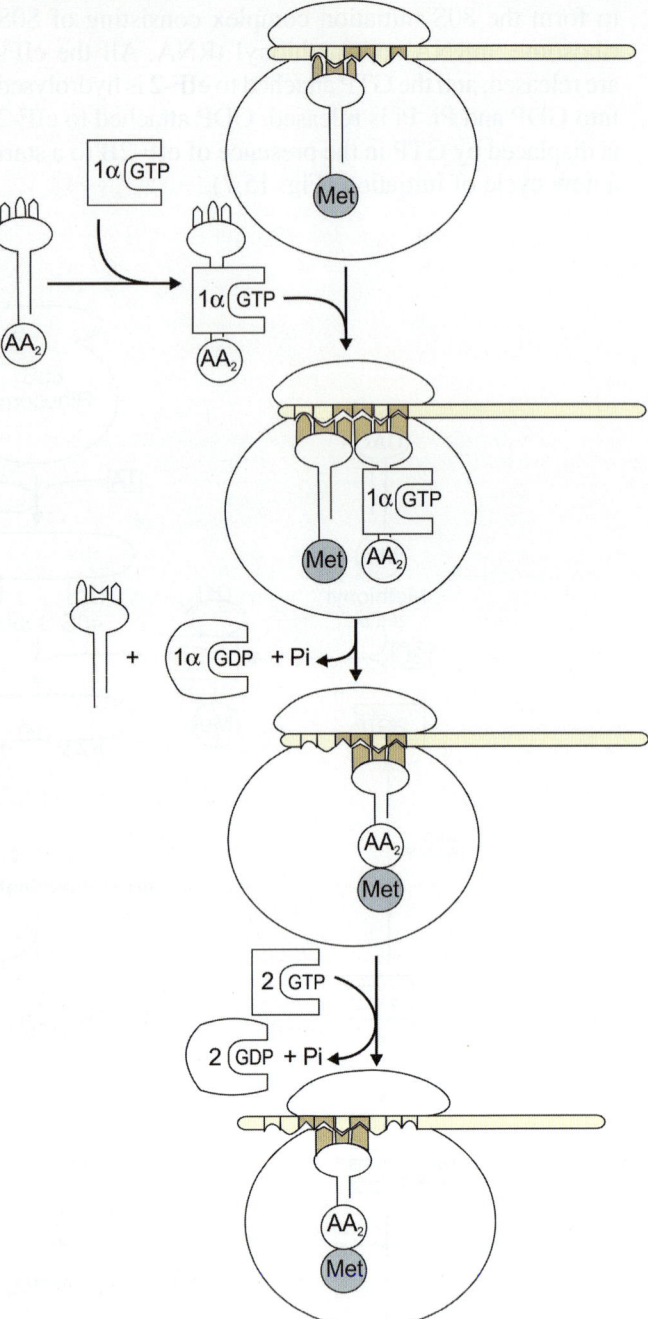

Fig. 15.8: Elongation of peptide chain. 1α and 2 are eukaryotic elongation factors, eEF-1α and eEF-2 respectively

also. The prokaryotic ribosomes are smaller.The rRNAs present in prokaryotic ribosomes are different.The prokaryotic initiation factors, elongation factors and releasing factors are different. Prokaryotic translation differs from eukaryotic translation in following important respects:

1. In prokaryotes, the primary transcript of any structural gene is mRNA which doesn't require any post-transcriptional modification, and is directly translated. The translation can begin even before the transcription

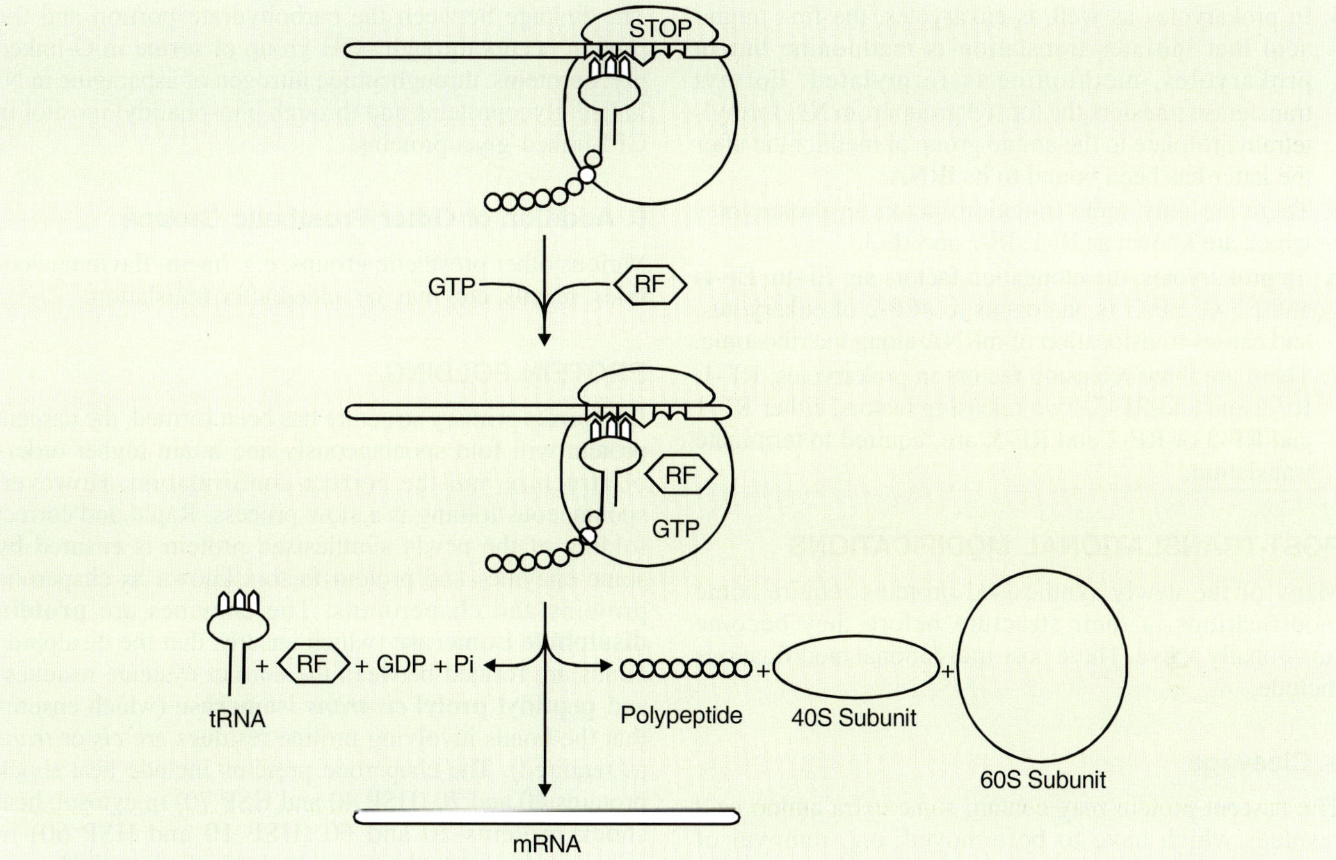

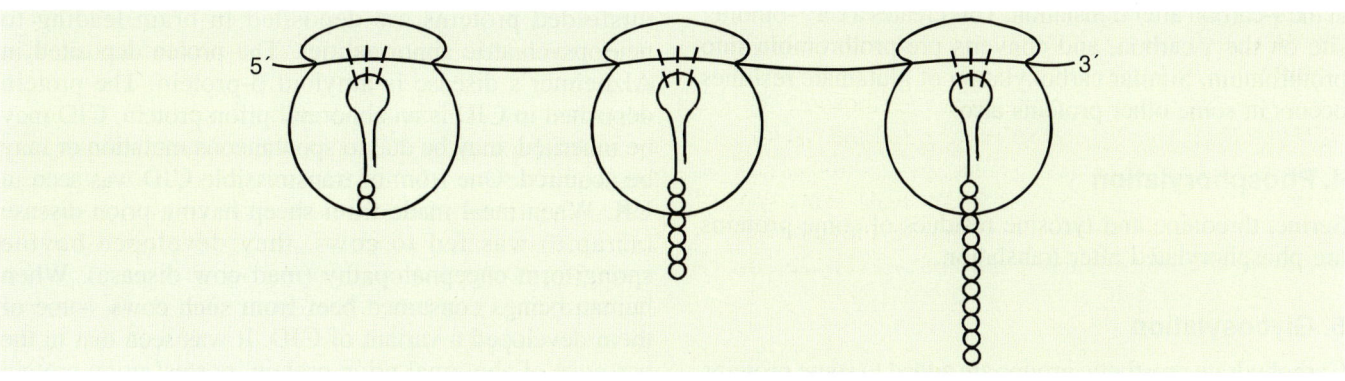

Fig. 15.9: Termination of translation. Binding of eukaryotic releasing factor (RF) and GTP to A site terminates translation

is complete, i.e. the partially synthesised mRNA can bind to a ribosome, and protein synthesis can begin.

2. Some of the prokaryotic mRNAs are **polycistronic** (a cistron is the coding unit for one polypeptide). Therefore, a number of polypeptides can be synthesised from the same mRNA.

3. Since more than one polypeptides may be synthesised from a single mRNA, there may be more than one initiation sites on a single mRNA. AUG is the initiator codon in prokaryotes also. Besides the initiator AUG, there may be AUG codons for internal methionine

residues also. The protein-synthesising machinery has to distinguish between the initiator AUG and the AUG codons for internal methionine residues. This distinction is facilitated by the presence of a short purine-rich sequence (Shine-Dalgarno sequence) on mRNA slightly upstream of the initiator AUG. A sequence of 3-9 bases, which is complementary to Shine-Dalgarno sequence, is present near the 3'-end of 16S rRNA of prokaryotic ribosomes. Therefore, the 16S rRNA binds to the Shine-Dalgarno sequence of mRNA and positions it correctly on the ribosome for initiation of translation.

Fig. 15.10: Polysome (different ribosomes have translated the same mRNA to different extents)

4. In prokaryotes as well as eukaryotes, the first amino acid that initiates translation is methionine but in prokaryotes, methionine is formylated. Formyl transferase transfers the formyl group from N^{10}-formyl-tetrahydrofolate to the amino group of methionine after the latter has been bound to its tRNA.

5. There are only three initiation factors in prokaryotes which are known as IF-1, IF-2 and IF-3.

6. In prokaryotes, the elongation factors are EF-tu, EF-ts and EF-G. EF-G is analogous to eEF-2 of eukaryotes, and causes translocation of mRNA along the ribosome.

7. There are three releasing factors in prokaryotes, RF-1, RF-2 and and RF-3. Two releasing factors, either RF-1 and RF-3 or RF-2 and RF-3, are required to terminate translation.

POST-TRANSLATIONAL MODIFICATIONS

Many of the newly-synthesised proteins require some modifications in their structure before they become functionally active. These post-translational modifications include:

1. Cleavage

The nascent protein may contain some extra amino acid residues which have to be removed, e.g. removal of connecting peptide from proinsulin to form insulin.

Alternative cleavage of precursor protein may yield different products, e.g. eight different proteins or peptides can be formed from pro-opiomelanocortin (POMC) by cleavage at different sites.

2. Hydroxylation

Some amino acid residues, e.g. proline and lysine, may be hydroxylated after translation. Hydroxylation of proline and lysine residues is important in the conversion of pro-collagen into collagen.

3. Carboxylation

Glutamate residues of pre-prothrombin are carboxylated at the γ-carbon after translation. This creates a Ca^{++}-binding site on the γ-carbon, and converts pre-prothrombin into prothrombin. Similar carboxylation of glutamate residues occurs in some other proteins also.

4. Phosphorylation

Serine, threonine and tyrosine residues of some proteins are phosphorylated after translation.

5. Glycosylation

Carbohydrate prosthetic groups are added to some proteins to form O-linked, N-linked and GPI-linked glycoproteins.

The linkage between the carbohydrate portion and the protein occurs through –OH group of serine in O-linked glycoproteins, through amide nitrogen of asparagine in N-linked glycoproteins and through phosphatidyl inositol in GPI-linked glycoproteins.

6. Addition of Other Prosthetic Groups

Various other prosthetic groups, e.g. haem, flavin nucleo-tides, metals, etc. may be added after translation.

PROTEIN FOLDING

If a correct primary structure has been formed, the nascent protein will fold spontaneously and attain higher orders of structure and the correct conformation. However, spontaneous folding is a slow process. Rapid and correct folding of the newly-synthesised protein is ensured by some enzymes and protein factors known as chaperone proteins and chaperonins. The enzymes are **protein disulphide isomerase** (which ensures that the disulphide bonds are formed between the correct cysteine residues) and **peptidyl prolyl *cis-trans* isomerase** (which ensures that the bonds involving proline residues are *cis* or *trans* as required). The chaperone proteins include heat shock proteins 40 and 70 (HSP 40 and HSP 70) in cytosol, heat shock proteins 10 and 60 (HSP 10 and HSP 60) in mitochondria, and calnexin and calreticulin in endoplasmic reticulum. The chaperonins include BiP, TriC, etc.

These enzymes and protein factors are also required to refold the proteins after they have passed through a membrane in the unfolded form.

Misfolding of proteins can be brought about by a change in the primary structure, defects in molecular chaperones or exogenous agents. A misfolded protein is usally degraded. Some of the misfolded proteins, e.g. amyloid protein, are resistant to degradation. Misfolded proteins may be deviod of function, may not reach their intended destination (e.g. cell membrane) or may be toxic.

Examples of human diseases that occur due to misfolding of proteins are Alzheimer's disease and Creutzfeldt-Jacob disease (CJD). In both these diseases, misfolded proteins are deposited in brain leading to neuropsychiatric abnormalities. The proten deposited in Alzheimer's disease is amyloid β-protein. The protein deposited in CJD is an abnormal prion protein. CJD may be inherited, may be due to spontaneons mutation or may be acquired. One from of transmissible CJD was seen in UK. When meal made from sheep having prion disease (scrapie) was fed to cows, they developed bovine spongiform encephalopathy (mad cow disease). When human beings consumed beef from such cows, some of them developed a variant of CJD. It was seen that in the presence of abnormal prion protein, normal prion protein is also misfolded.

PROTEIN TARGETING

The proteins synthesised on the ribosomes may have different **destinations**. Some remain in cytosol, some go to mitochondria, lysosomes or nucleus, some are incorporated in cell membrane and some are exported from the cell. The signal that directs the protein to its destination is inbuilt in the protein molecule. For example, addition of **mannose-6-phosphate** to the protein during post-translational modification directs it to **lysosomes**. In the absence of mannose-6-phosphate prosthetic group, the lysosomal enzymes fail to reach the lysosomes (in I-cell disease).

Proteins which are destined for **export or incorporation in the cell membrane** have a short **signal sequence (leader peptide)** of 15 to 30 amino acids at their amino terminus. As the signal sequence emerges from the ribosome, it is recognised and bound by **signal recognition particle (SRP)** made up of six polypeptides and 7S RNA. SRP binds to **SRP receptor** (docking protein made up of α and β subunits) present on the external side of endoplasmic reticulum (ER). The ribosome synthesising the protein is bound to a **ribosome receptor** present on the external side of ER. The signal sequence is directed into ER through a protein conducting channel **(translocon)**. The rest of the protein also follows the signal sequence. The signal sequence is split off by **signal peptidase** present in ER. The nascent protein is usually glycosylated and transferred to Golgi apparatus from where it is either directed to the cell membrane or is exported from the cell (Fig. 15.11).

INHIBITORS OF PROTEIN SYNTHESIS

Protein synthesis (translation) is inhibited by a number of compounds. Some inhibitors act selectively on prokaryotes or eukaryotes while others act on both. Inhibitors which act selectively on prokaryotes can be used as antibiotics. Some important **inhibitors** of **prokaryotic translation** which are used as **antibiotics** are:

1. **Streptomycin:** In prokaryotes, translation is initiated by binding of formylmethionyl tRNA to the 30S subunit of ribosomes. Streptomycin inhibits this binding and prevents initiation. It also causes misreading of codons on mRNA. Neomycin, kanamycin and gentamycin also inhibit initiation.

2. **Tetracyclines:** Tetracyclines bind to 50S ribosomal subunit of prokaryotes, and prevent binding of amino acyl tRNA to the A site.

3. **Chloramphenicol:** It inhibits peptidyl transferase activity of 50S ribosomal subunit in prokaryotes.

4. **Erythromycin:** It inhibits translocation of mRNA along the ribosome in prokaryotes by inhibiting EF-G (analogous to cEF-2 of eukaryotes).

Some inhibitors of translation act selectively on eukaryotes. **Cycloheximide** inhibits peptidyl transferase

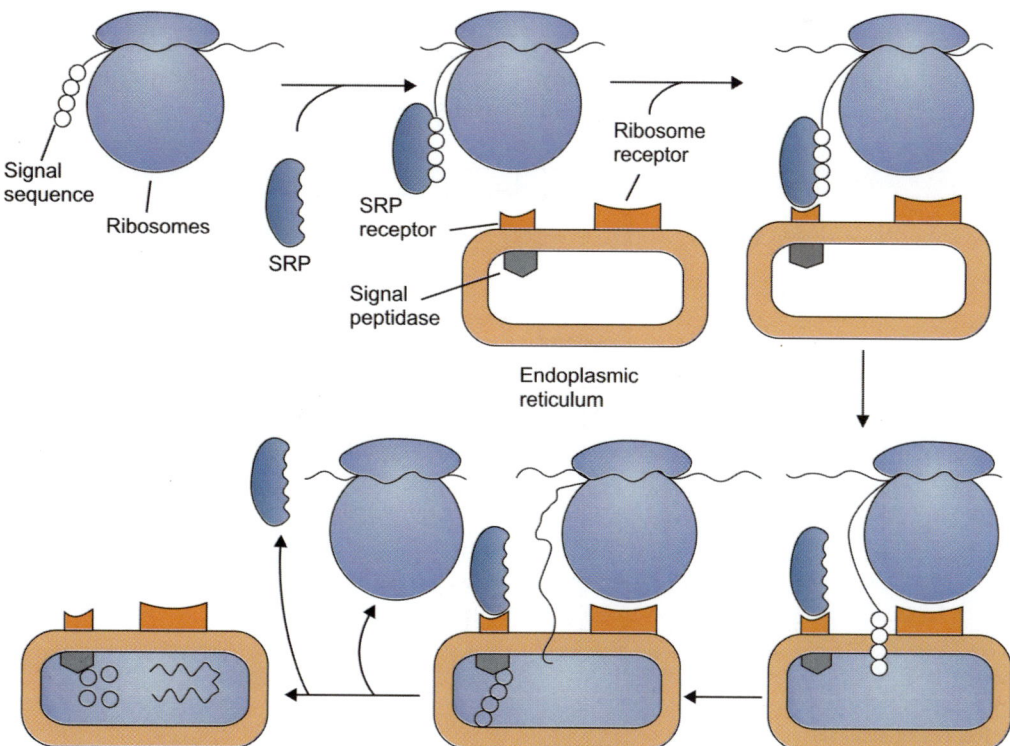

Fig. 15.11: Proteins destined for export or incorporation into cell membrane are first directed into endoplasmic reticulum with the help of their signal sequence, signal recognition particle (SRP) and SRP receptor

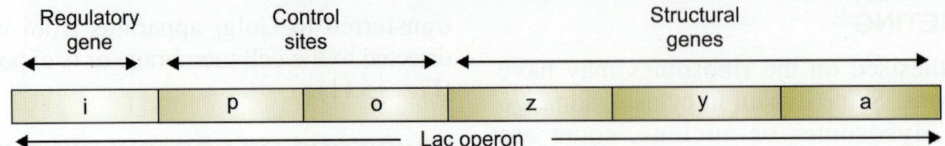

Fig. 15.12: Lac operon of *E.coli*

activity of 60S ribosomal subunit of eukaryotes. **Diphtheria toxin** inhibits translation in eukaryotes by **ADP-ribosylation** and inhibition of **eEF-2**. Puromycin inhibits translation in both prokaryotes and eukaryotes. It resembles the 3'-end of amino acyl tRNA, and binds to the A site of ribosome. A peptide bond is formed between puromycin and the last amino acid. Peptidyl puromycin is released from the ribosome, and translation is terminated prematurely.

REGULATION OF GENE EXPRESSION

A large number of genes is present in the genome of every organism but the proteins encoded by these genes are not required all the time. Moreover, the quantitative requirement for different proteins keeps on changing in response to internal and external stimuli. In higher organisms, certain genes are expressed selectively in certain tissues. Therefore, there must be mechanisms for regulating the expression of genes precisely in accordance with the changing requirements of the organism.

Regulation of Prokaryotic Gene Expression

The first insights into regulation of gene expression were provided by Jacob and Monod in 1961 in *E.coli*. They found that the key enzymes involved in the **metabolism** **of lactose** in *E.coli* are encoded by a cluster of genes called the **lac operon**. The enzymes, β-galactosidase, galactoside permease and galactoside transacetylase, are encoded by z, y and a genes respectively. These three structural genes are preceded by an operator (o) site, a promoter (p) site and a regulatory (i) gene. The entire cluster constitutes the lac operon (Fig. 15.12).

E.coli can use lactose as well as other sources of energy. When lactose is not available, the enzymes required to metabolise lactose are not synthesised. When lactose enters the cell, it induces the synthesis of enzymes encoded by z, y and a genes. The **i gene** encodes a repressor subunit, and its expression is **constitutive,** i.e. the repressor subunits are synthesised continuously. Four subunits combine to form the **repressor tetramer** which attaches to the **operator site** and **prevents the transcription** of z, y and a genes by RNA polymerase (Fig. 15.13).

When lactose enters the cell, it is converted into the inducer, allo-lactose. One **allo-lactose** molecule **binds** to each **repressor subunit**. This prevents the formation of the repressor tetramer. The operator site remains free. RNA polymerase transcribes the z, y and a genes to form a polycistronic mRNA. The mRNA is translated to form β-galactosidase, galactoside permease and galactoside transacetylase.

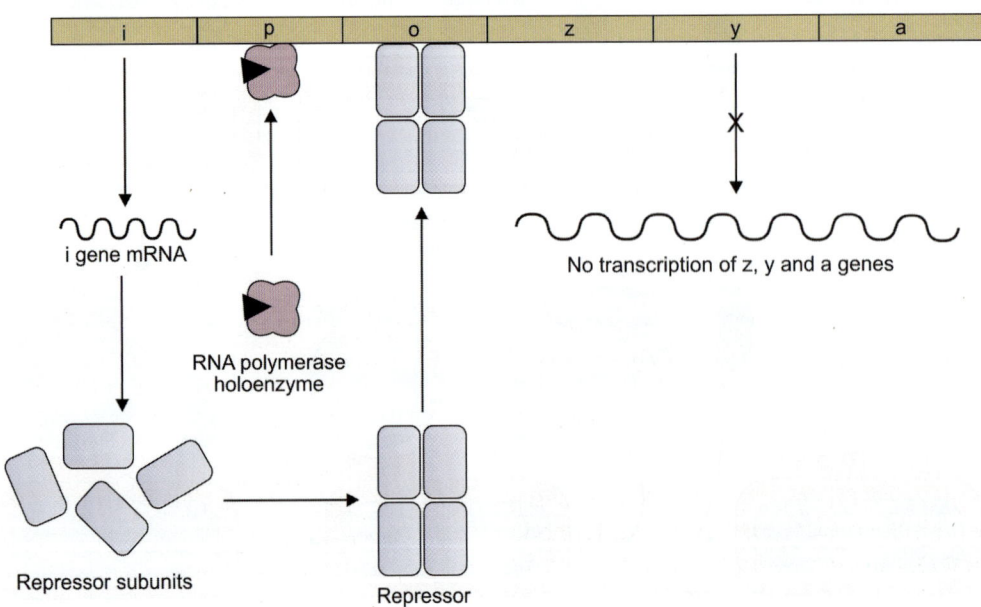

Fig. 15.13: The i gene is continuously transcribed and translated. The repressor tetramer attaches to the operator site and prevents the transcription of z, y and a genes by RNA polymerase

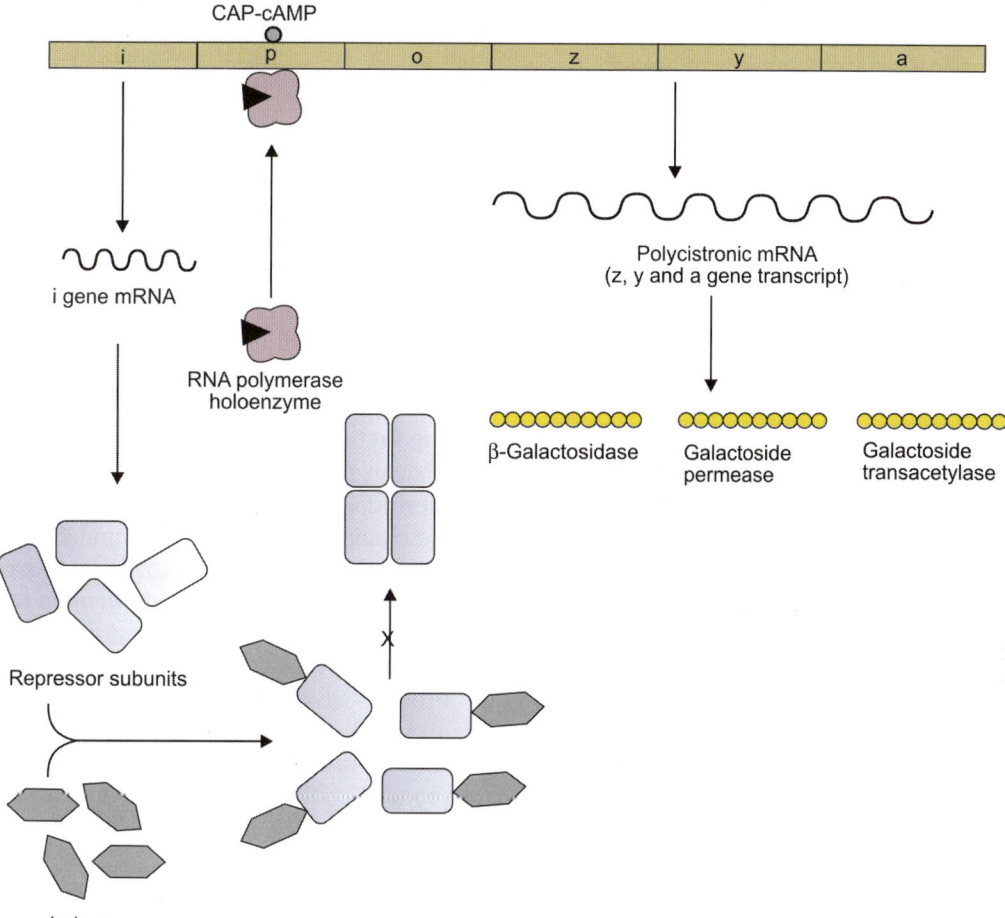

Fig. 15.14: Induction of enzyme synthesis. When inducer (allo-lactose) is present, it attaches to repressor subunits and prevents the formation of repressor tetramer. Operator site remains unoccupied. RNA polymerase transcribes the structural genes. A polycistronic mRNA is formed which is translated to form the three enzymes encoded by the z, y and a genes. CAP-cAMP (catabolite gene activator protein - cyclic AMP) complex binds to p site and facilitates the attachment of RNA polymerase holoenzyme

Lac operon has a **positive regulator** also. cAMP is an ancient hunger signal. When the bacterial cell is starved of energy, concentration of cAMP rises. **cAMP** forms a complex with **catabolite gene activator protein (CAP). CAP-cAMP complex** binds to the promoter site and **facilitates** the attachment of RNA polymerase holoenzyme to the promoter site(Fig. 15.14) . When energy is abundant, cAMP concentration falls, and CAP-cAMP complex is not formed.

A somewhat more complex regulatory mechanism is seen in the virus, **lambda phage.** When lambda phage infects *E.coli*, it can follow:

a. **Lysogenic pathway** in which the viral DNA is integrated in the bacterial genome, or

b. **Lytic pathway** in which the viral DNA replicates independently until the host cell is destroyed. Lambda phage DNA contains an operator region known as right operator (O_R) which is sub-divided into O_R1, O_R2 and O_R3. The right operator is flanked on the left side by a repressor gene, and on the right side by a cro gene.

In the lysogenic pathway, repressor gene is expressed forming a repressor dimer which bind to O_R1 and promotes the expression of repressor gene, at the same time repressing the expression of cro gene (Fig.15.15).

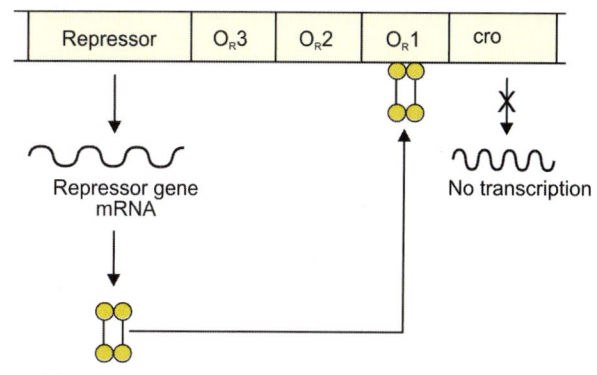

Fig. 15.15: In lysogenic pathway, repressor gene of lambda phage is expressed. The repressor protein binds to O_R1 and promotes the expression of repressor gene while repressing the expression of cro gene

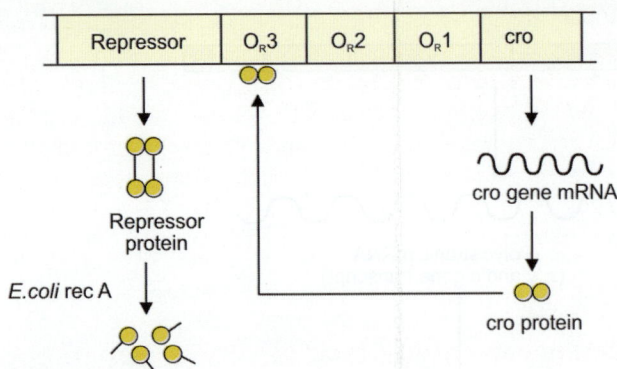

| Repressor | O$_R$3 | O$_R$2 | O$_R$1 | cro |

Fig. 15.16: In the lytic pathway, bacterial protease, rec A hydrolyses the repressor protein which cannot bind to O$_R$1. cro gene is expressed. cro protein binds to O$_R$3, and promotes the expression of cro gene while inhibiting the expression of repressor gene

In the lytic pathway, a host cell protease (rec A) becomes activated and hydrolyses the repressor which can no longer repress the cro gene. cro gene is expressed forming cro protein which binds to O$_R$3. This binding promotes the expression of cro gene and, at the same time, represses the expression of repressor gene (Fig.15.16).

Regulation of Eukaryotic Gene Expression

In eukaryotes, gene expression is more complex and therefore, regulation can occur at several stages. Regulatory strategies in eukaryotes include:

Gene Amplification

Gene amplification means formation of multiple copies of a gene. Certain genes can become amplified to permit increased synthesis of some proteins. Amplification may be spontaneous or secondary to some exogenous signals such as drugs. Amplification of genes forming tissue proteins has been seen during growing age in *Drosophilia*. Amplification of dihydrofolate reductase gene has been demonstrated in cancer cells on administration of amethopterin (a competitive inhibitor of dihydrofolate reductase).

Gene re-arrangement

Antibody diversity arises from gene re-arrangement. Different segments of light chains (variable, joining and constant segments) and heavy chains (variable, joining, diversity and constant segments) of antibodies are encoded at different locations on the DNA in a small number of copies. By joining these segments in different combinations and permutations, a huge variety of antibodies having different antigen specificities can be formed (see Chapter 19 for more details).

Regulation of Transcription

When a gene is to be transcribed, how often it is to be transcribed and in which tissues it is to be transcribed is

regulated by a number of factors most of which are proteins that act on some specific sequences present in the DNA having the gene. The intra-DNA sequences that affect transcription are known as *cis*-acting elements. These include **enhancer elements** that increase the rate of transcription, **silencer elements** that decrease or suppress transcription, **hormone response elements** that increase transcription when hormone-receptor complexes bind to them, **heat shock elements** that respond to heat and so on. Even **promoters** are intra-DNA sequences that are required for binding of RNA polymerase to the correct site on DNA for initiation of transcription. The extra-DNA factors that act on the *cis*-acting elements are called ***trans*-acting factors**. These include **inducers, repressors** and a number of **protein factors**.

Steroid hormones, thyroid hormones, calcitriol and retinoic acid are examples of regulatory compounds that bind to their receptors to form hormone-receptor complexes. A DNA-binding domain on the receptor binds to a specific hormone response element on DNA, and increases the transcription of certain structural genes.

Proteins which interact with DNA and affect the rate of transcription have been found to possess some distinct **structural motifs** which help them to bind to specific DNA sequences with high affinity. These structural motifs include **helix-turn-helix, zinc finger** and **leucine zipper motifs**.

DNA binding proteins having helix-turn-helix motif consist of two identical monomers. The DNA recognition domain (helix) of each monomer binds to five base pairs of DNA in a major groove (Fig. 15.17). An example is catabolite gene activator protein (CAP) of *E.coli*. DNA binding proteins having zinc finger motif have two to nine zinc fingers (Fig.15.18). Each zinc finger binds five base pairs of DNA in a major groove. Examples are steroid hormone receptors, thyroid hormone receptors, calcitriol receptor, etc. DNA binding proteins having leucine zipper motif consist of two identical monomers. In helical region

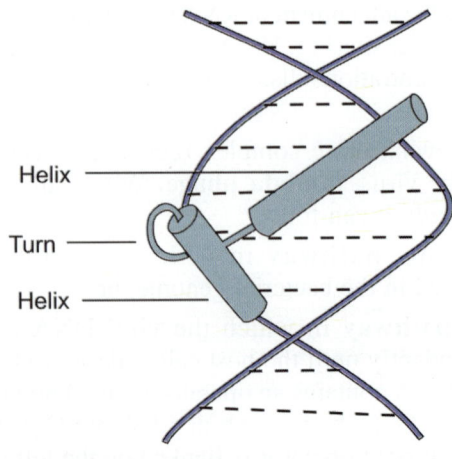

Fig. 15.17: Helix-turn-helix motif

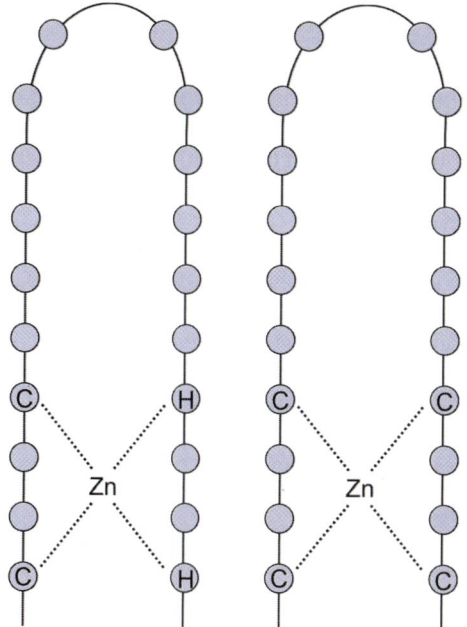

Fig. 15.18: Zinc finger motif (zinc may be bonded to two cysteine and two histidine residues or to four cysteine residues)

of each monomer, leucine residues are present at every seventh position. Leucine residues of the two monomers form a zipper (Fig.15.19). An example is cAMP response element binding protein (CREB).

MUTATIONS

Mutations are **changes** in **base sequence** of genes. Such changes can occur due to accidental errors during replication and can also be brought about by external agents, e.g. ultraviolet light, ionising radiation and mutagenic chemicals. Fortunately, repair mechanisms can correct most of these errors and defects. Rarely, some errors or defects escape correction or repair and, then, the changed base sequence becomes stably incorporated in the genome. These stable changes in base sequence are known as mutations. Mutations can be of two types: (a) point mutations and (b) frameshift mutations.

Point Mutations

Substitution of a single base by another is known as point mutation. If a purine base is replaced by another purine base or if a pyrimidine base is replaced by another pyrimidine base, it is known as **transition**. Substitution of a purine base by a pyrimidine base or vice versa is known as **transversion**. A point mutation will affect only **one codon**. Point mutations can be of following types:

i. *Silent Mutations*

If the substitution occurs in the third base of a codon, the code word may remain unchanged due to degeneracy of the genetic code. For example, if GGC changes to GGG, there will be **no change in amino acid sequence** as both are code words for glycine. This type of mutations which do not change the code words are known as silent mutations.

ii. *Mis-sense Mutations*

If the base substitution changes the code word, the amino acid sequence of the encoded protein will change. The effect of **amino acid substitution** is variable. If the

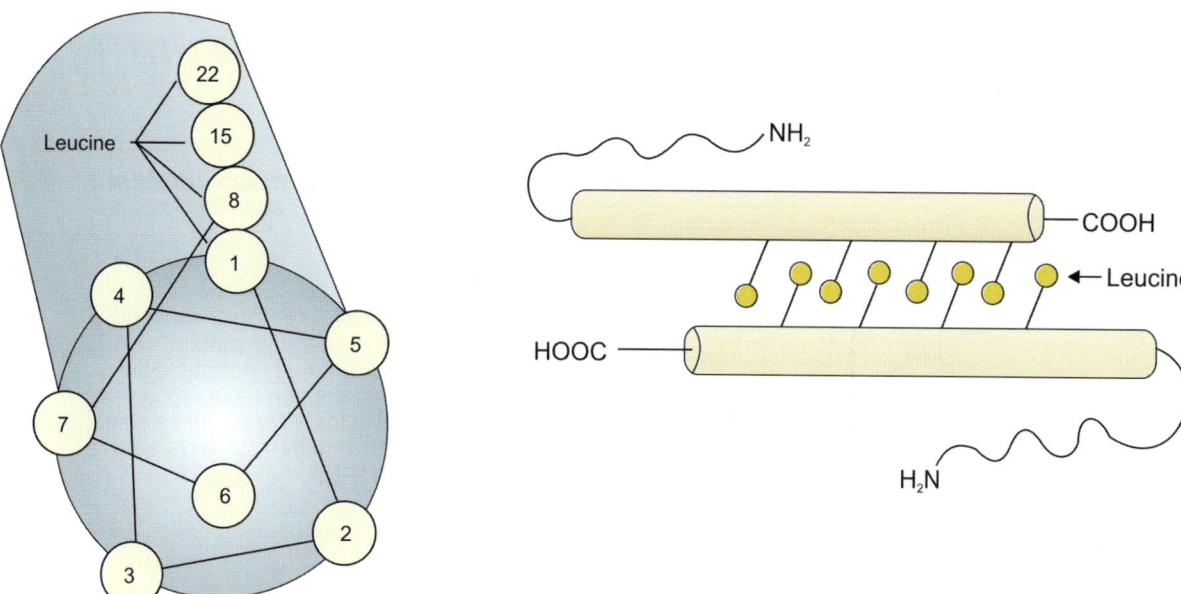

Fig. 15.19: Leucine zipper motif. Every seventh residue is leucine. The leucine residues are stacked upon each other. Leucine residues of two polypeptides jut against each other and form a zipper

structure of the substituted amino acid is similar to that of the original amino acid, the effect may be minimal. The effect also depends upon the site where the substitution has occurred. If the substitution occurs in an area of the protein molecule which is critical for its functioning, the effect will be severe. Accordingly, mis-sense mutations may be:

a. **Acceptable**,

b. **Partially acceptable** or

c. **Unacceptable**.

Haemoglobin Bristol and **Haemoglobin Sydney** are examples of acceptable mis-sense mutations in which the amino acid substitution occurs in a non-critical area of the molecule and, therefore, the haemoglobin is capable of functioning normally. **Haemoglobin S** is an example of **partially acceptable** mis-sense mutation. Substitution of glutamate by valine at position six in the β chain partially impairs the functioning of Hb S. It is able to function normally at high oxygen tension but gets precipitated at low oxygen tension. **Haemoglobin M** is an example of an **unacceptable** mis-sense mutation. Replacement of histidine by tyrosine at position 58 of α chain makes Hb M incapable of combining with oxygen.

iii. *Nonsense Mutations*

Sometimes, base substitution changes a **sense codon** into a **nonsense (stop) codon**. In such cases, protein synthesis will be terminated prematurely, and the resulting protein will be usually non-functional.

Frameshift Mutations

Frameshift mutations occur due to **insertion** or **deletion** of bases. Insertion or deletion of **one or two bases** would change the **reading frame** distal to the mutation. As a result, the protein will have a **garbled amino acid sequence** distal to the mutation, and it will be generally **non-functional**. **Premature termination** can also occur due to conversion of a sense codon into a nonsense codon. Conversely, a nonsense codon may be changed into a codon for an amino acid. This will result in the synthesis of an **abnormally large protein** which is usually devoid of function.

If bases are inserted in **multiples of three**, a corresponding number of extra amino acids would be incorporated in the protein. Similarly, if bases are deleted in multiples of three, a corresponding number of amino acids would be missing from the protein.

Suppressor Mutations

In prokaryotes and lower eukaryotes, mutations have been seen in **anticodons** of tRNA molecules which may sometimes **neutralise** the effect of mutations in structural genes. This type of mutations are known as suppressor mutations. tRNA molecules having this type of mutations are known as **suppressor tRNAs**. For example, if the codon UAC (tyrosine) changes to UAG (stop) as a result of a point mutation in a structural gene, translation will be prematurely terminated. But if the anticodon of tRNA$_{TYR}$ changes from GUA to CUA as a result of a point mutation, this mutant tRNA will read UAG as a codon for tyrosine. However, a normal tRNA is needed to translate the normal codon for tyrosine. This is not impossible as tRNA genes are present in multiple copies.

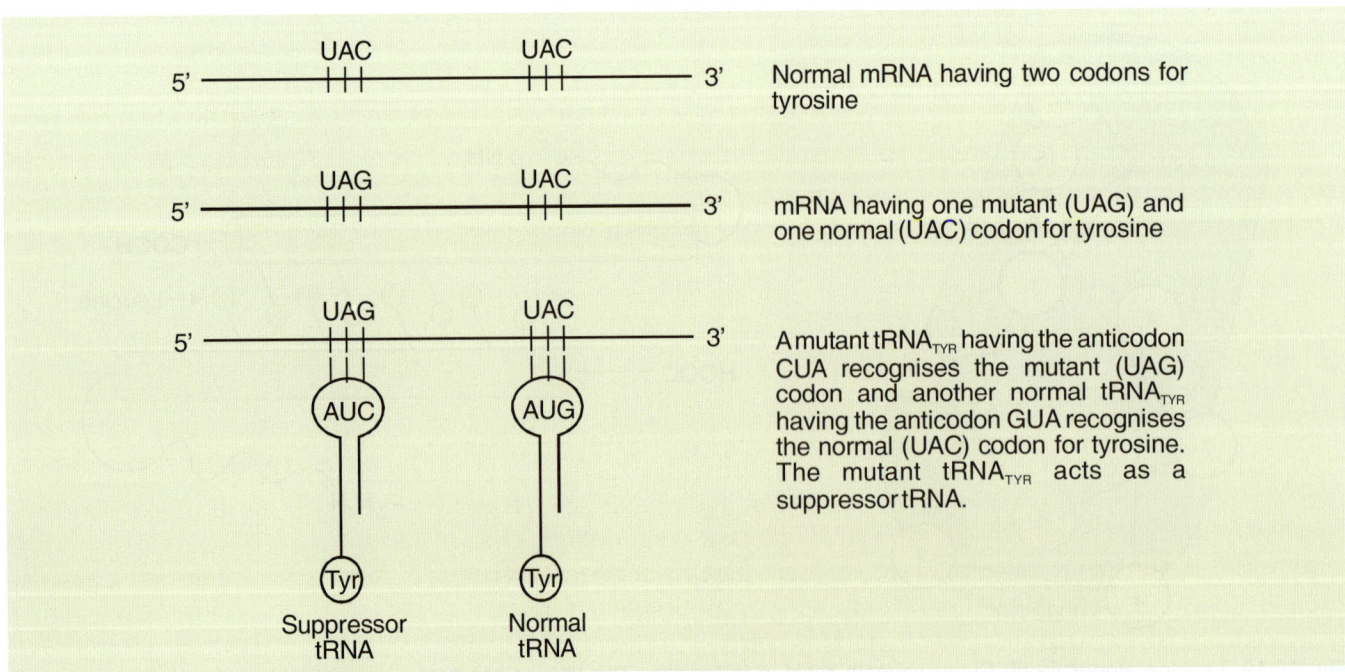

Fig. 15.20: A mutant tRNA$_{TYR}$ suppresses the effect of mutation in the structural gene.

EXERCISE

1. Describe the process of protein synthesis is eukaryotes. Explain post-translational modifications with examples.

2. Explain the regulation of gene expression in prokaryotes and eukaryotes.

3. Write short notes on:
   a. Genetic code
   b. Protein folding
   c. Signal sequence
   d. Inhibitors of translation
   e. Lac operon
   f. Gene amplification
   g. *cis*-Acting elements
   h. Point mutations
   i. Frameshift mutations
   j. Suppressor mutations

4. Write 'true' or' false':
   a. Nonsense codons have no function.
   b. There are more than one codons for some amino acids.
   c. Degeneracy of genetic code can cause mutations.
   d. One codon encodes only one amino acid.
   e. Genetic code is universal except for some differences in mitochondrial codons.
   f. One tRNA can be charged only with one specific amino acid.
   g. The anticodon on tRNA recognises the amino acid.
   h. Both ATP and GTP are required for translation.
   i. Chaperonins are required to transport proteins out of cells.
   j. Presence of mannose-6-phosphate in the protein directs it to lysosomes.
   k. Proteins meant for transport out of the cell or incorporation into cell membrane are first directed into endoplasmic reticulum.
   l. Signal peptidase is present in Golgi apparatus.
   m. Inhibitors of prokaryotic translation can be used as antibiotics.
   n. Streptomycin inhibits initiation of translation in eukaryotes.
   o. Diphtheria toxin inhibits translation in eukaryotes.
   p. Enhancer elements and silencer elements are *cis*-acting elements.
   q. Substitution of one base by another is known as transversion.
   r. Suppressor mutations occur in genes for tRNA.

5. Fill in the blanks:
   a. Anticodons are present on ....
   b. .... codons have no complementary anticodons.
   c. Non-coding sequences in a gene are known as ....
   d. .... are removed during splicing.
   e. Eukaryotic promoters have a .... box about 25 bp upstream of the transcription start site.
   f. Imprecise recognition of the third base of a codon by anticodon is known as ....
   g. .... tRNA initiates translation in eukaryotes.
   h. Binding of formylmethionyl tRNA to 30S subunit of ribosomes is inhibited by ....
   i. Chloramphenicol inhibits the .... activity of 50S ribosomal subunit.
   j. SRP receptors are present on ....
   k. Signal sequence of proteins is removed in ....
   l. Half-life of a protein depends upon its .... amino acid.
   m. Nitrosamine can deaminate cytosine to form ....
   n. Xeroderma pigmentosum results from a defect in the .... repair system.
   o. Substitution of a purine base by a pyrimidine base is known as ....
   p. A mutation resulting from substitution of one base by another is known as a .... mutation.
   q. .... mutations occur due to insertion or deletion of bases.
   r. Leucine zipper motif is seen in proteins having leucine residues at every ....position.

ANSWERS TO SHORT QUESTIONS

4. a. False
   b. True
   c. False
   d. True
   e. True
   f. True
   g. False
   h. True
   i. False
   j. True
   k. True
   l. False
   m. True
   n. False
   o. True
   p. True
   q. False
   r. True

5. a. tRNA
   b. Nonsense
   c. Introns
   d. Introns
   e. TATA
   f. Wobble
   g. Methionyl
   h. Streptomycin
   i. Peptidyl transferase
   j. Endoplasmic reticulum
   k. Endoplasmic reticulum
   l. N-terminus
   m. Uracil
   n. Nucleotide excision
   o. Transversion
   p. Point
   q. Frameshift
   r. Seventh

16

Recombinant DNA Technology

Recombinant DNA technology came into existence in the 1970s, and has revolutionised biochemistry. As the name suggests, recombinant DNA is formed by joining two (or more) different DNA molecules or fragments of DNA molecules. Such DNA, having unrelated genes, is known as **chimeric DNA**, named after a mythological creature, chimera having the head of a lion, the trunk of a goat and the tail of a snake. Recombinant DNA technology has proved to be of immense value in medicine, agriculture, animal husbandry, industry, etc.

RESTRICTION ENDONUCLEASES

Restriction endonucleases (or restriction enzymes) are among the most important tools of recombinant DNA technology. In fact, it was the discovery of restriction enzymes by Arber, Smith and Nathans in the early 1970s that opened the doors of recombinant DNA research. Restriction enzymes are found in bacteria, and protect the bacterial cells against viral infections. When a virus infects a bacterial cell, viral DNA is split by bacterial restriction enzymes and, thus, the virus is destroyed.

Hundreds of restriction enzymes have been discovered so far. These are named after the bacterium in which they are found, e.g. Hin I, Hae III, Eco RI, etc. The three-letter abbreviation stands for the bacterium, e.g. Hin for *Haemophilus influenzae*, Hae for *Haemophilus aegyptius*, Eco for *Escherichia coli*. Sometimes, a strain designation is also included in the name, e.g. R after Eco means strain R of *E.coli*. The numerals I, II, III, etc. indicate the serial numbers of the enzymes from the same bacterium in the order of discovery.

Each restriction enzyme recognises and splits a particular base sequence in **double-stranded DNA**. The sequence recognised by a restriction enzyme extends over **4-8 base pairs**, and is **palindromic** (a palindrome is a word or a sentence which reads the same from left to right and from right to left, e.g. DAD, MADAM, etc.). In DNA, the base sequences are read in 5' to 3' direction. If a sequence reads the same on both the strands in 5' to 3' direction, it is known as a palindromic sequence (Fig. 16.1).

5' GGCGCC 3'	5' CGATCG 3'
3' CCGCGG 5'	3' GCTAGC 5'

Fig. 16.1: Double-stranded palindromic sequences

Restriction enzymes split both the strands producing either **blunt** (even or non-overlapping) ends or **sticky** (overlapping or cohesive) ends. Sticky ends are more useful in recombinant DNA technology as these can be easily ligated to the complementary sticky ends of another fragment of DNA produced by the same restriction enzyme (Fig. 16.2).

The site cleaved by a particular restriction enzyme is known as its **restriction site**. The DNA fragments produced by restriction enzymes are known as **restriction fragments**. A DNA, generally, has several restriction sites for a number of restriction enzymes (Fig. 16.3).

RECOMBINANT DNA

Restriction fragments obtained from different sources can be joined together by DNA ligase to produce recombinant DNA having a base sequence different from that of the original DNA. For example, a foreign gene can be inserted into DNA by this method (Fig.16.4).

After preparing recombinant DNA, **amplification** is often required to prepare multiple copies of the DNA. Amplification can be done either by **cloning** the DNA or by **polymerase chain reaction**.

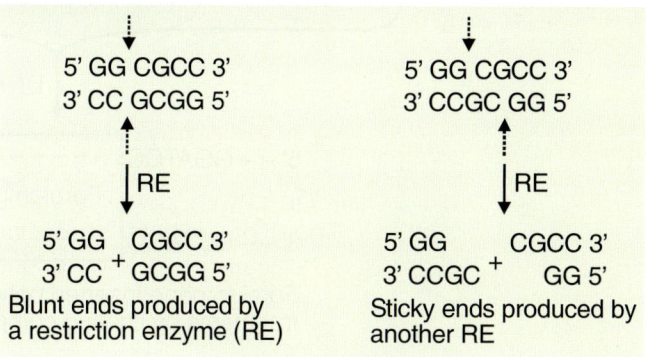

Fig 16.2: Blunt and sticky ends

235

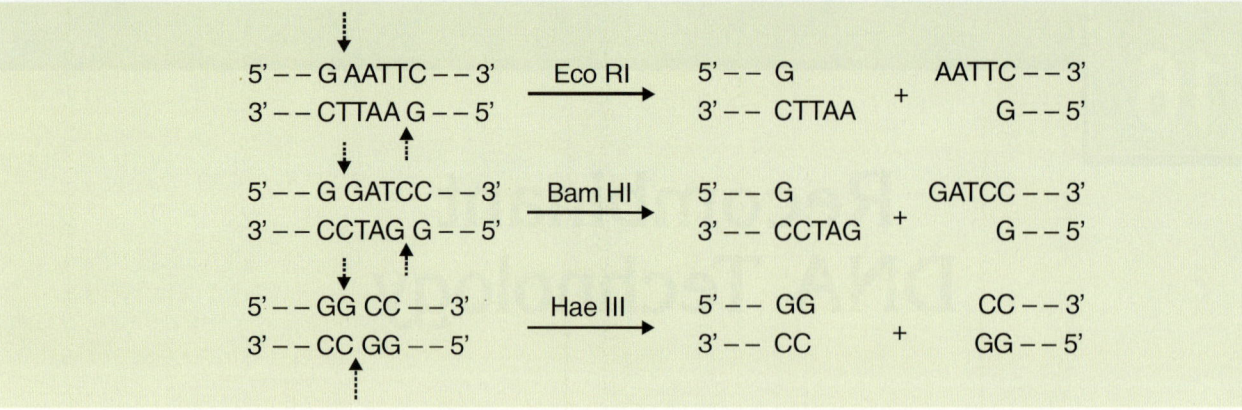

Fig. 16.3: Restriction sites of some restriction enzymes. Broken arrows show cleavage sites

CLONING OF RECOMBINANT DNA

A clone is a population of identical organisms or cells or molecules. Recombinant DNA can be cloned in living cells using suitable vectors to transfer the recombinant DNA into the cells. Some useful **cloning vectors** are plasmids, bacteriophages, cosmids and yeast artificial chromosomes.

Plasmid

Many prokaryotes possess a small circular double-stranded DNA in addition to the chromosomal DNA. This extra-chromosomal DNA is known as a plasmid. Plasmids may replicate independently of the chromosomes. One or more

antibiotic-resistance genes are often present in plasmids which provide antibiotic resistance to the micro-organisms. Bacterial plasmids can be transferred from one bacterium to another. DNA fragments up to 10 kb (kilobases) in size can be easily inserted into plasmids, and cloned in bacteria, e.g. *E.coli*. The plasmid is nicked by a suitable restriction enzyme to generate sticky ends. The foreign DNA having complementary sticky ends is joined to the nicked plasmid by DNA ligase. The plasmid is introduced into a bacterial cell. Multiplication of the plasmid and the bacterial cell produces multiple copies of the foreign gene (Fig. 16.5).

pSC 101 is a plasmid naturally present in *E. coli*. It was the first vector used for cloning. It has only one restriction

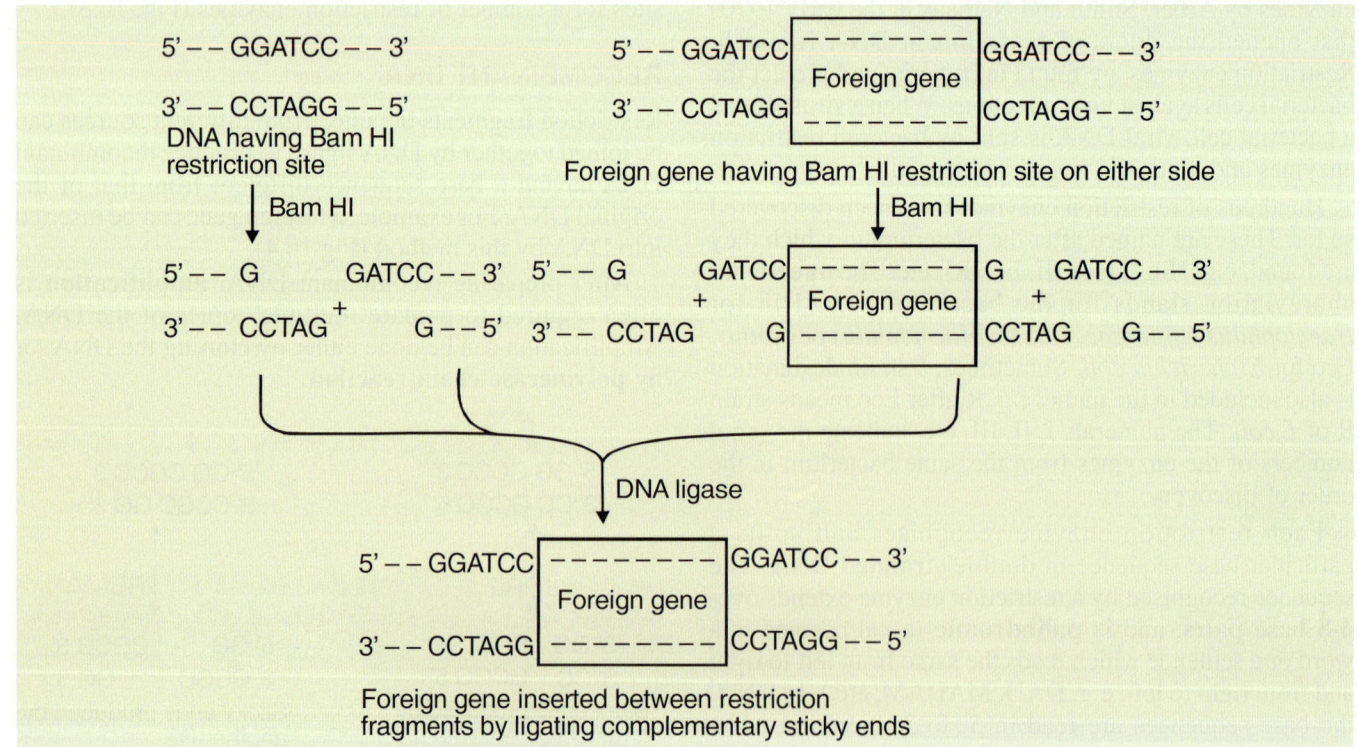

Fig. 16.4: Production of recombinant DNA containing a foreign gene

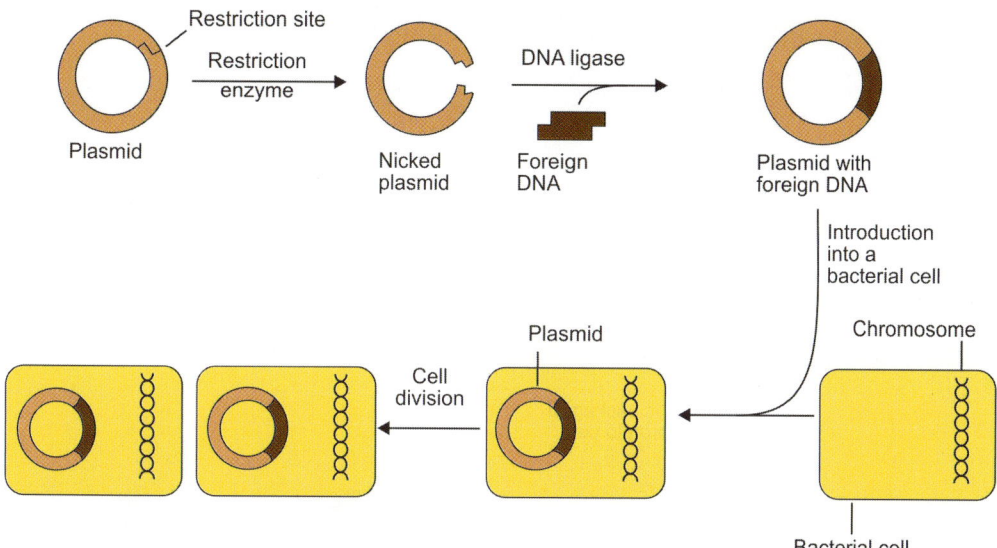

Fig. 16.5: Cloning of DNA by a plasmid vector

site (for Eco RI), only one antibiotic-resistance gene and replicates poorly. An ideal vector should replicate rapidly, should have several restriction sites for different restriction enzymes and more than one **antibiotic-resistance genes**. Several plasmid vectors having these characteristics have been constructed in the laboratory, e.g. pBR 322, pBR328, pUC18, etc.

Plasmids can be introduced into bacteria by exposing them to high concentration of divalent cations which increase the permeability of bacterial cell membrane so as to allow plasmids to enter the bacterial cells. However, plasmids may not enter all the bacterial cells and some plasmids might not have taken up the foreign DNA. To select bacterial cells harbouring recombinant plasmids, use may be made of antibiotic-resistance genes. For example, plasmid pBR322 possesses genes for ampicillin-resistance as well as tetracycline-resistance. Each of these two genes has a number of restriction sites. A foreign gene (or a DNA fragment) can be inserted in the middle of, say, tetracycline-resistance gene. In that case, the bacterial cells harbouring the recombinant plasmid would be resistant to ampicillin but not to tetracycline. By growing the bacteria on an agar plate containing ampicillin, the bacterial cells which have not taken up the plasmid are destroyed. By partially transferring the bacterial colonies on a replica plate containing tetracycline, the colonies on the original plate having the recombinant plasmid can be identified.

Bacteriophages

Bacteriophages are viruses having a DNA genome surrounded by a protein coat. The virus infects a bacterial cell by injecting its DNA into the bacterial cell. The viral DNA may enter one of the two alternate pathways. In one pathway, known as the lysogenic pathway, the viral DNA gets incorporated into the bacterial genome, and becomes

dormant (provirus). The proviral DNA replicates only when the bacterial cell divides. In the second pathway, known as the lytic pathway, the viral DNA remains separate, and replicates independently. The proteins encoded by the viral DNA are synthesised by the bacterial cell, and each DNA molecule is packaged into a protein coat forming a new virus particle. When the number of virus particles becomes very large, the bacterial cell ruptures. The provirus can break out of the bacterial DNA and enter lytic pathway if the bacterial cell is exposed to some DNA damaging agent, e.g. ultraviolet light.

Bacteriophages can be used as vectors for cloning. A portion of the viral DNA which is not essential for its replication and packaging is clipped out by restriction enzymes, and the foreign DNA to be cloned is inserted in the viral DNA. The virus infects a bacterial cell, multiplies inside it, and a large number of copies of foreign DNA are formed in the bacterial cell. Lambda phage and M13 phage are commonly used as cloning vectors. DNA fragments up to 20 kb in size can be inserted in phage vectors, and can be cloned in *E.coli*. Moreover, it is easier to infect *E.coli* with a bacteriophage than with a plasmid (Fig. 16.6).

Cosmids

Cosmids are hybrids of plasmids and lambda phage. Lambda phage DNA possesses sticky ends known as **cos sites** on either side. These cos sites are necessary for packaging the phage DNA into the protein coat. Cosmids are prepared by inserting the cos sites of phage DNA in plasmids. Cosmids can infect *E.coli* just like plasmids. DNA fragments upto 45 kb in size can be inserted in cosmids.

Yeast Artificial Chromosomes

Yeast artificial chromosomes (YACs) are linear double-stranded DNA molecules having the genes necessary for

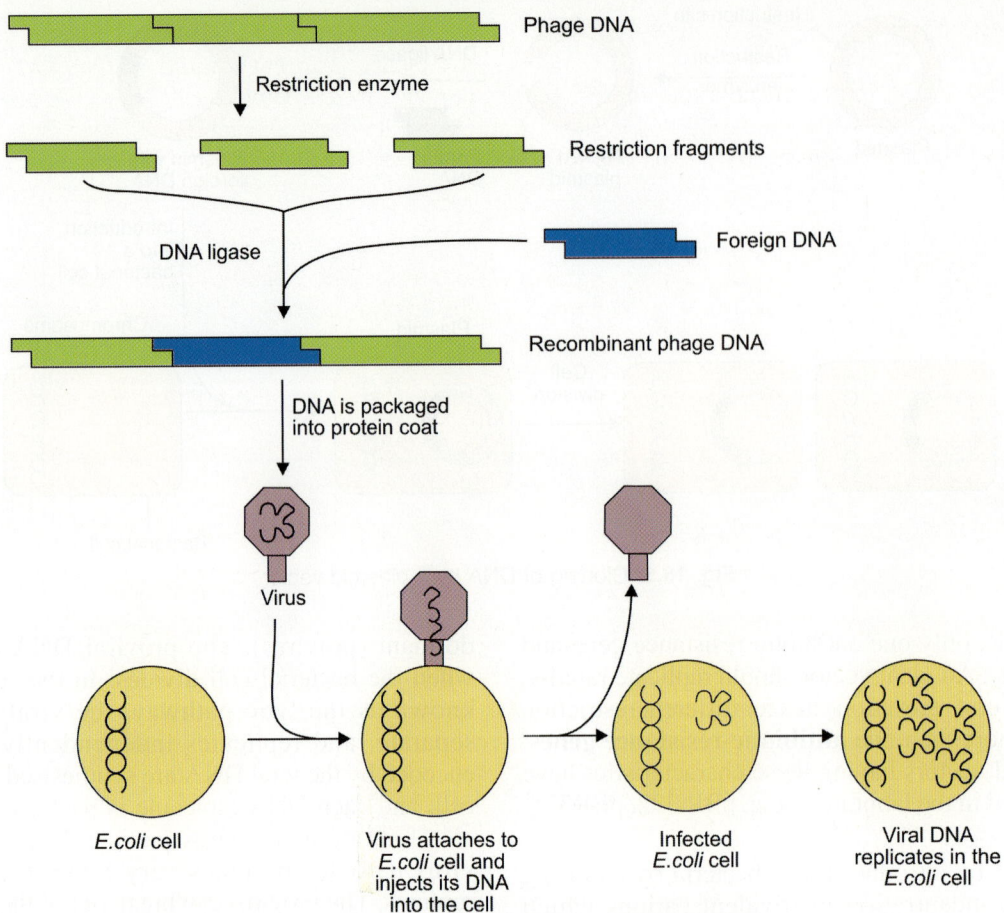

Fig. 16.6: Cloning of foreign DNA using a phage vector

replication. Large pieces of foreign DNA (up to 3,000 kb) can be inserted in YACs, and cloned in yeast cells.

POLYMERASE CHAIN REACTION

Polymerase chain reaction (PCR) is a technique for amplification of DNA devised by Mullis(1984).This technique is far quicker, easier and inexpensive than cloning. The only limitation of PCR is the size of DNA that can be amplified (up to 3 kb). In PCR, the DNA to be amplified is replicated by DNA polymerase of **Thermus aquaticus (Taq)**, a bacterium found in hot water springs. The optimum temperature of **Taq polymerase** is 72°C, and it is not denatured at temperatures upto 95°C. This property is important because DNA has to be heated to 94° to 95°C for separation of strands, and Taq polymerase is not destroyed at this temperature.

For amplifying a desired sequence in DNA, we have to know short flanking sequences on either side of the target sequence so that complementary primers can be prepared. Primers made up of deoxyribonucleotides are preferred. The reaction mixture consists of the DNA to be amplified, a large quantity of primers and deoxyribo-nucleotides (dATP, dGTP, dCTP and dTTP), and Taq polymerase. Amplification occurs in three steps (Fig. 16.7).

1. The temperature is raised to 95°C for a short period (30 seconds) so that the two strands of DNA separate.
2. The temperature is lowered to 56°C for a short period (30 seconds) so that primers can bind (anneal) to complementary sequences on both the strands of DNA.
3. The temperature is raised to 72°C for 2 to 5 minutes so that Taq polymerase can replicate the two strands.

By repeating these steps again and again, enormous amplification of the target sequence of DNA can be achieved. After twenty cycles, nearly one million copies

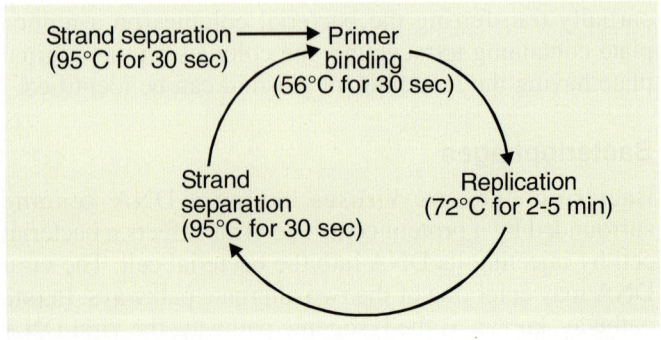

Fig. 16.7: Temperature cycles for polymerase chain reaction

are formed. The number rises to nearly one billion after thirty cycles.

Since sufficient quantities of primers and deoxyribo-nucleotides have been added to the reaction mixture in the beginning and since Taq polymerase is not destroyed during the reactions, the only thing one has to do to repeat the cycles is to change the temperature cyclically. This can be done automatically in instruments known as **thermocyclers**. A example of amplification of a target sequence by polymerase chain reaction is shown in Fig. 16.8.

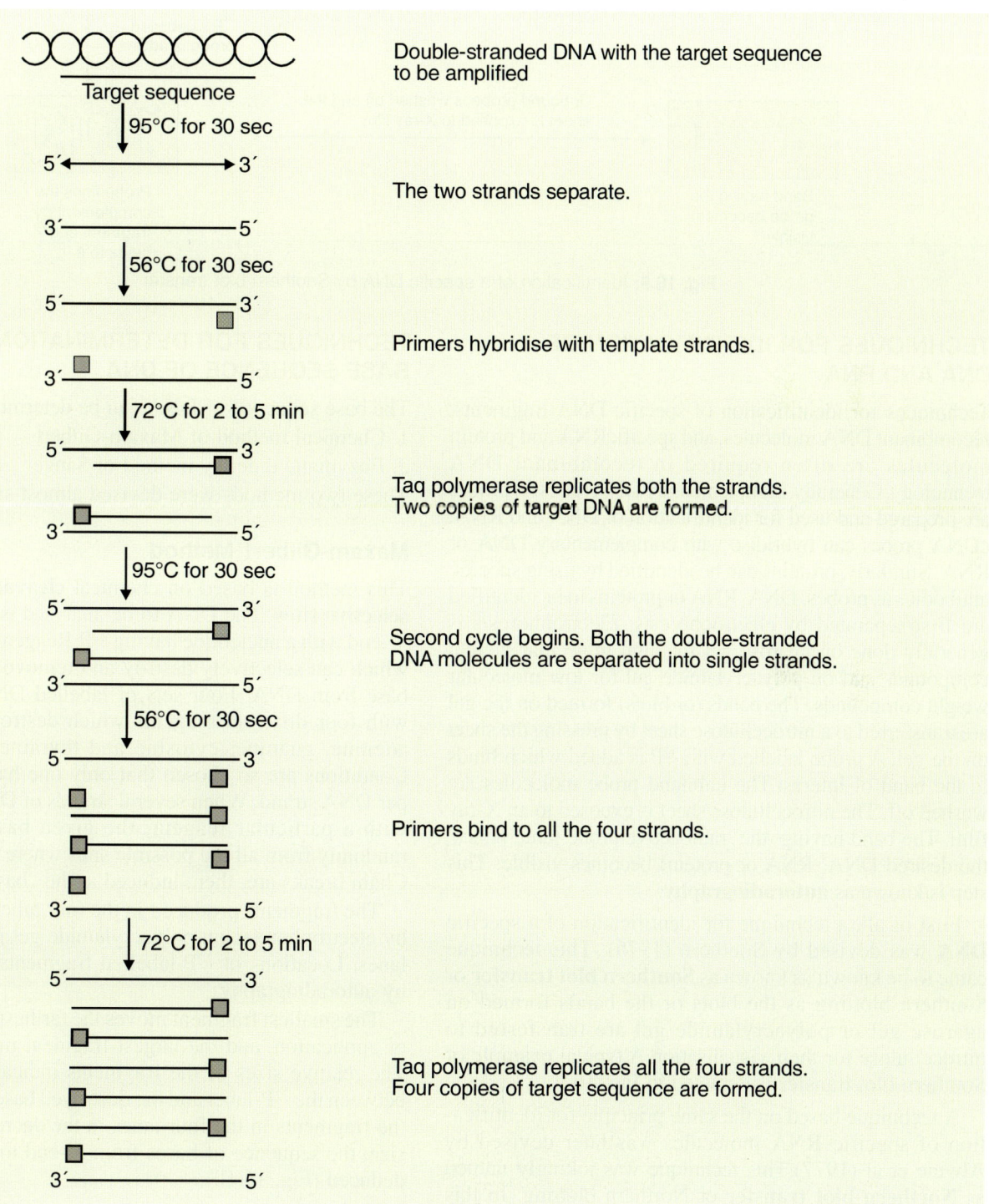

Fig.16.8: Polymerase chain reaction

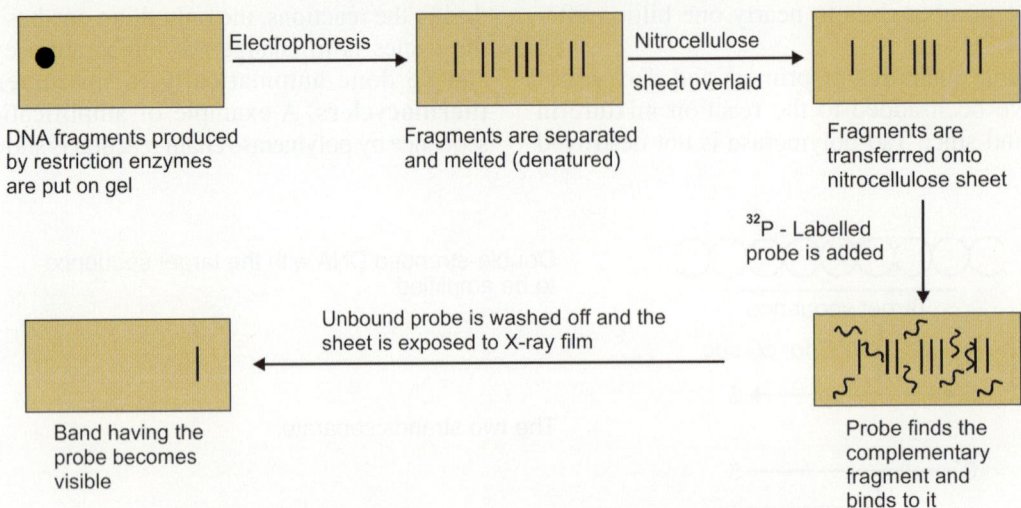

Fig. 16.9: Identification of a specific DNA by Southern blot transfer

TECHNIQUES FOR IDENTIFICATION OF DNA AND RNA

Techniques for identification of specific DNA fragments, recombinant DNA molecules, and specificRNA and protein molecules are often required in recombinant DNA technology. Generally, complementary DNA (cDNA) probes are prepared and used for identification of DNA and RNA. cDNA probes can hybridise with complementary DNA or RNA. Similarly, proteins can be identified by using specific antibodies as probes. DNA, RNA or proteins to be identified are first separated by electrophoresis. Electrophoresis is generally done on agarose gel for high molecular weight compounds and on polyacrylamide gel for low molecular weight compounds. The bands (or blots) formed on the gel are transferred to a nitrocellulose sheet by pressing the sheet on the gel. A probe labelled with ^{32}P is added which binds to the band of interest.The unbound probe molecules are washed off. The nitrocellulose sheet is exposed to an X-ray film. The band having the radioactive probe (and, hence, the desired DNA, RNA or protein) becomes visible. This step is known as **autoradiography**.

First of all, a technique for identification of a specific **DNA** was devised by Southern (1975). This technique came to be known as known as **Southern blot transfer** or Southern blotting as the blots or the bands formed on agarose gel or polyacrylamide gel are transferred to nitrocellulose for their visualisation A typical example of Southern blot transfer is depicted in Fig. 16.9.

A technique based on the same principle for identification of specific **RNA** molecules was later devised by Alwine et al (1977).This technique was jokingly named as **Northern blot transfer** or Northern blotting. In this technique, a cDNA–RNA hybrid is formed. A similar technique for identification of **proteins** with the help of labelled antibody probes was devised later, and was named **Western blot transfer** or Western blotting.

TECHNIQUES FOR DETERMINATION OF BASE SEQUENCE OF DNA

The base sequence of DNA can be determined by:
1. Chemical method of Maxam-Gilbert
2. Enzymatic dideoxy method of Sanger
These two methods were devised almost simultaneously.

Maxam-Gilbert Method

This method is based on chemical **cleavage of DNA at selective sites**. The DNA to be analysed is labelled at its 3'-end with a nucleotide having ^{32}P. Reagents are available which can selectively destroy and remove one particular base from DNA. Four sets of labelled DNA are treated with four different reagents which destroy and remove adenine, guanine, cytosine and thymine respectively. Conditions are so chosen that only one base is removed per DNA strand. When several strands of DNA are treated with a particular reagent, the given base is removed randomly from all the possible sites where it was present. Chain breaks are, then, induced at the "base-less" sites.

The fragments produced in the four tubes are separated by electrophoresis on polyacrylamide gel in four parallel lanes. Locations of ^{32}P-labelled fragments are identified by autoradiography.

The smallest fragment moves the farthest from the point of application, and the largest fragment moves the least. The relative sizes of the fragments indicate the distance between the ^{32}P-label and the destroyed base. By arranging the fragments in the four lanes in the decreasing order of size, the sequence of bases from 5'-end to 3'-end can be deduced (Fig. 16.10).

Sanger's Dideoxy Method

This method is based on **controlled interruption of replication**. Replication is interrupted by incorporating

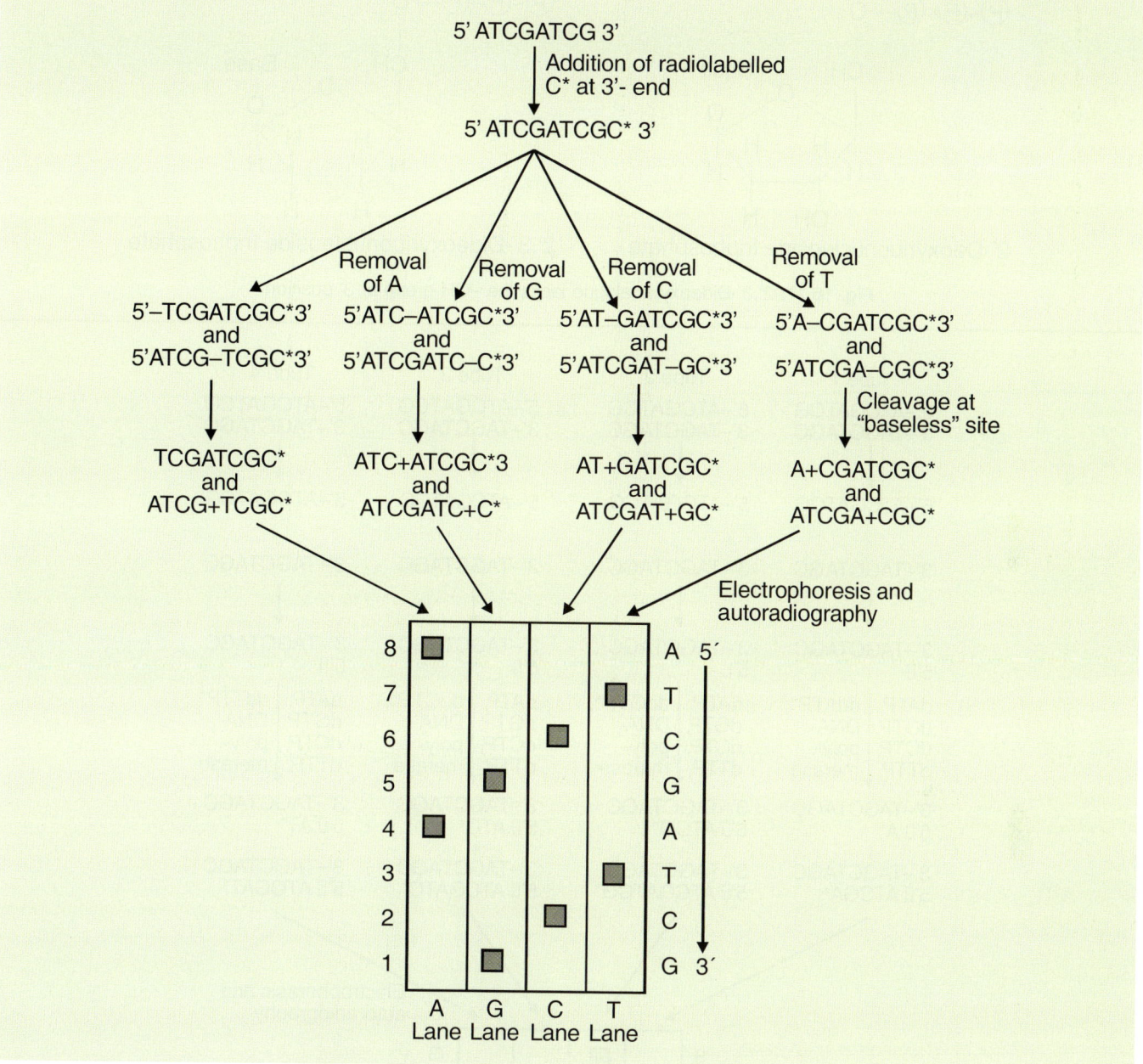

Fig. 16.10: DNA sequencing by Maxam-Gilbert method

the **dideoxy analogue** of a nucleotide in the growing DNA chain. Since the dideoxy analogue lacks the –OH group at 3' position, it can not form an ester bond with the next incoming nucleotide (Fig. 16.11).

The DNA strand to be sequenced is used as a template for replication. Four tubes are set up in each of which, the template strand, ^{32}P-labelled primer, dATP, dGTP, dCTP, dTTP and DNA polymerase are added. In each tube, one dideoxynucleotide (ddATP, ddGTP, ddCTP or ddTTP) is added. The dideoxynucleotide competes with the normal nucleotide. If a normal nucleotide enters the growing chain, replication continues. If a dideoxynucleotide enters the

growing chain, replication stops. The relative concentrations of the two are such that the dideoxy analogue enters randomly at different sites in different cycles of replication. After several cycles of replication, chains of different lengths, each ending with a dideoxynucleotide, are formed. The chains formed in four tubes are separated by electrophoresis on polyacrylamide gel in four parallel lanes, and are autoradiographed. The pattern of bands on the autoradiogram gives the sequence of bases which is complementary to the template strand (Fig.16.12). Automation of Sanger's method has made DNA sequencing much faster.

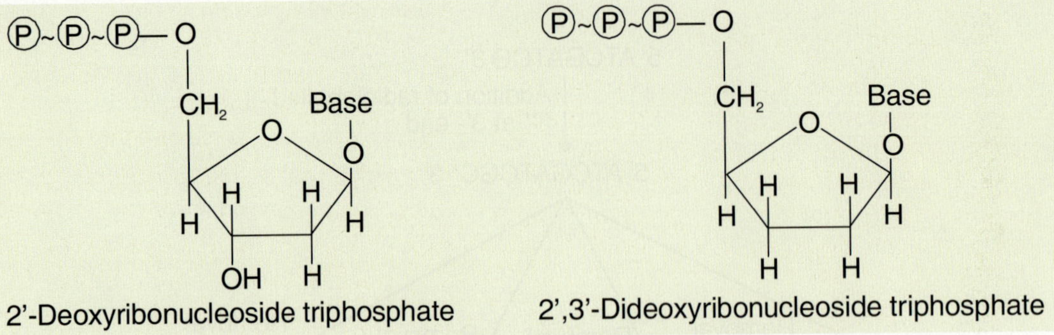

2'-Deoxyribonucleoside triphosphate

2',3'-Dideoxyribonucleoside triphosphate

Fig. 16.11: 2',3'-Dideoxy analogue lacks the –OH group at 3' position

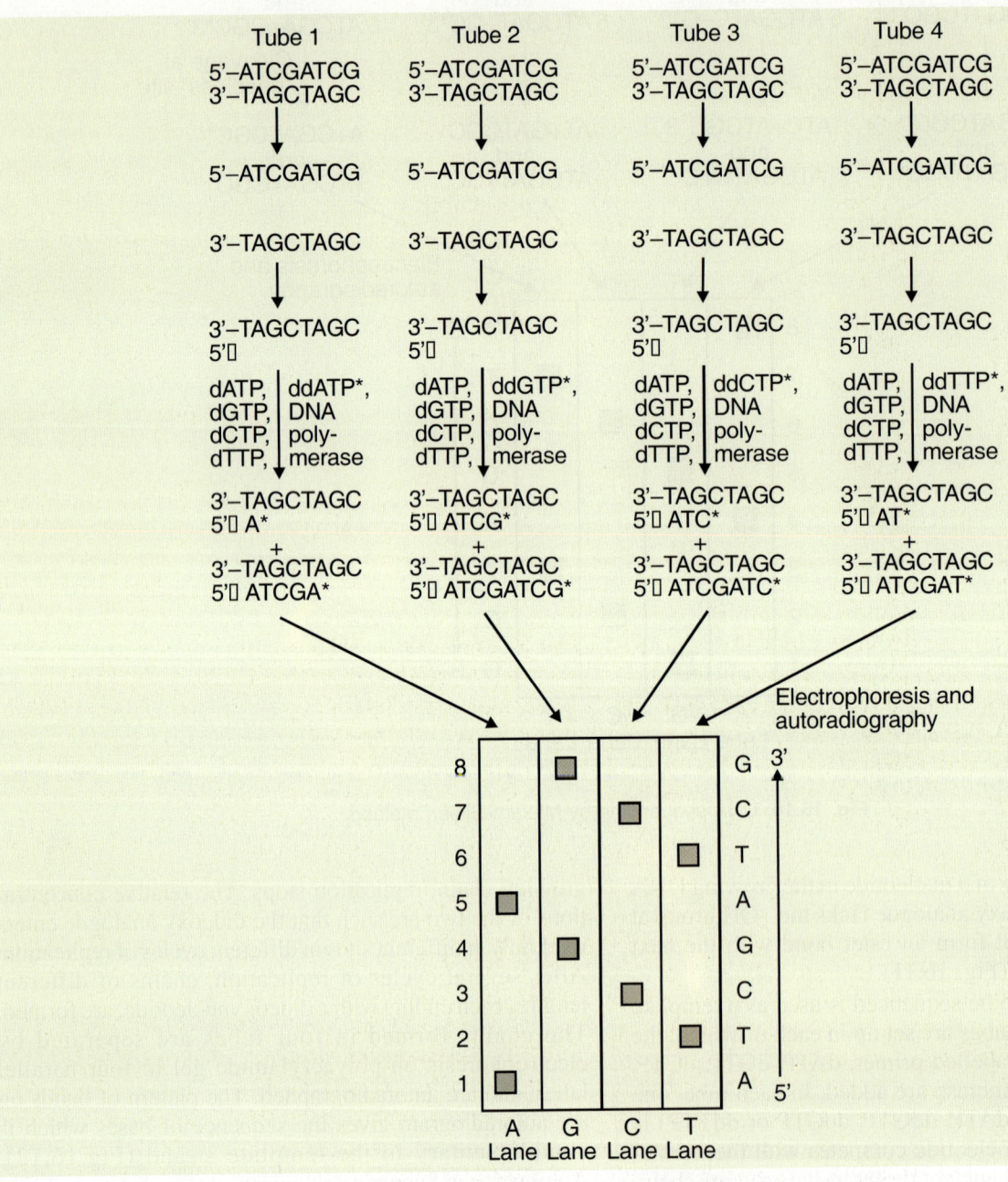

Fig. 16.12: DNA sequencing by Sanger's method

APPLICATIONS OF RECOMBINANT DNA TECHNOLOGY

Recombinant DNA technology finds applications in all branches of life sciences and industry. Advent of recombinant DNA technology has led to spectacular advances in medical science, and the future holds promise of even greater achievements. Some of the applications of recombinant DNA technology in medicine are:

1. Mapping of Genomes

Mapping of genome means determining the base sequence of entire DNA of an organism. Since the size of DNA is very big, it has to be broken up into small fragments so that the sequencing becomes easier. Fragments of DNA obtained from a genome are amplified and maintained in what is known as a library.

Genomic Library

The total DNA in a cell is hydrolysed by restriction enzymes to yield fragments of 15–25 kb. The fragments are separated by electrophoresis. Each fragment is ligated to a bacteriophage vector, e.g. phase lgt 10 or lgt 11. The vector is allowed to infect *E. coli*. Multiple copies of different DNA fragments will be formed in different *E. coli* cells. Each clone of the vector would contain one DNA fragment. A collection of such clones is known as genomic library of the organism. The number of clones required to represent the total DNA of the organism depends upon the size of its genome. It has been estimated that about half a million clones are required to prepare a genomic library of man.

cDNA Library

The genomic library is made from total DNA which includes coding sequences as well as non-coding sequences. Non-coding sequences are present in genes in the form of introns and as long stretches in between the genes. If a library of only structural genes is desired, one can prepare a cDNA (complementary DNA) library. cDNA library is prepared from mRNA templates. Total RNA is isolated from a cell or a tissue. It is passed through a column having poly-T oligonucleotides fixed to an inert gel. The poly-T oligonucleotides bind the poly-A tails of mRNA molecules while the other types of RNA pass through the column. The mRNA molecules are later eluted and used as templates for synthesizing a cDNA strand by reverse transcriptase. The RNA template is hydrolysed by ribonuclease H. The cDNA strand is than used as a template to synthesise the second strand of DNA by DNA polymerase. Such double-stranded DNA molecules are ligated to a vector, e.g. a plasmid, and amplified and maintained in *E. coli* cells. The entire collection of these vectors constitutes a cDNA library.

Whether it is a genomic library or a cDNA library, we need techniques to locate a particular colony having a desired DNA insert in the vector. This can be done by one of the following methods:

i. If the base sequence of the desired DNA insert is known, a radio-labelled cDNA probe can be used to identify the particular vector by autoradiography.

ii. If the base sequence is not known, we can look for the protein encoded by the DNA insert. The protein can be detected either with the help of an antibody or by assaying its function.

With advent of automated DNA sequencing and other advancements in recombinant DNA technology, it became possible to map the genomes . The work started with small organisms but culminated into successful conclusion of the ambitious human genome project.

Human Genome Project

Mapping of the human genome could provide valuable insights into human health and disease. Genes, unknown so far, could be discovered. Diagnosis of genetic diseases could improve. Understanding of polygenic disorders could improve. New targets for pharmacological intervention could be found. Drug-designing could improve. Comparison of base sequence of genes from different species could lead to a better understanding of evolution.

However, mapping of genome is an extremely labour-intensive, time-consuming and expensive exercise. Given the size of the human genome, it was realised in 1980s that a collaborative and co-operative effort was required if the human genome was to be mapped in reasonable time at a reasonable cost. The human genome project (HGP) was launched in 1990 under the leadership of James D. Watson by the U. S. Department of Energy and National Institute of Health with participation of several laboratories worldwide. A budget of three billion dollars was allotted for the project. The project was planned to be completed in 15 years.

The Aims and Objects of the Project were

1. To determine the base sequence of entire human DNA.
2. To locate and sequence all the genes in human DNA.
3. To analyse sequence variations (polymorphism) in human genome.
4. To sequence the genomes of some other organisms for comparison of base sequences of genes.
5. To improve sequencing techniques.
6. To store the information obtained in databases freely accessible to everyone.
7. To consider and debate ethical, social and legal issues arising from the project.

The project was split into three phases of five years each. The first phase comprised the preparation of a genetic map of the human genome. The second phase comprised the preparation of a physical map of the human genome. The final phase comprised base-by-base sequencing of the entire genome.

The work began simultaneously in several laboratories. Cells donated by several anonymous individuals belonging to different ethnic groups were used as sources of DNA. Though there were some differences in the methodologies used in different laboratories, the basic steps were:

1. Separation of chromosomes from cultured cells arrested in metaphase by fluorescence-activated cell sorter.
2. Micro-dissection of chromosomes into large fragments by ultra-fine glass needles.
3. Restriction enzyme digestion of fragments to prepare smaller fragments.
4. Ligation of fragments to linkers of known sequence so as to prepare complementary primers.
5. Amplification of fragments by polymerase chain reaction.
6. Cloning of fragments in suitable vectors.
7. Identification of cloned fragments by sequence-tagged sites (sequence-tagged sites are 200–500 bp unique sequences present at known locations).
8. Sequencing of individual DNA fragments.
9. Arranging the base sequence of different fragments in correct order on the basis of their sequence-tagged sites.
10. Feeding the information generated into databases.

Collaborative efforts of the multi-national group resulted in rapid progress in mapping the human genome. A genetic map was prepared by 1995. Sequence-tagged sites were also identified by 1995. Individual chromosomes began to be mapped thereafter. In 1997, a private company, Celera Genomics led by Craig Venter entered the race with the aim of completing the project ahead of the publicly-funded multi-national group. This led to intense competition. On June 26, 2000, both the groups simultaneously released a working draft of the human genome. In April, 2003, the final draft of the human genome was released.

Before the beginning of the human genome project, it was speculated that the human genome is made up of about three billion base pairs, has about 100,000 genes, and 90% of the DNA is non-coding. Mapping of the human genome revealed that human genome is made up of 3.2 billion base pairs, has about 30,000 genes, and 95% of the DNA is non-coding. Comparison of base sequence of DNA from different persons revealed that individual variations in base sequence are only 0.1%.

Human genome project has opened up a new science of **genomics**. Genomes of several other organisms have been, and are being, mapped. The next step is **proteomics,** i.e. study of structure and functions of all the proteins synthesised in a cell.

Mapping of the human genome is one of the most important milestones in human biology. The benefits likely to accrue from the project are tremendous. At the same time, the project has thrown up some ethical, legal and social issues. For instance, the genome of an individual is private, and measures are required to prevent it from becoming public. Unauthorised access to genomic information may create piquant situations. If the genome of an individual shows the likelihood of a disease in later life and a prospective employer gets access to it, the employer may refuse to employ him. Likewise, an insurance company may refuse to insure him or hike the premium. Though hypothetical at present, these issues may assume importance in future, and may warrant enactment of suitable laws.

2. Production of Recombinant Proteins

Proteins of diagnostic, therapeutic, nutritional or industrial importance can be produced in large quantities by recombinant DNA technology.

Human insulin was the first protein to be synthesised in *E.coli* by this technology. Human growth hormone, interferon, tissue plasminogen activator, Factor VIII, erythropoietin, etc are being synthesised by this technology. All these are being used as drugs.

Bovine growth hormone and subtilisin, a proteolytic enzyme used in detergents, are being produced by recombinant DNA technology. Efforts are on to produce human proteins in plants and animals. Human albumin and enkephalin genes have been transferred into plants. Recombinant vaccines and antibodies are being synthe-sised for laboratory and clinical use. By site-directed mutagenesis, specific alterations can be made in the amino acid sequence of a protein.

The vectors used to introduce genes into cells for the purpose of **protein synthesis** are known as **expression vectors** which include **plasmids, phages, baculovirus, vaccinia virus**, etc.

A scheme outlining the synthesis of human insulin in *E.coli* is depicted in Fig.16.13. Human insulin gene is constructed by reverse transcription of mRNA for insulin. Natural insulin gene is not used as it contains introns which cannot be removed by bacteria. The constructed insulin gene is introduced into *E.coli* with the help of a plasmid vector. *E.coli* multiplies and synthesises vast quantitites of insulin which can be extracted and purified.

A vaccine against hepatitis B has been prepared in yeast. Vaccines against a variety of infectious diseases are traditionally prepared from killed or live attenuated micro-organisms. In either case, there is some risk of infection if some potent, infectious micro-organisms remain in the vaccine. This risk can be eliminated if the vaccine contains only the antigenic protein and not the DNA or RNA of the micro-organism. Such a vaccine is known as a subunit

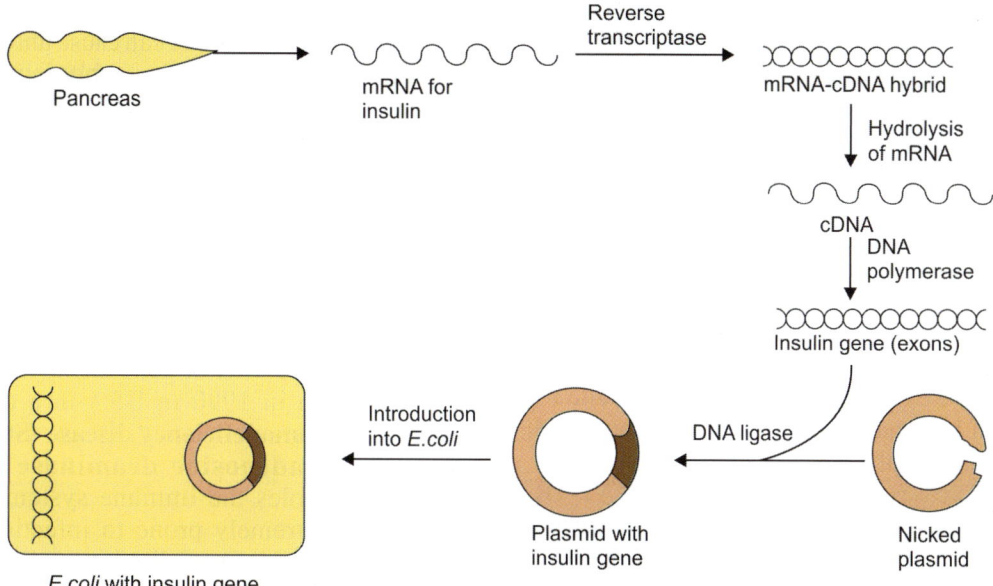

Fig. 16.13: Synthesis of human insulin in *E.coli*

vaccine. Hepatitis B virus has a surface antigen (HbsAg) in its coat which is antigenic but not infectious. The gene for HbsAg is isolated from the viral genome, and is ligated to yeast plasmid. The plasmid is introduced into yeast which multiplies and synthesises large quantities of HbsAg. HbsAg is isolated and is used as a vaccine.

3. Diagnosis of Genetic Diseases

Genetic diseases result from mutations, e.g. substitution, insertion or deletion. Mutations can occur in non-coding as well as coding regions of DNA. Mutations in non-coding regions do not impair function but result in polymorphism. If DNA of normal individuals is treated with a restriction enzyme, restriction fragments of varying length are formed depending on the number of restriction sites in the DNA. The restriction pattern is inherited, and results in **restriction fragment length polymorphism (RFLP)**. A mutation in coding region can create a new restriction site or can obliterate a restriction site, thus, changing the number and length of restriction fragments. For example, three restriction sites for Mst II are normally present in the β-globin gene. Therefore, Mst II produces two restriction fragments. In sickle cell anaemia, the single base substitution obliterates one of the restriction sites for Mst II with the result that only one, larger fragment will be produced by Mst II (Fig. 16.14). Thus, the change in RFLP pattern can be used to diagnose the disease. Several genetic diseases can be diagnosed pre-natally by obtaining DNA from amniotic fluid, amplifying it by PCR and studying its RFLP pattern.

In future, it may be possible to diagnose infectious diseases by detecting specific bacterial or viral genes in a biological sample with the help of complementary probes.

Even if the number of micro-organisms in the sample is very small, PCR can be used to amplify the DNA.

4. Medicolegal Applications

Genomes of higher organisms, including human beings, contain some short repetitive sequences in the non-coding regions which are scattered throughout the genome. Such sequences are called **tandem repeats**. The number of repeats varies in different persons. This phenomenon is called **variable number of tandem repeats (VNTR)**. VNTR pattern is inherited from parents in a Mendelian fashion. VNTR pattern is unique for each individual, and there are striking resemblances between close blood relations, e.g. parents and offsprings.

Restriction sites for various restriction enzymes are present on the flanks of many tandem repeats. cDNA probes have been developed for several tandem repeats. When the DNA is treated with suitable restriction enzymes,

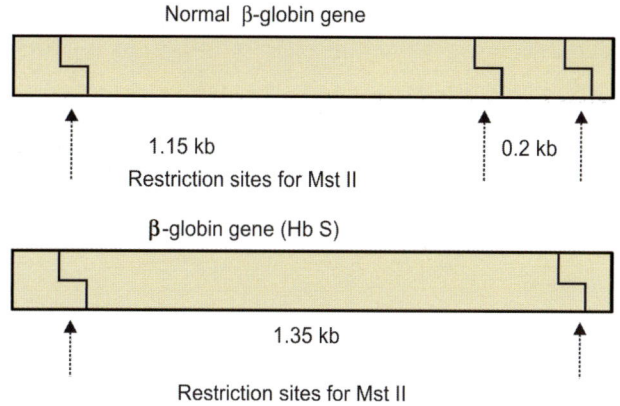

Fig. 16.14: RFLP pattern of β-globin gene in normal Hb and Hb S

a number of fragments having tandem repeats will be formed. The relative lengths of the fragments will depend upon the number of tandem repeats. The fragments can be separated by electrophoresis and, using suitable cDNA probes, their positions can be seen on autoradiograms. If three or four different repetitive sequences are identified by cDNA probes, the autoradiographic pattern becomes unique for each individual. The pattern is so unique that it is called as the **DNA finger-print** of the individual. DNA finger printing has tremendous applications in forensic medicine. If a criminal has left behind some biological material, e.g. hair, blood stain, semen stain, etc. at the scene of crime, DNA can be extracted, amplified by PCR and its VNTR pattern can be established. This can be compared with the VNTR pattern of suspects, and the real culprit can be identified. In cases of disputed parenthood, VNTR pattern of the child can be compared with that of suspected father/mother, and paternity/maternity can be established.

5. Gene Therapy

Treatment of genetic diseases by introducing normal genes into the DNA of patients was an impossible task before the advent of recombinant DNA technology. With the development of techniques for DNA sequencing, cloning of genes and availability of expression vectors, gene therapy has now become a practical reality. Gene therapy may be tried in an embryo if pre-natal diagnosis can be made or in a patient in whom a genetic disease has been diagnosed. Some successful experiments of both types have been done in animals in diseases like cystic fibrosis, Lesch-Nyhan syndrome, Duchenne muscular dystrophy, thalassaemia, etc. Initial trials of gene therapy were done in **transgenic animals** and **knock out animals**. Transgenic animals are prepared by micro-injecting a foreign gene into a fertilised ovum. The gene gets stably incorporated in the genome of the animal, and is transmitted to future generations as well. Knock out animals are prepared by deleting a particular gene from a fertilised ovum. In this way, a particular genetic disease can be produced in the knock out animal.

Gene therapy in human embryos poses some problems. Introduction of foreign DNA can cause unforeseen changes in host DNA which would be stably incorporated in the genome of germ cells, and would be transmitted to the future offsprings. Genetic manipulations in somatic cells do not pose this problem as the change would affect only one individual. However, targeting the foreign gene to a specific destination, e.g. brain, liver, pancreas, etc. is still a problem. Gene therapy of blood cells and bone marrow cells doesn't pose this problem as the gene-treated cells can be easily introduced in circulation or bone marrow.

The first clinical trial of gene therapy in human beings was undertaken in 1990 in USA in a disease, **severe combined immunodeficiency disease (SCID)** caused by deficiency of **adenosine deaminase (ADA)**. ADA deficiency cripples the immune system. The affected children are extremely prone to infections, and rarely survive long without specialised care. Gene therapy was started in two children suffering from SCID. T lympho-cytes were isolated from their blood. Normal ADA gene was introduced in these cells with the help of a **disabled retroviral vector**, and the cells were put back into circulation. Since the lifespan of these cells is limited, the treatment was repeated every month. The children showed a significant increase in their T cell count and increased ADA levels in T cells. Their immune system showed significant improvement, and they were able to fight infections. The treatment was stopped after two years but clinical improvement persisted even after cessation of gene therapy. Since then, several more children with SCID have been successfully treated by gene therapy.

The success of gene therapy in SCID has opened new vistas for the treatment of genetic and even non-genetic diseases. Advanced clinical trials are in progress in human beings for gene therapy of ischaemic vascular diseases. The introduction of the gene for **vascular endothelial growth factor** (VEGF) has given promising results so far. With refinements in technology and further research, gene therapy is expected to be used successfully in many human diseases in future.

EXERCISE

1. Describe the preparation and cloning of recombinant DNA.

2. Explain polymerase chain reaction and its applications in medical science.

3. Give a brief account of applications of recombinant DNA technology in medical science.

4. Write short notes on:
   a. Restriction enzymes
   b. Plasmids
   c. PCR
   d. Southern blotting
   e. Human genome project
   f. DNA finger printing
   g. Transgenic animals
   h. Gene therapy

5. Write 'true' or 'false':
   a. Restriction enzymes split double-stranded DNA.
   b. Overlapping ends of restriction fragments are known as blunt ends.
   c. A plasmid is a double-stranded circular DNA.
   d. DNA fragments can be identified by Northern blotting.
   e. A radioactive isotope-labelled cDNA probe is used in Western blotting.
   f. Chimeric DNA contains unrelated genes.
   g. Cosmids can be used as cloning vectors.
   h. Yeast artificial chromosome can be used to clone DNA upto 1,000 kb in size.
   i. As compared to cosmids, plasmids can take up foreign DNA of larger size.
   j. Sanger's dideoxy method of DNA sequencing is based upon chemical cleavage of DNA at selective sites.

6. Fill in the blanks:
   a. Restriction endonucleases are present in ....
   b. Restriction enzymes recognise ....sequences.
   c. Sites recognised by restriction enzymes are known as .... sites.
   d. Restriction sites are ....bp in length.
   e. Phage DNA has .... sites which are necessary for packaging of phage DNA in .... coat.
   f. Cosmids are prepared by inserting cos sites of .... into plasmids.
   g. Foreign DNA upto ....kb in size can be inserted into plasmids.
   h. Bacteriophages can be used to clone foreign DNA upto ....kb in size.
   i. Optimum temperature of Taq polymerase is ....
   j. PCR can be used to amplify DNA upto ....kb in size.
   k. .... was the first protein to be synthesised by recombinant DNA technology.
   l. A DNA fragment of interest can be identified by .... blotting.
   m. Northern blotting is used to identify a specific ....
   n. DNA finger printing is based on the presence in DNA of variable number of ....
   o. .... method of DNA sequencing is based upon controlled interruption of replication.

ANSWERS TO SHORT QUESTIONS

5. a. True
   b. False
   c. True
   d. False
   e. False
   f. True
   g. True
   h. True
   i. False
   j. False

6. a. Bacteria
   b. Palindromic
   c. Restriction
   d. 4 to 8
   e. Cos, protein
   f. Phage DNA
   g. 10
   h. 20
   i. 72°C
   j. Three
   k. Insulin
   l. Southern
   m. RNA
   n. Tandem repeats
   o. Sanger's dideoxy

17

Hormones

Multicellular organisms require mechanisms by which different cells can communicate with each other. Higher animals and human beings possess a diversity of cells, tissues, organs and systems for specialised functions. Intercellular communication is all the more important in these organisms so that the organism as a whole can respond in a coordinated manner to changes in environment. Communication can occur through:

i. **Nervous system** which employs electrical-chemical signals transmitted through fixed structural routes and

ii. **Endocrine system** which employs chemical signals transmitted in the form of mobile signal molecules (**hormones**) which circulate in blood. Nervous system and endocrine system also communicate with each other (Fig. 17.1).

Hormones are present in blood in very small concentrations yet they produce profound biological effects. The action of a hormone occurs through a cascade of events in which the **signal is amplified** at a number of stages. For example, in the glucagon-stimulated glycogenolysis, binding of glucagon to its receptor activates adenylate cyclase, each molecule of adenylate cyclase can convert several molecules of ATP into cAMP, each molecule of protein kinase A can activate several molecules of phosphorylase b kinase, each molecule of phosphorylase b kinase can activate several molecules of phosphorylase and each molecule of phosphorylase can release several molecules of glucose from glycogen (Fig. 17.2).

DEFINITION

A hormone is a molecule secreted by a cell or a group of cells into circulation which produces its effects on its **target cells** or tissues which possess specific **receptors** for the hormone. The target cells may be distant or nearby. Depending upon the distance between the target cell and the hormone-secreting cell, the hormone may be:

a. **Endocrine**,

b. **Paracrine** or

c. **Autocrine**.

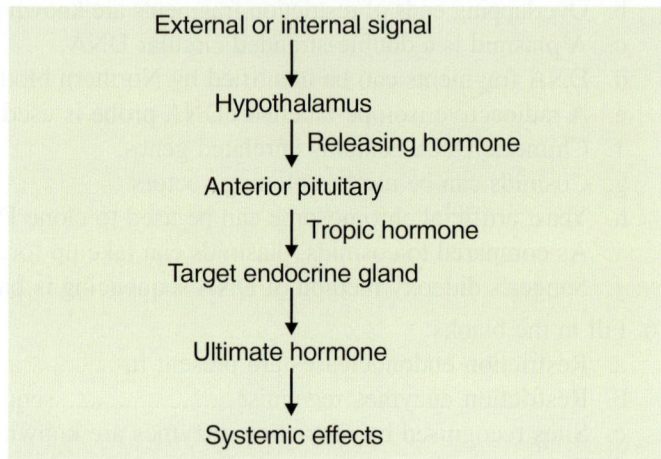

Fig. 17.1: Communication between nervous and endocrine systems

The endocrine hormones are secreted by endocrine (ductless) glands, and act on distant cells. The paracrine hormones act on cells in near vicinity of the hormone-secreting cells. The autocrine hormones act on the cells secreting the hormone.

HORMONE RECEPTORS

The target cells possess receptors for hormones. Chemically, the receptors are proteins. Each receptor is specific for a particular hormone. It has at least two domains, a **recognition domain** and a **signal domain**. The receptor may be located in the membrane or inside the cell. The intracellular receptors may be located in the cytosol or in the nucleus. The receptors can undergo **upregulation** (increase in the number of receptors) and **downregulation** (decrease in the number of receptors). A given cell may possess receptors for several hormones (Fig. 17.3).

CLASSIFICATION OF HORMONES

Hormones may be classified on the basis of their chemical nature, on the basis of their solubility or on the basis of location of their receptors in the target cells and the nature

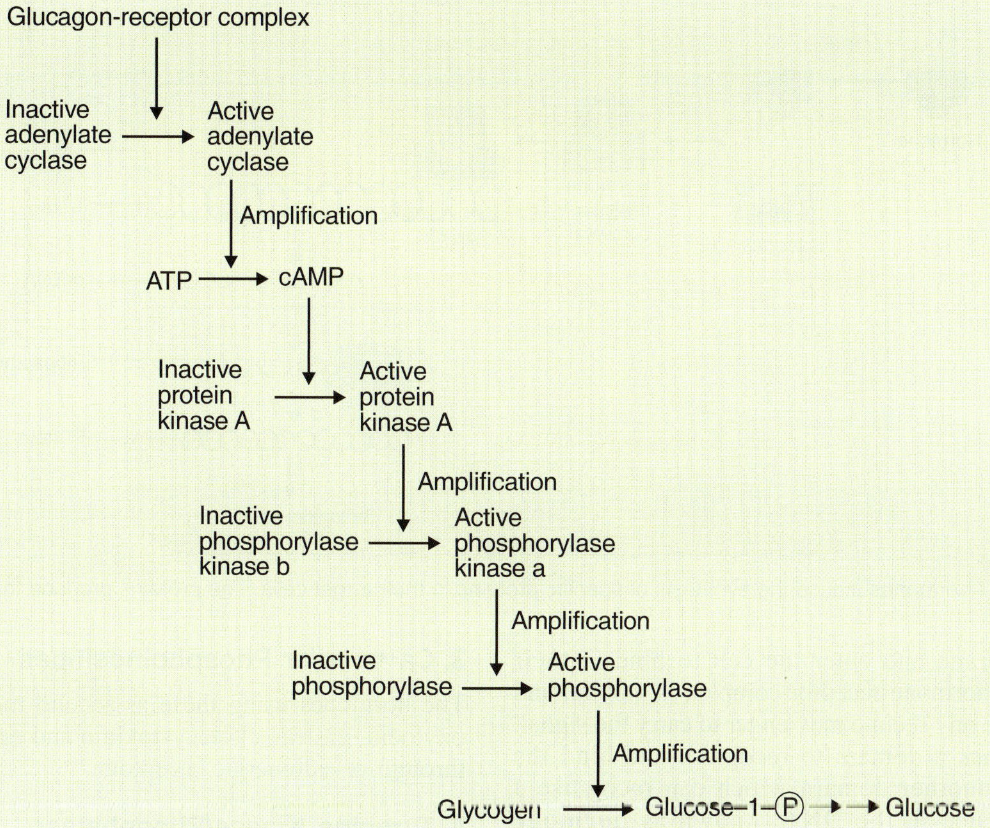

Glucagon-receptor complex

Inactive
adenylate → Active
cyclase   adenylate
        cyclase

Amplification

ATP ——→ cAMP

Inactive
protein —→ Active
kinase A   protein
      kinase A

Amplification

Inactive
phosphorylase —→ Active
kinase b   phosphorylase
        kinase a

Amplification

Inactive
phosphorylase —→ Active
         phosphorylase

Amplification

Glycogen ——→ Glucose–1–(P) –→ –→ Glucose

Fig. 17.2: Sites of amplification in glucagon-stimulated glycogenolysis

of their second messengers. On chemical basis, they can be divided into:

  i. Proteins, peptides and amino acid derivatives and
  ii. Steroids.

On the basis of solubility, they can be divided into:

  i. Hydrophilic hormones, e.g. proteins, peptides and catecholamines, and
  ii. Hydrophobic hormones, e.g. steroid hormones and thyroid hormones.

The classification based on the location of receptors and nature of second messengers is more comprehensive. On this basis, the hormones may be divided into Group I and Group II hormones.

GROUP I HORMONES

Their receptors are **intracellular** and they do not require any second messenger. Examples are steroid hormones, thyroid hormones, calcitriol, etc. The receptors for glucocorticoids and mineralocorticoids are present in the cytosol while those for oestrogen, progesterone, thyroid hormones and calcitriol are present in the nucleus.

Mechanism of Action of Group I Hormones

These hormones are chemically steroids and iodo-thyronines. They are lipophilic and, hence, require **carrier**

proteins to transport them in circulation. Their receptors are intracellular. Being lipophilic, they can easily traverse

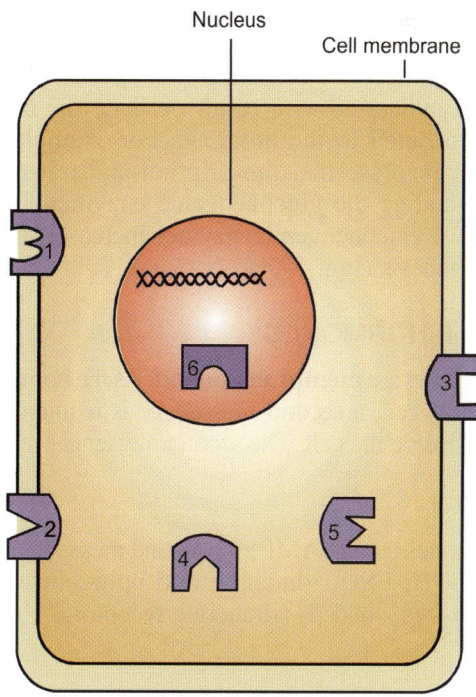

Fig. 17.3: Membrane-bound receptors (1,2 and 3), cytosolic receptors (4 and 5) and nuclear receptor (6) in a cell

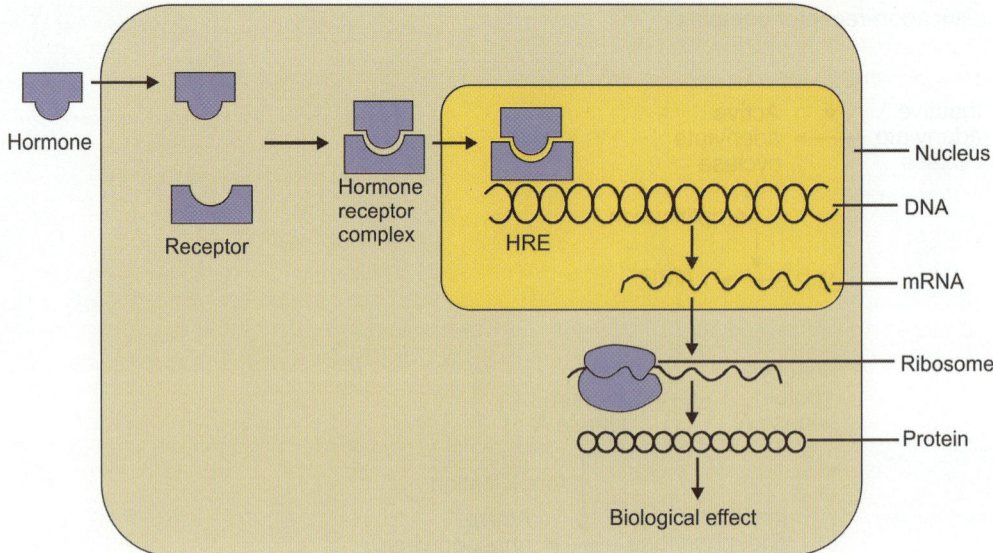

Fig. 17.4: Group I hormones induce the synthesis of specific proteins in their target cells. The proteins produce the biological effects

the cell membrane and enter the cell to bind to their receptors. The hormone-receptor complex is mobile, and does not require any second messenger to carry the signal. The receptor has a domain to recognise and bind the hormone and another domain which can recognise a specific sequence in the DNA, known as **hormone response element** (HRE). There are different response elements for different hormones, e.g. glucocorticoid response element (GRE), mineralocorticoid response element (MRE), thyroid hormone response element (TRE), etc. The HREs are located just upstream of some structural genes and their promoters. The hormone-receptor complex goes to the nucleus and binds to the HRE. This increases the **transcription** and **translation** of specific genes. The proteins synthesised as a result produce the biological effects attributed to the hormone. For example, glucocorticoids increase the transcription and translation of genes encoding the gluconeogenic enzymes. Increased synthesis of gluconeogenic enzymes increases the rate of gluconeogenesis (Fig. 17.4).

GROUP II HORMONES

Their receptors are **membrane-bound.** As the hormone does not enter the cell, a **second messenger** is required to carry the signal inside the cell. The second messenger may be:

1. cAMP

The hormones using cAMP as a second messenger include TSH, ACTH, FSH, glucagon and epinephrine acting through α_2-, β_1- and β_2-adrenergic receptors.

2. cGMP

The hormones using cGMP as a second messenger include atrial natriuretic peptide, nitric oxide, etc.

3. Ca++ and/or Phosphoinositides

The hormones using these as second messenger include oxytocin, gastrin, cholecystokinin and epinephrine acting through α_1-adrenergic receptors.

4. Tyrosine Kinase/Phosphatase

These hormones act through phosphorylation/dephosphorylation of tyrosine residues of some target proteins in the cell. These hormones include insulin, growth hormone, prolactin and a number of growth factors, e.g. insulin-like growth factor-1 (IGF-1), insulin-like growth factor-2 (IGF-2), nerve growth factor (NGF), epidermal growth factor (EGF), platelet-derived growth factor (PDGF), etc.

Mechanism of Action of Group II Hormones

These hormones are chemically proteins, peptides and catecholamines. They are hydrophilic and do not require carriers to transport them in circulation. Their receptors are transmembrane proteins. The hormone binds to its receptor on the cell surface, and does not enter the cell. The biological effect inside the cell is produced by a second messenger generated by an **effector**. Different hormones use different second messengers.

Hormones using cAMP as Second Messenger

cAMP is produced in the cell from ATP by adenylate cyclase, a membrane-bound enzyme that is normally inactive. Binding of the hormone to its receptor activates adenylate cyclase. Concentration of cAMP in the cell increases producing biological effects. Most of these effects occur due to cAMP-induced activation of **protein kinase A,** e.g. increased hepatic glycogenolysis and decreased glycogenesis on binding of glucagon to its receptors on the liver cells (Fig. 17.5).

Adenylate cyclase is not contiguous with the hormone receptor. Therefore, a **signal transducer** is required to carry the signal from the receptor to the effector (**receptor-effector coupling**). The signal transducer is a **G-protein**. G-protein is a trimer made up of an α-subunit, a β- subunit and a γ-subunit. The α-subunit has a site which can be occupied by GDP or GTP. Normally, it is occupied by GDP.

When the hormone binds to its receptor, GDP is displaced by GTP. The GTP-bearing α-subunit dissociates from the β- and γ-subunits, and goes and binds to adenylate cyclase which is, then, activated. Active adenylate cyclase produces cAMP. The α-subunit also has intrinsic **GTPase** activity which slowly hydrolyses GTP into GDP. The GDP-bearing α-subunit dissociates from adenylate cyclase and

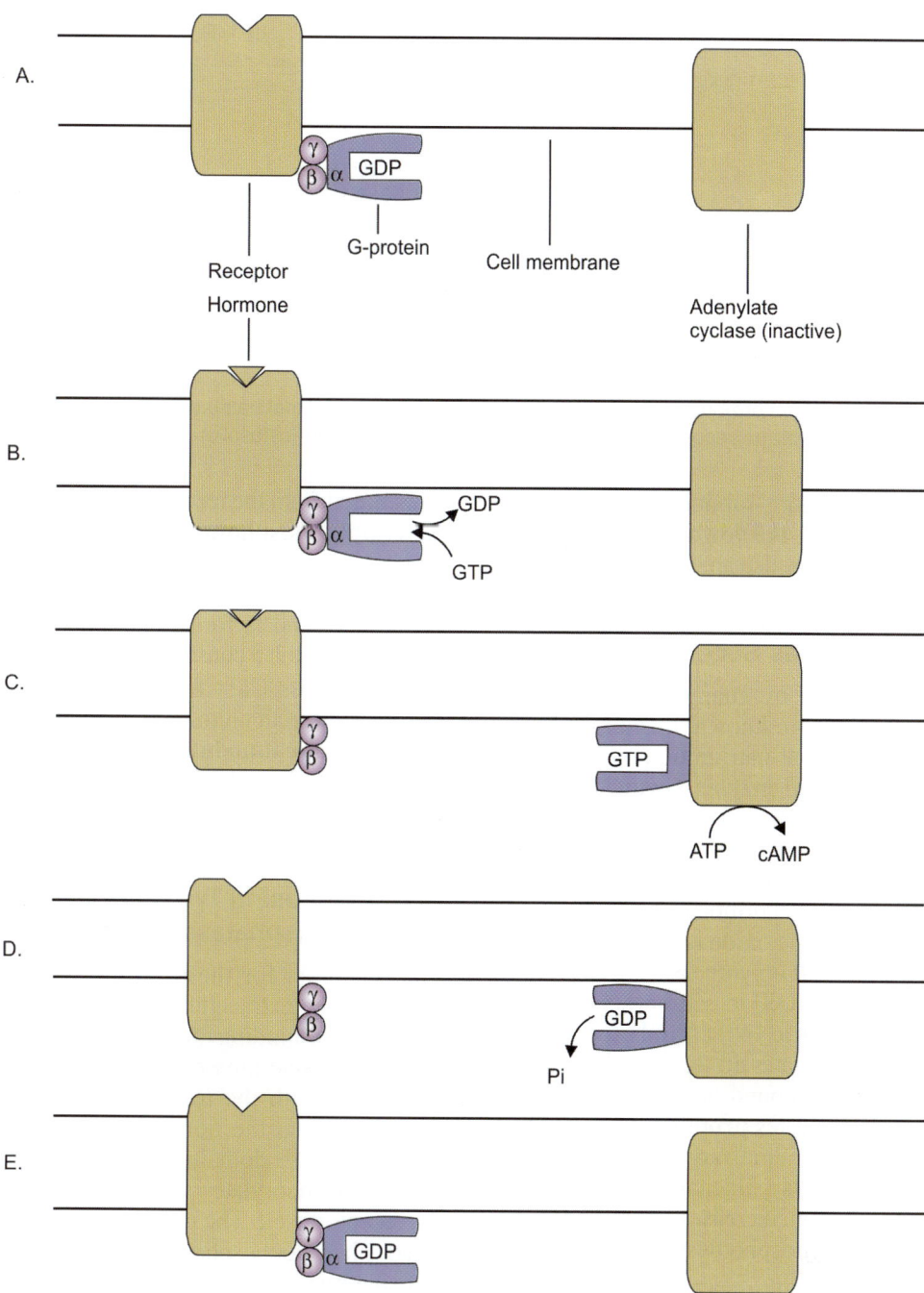

Fig. 17.5: Mechanism of action of hormones using cAMP as second messenger. A. Receptor is free, α-subunit of G-protein is occupied by GDP and adenylate cyclase is inactive. B. Hormone binds to the receptor and GTP displaces GDP in the α-subunit of G-protein. C. GTP-bearing α-subunit binds to adenylate cyclase which becomes active and converts ATP into cAMP. D.Hormone dissociates from the receptor and the GTPase activity of α-subunit converts GTP into GDP. E. GDP-bearing α-subunit dissociates from adenylate cyclase and re-associates with the β- and γ-subunits

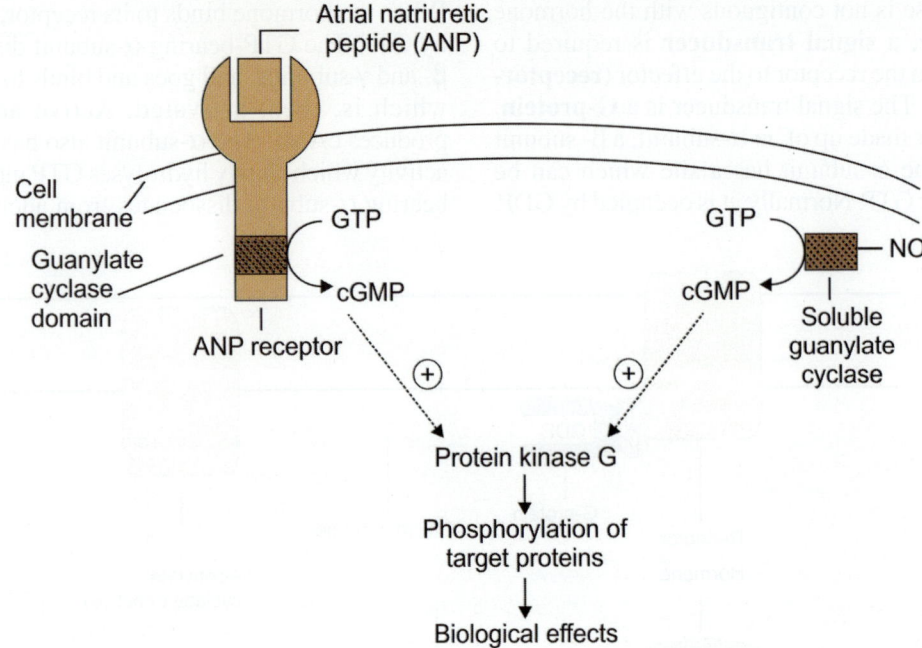

Fig. 17.6: Mechanism of action of hormones using cGMP as second messenger. Atrial natriuretic peptide (ANP) activates guanylate cyclase domain of its transmembrane receptor. Nitric oxide (NO) activates soluble (cytosolic) guanylate cyclase

goes back to join the β- and γ-subunits. The G-protein which stimulates the effector is known as stimulatory G-protein or **G_s-protein**. There is also an inhibitory G-protein or **G_i-protein** which inhibits the effector.

Hormones Using cGMP as Second Messenger

cGMP is formed from GTP by guanylate cyclase. Two forms of guanylate cyclase are known, membrane-bound and cytosolic (soluble). Atrial natriuretic peptide (ANP) activates the membrane-bound enzyme. Guanylate cyclase activity is present in the cytoplasmic portion of the ANP receptor which is switched on by binding of ANP to its receptor on the cell surface (Fig.17.6).

Nitric oxide (NO) is another hormone which uses cGMP as its second messenger. Nitric oxide is the only hormone known so far which is a gas. It is synthesised from arginine by nitric oxide synthetase (NOS) in neurones, endothelial cells and macrophages. Nitric oxide binds to cytosolic guanylate cyclase, and activates it. Activated guanylate cyclase, whether membrane-bound or cytosolic, converts GTP into cGMP. cGMP activates **protein kinase G** which causes phosphorylation of some target proteins which produce the biological effects (sildenafil, a drug used to treat male erectile dysfunction, increases cGMP concentration by inhibiting cGMP phosphodiesterase, an enzyme that degrades cGMP to GMP).

Hormones using Ca++ and/or Phosphoinositides as Second Messenger

Binding of these hormones to their receptors causes activation of membrane-bound **phospholipase C**. Signal is transmitted from the receptor to the enzyme by a G-protein. Activated phospholipase C hydrolyses **phosphatidyl inositol-4,5-biphosphate (PIP$_2$)** into **inositol triphosphate (IP$_3$)** and **diacylglycerol (DAG)**. PIP$_2$ is present in the cell membrane, and is formed by phosphorylation of phosphatidyl inositol, a constituent of the membrane (Fig. 17.7).

IP$_3$ releases Ca++ from its intracellular stores, e.g. endoplasmic reticulum. Ca++ combines with calmodulin, and activates **calmodulin kinase**. DAG activates **protein kinase C**. Activated calmodulin kinase and protein kinase C cause phosphorylation of some target proteins which produce the biological effects (Fig. 17.8).

Hormones using Tyrosine Kinase/Phosphatase as Second Messenger

The receptors for these hormones are transmembrane proteins. The extracellular portion of the receptor has got the hormone-binding domain, and the cytoplasmic portion has got tyrosine kinase domain. In some cases, a protein associated with the receptor possesses tyrosine kinase domain. When the hormone binds to the receptor, the tyrosine kinase domain becomes active. Active tyrosine kinase phosphorylates some tyrosine residues present in the receptor itself. The receptor becomes **autophosphorylated**. The autophosphorylated receptor phosphorylates the tyrosine residues of some other target proteins present in the cell which become active and produce the biological effects.

An example of this subgroup of hormones is insulin. The insulin receptor is a tetramer made of two identical α-subunits and two identical β-subunits. The α-subunits

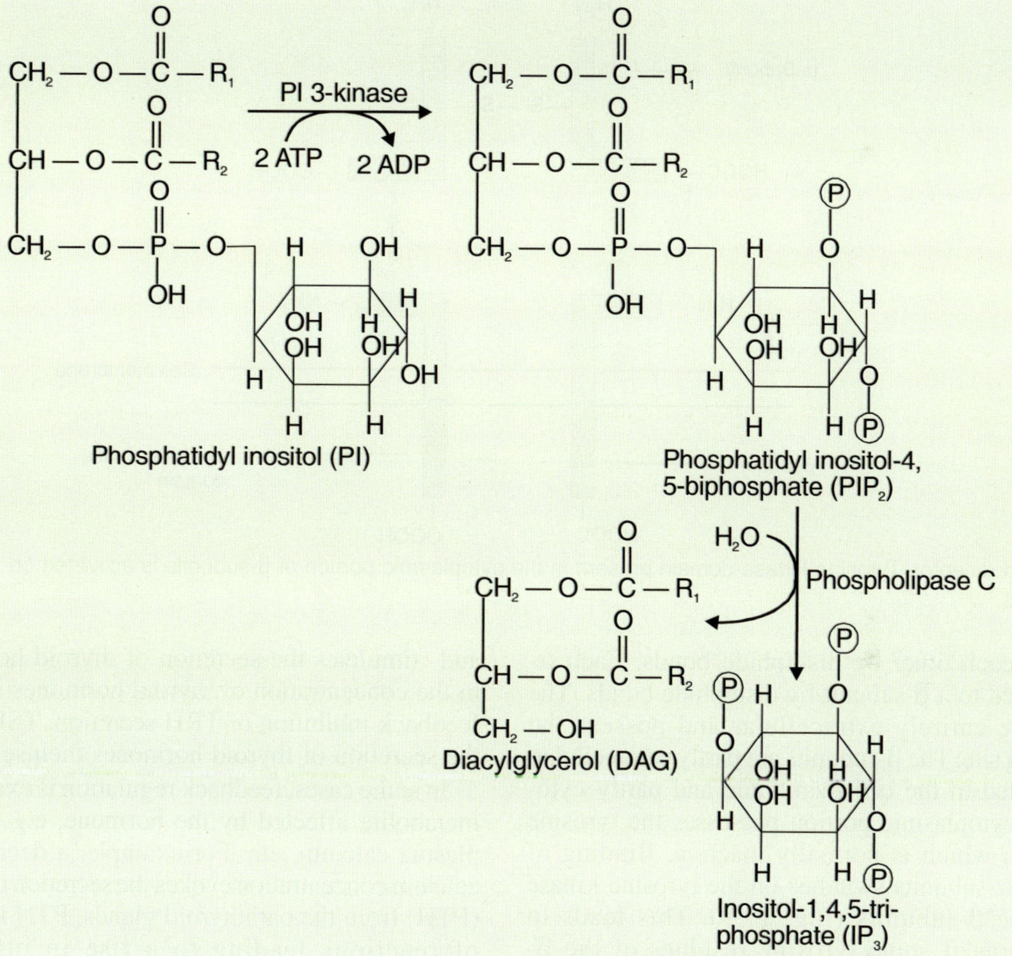

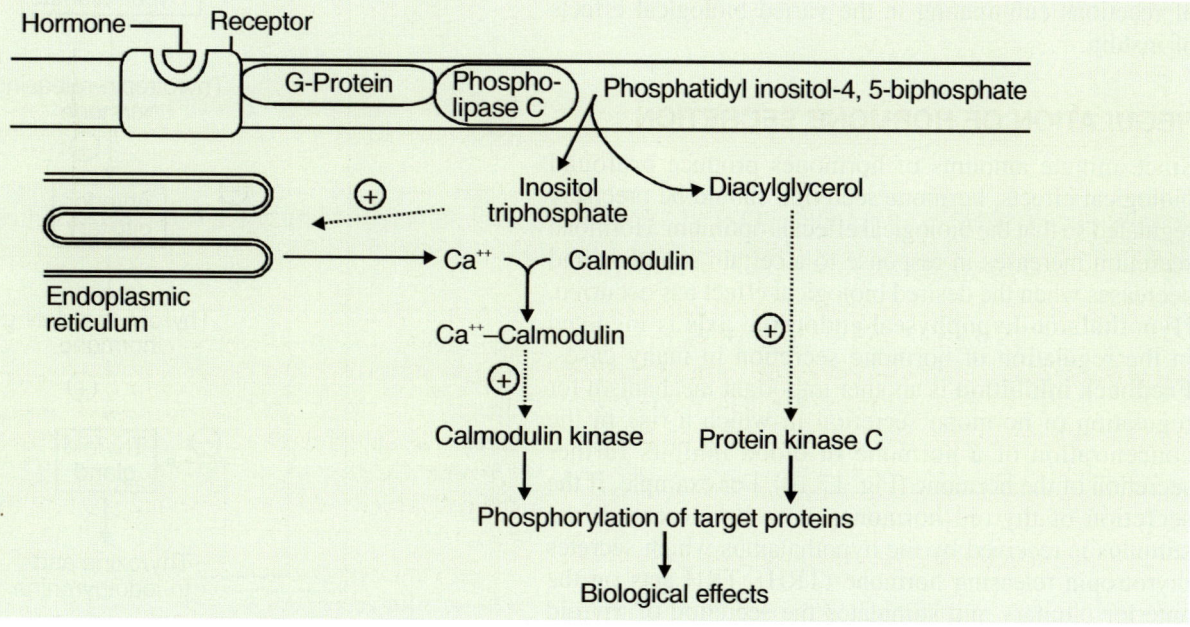

Fig.17.7: Formation and hydrolysis of phosphatidyl inositol-4, 5-biphosphate

Fig.17.8: Mechanism of action of hormones acting via Ca⁺⁺/phosphoinositide cascade

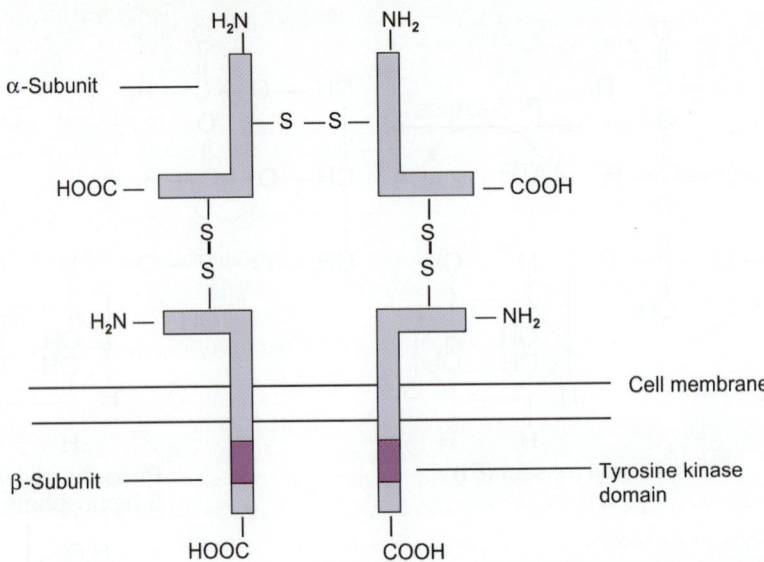

Fig. 17.9: Insulin receptor. Tyrosine kinase domain present in the cytoplasmic portion of β-subunits is activated on binding of insulin to the α-subunits

are linked to each other by disulphide bonds. Each α-subunit is linked to a β-subunit by disulphide bonds. The α-subunits are entirely extracellular and possess the insulin-binding site. The β-subunits are partly extracellular, partly embedded in the cell membrane and partly cytoplasmic. The cytoplasmic portion possesses the tyrosine kinase domain which is normally inactive. Binding of insulin to the α-subunits switches on the tyrosine kinase activity of the β-subunits (Fig. 17.9). This leads to phosphorylation of some tyrosine residues of the β-subunits themselves. The autophosphorylated receptor phosphorylates the tyrosine residues of some target proteins, e.g. insulin receptor substrate-1 (IRS-1), insulin receptor substrate-2 (IRS-2), etc. This initiates a cascade of reactions culminating in the varied biological effects of insulin.

REGULATION OF HORMONE SECRETION

Since minute amounts of hormones produce profound biological effects, hormone secretion should be precisely regulated so that the biological effect is optimum. Hormone secretion increases in response to a certain stimulus, and decreases when the desired biological effect has occurred. **Hypothalamo-hypophyseal-endocrine axis** is involved in the regulation of hormone secretion in many cases. **Feedback inhibition** is another important mechanism for regulation of hormone secretion in which a rise in the concentration of a hormone in blood inhibits further secretion of the hormone (Fig. 17.10). For example, if the secretion of thyroid hormones is to be increased, the stimulus is received by the hypothalamus which secretes thyrotropin releasing hormone (TRH). TRH acts on the anterior pituitary and stimulates the secretion of thyroid stimulating hormone (TSH). TSH acts on the thyroid gland

and stimulates the secretion of thyroid hormones. A rise in the concentration of thyroid hormones in blood causes feedback inhibition of TRH secretion, TSH secretion and the secretion of thyroid hormones themselves.

In some cases, feedback regulation is exercised by some metabolite affected by the hormone, e.g. blood glucose, plasma calcium, etc. For example, a decrease in plasma calcium concentration evokes the secretion of parathormone (PTH) from the parathyroid glands. PTH initiates a series of reactions leading to a rise in plasma calcium concentration. Raised plasma calcium concentration causes feedback inhibition of PTH secretion (Fig. 17.11).

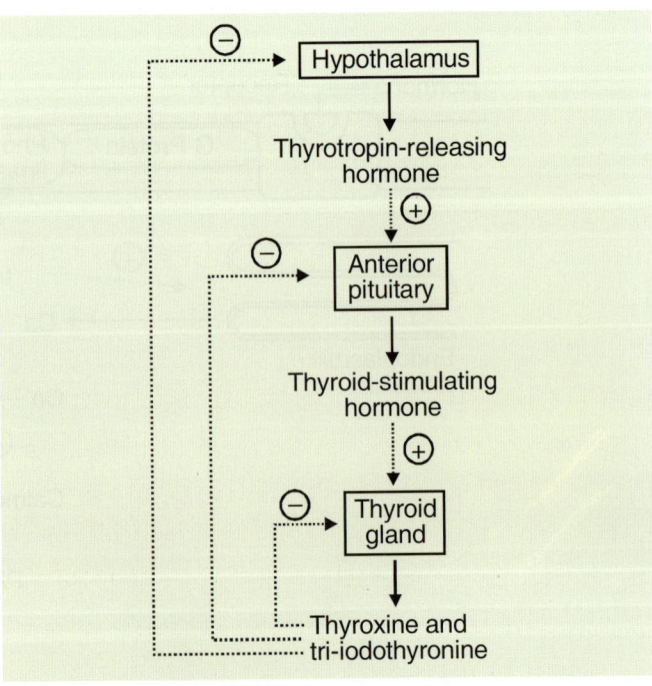

Fig. 17.10: Regulation of thyroid hormone secretion

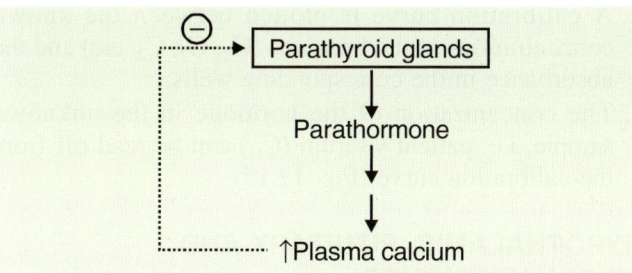

Fig. 17.11: Regulation of parathormone secretion

MEASUREMENT OF HORMONE CONCENTRATIONS

Hormones are present in blood in very minute concentrations. Therefore, the usual techniques of measurement, e.g. colorimetry, are not suitable for measurement of hormone concentrations. Yet measurement of hormone concentrations is important because diagnosis of endocrine disorders can be established only by measuring hormone concentrations. In the past, hormone concentrations were measured by bioassay which lacked sensitivity. Modern techniques of hormone measurement include radio-immuno-assay and enzyme-immuno-assay which are quick, accurate and highly sensitive.

Radio-Immuno-Assay (RIA)

Radio-immuno-assay is based on competition between unlabelled hormone and the hormone labelled with a radioactive isotope to bind to a limited amount of the antibody against the hormone. Antibody against the hormone is prepared in animals. The hormone to be assayed is labelled with a radioactive isotope, e.g. ^{125}I. Briefly, the steps are:

a. A series of tubes, marked S_1, S_2, S_3, S_4 (standards) and U (unknown) is set up.

b. A fixed, and relatively small, amount of antibody (Ab) is added to each tube.

c. A fixed amount of the labelled hormone (Ag*) is added to each tube.

d. Unlabelled hormone (Ag) is added in increasing amounts (C_1, C_2, C_3 and C_4) to tubes marked S_1, S_2, S_3 and S_4.

e. Patient's serum having an unknown amount of unlabelled hormone (C_U) is added to the tube marked U (Fig. 17.12).

f. The tubes are incubated for a fixed period. Ag and Ag* compete with each other to bind to the limited amount of Ab. If the amount of Ag in a tube is less than that of Ag*, less Ag-Ab complex will be formed than Ag*-Ab complex. As the amount of Ag increases, more Ag-Ab and less Ag*-Ab complex will be formed. The concentration of Ag*-Ab complex in different tubes will be inversely proportional to the concentration of Ag. Since the concentrations of Ag and Ag* are relatively high, some unbound Ag and Ag* will also remain in each tube.

$$Ag + Ag^* + Ab \longrightarrow Ag\text{--}Ab + Ag^*\text{--}Ab + Ag + Ag^*$$

g. The tubes are centrifuged so that the Ag-Ab and Ag*-Ab complexes settle at the bottom. The supernatant containing unbound Ag and Ag* is removed. Radioactivity is measured in each tube. A calibration curve is prepared by plotting radioactivity in S_1, S_2, S_3, etc against the concentrations of Ag (C_1, C_2, C_3, etc). The concentration of the hormone in the patient's serum (C_U) can be read off from the calibration curve (Fig. 17.13).

Enzyme-Immuno-Assay (EIA)

The principle of EIA is similar to that of RIA. Instead of a radioactive isotope, an enzyme (usually peroxidase or alkaline phosphatase) is used as a label. Instead of measuring radioactivity, the enzyme concentration is measured by adding the substrate and determining the amount of the product. A widely used form of EIA is **enzyme-linked immunosorbent assay (ELISA)**. In ELISA, the antibody is fixed on a solid support, e.g. in wells molded in a plastic plate. The antibody concentration

	S_1	S_2	S_3	S_4	U
Amount of antibody (Ab)	x	x	x	x	x
Amount of labelled hormone (Ag*)	y	y	y	y	y
Amount of unlabelled hormone (Ag)	C_1	C_2	C_3	C_4	–
Amount of hormone in patient's serum	–	–	–	–	C_U

Fig. 17.12: Experimental set-up for radio-immuno-assay

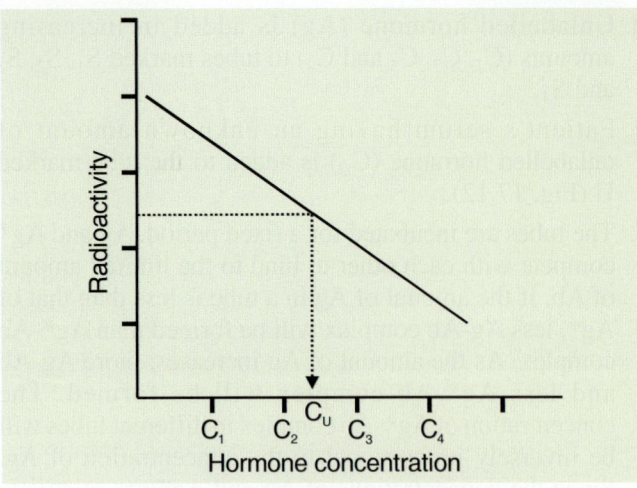

Fig. 17.13: Calibration curve for RIA

is higher than that of the antigen (hormone). The steps are:

a. Standard solutions having different concentrations of the hormone (C_1, C_2, C_3, etc) are added to different wells (S_1, S_2, S_3, etc.). Serum of the patient having an unknown concentration of the hormone (C_U) is added to the well, U. The hormone molecules bind to the antibody molecules fixed in the wall of the wells.

b. A second antibody, which is tagged with an enzyme and which recognises a different epitope of the antigen (hormone), is added to each well in a relatively large amount. The enzyme-linked antibody also binds to the hormone (Fig. 17.14).

c. The unbound enzyme-linked antibody molecules are washed off. Each well now contains complexes of the fixed antibody, the antigen and the enzyme-linked antibody.

d. Substrate of the enzyme is added to each well. After a fixed incubation period, a coloured product is formed.

e. Intensity of the colour (absorbance) is measured in each well. The absorbance is proportional to the enzyme concentration which, in turn, is proportional to the hormone concentration.

f. A calibration curve is plotted between the known concentrations of the hormone (C_1, C_2, C_3, etc) and the absorbance in the corresponding wells.

g. The concentration of the hormone in the unknown sample, i.e. patient's serum (C_U) can be read off from the calibration curve (Fig. 17.15).

HYPOTHALAMIC, PITUITARY AND PINEAL HORMONES

Pituitary gland or hypophysis is a small gland located at the base of brain. It is connected to hypothalamus by a stalk. It comprises anterior lobe (adenohypophysis), posterior lobe (neurohypophysis) and intermediate region (pars intermedia). The anterior pituitary is said to be the master endocrine gland as it controls the activity of several other endocrine glands through its tropic hormones. The secretion of anterior pituitary hormones like growth hormone, thyroid stimulating hormone, adrenocorticotropic hormone, prolactin, follicle stimulating hormone and luteinising hormone is, in turn, regulated by hypothalamus.

HYPOTHALAMIC HORMONES

Hypothalamus receives signals, internal and external, and responds to them by secreting various hormones which reach the anterior pituitary through hypothalamo-hypophyseal portal system. Hypothalamic hormones are peptides (or polypeptides) which increase or decrease the secretion of various anterior pituitary hormones.

Calcium-phosphoinositide system mediates the actions of the hypothalamic hormones on their target cells in the anterior pituitary. The secretion of hypothalamic hormones is pulsatile, and is under the feedback control of the ultimate hormones affected by them. Important features of hypothalamic hormones are listed in Table 17.1.

ANTERIOR PITUITARY HORMONES

Several hormones have been isolated from the anterior pituitary. The major anterior pituitary hormones are growth

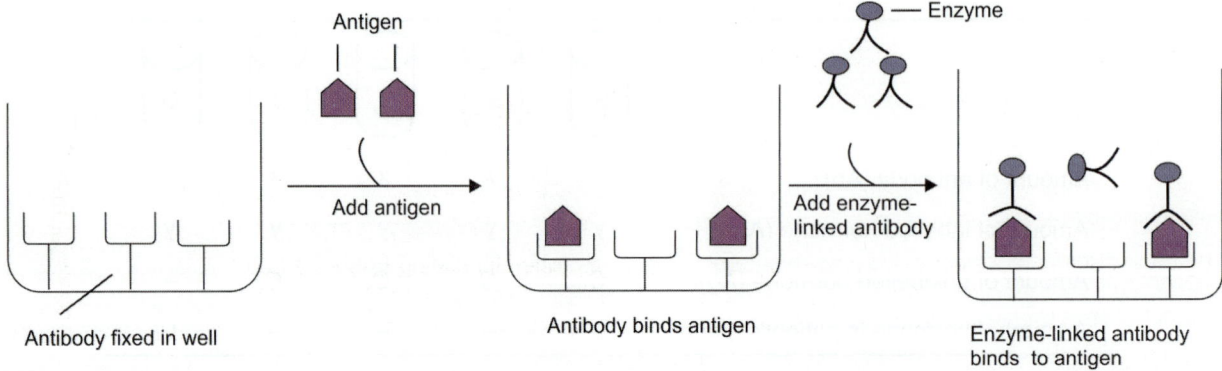

Fig. 17.14: Antigen-antibody binding in ELISA

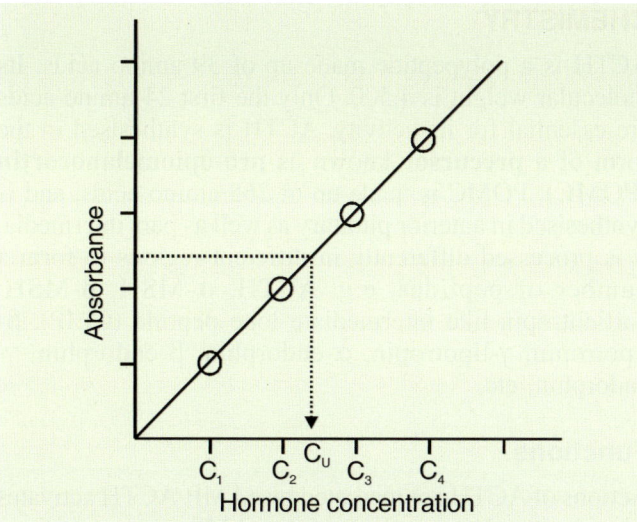

Fig. 17.15: Calibration curve for ELISA

hormone (GH), prolactin (PRL), adrenocorticotropic hormone (ACTH), thyroid stimulating hormone (TSH), follicle stimulating hormone (FSH) and leutinising hormone (LH). The first two are ultimate hormones. The last four are tropic hormones, which stimulate the secretory activity of other endocrine glands.

GROWTH HORMONE

Growth hormone is the major hormone secreted by anterior pituitary. It is also known as somatotropic hormone or somatotropin.

Chemistry

Human growth hormone is a polypeptide having 191 amino acid residues. There are two intra-chain disulphide bonds in the polypeptide chain. Its molecular weight is about 21,500. Its plasma concentration is 1 to 5 ng/ml.

Functions

The major function of GH is to promote growth. It also affects the metabolism of proteins, lipids, carbohydrates and minerals. It has some prolactin-like effects also.

Growth

GH acts on different tissues, e.g. bones, cartilages, muscles, adipose tissue, liver, etc. and promotes their growth. Deficiency of GH in growing age retards growth. Excess of GH during growing age leads to abnormally excessive growth. The growth-promoting effects of GH are mediated by two peptides synthesised in liver and other tissues under the influence of GH. These are known as insulin-like growth factor-1 (IGF-1) and insulin-like growth factor-2 (IGF-2). IGF-1 is made up of 70 amino acids, and IGF-2 is made up of 67 amino acids. IGF-1 is more active than IGF-2. IGFs have some structural resemblance with proinsulin. Their receptors are also similar to insulin receptors. IGF-1 was earlier known as sulphation factor and somatomedin C.

Protein Metabolism

GH increases the uptake of amino acids by various cells. Protein synthesis is increased. Concentrations of amino acids in plasma are decreased. Serum urea is decreased. The nitrogen balance becomes positive.

Lipid Metabolism

GH increases lipolysis in the adipose tissue. The concentration of free fatty acids in plasma is increased. Oxidation of fatty acids in liver is increased.

Carbohydrate Metabolism

GH decreases the utilisation of glucose in muscles and other tissues. It promotes gluconeogenesis and

Table 17.1: Salient features of hypothalamic hormones			
Hypothalamic hormone	No.of amino acid residues	Anterior pituitary hormone affected	Action
Growth hormone-releasing hormone (GHRH or GRH)	44	Growth hormone	Stimulation of secretion
Growth hormone release-inhibiting hormone (GHRIH or somatostatin)	14	Growth hormone	Inhibition of secretion
Thyrotropin-releasing hormone (TRH)	3	Thyroid-stimulating hormone	Stimulation of secretion
Corticotropin-releasing hormone (CRH)	41	Adrenocorticotropic hormone	Stimulation of secretion
Gonadotropin-releasing hormone (GnRH)	10	Follicle-stimulating hormone and leutinising hormone	Stimulation of secretion
Prolacting release-inhibiting hormone (PRIH)	56	Prolactin	Inhibition of secretion

Note: GnRH and PRIH activities are probably present together in a single polypeptide, GnRH associated peptide (GAP).

glycogenesis in liver. It increases the blood glucose concentration. Therefore, it is a diabetogenic hormone.

Mineral Metabolism

Retention of calcium, magnesium, sodium, potassium, phosphate and chloride is increased. Incorporation of calcium and phosphate in growing bones is increased. Incorporation of sulphate in cartilages is increased.

Prolactin-like Effect

GH shares some of the properties of prolactin because of similarities in their structures. It stimulates the production of milk in the mammary glands.

Regulation

Release of GH is regulated by two hormones secreted by the hypothalamus. GHRH promotes the secretion of GH. GHRIH or somatostatin inhibits GH secretion. IGF-1 inhibits the release of GHRH, and promotes the release of GHRIH.

PROLACTIN

Prolactin is also known as mammotropin, lactogenic hormone or luteotropic hormone (LTH).

Chemistry

PRL is a polypeptide made up of 198 amino acids. It has three intra-chain disulphide bonds. Its molecular weight is about 23,000. In certain regions of PRL, the amino acid sequence is similar to that in GH.

Functions

1. PRL stimulates the development of mammary glands during pregnancy. It increases the production of milk. Synthesis of lactose, lipids and proteins in the mammary gland is increased.
2. PRL increases protein synthesis in various tissues but not to the same extent as GH does.

Regulation

Secretion of prolactin is regulated by a hypothalamic hormone, PRIH which inhibits the secretion of PRL. PRIH is a peptide, which is associated with another hypothalamic hormone, GnRH. Thus, PRIH activity is present alongwith GnRH activity in a single peptide made up of 56 amino acids, which is known as GnRH associated peptide (GAP).

ADRENOCORTICOTROPIC HORMONE

This hormone is also known as adrenocorticotropin or corticotropin. It stimulates the secretory activity of adrenal cortex.

CHEMISTRY

ACTH is a polypeptide made up of 39 amino acids. Its molecular weight is 4,500. Only the first 24 amino acids are essential for its activity. ACTH is synthesised in the form of a **precursor** known as **pro-opiomelanocortin (POMC)**. POMC is made up of 265 amino acids, and is synthesised in anterior pituitary as well as pars intermedia. It is processed differently in different regions to form a number of peptides, e.g. ACTH, α-MSH, β-MSH, corticotropin-like intermediate lobe peptide (CLIP), β-lipotropin, γ-lipotropin, α-endorphin, β-endorphin, γ-endorphin, etc.

Functions

Actions of ACTH are mediated by cAMP. ACTH activates adenylate cyclase , and increases cAMP concentration in its target cells. Its effects are:

1. Synthesis of steroid hormones in the adrenal cortex is increased. Conversion of cholesterol into pregnenolone, which is the first reaction in the synthesis of steroid hormones, is increased. Synthesis of glucocorticoids is increased to a greater extent than the synthesis of other steroid hormones.
2. Release of steroid hormones from the adrenal cortex is increased.
3. Protein synthesis in the adrenal cortex is increased. Prolonged exposure of adrenal cortex to high concentrations of ACTH may cause hypertrophy of adrenal cortex.
4. High concentrations of ACTH increase lipolysis in adipose tissue and increase insulin secretion from pancreas.

Regulation

Secretion of ACTH is regulated by hypothalamus as well as by feedback mechanism.

Hypothalamic Regulation

Hypothalamus secretes CRH which increases the release of ACTH from anterior pituitary. Secretion of CRH from hypothalamus is increased by physical or mental stress.

Feedback Regulation

High concentrations of glucocorticoids, particularly cortisol, inhibit the secretion of ACTH from anterior pituitary, and of CRH from hypothalamus, by feedback mechanism. A high level of ACTH in blood also inhibits the secretion of CRH from hypothalamus by feedback mechanism.

THYROID-STIMULATING HORMONE

Thyroid-stimulating hormone increases the secretory activity of the thyroid gland. It is also known as thyrotropic hormone or thyrotropin.

Chemistry

There is a lot of similarity in the structures of TSH, FSH and LH. All the three are glycoproteins. The carbohydrate portion of all the three is made up of hexoses, hexosamines and sialic acid. The protein portion is made up of an α-subunit and a β-subunit. The α-subunit is identical in all the three, and is made up of 89 amino acids. The β-subunit is different in each of the three. The biological specificity resides in the β-subunit but the presence of the α-subunit is essential for biological activity. The β-subunit of TSH is made up of 113 amino acids. The molecular weight of TSH is about 30,000.

Functions

TSH activates adenylate cyclase in its target cells in the thyroid gland, and increases the intracellular concentration of cAMP. The effects occuring in the thyroid cells are due to increased cAMP concentration in the cells. The effects are:

1. Iodide uptake by the thyroid cells increases.
2. Oxidation of iodide to iodine is increased.
3. Incorporation of iodine into tyrosine is increased.
4. Synthesis of thyroid hormones increases.
5. Release of thyroid hormones into circulation is increased.
6. Metabolic activity of the thyroid gland is increased. This is evident from increased uptake and oxidation of glucose, and increased oxygen utilisation.
7. Excessive TSH secretion can cause hypertrophy of the thyroid gland.

Regulation

Secretion of TSH is regulated by hypothalamus as well as by feedback mechanism.

Hypothlamic Regulation

Hypothalamus secretes TRH which increases the secretion of TSH from the anterior pituitary.

Feedback Regulation

The circulating thyroid hormones regulate the secretion of TSH by feedback mechanism. A high concentration of thyroid hormones in blood inhibits the secretion of TSH.

GONADOTROPINS

Follicle stimulating hormone (FSH) and luteinising hormone (LH) are known as gonadotropic hormones or gonadotropins as they stimulate the development and secretory activity of gonads (testes and ovaries). These two hormones act in concert. LH is also known as interstitial cell stimulating hormone (ICSH).

Chemistry

FSH and LH have a structure similar to that of TSH. The α-subunit of all the three is identical. The β-subunit is different, and is made up of 118 amino acids in FSH, and 119 amino acids in LH. The molecular weight of FSH and LH is about 32,000.

A **hormone similar to LH** in structure and function is secreted by placenta, and is known as **chorionic gonadotropin** (CG). Its secretion begins immediately after the implantation of fertilised ovum. CG is excreted in urine. Many tests for pregnancy are based on the detection of chorionic gonadotropin in urine.

Functions

FSH and LH activate adenylate cyclase in their target cells, and produce their effects through increased cAMP concentration. In males, LH acts on Leydig cells (interstitial cells), and stimulates them to secrete testosterone. FSH acts on Sertoli cells in seminiferous tubules, and promotes the synthesis of androgen-binding protein (ABP) which is released into the lumen of the tubules. ABP binds testosterone, and provides a high concentration of testosterone in the lumen of seminiferous tubules which is necessary for spermatogenesis. Thus, these two hormones act in concert to promote testosterone production and spermatogenesis in testes.

In females, these two hormones regulate the menstrual cycle and the secretion of oestrogen and progesterone. FSH secretion begins to increase in the beginning of a menstrual cycle, and promotes the development of a graafian follicle in one of the ovaries. The graafian follicle secretes oestrogen. As the follicle develops, the oestrogen secretion increases. When the blood oestrogen level reaches a certain critical level, usually in the middle of the menstrual cycle, it causes a spurt in the secretion of LH, and a smaller increase in the secretion of FSH, from anterior pituitary. This leads to rupture of the graafian follicle, and release of the ovum (ovulation). LH and FSH secretion declines after ovulation. Oestrogen secretion also declines to the basal level.

The ruptured graafian follicle is converted into corpus luteum. LH stimulates the secretion of progesterone from the corpus luteum. Thus, progesterone level in blood begins to rise after ovulation. The corpus luteum degenerates after about two weeks. The progesterone level declines, and the endometrium is shed off in the form of menstrual flow. A new cycle begins with development of another graafian follicle under the influence of FSH.

If ovulation is followed by fertilisation and the fertilised ovum is implanted, it begins to secrete CG. CG takes over the function of LH and maintains a high level of progesterone. This prevents menstruation.

Regulation

Secretion of FSH and LH is regulated by a hypothalamic hormone and by feedback mechanism.

Hypothalamic Regulation

Hypothalamus secretes a decapeptide known as gonadotropin releasing hormone (GnRH) which increases the secretion of both FSH and LH.

Feedback Regulation

In males, the secretion of LH is inhibited by a high concentration of testosterone in blood. A high testosterone concentration also inhibits the secretion of GnRH. The secretion of FSH is inhibited by a high blood level of inhibin. Inhibin is a peptide synthesised in the Sertoli cells under the influence of FSH.

In females, the concentration of oestrogen in blood regulates the secretion of LH. The feedback is positive. A high oestrogen concentration evokes the release of LH. Secretion of FSH is inhibited by inhibin, a peptide synthesised in the granulosa cells of graafian follicles.

DYSFUNCTION OF ANTERIOR PITUITARY

Adenohypophyseal dysfunction may involve either an overproduction or an underproduction of various hormones. Overproduction (hyperpituitarism) may result from a tumour of hormone-producing cells. Underproduction (hypopituitarism) may be due to pressure upon or atrophy of the hormone-producing cells.

Hyperpituitarism

Three syndromes may result from overproduction of adenohypophyseal hormones:

1. Acromegaly

This results from a tumour of α_1-eosinophilic cells. The secretion of growth hormone is excessive. Acromegaly occurs when the excessive secretion of GH begins after the fusion of epiphyses. The clinical features include:

   i. Overgrowth of the bones of face, hands and feet,
   ii. Kyphosis,
   iii. Enlargement of viscera, e.g. heart, lungs, liver, spleen, thymus, tongue, etc. and
   iv. Impaired glucose tolerance.

2. Gigantism

This is due to a tumour of the α_1-eosinophilic cells that develops before the fusion of epiphyses. This results in a generalised overgrowth of the skeleton. The stature becomes unusually large. The limbs are disproportionately long. Glucose tolerance may be impaired.

3. Cushing's Disease

This results from a tumour of the β_1-basophilic cells. There is excessive production of ACTH. This leads to an excessive secretion of adrenocortical hormones, particularly glucocorticoids. The clinical picture is similar to that of Cushing's syndrome which is caused by a tumour or hyperplasia of adrenal cortex.

Hypopituitarism

Two syndromes result from underproduction of adeno-hypophyseal hormones:

1. Dwarfism

Deficient production of growth hormone before puberty leads to dwarfism. Physical growth is stunted. Mental development is normal. Sexual development is usually impaired. The patient is short-statured. The height is less than 3 or 4 feet. Relative proportions of different parts of the skeleton are normal.

2. Simmond's Disease

This results from atrophy or degeneration of anterior pituitary in adult life. The secretory activity of thyroid, adrenal cortex and gonads is impaired. The clinical features include loss of weight, wasting of tissues, muscular weakness, anaemia, amenorrhoea or impotence, mental degeneration, loss of hair, premature greying of hair, wrinkling of skin, low BMR, etc. Hypoglycaemia may occur in some patients.

POSTERIOR PITUITARY HORMONES

Posterior pituitary or neurohypophysis secretes oxytocin and vasopressin. These hormones are actually synthesised in paraventricular and supra-optic nuclei of hypothalamus. They are transported along the hypothalamo-hypophyseal tract to the posterior pituitary where they are stored. They are secreted by the posterior pituitary in response to specific stimuli. Oxytocin and vasopressin are released alongwith **neurophysin I** and **neurophysin II** respectively. Neurophysins are peptides which stabilise the posterior pituitary hormones. Neurophysin I is encoded together with oxytocin by a single gene. The two peptide products are split out of a single polypeptide precursor. Likewise, vasopressin and neurophysin II are split out of another polypeptide precursor encoded by a single gene.

OXYTOCIN

Oxytocin is a cyclic nonapeptide that is secreted in response to the suckling reflex and a high oestrogen concentration.

Functions

1. The main function of oxytocin is to stimulate contraction of smooth muscles in the mammary glands leading to expulsion of milk in response to suckling.

2. Oxytocin also stimulates contraction of uterine smooth muscles at term, and helps in parturition. Some synthetic analogues of oxytocin have also been prepared, and are used to strengthen uterine contractions during labour.

VASOPRESSIN

Vasopressin (arginine-vasopressin or AVP) is also known as **anti-diuretic hormone (ADH)**. It is a cyclic nonapeptide. It is secreted in response to increased osmolality of plasma perceived by osmoreceptors located in the hypothalamus.

Functions

1. The main function of vasopressin is to stimulate reabsorption of water from distal convoluted tubules and collecting ducts.Hence, ADH is a more apt name of this hormone. The cell membrane of the cells of distal convoluted tubules and collecting ducts is impermeable to water in the absence of ADH. ADH increases the concentration of **cAMP** in these cells which makes the membrane permeable to water. This is known as facultative reabsorption of water. ADH helps in maintaining the fluid balance of the body by adjusting the facultative reabsorption of water according to the requirements of the body (*see* Chapter 24 for more details).

2. High concentrations of ADH cause peripheral vaso-constriction resulting in a rise in blood pressure. The name vasopressin derives from this effect. This extra-renal effect in mediated by **inositol triphosphate** and **diacylglycerol.**

Deficient secretion of ADH leads to **diabetes insipidus** in which urine output is greatly increased. Total absence of ADH can lead to excretion of 25–30 litres of urine per day.

PINEAL HORMONES

Pineal gland is located on the posterior aspect of midbrain. It is a small gland which generally calcifies after puberty in human beings.

Several hormones have been isolated from the pineal gland, e.g. melatonin, serotonin, histamine, norepinephrine, etc. Of these, melatonin is synthesised only in the pineal gland. It is synthesised from tryptophan. Serotonin is formed as an intermediate in the synthetic pathway. In the presence of light, the pathway progresses upto serotonin. In dark, it progresses upto melatonin (Fig. 17.16).

Functions

Melatonin can be considered as the true pineal hormone. The exact function of melatonin in human beings is uncertain. Recent evidence suggests that melatonin has an anti-gonadotropic effect. It has also been proposed that melatonin and serotonin regulate the sleep-wakefulness cycle.

THYROID HORMONES

The glandular tissue of the thyroid gland is composed of spherical follicles. The follicles are made up of a single layer of cuboidal (follicular) cells enclosing a hollow space within. This space is filled up with a colloidal substance which contains the stored hormones.

Chemistry

The thyroid gland synthesises two main hormones, **thyroxine** and **tri-iodothyronine** (thyrocalcitonin or calcitonin, a hormone regulating calcium metabolism, is also synthesised in the thyroid gland but will be discussed later) (Fig. 17.17).

Synthesis

Circulating iodide is taken up by the thyroid gland by an active transport process. It is released by the follicular cells into the follicular space where it is oxidised in the presence of hydrogen peroxide by a peroxidase (thyroperoxidase). A glycoprotein, thyroglobulin (MW 660,000) is also present in the follicular space. Thyro-globulin is made up of about 5,000 amino acid residues of which more than a hundred are tyrosine residues.

The tyrosine residues of thyroglobulin are iodinated first at position 3 and then at position 5 to form 3-mono-iodo-tyrosine (**MIT**) and 3,5-di-iodo-tyrosine (**DIT**) respectively. Two DIT residues are coupled to form a tetra-iodo-thryonine (thyroxine or T_4) residue. One MIT residue may be coupled with a DIT residue to form a tri-iodo-thyronine (T_3) residue. The iodination and coupling reactions are also probably catalysed by thyroperoxidase (Fig. 17.18).

T_4 and T_3 synthesised in the follicular space are still part of the thyroglobulin molecule, and are stored there until they are needed in circulation. When the hormones are to be secreted, thyroglobulin enters the follicular cells by endocytosis. The lysosomal proteolytic enzymes hydrolyse thyroglobulin and release T_4 and T_3 which are secreted into blood. They are transported in blood by two specific carrier proteins,**thyroxine-binding globulin (TBG)** and **thyroxine-binding prealbumin (TBPA)**. Very small amounts of T_4 and T_3 are present in unbound, free form in the blood. All the physiological functions are performed by free T_4 and T_3. Plasma level of T_4 is much higher than that of T_3 but T_3 is biologically much more powerful than T_4. Some of the circulating T_4 is converted into T_3 in peripheral tissues by removal of one iodine atom from T_4.

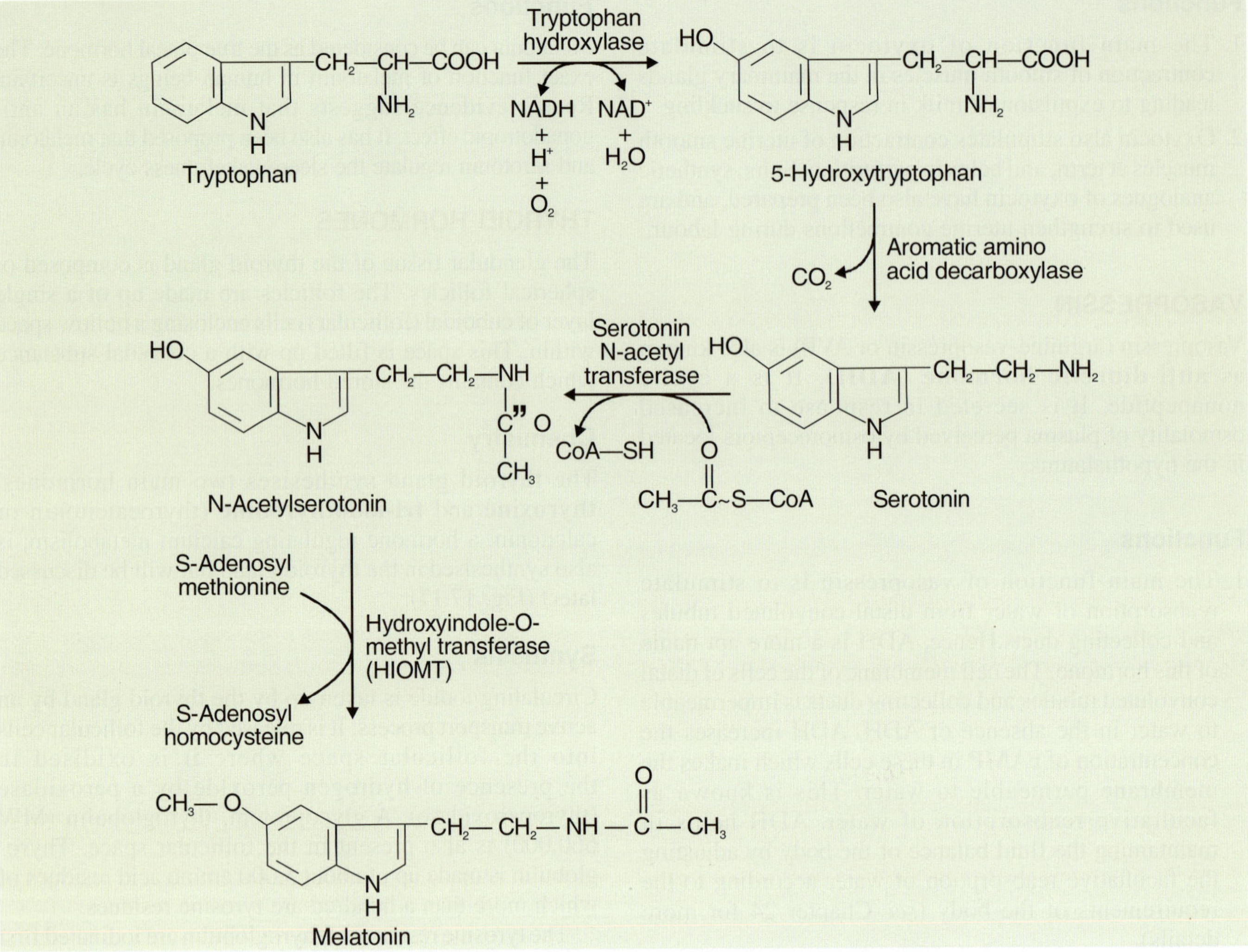

Fig. 17.16: Synthesis of serotonin and melatonin from tryptophan

Functions

Effect on Metabolic Rate

Thyroid hormones increase the metabolic activities in nearly all the cells in the body resulting in an increase in the basal metabolic rate (BMR).

Effect on Protein Metabolism

Thyroid hormones stimulate the synthesis of proteins in various tissues resulting in a positive nitrogen balance. Their presence is essential for normal growth as they increase the synthesis of structural proteins. Very high concentrations of thyroid hormones increase the catabolism of proteins.

Effect on Carbohydrate Metabolism

Thyroid hormones increase the intestinal absorption of glucose and utilisation of glucose by various tissues. They increase gluconeogenesis.

Effect on Lipid Metabolism

Thyroid hormones increase lipolysis in adipose tissue resulting in an increase in the concentration of free fatty acids in plasma. They also increase the oxidation of fatty acids.

Physiological Effects

Thyroid hormones stimulate physical **growth** by increasing the synthesis of growth hormone and by increasing the synthesis of structural proteins. They are also essential for **mental development**. They increase the force of contraction of heart muscle and cardiac output. Other effects include increase in heart rate, increase in rate and depth of respiration, increase in the secretion of digestive juices, increase in gastrointestinal motility, etc.

Regulation
Hypothalamic Regulation

Hypothalamus secretes thyrotropin-releasing hormone (TRH) which acts on anterior pituitary, and increases the secretion of thyroid-stimulating hormone (TSH).

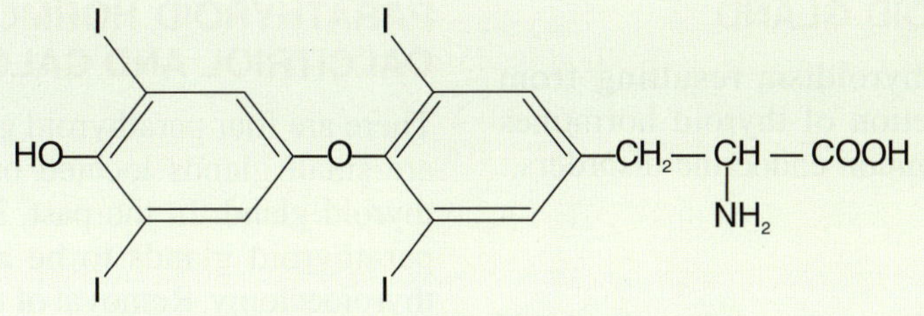

3,5,3',5'–Tetraiodothyronine (thyroxine or T_4)

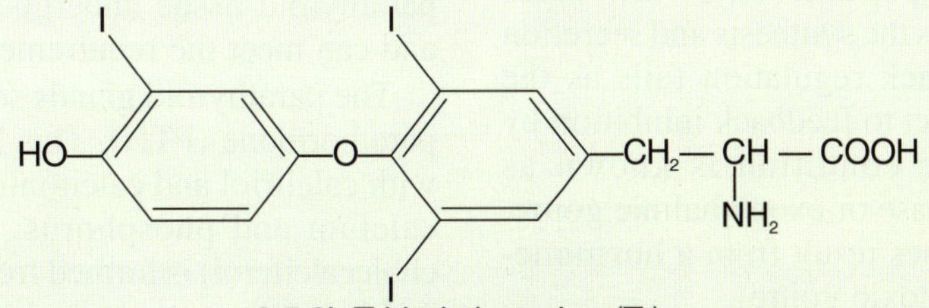

3,5,3'–Tri-iodothyronine (T_3)

Fig. 17.17: Thyroid hormones

Adenohypophyseal Regulation

TSH secreted by the anterior pituitary increases the secretion of thyroid hormones.

Feedback Regulation

Circulating T_4 and T_3 regulate their own secretion. Increased levels of T_4 and T_3 in plasma inhibit their own secretion as well as the secretion of TSH and TRH by feedback mechanism.

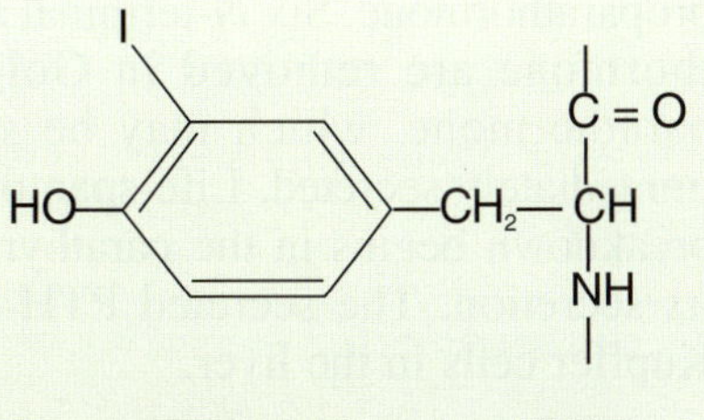

3-Mono-iodo-tyrosyl (MIT) residue

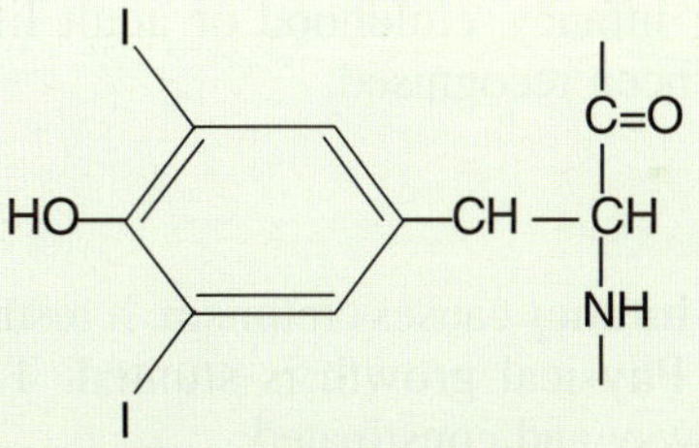

3, 5-Di-iodo-tyrosyl (DIT) residue

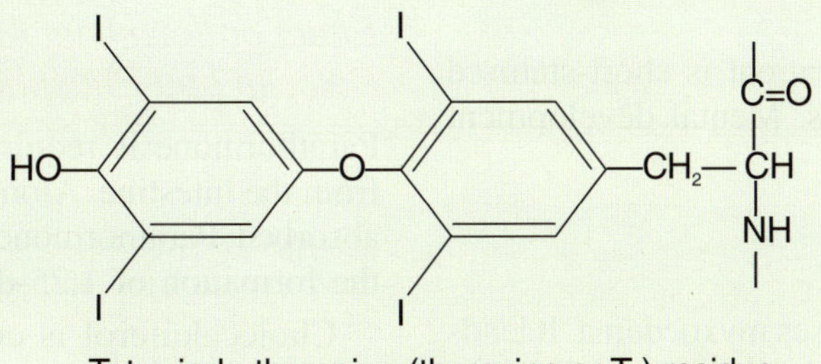

Tetra-iodo-thyronine (thyroxine or T_4) residue

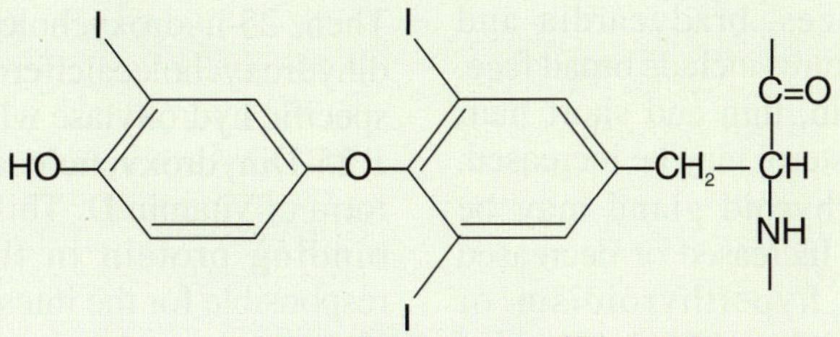

Tri-iodo-thyronine (T_3) residue

Fig. 17.18: Mono-iodo-tyrosine, di-iodo-tyrosine, tetra-iodo-thyronine and tri-iodo-thyronine residues in thyroglobulin

DYSFUNCTION OF THYROID GLAND

Hyperthyroidism and hypothyroidism resulting from excessive and deficient secretion of thyroid hormones respectively are relatively common endocrine disorders.

Hyperthyroidism

A common cause of hyperthyroidism is synthesis of **thyroid stimulating immunoglobulin** (TSI) which binds to TSH receptors, and increases the synthesis and secretion of thyroid hormones. Feedback regulation fails as the production of TSI is not subject to feedback inhibition by the thyroid hormones. The condition is known as thyrotoxicosis or Graves' disease or exophthalmic goitre. Hyperthyroidism can sometimes result from a **hormone-secreting adenoma** (nodular toxic goitre).

Hyperthyroidism causes tiredness, nervousness, anxiety, palpitations, dyspnoea on exertion, muscular weakness, tremors, diarrhoea, excessive sweating, heat intolerance, loss of weight despite increased appetite, tachycardia, exophthalmos and enlargement of the thyroid gland (diffuse in Graves' disease and localised in nodular toxic goitre). Osteoporosis can occur. Hyperglycaemia and hypocholesterolaemia may also occur.

Hypothyroidism

This may occur during infancy, childhood or adult life. Three syndromes have been recognised:

1. Cretinism

Hypothyroidism during **infancy** causes cretinism. It results in mental retardation. Physical growth is stunted. The patient is lethargic, drowsy and constipated.

2. Juvenile Myxoedema

This occurs in **childhood**. The patient is short-statured with infantile skeletal proportions. Mental development is normal.

3. Myxoedema

Hypothyroidism in **adulthood** causes myxoedema. It leads to tiredness, lethargy, cold intolerance, constipation, menorrhagia, mental disturbances, bradycardia and sluggish tendon reflexes. Other features include broad face, puffy eyelids, dry and coarse skin, thin and short hair, scanty sweating, etc. Serum cholesterol may be increased.

Sometimes, dysfunction of thyroid gland may be secondary to a pituitary disorder. Increased or decreased secretion of TSH may cause hyperthyroidism or hypothyroidism respectively. Therefore, measurement of serum TSH is often required alongwith that of T_3 and T_4 to reach a diagnosis (*see* Chapter 28).

PARATHYROID HORMONE, CALCITRIOL AND CALCITONIN

There are four parathyroid glands in human beings. These are small glands located on the posterior aspect of the thyroid gland. In the past, it was not uncommon for the parathyroid glands to be accidentally removed during thyroidectomy. Removal of two, or even three, parathyroid glands may not produce any abnormality as the remaining parathyroid tissue undergoes compensatory hypertrophy, and can meet the requirement of parathyroid hormone.

The parathyroid glands secrete parathyroid hormone or parathormone (PTH). This hormone, in close association with calcitriol and calcitonin, regulates the metablosim of calcium and phosphorus. Calcitriol (1,25-dihydroxy-cholecalciferol) is formed from vitamin D (cholecalciferol), and is now regarded as a hormone.

PARATHORMONE

Chemistry

Parathyroid hormone is a polypeptide made up of 84 amino acids. Its molecular weight is about 9,500. Only the first 34 amino acids are essential for its activity. The hormone is initially synthesised as a precursor (pre-proparathormone) containing 31 extra amino acids. Twenty-five N-terminal amino acids are removed in endoplasmic reticulum to form proparathormone. Six N-terminal amino acids of proparathormone are removed in Golgi apparatus to form parathormone, which may be stored in the gland or immediately secreted. Life-span of PTH is very short. Its breakdown begins in the parathyroid glands even before its secretion. The secreted PTH is rapidly degraded in Kupffer cells in the liver.

Functions

Effect on Intestinal Absorption of Calcium and Phosphorus

Parathormone is required for the absorption of calcium from the intestine. Alongwith calcium, phosphorus is also absorbed. Parathormone produces this effect by promoting the formation of 1,25-dihydroxycholecalciferol.

Cholecalciferol is converted into 25-hydroxy-chole-calciferol by microsomal hydroxylase system in liver. Then, 25-hydroxycholecalciferol is converted into 1,25-dihydroxycholecalciferol (calcitriol) in the kidneys by a specific hydroxylase which is activated by parathormone. 1,25-Dihydroxycholecalciferol is the active (hormone) form of vitamin D. This induces the synthesis of calcium binding protein in the intestinal mucosa which is responsible for the intestinal absorption of calcium. When plasma calcium level rises as a result of increased intestinal absorption of calcium, the secretion of parathormone is inhibited (Fig.17.19).

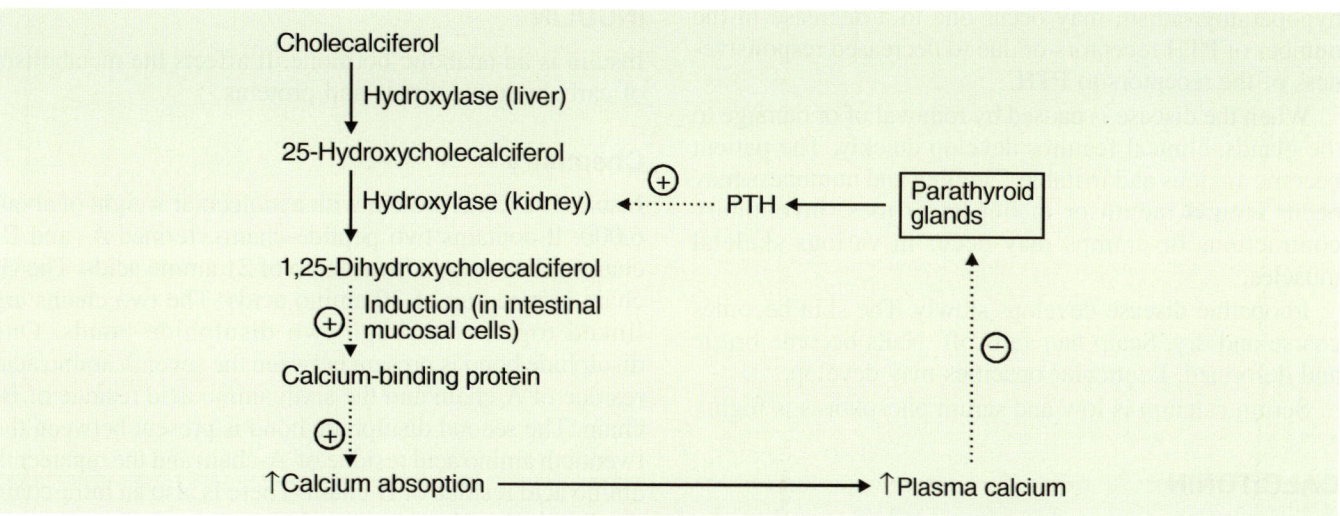

Fig. 17.19: Role of parathormone (PTH) in calcium absorption in intestine

Effect on Bone Resorption

Parathormone increases the activity of osteoclasts in the bones. It also triggers an increase in the number of osteoclasts. This results in demineralisation of bones with release of calcium into circulation.

Effect on Renal Excretion of Calcium and Phosphorus

Parathormone increases the renal tubular reabsorption of calcium, and decreases that of phosphate. Therefore, excretion of calcium is decreased, and that of phosphorus is increased.

Effect on Plasma Calcium and Phosphorus

Plasma calcium is increased due to greater absorption from intestine, demineralisation of bones and decreased renal excretion. Plasma phosphorus is decreased due to its greater excretion in urine.

Regulation

The plasma concentration of **ionised calcium** regulates the secretion of parathormone by **feedback mechanism**. A high concentration of ionised calcium in plasma inhibits the secretion of parathormone which decreases the plasma calcium concentration. When the concentration falls below normal, the inhibition is relieved, and plasma calcium begins to rise again in response to the secretion of parathormone.

DYSFUNCTION OF PARATHYROID GLANDS

Increased secretion of parathormone results in hyperparathyroidism. Decreased secretion results in hypoparathyroidism.

Hyperparathyroidism

This may be primary or secondary.

Primary Hyperparathyroidism

This disease affects women more commonly than men. It usually develops between the ages of 30 and 60. There are three common clinical presentations:

1. The commonest presentation is recurrent renal stones which may ultimately damage the kidneys.
2. Some patients present with bone disease in the form of pathological fractures, backache, bone pains and skeletal deformities.
3. In some patients, the signs and symptoms are attributable to hypercalcaemia. There is loss of weight, loss of appetite, nausea, weakness, drowsiness, polydipsia, polyuria, anxiety, depression, etc. Indigestion and peptic ulcers may also occur.

   High serum calcium and low serum phosphorus are seen in all the patients. Serum alkaline phosphatase may be elevated if bones are affected.

Secondary Hyperparathyroidism

Secondary hypersecretion of parathormone may occur in response to prolonged hypocalcaemia due to chronic renal disease or intestinal malabsorption.

The clinical picture is dominated by the primary disease. Skeletal deformities and bone pains may be present. Serum calcium is low or normal. Serum alkaline phosphatase is high. Serum phosphorus is normal or high.

Hypoparathyroidism

Hypoparathyroidism is most commonly due to accidental removal of or damage to parathyroid glands during thyroidectomy. Some cases are of idiopathic origin. Pseudohypoparathyroidism may occur due to a decrease in the number of PTH receptors or due to decreased responsiveness of the receptors to PTH.

When the disease is caused by removal of or damage to the glands, clinical features develop quickly. The patient become anxious and irritable. Tingling and numbness may occur around mouth or in fingers or toes. Involuntary contractions or cramps may occur in various skeletal muscles.

Idiopathic disease develops slowly. The skin becomes coarse and dry. Scalp hair falls off. Nails become brittle and deformed. Lenticular opacities may develop.

Serum calcium is low and serum phosphorus is high.

CALCITONIN

Calcitonin or thyrocalcitonin is a hormone synthesised in parafollicular cells of the thyroid gland.

Chemistry

Calcitonin is a polypeptide made up of 32 amino acids. Its molecular weight is 3,600. The complete molecule is required for biological activity. Its life-span is very short. Its half-life is 4 to 12 minutes.

Functions

The effects of calcitonin are opposite to those of parathormone. It decreases plasma calcium by decreasing demineralisation of bones and by increasing renal excretion of calcium. It also inhibits the formation of 1,25-dihydroxycholecalciferol. Plasma calcium level is maintained within the normal range by the opposing effects of parathormone and calcitonin.

Regulation

The secretion of calcitonin is regulated by feedback mechanism. An increase in the plasma concentration of ionised calcium evokes an immediate release of calcitonin. Decreased plasma calcium inhibits the secretion of calcitonin.

Following any alteration in plasma calcium concentration, immediate readjustments are made by calcitonin whereas the long-term readjustments are made by parathormone.

PANCREATIC HORMONES

The pancreas is both an exocrine and an endocrine gland. The endocrine portion is the islets of Langerhans. The islets are dispersed throughout the gland, and contain α-, β-, δ- and F-cells. The α-cells secrete glucagon, and β-cells secrete insulin. Both these hormones profoundly affect the carbohydrate metabolism. The δ-cells secrete somatastatin, and F-cells secrete pancreatic polypeptide.

INSULIN

Insulin is an anabolic hormone. It affects the metabolism of carbohydrates, lipids and proteins.

Chemistry

Insulin is a small protein with a molecular weight of about 6,000. It contains two peptide chains, termed A- and B-chains. The A-chain is made up of 21 amino acids. The B-chain is made up of 30 amino acids. The two chains are linked together through two disulphide bonds. One disulphide bond is present between the seventh amino acid residue of A-chain and the sixth amino acid residue of B-chain. The second disulphide bond is present between the twentieth amino acid residue of A-chain and the nineteenth amino acid residue of B-chain. There is also an intra-chain disulphide bond between the sixth and eleventh amino acid residues of A-Chain. If the disulphide bonds are broken by chemical treatment, there is complete loss of biological activity.

Insulin is first synthesised on rough endoplasmic recticulum in the form of a precursor, **preproinsulin** which is a single polypeptide made up of 103 amino acids. The N-terminal 19 amino acids constitute the **signal sequence**

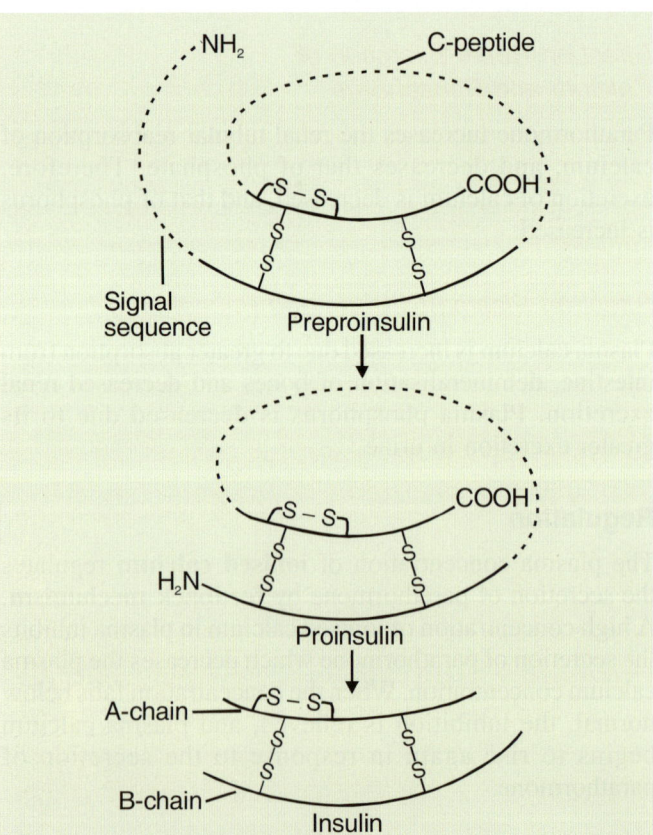

Fig. 17.20: Conversion of preproinsulin into insulin. Signal sequence is removed to convert preproinsulin into proinsulin followed by removal of connecting peptide to convert proinsulin into insulin

which is removed in the endoplasmic reticulum converting preproinsulin into **proinsulin**. A 33-amino acid **connecting peptide (C-peptide)** is removed in the secretory granules converting proinsulin into insulin (Fig.17.20). Crystallisation of insulin requires zinc which is easily available in the islets of Langerhans.

Variations in Primary Structure of Insulin

Primary structure of insulin is highly conserved. Only minor variations are found in the amino acid sequence of insulin in different species. Porcine insulin and bovine insulin are used commonly for the treatment of diabetes mellitus. Porcine insulin differs from insulin only with respect to position 30 in the B chain. Bovine insulin has different amino acid residues at positions 8 and 10 in the A chain and at position 30 in the B chain. **Lispro insulin** and **aspart insulin** are genetically-engineered human insulins synthesised by recombinant DNA technology. In lispro insulin, positions of proline (B 28) and lysine (B 29) are interchanged. In aspart insulin, proline (B 28) is replaced by aspartate (Table 17.2). These variations or substitutions do not affect the biological activity of insulin showing thereby that positions 8, 9 and 10 in A chain and positions 28, 29 and 30 in B chain are not critical for the biological activity of insulin.

Natural insulin has a tendency to polymerise. Hydrogen bonds are formed between the B chains of two insulin molecules forming a dimer. At high insulin concentrations, three dimers come together along with some zinc ions to form a hexamer. Only the monomeric form of insulin is biologically active. In lispro and aspart insulins, hydrogen bonds can not be formed between B chains because of amino acid switching/substitution. Therefore, lispro and aspart insulins remain in the monomeric form. They act rapidly and for a shorter period as compared to natural insulin.

FUNCTIONS

Insulin binds to its receptors on the cell membrane of the target cells. The insulin receptor is a transmembrane glycoprotein made of **two α-** and **two β-subunits.**

The α-subunits are present outside the cell membrane. The β-subunits traverse the membrane. Cytosolic portion of each β-subunit possesses a **tyrosine kinase** domain which is activated on **binding of insulin to the α-subunits** (Fig. 17.9). The activated tryosine kinase domain phosphorylates some tyrosine residues in the β-subunit itself. The autophosphorylated receptor phosphorylates the tyrosine residues of some target proteins, **insulin receptor substrates**. This initiates a phosphorylation/dephosphorylation cascade resulting in the ultimate effects of insulin.

Insulin produces a variety of physiological and biochemical effects which can be broadly divided into growth-promoting effects and metabolic effects. Two different cascades are involved in these two effects. A number of molecules are involved in these cascades several of which are yet to be identified.

Phosphorylation of tyrosine residues of insulin receptor substrate-1 (IRS-1) initiates the **growth-promoting effects**. Several proteins having src homology 2 (SH2) domains are involved in this cascade including growth factor receptor binding protein 2 (GRB2). p21, the protein encoded by ras proto-oncogene, mitogen-activated protein kinase (MAP kinase) and raf proto-oncogene are also involved in this cascade.

Phosphorylation of tyrosine residues of insulin receptor substrate-2 (IRS-2) initiates the second cascade involving activation/inactivation of some enzymes, induction of some enzymes and translocation of GLUT 4 from cytosol to the cell membrane. This cascade results in the **metabolic effects** of insulin.

Effect on Growth

Insulin promotes growth by stimulating cell division, tissue differentiation and organogenesis.

Effect on Carbohydrate Metabolism

Insulin produces profound effects on various facets of carbohydrate metabolism. It increases the uptake of glucose by muscles, myocardium and adipose tissue by translocating GLUT 4 from cytosol to the cell membrane in these tissues. It activates/inactivates several enzymes

Table 17.2: Variations in amino acid sequence of insulin.

	Amino acid at position					
	A8	A9	A10	B28	B29	B30
Human insulin	Thr	Ser	Ile	Pro	Lys	Thr
Porcine insulin	Thr	Ser	Ile	Pro	Lys	Ala
Bovine insulin	Ala	Ser	Val	Pro	Lys	Ala
Lispro insulin	Thr	Ser	Ile	Lys	Pro	Thr
Aspart insulin	Thr	Ser	Ile	Asp	Lys	Thr

and induces/represses some others. This results in activation of pathways which utilise glucose, e.g. glycolysis, HMP shunt and glycogenesis. Pathways which produce glucose, e.g. gluconeogenesis and glycogenolysis, are deactivated. As a result, the blood glucose concentration is decreased.

Effects on Lipid Metabolism

Insulin decreases lipolysis and increases lipogenesis. It increases the conversion of glucose into fatty acids.

Effects on Protein Metabolism

Insulin increases the uptake of amino acids by the cells. It increases the synthesis of proteins.

Regulation

Secretion of insulin is regulated by feedback mechanism by the concentration of glucose in blood. A rise in blood glucose, for example after a meal, stimulates the secretion of insulin. This leads to increased utilisation of glucose and lowering of blood glucose level. A fall in blood glucose, for example during fasting, inhibits the secretion of insulin. This leads to decreased utilisation and increased production of glucose. Thus, insulin secretion is regulated in such a way that the blood glucose concentration is maintained within the normal range.

DISORDERS OF INSULIN SECRETION

Decreased secretion or action of insulin results in diabetes mellitus which is the commonest endocrine disorder. Increased secretion of insulin, i.e. hyperinsulinism, is very rare.

Diabetes Mellitus

This results from deficient secretion of insulin or unresponsiveness of target cells to insulin. Two types of diabetes mellitus are clinically recognised, **juvenile diabetes** and **maturity-onset diabetes**. Juvenile diabetes (insulin-dependent diabetes mellitus or IDDM or type I diabetes) occurs in childhood, and is associated with severe deficiency or total absence of insulin production. This is usually due to **destruction of β-cells** by an **autoimmune disorder**.

Maturity-onset diabetes (non-insulin-dependent diabetes mellitus or NIDDM or type II diabetes) is far more common. Several causes have been suggested of which heredity and obesity appear to be the most important. Maturity-onset diabetes is usually due to **unresponsiveness** of target cells to insulin. The unresponsiveness may be due to **decreased number of insulin receptors** or due to the presence of **antibodies against insulin receptors.**

The following biochemical disturbances occur in diabetes mellitus.

1. *Decreased utilisation of glucose:* As insulin is essential for the uptake and utilisation of glucose by several of the body cells, deficiency of insulin leads to decreased utilisation of glucose by the body cells. Blood glucose concentration is, therefore, raised.

2. *Increased utilisation of lipids:* To meet the energy requirements of the body, fats are mobilised from fat depots and oxidation of fatty acids is increased. Production of ketone bodies and cholesterol is also increased.

3. *Depletion of proteins:* Protein synthesis is decreased. Proteins are broken down to provide energy. Amino acids are diverted to synthesise glucose (gluco-neogenesis). All this results in depletion of body proteins.

Clinically, the classical symptoms of diabetes mellitus include polyuria, polydipsia and polyphagia. Tiredness and loss of weight may also occur. However, these symptoms are usually seen only in type I diabetes.

Type II diabetics may be free of signs and symptoms until very late when ophthalmological, cardiovascular, neurological or renal complications may lead to the diagnosis of diabetes mellitus.

As stated earlier, blood glucose concentration is raised in diabetes. When it exceeds the renal threshold for glucose (about 180 mg/dl), glucose is excreted in urine. To dissolve this extra glucose, urine volume is increased (polyuria). Increased loss of water leads to increased thirst (polydipsia). Decreased utilisation of glucose leads to excessive eating (polyphagia) and tiredness. Decreased utilisation of glucose and increased breakdown of proteins causes loss of weight.

Excessive breakdown of fatty acids leads to excessive production of ketone bodies which, in turn, disturbs the acid-base balance of the body fluids causing acidosis (diabetic ketoacidosis). Severe deficiency of insulin may cause diabetic coma and death. This occurs more frequently in type I diabetes mellitus. Diabetics usually have an increased susceptibility of infections and delayed wound healing.

The following laboratory investigations are commonly employed for diagnosis of diabetes mellitus and for monitoring the efficacy of treatment.

1. *Urine glucose:* The urine of normal persons does not contain detectable amount of glucose. Diabetic patients often excrete detectable amounts of glucose in their urine. However, a negative test does not rule out diabetes and a positive test may sometimes be due to conditions other than diabetes.

2. *Blood glucose:* Measurement of blood glucose concentration after an overnight fast is the most definitive method of establishing the diagnosis of diabetes mellitus. A fasting hyperglycaemia is characteristic of diabetes mellitus.

3. *Glucose tolerance test:* This test is sometimes performed when determination of fasting blood glucose is inconclusive. After measuring fasting blood glucose, oral glucose is given in the dose of 1.5 gm/kg of body weight subject to a maximum of 75 gm. Then, blood glucose is measured every half an hour for two hours. In normal subjects, fasting blood glucose is normal. After glucose ingestion, the blood glucose rises to 130 to 140 mg/dl, and returns to the fasting level or slightly below the fasting level within two hours. In diabetics, fasting blood glucose is usually raised. There is an excessive increase in blood glucose after glucose ingestion, and the blood glucose fails to return to normal in two hours. One or more urine samples passed during the test may contain glucose.

More commonly, a shortened version of glucose tolerance test is done in which only fasting blood glucose and two-hour post-glucose load blood glucose are measured. A fasting plasma glucose above 126 mg/dl on two occasions or a fasting plasma glucose above 126 mg/dl and two-hour post-glucose load plasma glucose above 200 mg/dl on the same occasion is considered to be diagnostic of diabetes.

4. *Glycosylated haemoglobin:* This measurement is cmployed to monitor long term control of diabetes (*see* Chapter 10).

Hyperinsulinism

This rare condition is caused by a tumour of β-cells of the islets of Langerhans. There is excessive production of insulin. Blood glucose is decreased. The patient complains of nervousness, trembling, excessive sweating and hunger. In severe cases, convulsions and coma may occur. Sometimes, a similar clinical picture may result from accidental overadministration of insulin to a diabetic patient. Administration of glucose by oral or intravenous route leads to an immediate improvement.

GLUCAGON

Glucagon acts in association with insulin to maintain the blood glucose concentration within the normal range.

Chemistry

Glucagon is a polypeptide containing 29 amino acid residues. Its molecular weight is about 3,500. Glucagon is synthesised mainly in α-cells of islets of Langerhans, but small amounts are also synthesised in the gastrointestinal tract.

Functions

Effect on Carbohydrate Metabolism

The most important effect of glucagon is to increase glycogenolysis and to decrease glycogenesis in liver.

Output of glucose from liver into the circulation is increased. The blood glucose concentration is raised.

Glucagon also increases the rate of gluconeogenesis in the liver. Therefore, blood glucose continues to be high even when the liver glycogen is completely depleted.

Effect on Lipid Metabolism

Glucagon increases lipolysis in fat cells and also possibly in liver. The free fatty acids which are released are used as a source of energy. The liberated glycerol is used as a substrate for gluconeogenesis.

Regulation

Secretion of glucagon is regulated by the blood glucose concentration. A decrease in blood glucose stimulates the secretion of glucagon. A raised blood glucose concentration inhibits the secretion of glucagon.

Since insulin and glucagon have opposite effects on blood glucose, they serve to maintain the blood glucose level within the normal range. After a meal, when blood glucose tends to rise, insulin decreases it by converting glucose into glycogen and lipids. In between meals, glucagon prevents a fall in blood glucose by stimulating glycogenolysis and gluconeogenesis.

ADRENAL MEDULLARY HORMONES

The adrenal or suprarenal glands are located above the kidneys, and consist of adrenal medulla and adrenal cortex. The hormones of adrenal medulla are synthesised in the chromaffin cells (phaeochromocytes) from phenylalanine or tyrosine. The adrenal medullary hormones are also termed as **catecholamines** as they resemble catechol (or pyrocatechol) in structure. Several catecholamines are synthesised in adrenal medulla of which epinephrine (adrenalin) and norepinephrine (noradrenaline) are predominant. Quantitatively, epinephrine is the major hormone of adrenal medulla.

Chemistry and Synthesis

Catecholamines are amino acid derivatives. They can be synthesised from phenylalanine or tyrosine. Phenylalanine is hydroxylated to tyrosine. Tyrosine is hydroxylated to dihydroxyphenylalanine (DOPA). DOPA is decarboxylated to dopamine. Dopamine is converted into norepinephrine, and the latter into epinephrine. The difference between norepinephrine and epinephrine is that norepinephrine lacks the methyl group attached to the side chain of epinephrine (Fig. 17.21).

Catecholamines are synthesised in some extra-adrenal tissues also, e.g. brain and sympathetic ganglia. Blood brain barrier is impermeable to norepinephrine and epinephrine. However, it is permeable to dopamine. Dopamine synthesised in the adrenal medulla can be

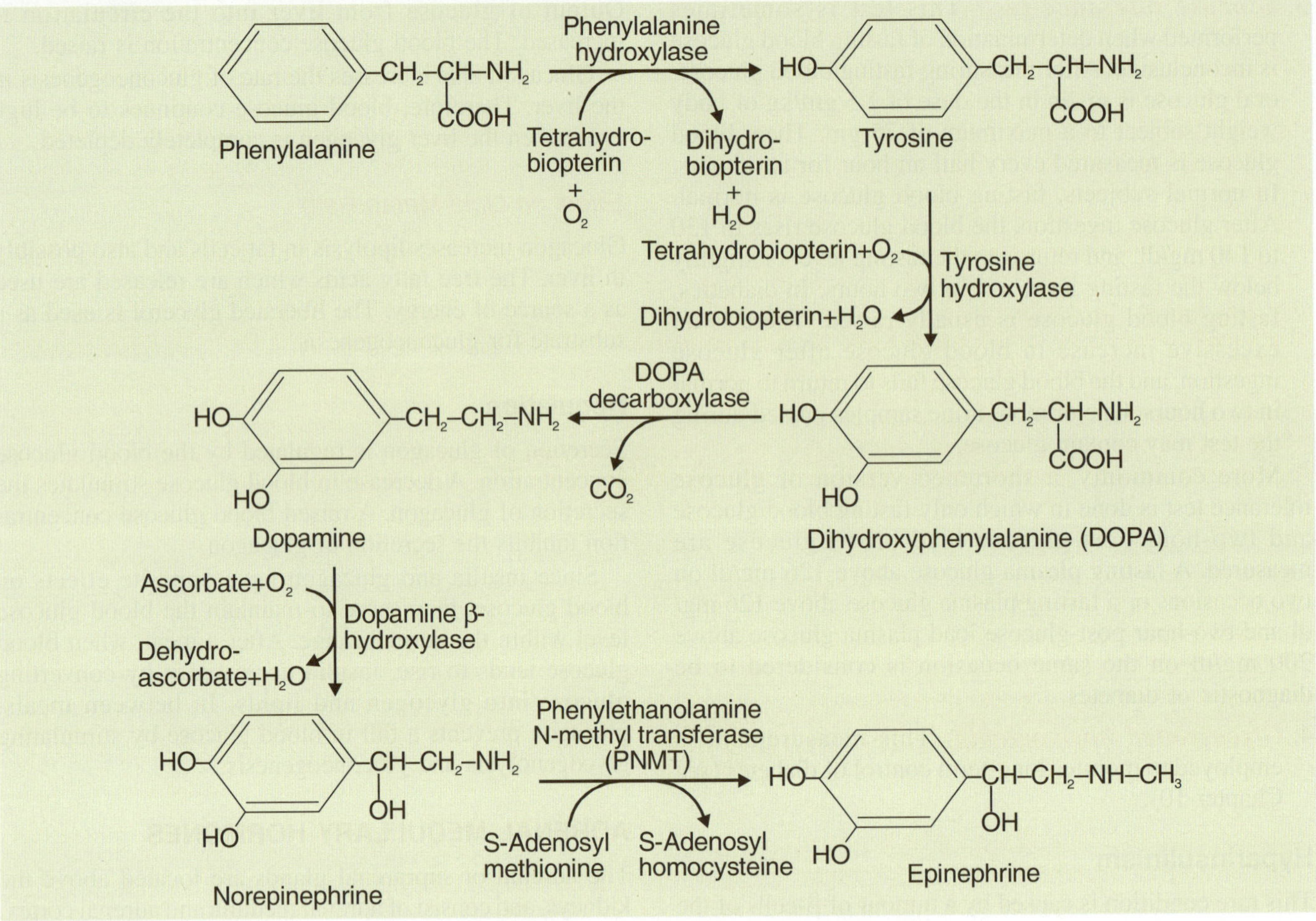

Fig. 17.21: Synthesis of norepinephrine and epinephrine

released into circulation. It can cross the blood-brain barrier, and can be converted into norepinephrine and epinephrine in the brain.

Catecholamines are stored in adrenal medulla in the form of chromaffin granules. Presence of calcium ions is required for their secretion.

Catabolism

Catabolism of epinephrine and norepinephrine occurs both in their target cells and in liver. Epinephrine is catabolised to vanillyl mandelic acid (**VMA**) via 3,4-dihydroxymandelic acid or metanephrine. Norepineph-rine is converted into normetanephrine and, then, into VMA. VMA is the main metabolite of catecholamines, and is excreted in urine. Small amounts of metanephrine and normetanephrine are also excreted in urine (Fig. 17.22).

Functions

Epinephrine and norepinephrine act upon structures innervated by sympathetic nerves or having adrenergic receptors. The receptors are of two types, α-adrenergic receptors and β-adrenergic receptors. The α-adrenergic receptors are sub-divided into α_1 and α_2. The β-adrenergic receptors are also sub-divided into β_1 and β_2. Norepine-phrine acts mainly on α-adrenergic receptors while epinephrine acts on both α-adrenergic and β-adrenergic receptors.

Binding of the hormones to α_1-**adrenergic receptors** activates **phospholipase C**. The biological effects are produced by diacylglycerol and inositol triphosphate which act as the second messengers. The second messenger in case of α_2-, β_1- and β_2- **adrenergic receptors** is **cAMP**. The signal transducer for α_2-adrenergic receptors is a G_i protein which inhibits adenylate cyclase. The signal transducer for β_1- and β_2- **adrenergic receptors** is a G_s protein which activates adenylate cyclase. The varied effects of catecholamines in different tissues depend upon the type of receptors present in different tissues.

Effect on Cardiovascular System

Epinephrine has a stimulatory effect on myocardium. It increases the rate and the force of contraction of heart resulting in an increase in the cardiac output. Norepine-phrine has much less effect on heart.

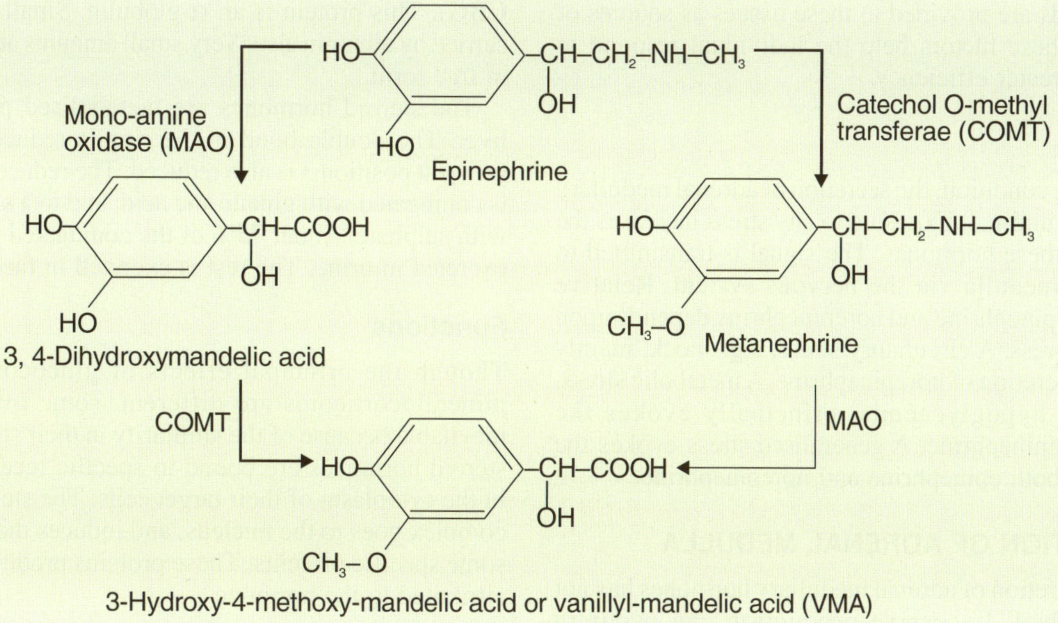

Fig. 17.22: Catabolism of epinephrine

Epinephrine constricts the blood vessels of skin, alimentary tract and kidneys. It dilates the blood vessels of muscles, liver and coronary arteries. The vasodilator effect is much greater than the vasoconstrictor effect. Therefore, the peripheral resistance is decreased. Systolic blood pressure is increased, and diastolic blood pressure is either decreased or remains unchanged.

Norepinephrine causes generalised vasoconstriction. Therefore, the peripheral resistance is increased, and blood pressure is raised. For this reason, norepinephrine is used pharmacologically to raise blood pressure in patients with shock.

Effect on Respiration

Both epinephrine and norepinephrine increase the rate and depth of respiration.

Effect on Smooth Muscles

Epinephrine relaxes the smooth muscles of stomach, intestine, bronchioles and urinary bladder. Because of its bronchodilator effect, epinephrine is used pharmacologically in bronchial asthma to relieve the bronchial spasm. Epinephrine constricts the sphincters of stomach and urinary bladder. The uterine muscle is also contracted. Norepinephrine also produces similar effects on smooth muscles of gastrointestinal tract but is much weaker than epinephrine in this respect. It stimulates contraction of smooth muscles of genitourinary tract.

Effect on Skeletal Muscles

Epinephrine increases the tone of skeletal muscles, and delays the onset of fatigue.

Metabolic Effects

Epinephrine produces more pronounced metabolic effects as compared to norepinephrine. Its effects are similar to those of glucagon but it acts predominantly on muscles, and to a smaller extent, on liver.

It increases oxygen consumption and raises the basal metabolic rate. The effect on basal metabolic rate is not mediated by thyroxine as it persists even after thyroidectomy.

Epinephrine decreases glycogenesis and increases glycogenolysis in muscles and liver. Its effect on hepatic glycogen metabolism is weaker than that of glucagon. Blood glucose concentration is raised due to increased glycogenolysis.

Epinephrine increases lipolysis in the adipose tissue. Free fatty acids are released and are used as a source of energy in various tissues, e.g. heart and skeletal muscles.

Epinephrine increases the secretion of insulin from the pancreas. Therefore, glucose utilisation is increased.

Other Effects

Epinephrine produces several other minor effects, e.g. increased salivation, increased lacrimation, increased sweating, contraction of spleen, increased coagulability of blood and increased secretion of ACTH.

In general, adrenal medulla, acting in concert with the sympathetic nervous system, helps the individual cope with stressful situations. Secretion of epinephrine is increased under stress. Epinephrine increases cardiac output. Supply of blood to more essential organs, e.g. brain, heart, liver and muscles, is increased at the expense of less essential organs. More oxygen is made available to these tissues by increasing the rate and depth of respiration. More glucose and fatty acids are provided to these tissues as sources of energy. All these factors help the individual respond to stress with greater efficiency.

Regulation

Under resting condition, the secretion of adrenal medullary hormones is minimal. Exposure to any stress increases the secretion of these hormones. The signal is transmitted to the adrenal medulla via the nervous system. Relative secretion of epinephrine and norepinephrine depends upon the type of stress. A circulatory stress, e.g. shock, mainly evokes the secretion of norepinephrine. A metabolic stress, e.g. sudden hypoglycaemia, principally evokes the secretion of epinephrine. A generalised stress evokes the secretion of both epinephrine and norepinephrine.

DYSFUNCTION OF ADRENAL MEDULLA

Deficient secretion of adrenal medullary hormones has not been described. Excessive production can occur in **phaeochromocytoma** which is a tumour of chromaffin cells. Initially, there are episodes of hypertension. At late stages, the **hypertension** becomes permanent. The tumour secretes more norepinephrine than epinephrine. The diagnosis can be confirmed by measuring the urinary excretion of **VMA**, which is increased in phaeochromocytoma.

ADRENOCORTICAL HORMONES

The adrenal cortex consists of zona glomerulosa, zona fasciculata and zona reticularis. Zona glomerulosa secretes mineralocorticoids. Zona fasciculata and zona reticularis secrete glucocorticoids and sex hormones. Mineralocorticoids produce their effects mainly on sodium and potassium metabolism. Glucocorticoids principally affect carbohydrate metabolism but also affect lipid and protein metabolism to a smaller extent. The sex hormones include androgens, oestrogen and progesterone but are quantitatively insignificant.

Chemistry and Synthesis

The adrenocortical hormones are steroids. Over 50 steroids have been isolated from the adrenal cortex. Only four of these are secreted in significant quantities, **cortisol, cortisone, aldosterone** and **deoxycorticosterone.** The first two are glucocorticoids. The latter two are mineralocorticoids. Cortisol and aldosterone are secreted in the largest quantities. All these hormones are synthesised from cholesterol. Ascorbic acid is required for steroid synthesis but its precise role is unknown (Fig. 17.23).

Transport, Metabolism and Excretion

The steroid hormones are transported by a specific carrier protein, **transcortin (corticosteroid binding globulin,**

CBG). This protein is an α-globulin. Small amounts are carried by albumin also. Very small amounts are transported in free form.

The steroid hormones are metabolised principally in liver. The double bond in the ring is reduced. The keto group at position 3 is also reduced. The reduced compound is conjugated with glucuronic acid, and to a smaller extent with sulphate. About 75% of the conjugated compound is excreted in urine. The rest is excreted in faeces.

Functions

Though the principal effects of glucocorticoids and mineralocorticoids are different, some overlapping is inevitable because of the similarity in their structures. The steroid hormones are bound to specific receptor proteins in the cytoplasm of their target cells. The steroid-receptor complex goes to the nucleus, and induces the synthesis of some specific proteins. These proteins produce the effects attributed to the hormone.

Functions of Glucocorticoids

Effect on Carbohydrate Metabolism

The main effect of glucocorticoids is to increase gluconeogenesis in liver. The synthesis of gluconeogenic enzymes is increased. The entry of amino acids into liver cells is increased. Amino acids, lactate and glycerol are converted into glucose and glycogen. The glycogen content of liver is increased.

The glucocorticoids also decrease the uptake and utilisation of glucose by the cells. As a result of increased formation and decreased utilisation of glucose, the blood glucose concentration is raised.

Effect on Protein Metabolism

Glucocorticoids decrease the synthesis, and increase the breakdown of proteins in extrahepatic tissues. Therefore, the plasma concentrations of amino acids are increased, and extrahepatic tissues are depleted of proteins.

On the other hand, the hepatic uptake of amino acids and protein synthesis are increased by glucocorticoids. The protein content of liver is increased. The concentrations of plasma proteins are also increased as the plasma proteins are synthesised mainly in the liver.

Effect on Lipid Metabolism

Glucocorticoids increase lipolysis and decrease lipogenesis in the adipose tissue. Concentration of free fatty acids in plasma is raised. Utilisation of fatty acids as a source of energy is also increased.

Other Effects

Glucocorticoids produce several other effects, many of which occur only when glucocorticoids are present in high

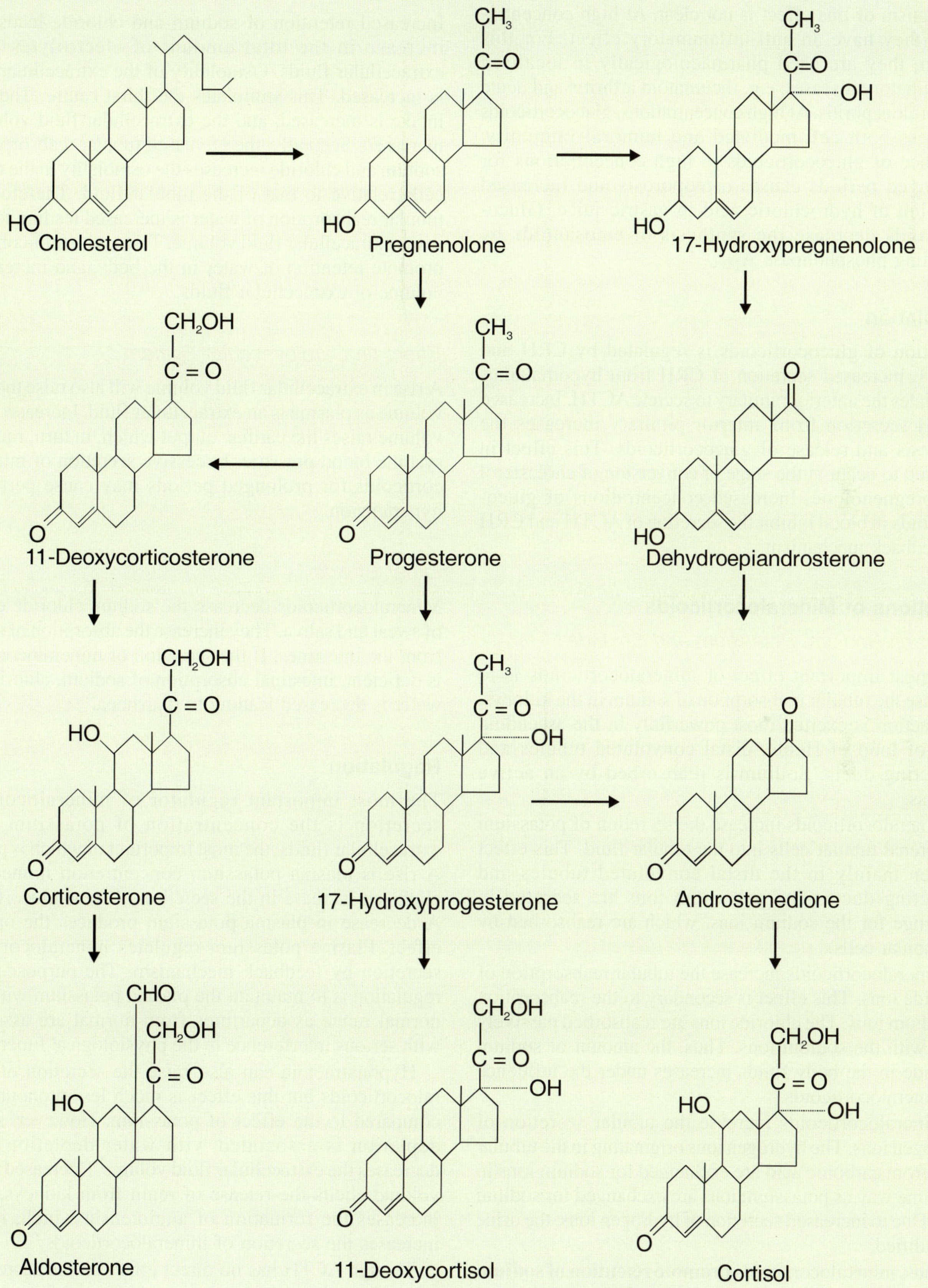

Fig. 17.23: Synthesis of adrenal corticoid hormones

concentrations. They help in combating stress though the mechanism of this effect is not clear. At high concentrations, they have an anti-inflammatory effect. For this reason, they are used pharmacologically in localised inflammatory diseases, e.g. rheumatoid arthritis and acute glomerulonephritis. At high concentrations, glucocorticoids suppress both cell-mediated and humoral immunity. Presence of glucocorticoids in high concentrations for prolonged periods causes osteoporosis and increased secretion of hydrochloric acid in gastric juice. Glucocorticoids decrease the synthesis of eicosanoids by inhibiting phospholipase A_2.

Regulation

Secretion of glucocorticoids is regulated by CRH and ACTH. Increased secretion of CRH from hypothalamus stimulates the anterior pituitary to secrete ACTH. Increased ACTH secretion from anterior pituitary increases the synthesis and release of glucocorticoids. This effect in believed to occur at the stage of conversion of cholesterol into pregnenolone. Increased concentrations of glucocorticoids in blood inhibit the secretion of ACTH and CRH by feedback mechanism.

Functions of Mineralocorticoids

Effect on Sodium, Potassium and Chloride

The most important effect of mineralocorticoids is to increase the tubular reabsorption of sodium in the kidneys. This action is exerted most powerfully in the ascending limb of loop of Henle, distal convoluted tubules and collecting ducts. Sodium is reabsorbed by an active process.

Mineralocorticoids increase the secretion of potassium from renal tubular cells into the tubular fluid. This effect is seen mainly in the distal convoluted tubules and collecting ducts. The potassium ions are secreted in exchange for the sodium ions, which are reabsorbed by the tubular cells.

Mineralocorticoids increase the tubular reabsorption of chloride ions. This effect is secondary to the reabsorption of sodium ions. The chloride ions are reabsorbed passively alongwith the sodium ions. Thus, the amount of sodium chloride in the body fluids increases under the influence of mineralocorticoids.

Mineralocorticoids increase the tubular secretion of hydrogen ions. The hydrogen ions originating in the tubular cells from carbonic acid are exchanged for sodium ions in the same way as potassium ions are exchanged for sodium ions. Due to increased secretion of hydrogen ions, the urine is acidified.

Thus, mineralocorticoids **promote retention of sodium** and chloride ions, and **excretion of potassium** and hydrogen ions.

Effect on Body Fluids

Increased retention of sodium and chloride leads to an increase in the total amount of electrolytes in the extracellular fluids. Osmolality of the extracellular fluids is increased. This stimulates the thirst centre. The water intake is increased, and the extracellular fluid volume is increased. Secondly, the increased tubular reabsorption of sodium and chloride increases the osmolality in the tubular cells relative to that of the tubular fluid. Therefore, the tubular reabsorption of water is increased leading to a rise in the extracellular fluid volume. Thus, mineralo-corticoids promote retention of water in the body, and increase the volume of extracellular fluids.

Effect on Cardiovascular System

A rise in extracellular fluid volume will also raise the blood volume as plasma is an extracellular fluid. Increased blood volume raises the cardiac output which, in turn, raises the systolic blood pressure. Excessive secretion of mineralocorticoids for prolonged periods may cause permanent hypertension.

Other Effects

Mineralocorticoids decrease the sodium chloride content of sweat and saliva. They increase the absorption of sodium from the intestines. If the secretion of mineralocorticoids is deficient, intestinal absorption of sodium, chloride and water is decreased leading to diarrhoea.

Regulation

The most important regulator of mineralocorticoid secretion is the concentration of potassium in the extracellular fluids, the most important of which is plasma. A rise is plasma potassium concentration immediately elicits an increase in the secretion of mineralocorticoids. A decrease in plasma potassium produces the opposite effect. Plasma potassium regulates mineralocorticoids secretion by feedback mechanism. The purpose of this regulation is to maintain the plasma potassium within the normal range as departures from normal are associated with serious interference in the physiological functioning.

Hyponatraemia can also raise the secretion of mineralocorticoids but this effect is much less pronounced as compared to the effect of potassium. However, sodium depletion is associated with water depletion which decreases the extracellular fluid volume. Decreased plasma volume elicits the release of renin from kidneys. Renin increases the formation of angiotensin which, in turn, increases the secretion of mineralocorticoids.

Though ACTH has no direct effect on the secretion of mineralocorticoids, its presence is essential for potassium and sodium to produce their effects.

DYSFUNCTION OF ADRENAL CORTEX

Deficient secretion of adrenocortical hormones results in hypoadrenocorticism. Excessive secretion results in hyperadrenocorticism.

Hypoadrenocorticism

Deficient production of adrenocortical hormones can occur due to atrophy of the gland or tuberculosis or cancer of the gland, and is known as **Addison's disease**. Production of both glucocorticoids and mineralocorticoids is decreased. The anterior pituitary responds by producing an excess of ACTH.

Deficient glucocorticoid production leads to hypoglycaemia in between meals. Mobilisation and utilisation of fats is also decreased. This leads to decreased availability of energy and muscular weakness. The ability to withstand stress is decreased.

Deficient production of mineralocorticoids leads to excessive loss of sodium, chloride and water in urine. Blood volume and cardiac output are decreased. There is a fall in blood pressure. Hyperkalaemia and acidosis develop due to decreased excretion of potassium and hydrogen ions. Hyperkalaemia can cause cardiac arrhythmias and death.

Increased production of ACTH, and possibly also of MSH, leads to increased pigmentation of mucous membranes and skin. Hyperpigmentation of skin usually occurs over face, neck and dorsum of hands.

Hyperadrenocorticism

Hyperactivity of adrenal cortex can produce three distinct syndromes:

1. Cushing's Syndrome

This results from hyperplasia or a tumour of the adrenal cortex. A similar clinical condition may occur due to excessive secretion of ACTH from anterior pituitary and is known as Cushing's disease.

Cushing's syndrome is clinically characterised by a centripetal distribution of fat, moon face, hyperglycaemia, tissue wasting, weakness, osteoporosis, acne and hirsutism.

2. Primary Aldosteronism

This results from a tumour of the zona glomerulosa. There is excessive secretion of mineralocorticoids. This leads to an increase in the extracellular fluid volume and blood volume, hypertension, polydipsia and polyuria. Hypokalaemia causes hyperpolarisation of the membranes of nerves and muscles leading to muscular weakness and fatigue.

Secondary aldosteronism can sometimes occur in patients with congestive heart failure, cirrhosis of liver, nephrotic syndrome, renal artery stenosis, etc. This is due to increased secretion of renin from the kidneys. Renin increases the formation of angiotensin, which acts on the adrenal cortex and increases the secretion of aldosterone.

3. Adrenogenital Syndrome

Adrenogenital syndrome or congenital adrenal hyperplasia can be considered to be an **inborn error of corticosteroid synthesis**. Some enzyme in the corticosteroid synthetic pathway is congenitally absent or deficient. This leads to a block in the pathway. The product is not synthesised, and the intermediates proximal to the block accumulate. The excess intermediates are channelised into alternate pathways.

The commonest disorder is **21-hydroxylase deficiency**. The production of glucocorticoids and mineralocorticoids is decreased. The intermediates are diverted to androgen synthesis. The syndrome is difficult to recognise in males. In females, it leads to the development of masculine features (female pseudohermaphroditism). In about a third of the patients, there is excessive sodium and water loss due to deficient aldosterone secretion.

The second commonest disorder is **11-β-hydroxylase deficiency** which leads to accumulation of 11-deoxycortisol and 11-deoxycorticosterone, and excessive production of androgens. Excess androgens cause masculinisation in females. Since 11-deoxycorticosterone possesses mineralocorticoid activity, its excess secretion leads to retention of sodium and water which, in turn, causes hypertension.

GONADAL HORMONES

Besides performing other functions concerned with reproduction, the gonads–testes in males, and ovaries in females–also secrete **sex hormones**. The male sex hormones are **androgens**. The females sex hormones are **oestrogens** and **progesterone**. Androgens are synthesised in the testes, oestrogens in ovaries, and progesterone in ovaries and placenta (Fig. 17.24).

MALE SEX HORMONES

The male sex hormones are testosterone, androsterone, androstenedione, epiandrosterone, dehydroepiandrosterone, etc. They are synthesised by the interstitial cells of Leydig in the testes, and are collectively known as androgens. Testosterone is the most potent and most abundant androgen. Testosterone circulates in blood in association with sex hormone binding globulin (SHBG) synthesied in the liver. The metabolic end products of androgens are 17-ketosteroids which are excreted in urine.

Functions

Secretion of androgens is insignificant before puberty. At puberty, the secretion of androgens increases markedly under the influence of LH of anterior pituitary. The androgens stimulate the development of primary and secondary sexual characteristics besides affecting some of the physiological and metabolic activities. The action occurs at the nuclear level. In many target cells, testosterone is converted into a more active compound, dihydrotestosterone (DHT) which is formed by reduction of the double bond between carbon atoms 5 and 6 of testosterone.

Effect on Sexual Characteristics

Androgens cause rapid development of testes, scrotum and penis at puberty. Secondary sexual characteristics such as deepening of voice and masculine distribution of body hair also appear under the influence of androgens. Normal spermatogenesis requires the presence of FSH and androgens. Androgens also increase the secretory activity of sebaceous glands which may lead to acne.

Effect on Nitrogen Balance

Androgens create a positive nitrogen balance. Synthesis of proteins is increased in various tissues including muscles. Muscular development which occurs after puberty is mainly due to androgens.

Effect on Bones

Androgens increase the size and the strength of bones. The primary effect is increased formation of matrix proteins. Calcium deposition is increased due to increased availability of bone matrix.

Effect on Basal Metabolic Rate

Androgens increase the basal metabolic rate.

Effect on Electrolytes

Androgens increase the retention of sodium though to a much smaller extent as compared to the mineralocorticoids.

Regulation

Secretion of androgens is regulated by feedback mechanism. LH increases the secretion of androgens. Excess of androgens inhibits further secretion of LH through inhibition of GnRH secretion from hypothalamus.

GONADAL DYSFUNCTION IN MALES

Deficient secretion of sex hormones causes hypogonadism. Excessive secretion causes hypergonadism.

Hypogonadism

This may be due to congenital absence of testes, undeveloped testes due to deficiency of gonadotropic hormones, undescended testes or castration. Hypogonadism developing before puberty leads to eunuchism. Primary and secondary sexual characteristics fail to develop. Sex organs remain infantile. Bones and muscles are weak.

When hypogonadism develops after puberty, there is some regression of secondary sexual characteristics. Sexual feelings are decreased. Behavioural changes, e.g. irritability, passivity and depression are common.

Sometimes, hypogonadism occurs due to a hypothalamic lesion which decreases the secretion of gonadotropic hormones from the anterior pituitary. The hypothalamic lesion also stimulates the feeding centre, and leads to overeating. The patient develops eunuchism and obesity.

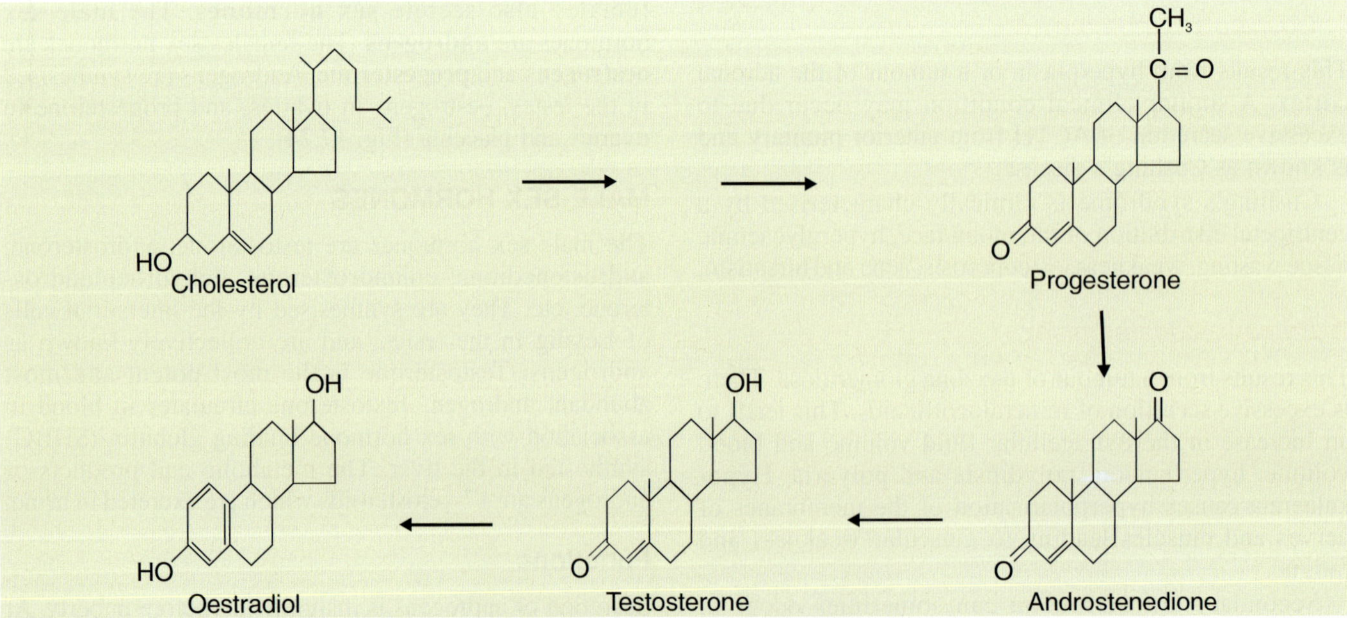

Fig. 17.24: Synthesis of sex hormones

This condition is known as adiposogenital syndrome or Frohlich's syndrome.

Hypergonadism

This is due to a tumour of the Leydig cells which secretes an excess of androgens. When it develops before puberty, it causes precocious pseudopuberty. There is excessive and premature development of sex organs and secondary sexual characteristics. But there is no spermatogenesis as FSH production is not increased. The growth of muscles and bones is accelerated. However, early union of epiphyses decreases the stature.

Development of Leydig cell tumour after puberty is difficult to diagnose because the primary and secondary sexual characteristics are already fully developed. However, increased excretion of 17-ketosteroids in urine will confirm the diagnosis.

FEMALE SEX HORMONES

A number of sex hormones are secreted by the ovaries. These can be broadly divided into oestrogens and progesterone. In pregnancy, placenta also secretes significant amounts of progesterone.

OESTROGENS

Several oestrogenic hormones are synthesised by graafian follicles in the ovaries. Only three of them are secreted in significant quantities, oestradiol, oestrone and oestriol. Oestradiol is the most potent of these. Oestrogens are metabolised in the liver, and excreted in bile.

Some synthetic oestrogenic compounds, e.g. ethinyl oestradiol, mestranol and diethylstilbestrol, are used pharmacologically, and are more potent than the naturally occurring oestrogens.

Functions

Effect on Sexual Organs

The secretion of oestrogens increases at puberty under the influence of gonadotropic hormones of anterior pituitary. The oestrogens stimulate the development of sexual organs. Fallopian tubes, uterus, vagina, labia majora and labia minora are enlarged. The cuboidal epithelium of vagina is changed into stratified epithelium. There is proliferation of endometrium and mucosal lining of fallopian tubes.

Effect on Secondary Sexual Characteristics

Oestrogens stimulate the development of secondary sexual characteristics. Breasts are enlarged.

Effect on Nitrogen Balance

The nitrogen balance becomes positive. Protein synthesis is increased. However, the protein anabolic effect of oestrogens is not as strong as that of androgens.

Effect on Fat Deposition

Oestrogens increase deposition of fat in subcutaneous tissues.

Effect on Bones

Oestrogens increase skeletal growth. The pelvis is broadened, and the size of the pelvic outlet is increased.

Effect on Electrolytes

Oestrogens increase the retention of sodium, chloride and water but are much weaker than mineralocorticoids in this respect. However, this effect may become significant in pregnancy.

Regulation

Regulation of oestrogen secretion is complex. There are cyclic changes in the secretion of oestrogens during menstrual cycle. These changes are essential for the occurrence of normal menstrual cycles. The cyclic changes are regulated by the gonadotropic hormones of the anterior pituitary which, in turn, are under the control of GnRH.

FSH increases the secretion of oestrogens from the graafian follicles in the first half of the menstrual cycle. When the concentration of oestrogens reaches a critical level, it inhibits the secretion of FSH acting through hypothalamus. The graafian follicle ruptures.Oestrogen secretion declines after the rupture of graafian follicle.

PROGESTERONE

Progesterone is secreted by the corpus luteum, placenta and adrenal cortex. In non-pregnant women, corpus luteum is the major source of progesterone. The secretion of progesterone is most abundant in the second half of the menstrual cycle. In pregnancy, placenta becomes the major source of progesterone. Progesterone is transported in blood by transcortin. The major metabolite of progesterone is pregnanediol, which is conjugated with glucuronic acid, and is excreted in urine.

Some synthetic progesterones, e.g. norethindrone and norethynodrel areused pharmacologically. These are more potent than natural progesterone.

Functions

Effect on Reproductive Organs

Progesterone is secreted in significant quantities in the second half of the menstrual cycle (after ovulation). In the first half of the cycle, oestrogen causes proliferation of the endometrium. After ovulation, progesterone causes secretory changes in the endometrium, and induces the secretion of mucus. This is essential for the implantation of the fertilised ovum. If pregnancy occurs, the corpus luteum continues to secrete progesterone. The placenta also secretes progesterone. Progesterone maintains pregnancy, and prevents ovulation and menstruation during pregnancy. If pregnancy does not occur, the secretion of progesterone declines around the twenty-sixth day of the cycle. The proliferated endometrium is shed off, and is lost with the menstrual bleeding.

Effect on Breasts

Alongwith oestrogens, progesterone stimulates the development of breasts.

Effect on Electrolytes

In high concentration, progesterone mimics the effect of mineralocorticoids on electrolytes.

Regulation

As with oestrogens, there are cyclic changes in the secretion of progesterone during each menstrual cycle in non-pregnant women. The secretion of progesterone is stimulated by LH. Excess of progesterone inhibits the secretion of LH.

GONADAL DYSFUNCTION IN FEMALES

As in males, deficient secretion of female sex hormones results in hypogonadism, and excessive secretion results in hypergonadism.

Hypogonadism

This may be due to hypopituitarism, gonadal agenesis or polycystic ovaries.

Depending upon the age of outset and severity of the disease, it may cause a variety of clinical features. These include sexual infantilism, delayed menarche, scanty menstrual bleeding, absence of menstrual bleeding, infertility, etc. Virilism may occur in some patients due to excessive secretion of androgens.

Hypergonadism

Excessive secretion of sex hormones may occur in early childhood due to hypothalamic disease or an unknown cause. This causes precocious puberty. Primary and secondary sexual characteristics and reproductive potential develop prematurely.

Some ovarian and adrenal tumours cause precocious pseudopuberty in which sexual development occurs prematurely but the patient is infertile due to lack of ovulation.

Some ovarian tumours occur in adult life. They may produce an excess of oestrogens or androgens. The oestrogen-secreting tumours cause increase in libido,

postmenopausal bleeding and endometrial hyperplasia. The androgen-secreting tumours cause amenorrhoea, sterility and masculinisation.

CHORIONIC GONADOTROPIN

Chorionic gonadotropin is secreted during pregnancy by the placenta. It is a glycoprotein, and its actions resemble those of LH. It maintains the corpus luteum during pregnancy.

Chorionic gonadotropin can be detected in the urine of pregnant women eight days after the first missed period. Most of the older pregnancy tests, e.g. Aschheim-Zondek test and Friedman test that lacked sensitivity, and the modern dry-reagent strip tests, are based on the detection of chorionic gonadotropin in urine. Secretion of chorionic gonadotropin reaches its peak 6 to 8 weeks after fertilisation and, then, declines.

RELAXIN

It is a polypeptide with a molecular weight of about 9,000. It is secreted during pregnancy by placenta and corpus luteum. It causes relaxation of pelvic ligaments and symphysis pubis, and facilitates the passage of the foetus during parturition. However, the exact role of relaxin in human beings is yet to be established.

PLACENTAL LACTOGEN

This is another polypeptide hormone secreted by the placenta. Its molecular weights is about 38,000. It is also known as chorionic somatomammotropin. Its actions partly resemble those of growth hormone and partly those of prolactin. But its function in human beings is still unknown.

GASTROINTESTINAL HORMONES

Cells of gastrointestinal mucosa secrete a number of hormones into circulation. The hormone-secreting cells are not organised into discrete anatomical structures but are dispersed in the gastrointestinal tract. The gastrointestinal hormones have short half-lives, and produce their effects on the gastrointestinal tract itself and on some closely related organs, e.g. pancreas and liver. The following are the important gastrointestinal hormones:

GASTRIN

Gastrin is a polypeptide made up of 17 amino acids, and has a molecular weight of 2,100. There are two closely related hormones, gastrin I and gastrin II. They have an identical amino acid sequence but the tyrosine residue at position 12 is sulphated in gastrin II. Only the last four amino acid residues are essential for biological activity. A synthetic compound having these four amino acids plus alanine is commercially available, and is known as pentagastrin.

Gastrin is secreted by gastric mucosa in response to the entry of food into stomach. Acetylcholine and vagal stimulation also evoke gastrin secretion. Gastrin stimulates the secretion of gastric juice which is rich in hydrochloric acid and pepsin.

SECRETIN

Secretin was the first hormone to be discovered. It is a polypeptide made up of 27 amino acids. It has a molecular weight of 3,000. It is secreted by the mucosa of duodenum and jejunum in response to the entry of food and hydrochloric acid into duodenum. It stimulates the secretion of pancreatic juice rich in bicarbonate. It inhibits gastric acid secretion and intestinal motility.

CHOLECYSTOKININ

Cholecystokinin or cholecystokinin-pancreozymin (CCK-PZ) is a polypeptide made up of 33 amino acids. Its molecular weight is about 4,000. It is secreted by the mucosa of small intestine in response to the entry of food in the gut. It stimulates the secretion of enzyme-rich pancreatic juice, and causes contraction of the gall bladder leading to expulsion of bile into the duodenum.

GASTRIC INHIBITORY PEPTIDE

Gastric inhibitory peptide (GIP) is made up of 43 amino acids, and has a molecular weight of about 5,100. It is secreted by the mucosa of duodenum and jejunum in response to the entry of carbohydrates and fat into the duodenum. It inhibits gastric acid secretion and gastric motility. It also evokes the secretion of insulin.

VASOACTIVE INTESTINAL PEPTIDE

Vasoactive intestinal peptide (VIP) is made up of 28 amino acids, and has a molecular weight of about 3,100. It is secreted by the mucosa of small intestine and colon. The stimulus for its secretion is not known. It inhibits gastric secretion and motility. It stimulates the secretion of pancreatic juice and succus entericus. It inhibits the contraction of gall bladder.

MOTILIN

Motilin is a peptide made up of 22 amino acids. Its molecular weight is about 2,700. It is secreted by the mucosa of duodenum and jejunum. It increases gastric motility.

PANCREATIC POLYPEPTIDE

This is a polypeptide made up of 36 amino acids. It is secreted by F cells of the islets of Langerhans. Its secretion is evoked by a protein-rich meal, fasting, hypoglycaemia and exercise. It decreases the bicarbonate and protein content of pancreatic juice.

SOMATOSTATIN

This is a peptide made up of 14 amino acids. It is secreted by D cells (δ cells) of islets of Langerhans. It is identical in structure to the hypothalamic somatostatin. Pancreatic somatostatin inhibits the secretion of gastrin, secretin, cholecystokinin-pancreozymin and pancreatic polypeptide.

LOCAL HORMONES

These hormones are produced in different tissues, and produce their effects in their immediate vicinity. Some of the hormones are produced in blood itself from some pre-existing precursors.

HISTAMINE

Histamine is synthesised in a variety of tissues, e.g. skin, intestines, lungs, etc. It is formed from histidine (Fig. 17.25).

Functions

Histamine acts by increasing the intracellular concentration of cAMP, and altering the permeability of the cell membrane to some ions. Histamine receptors are of two types, H_1 receptors and H_2 receptors. Some tissues, e.g. brain and blood vessels possess both types of receptors. Smooth muscles have only H_1 receptors. Secretory cells of gastric mucosa and leukocytes have only H_2 receptors.

Effect on Capillary Permeability

Histamine increases the permeability of capillaries. Colloidal substances pass out of the capillaries into the interstitial fluid. Colloid osmotic pressure of the interstitial fluid is increased. Water passes from blood vessels into the interstitial space. Blood volume is decreased.

Effect on Blood Vessels

Histamine causes dilatation of arterioles and capillaries. Peripheral resistance is decreased. Diastolic blood pressure falls. Decreased blood volume may cause a fall in systolic blood pressure as well. Heart rate is increased.

Effect on Smooth Muscles

Histamine causes contraction of smooth muscles of bronchioles, intestine and uterus.

Effect on Exocrine Glands

Histamine is a powerful stimulant of gastric secretion. The gastric juice secreted under the influence of histamine is rich in hydrochloric acid. Secretion of saliva, pancreatic juice, succus entericus and lacrimal fluid is also mildly stimulated by histamine.

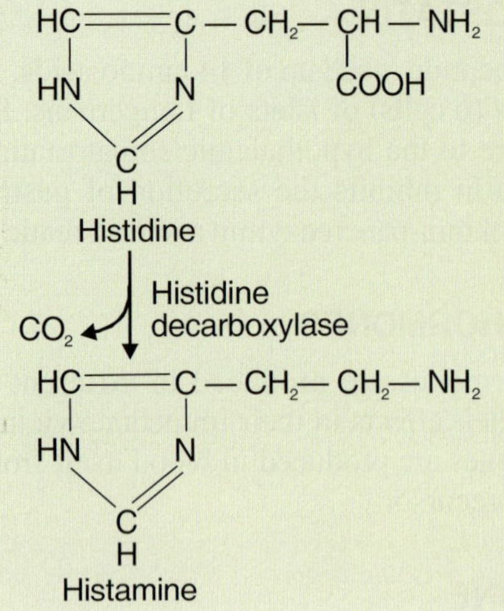

Fig. 17.25: Synthesis of histamine

Role in Allergic Response

The allergic reactions occur due to allergen-antibody reaction which releases histamine and some other chemicals from mast cells and basophils. The liberated histamine produces some of the manifestations of allergic reactions, e.g. hypotension, contraction of smooth muscles, itching, rash, etc.

Metabolism and Excretion

A small amount of histamine is excreted as such in urine. Some of the histamine is conjugated with acetic acid to from N-acetyl histamine which is excreted in urine. The rest is oxidised by histaminase into 4-imidazole acetic acid which is also excreted in urine.

Histamine Agonists and Antagonists

Some drugs, e.g. morphine, pethedine, tubocurarine, etc. stimulate the release of histamine from tissues. Epinephrine does not affect the secretion of histamine but acts as its antagonist by producing opposite physiological effects, e.g. vasoconstriction and relaxation of smooth muscles.

Certain drugs known as **anti-histamines** occupy the histamine receptors and prevent the attachment of histamine to the receptors. They, thus, block the effects of histamine. Drugs like diphenhydramine, mepyramine, pyrilamine and promethazine block the H_1 receptors.

Some more recent drugs, e.g. cimetidine and ranitidine, block the H_2 receptors. These drugs, known as H_2 blockers, are used to decrease gastric hydrochloric acid secretion.

SEROTONIN

Serotonin is synthesised in gastrointestinal mucosa and brain from tryptophan (Fig. 17.16).

Functions

1. *Effect on cardiovascular system:* Serotonin increases the force of contraction of heart, and causes vasoconstriction. Systolic and diastolic blood pressures are raised.
2. *Effect on respiration:* Rate of respiration is increased.
3. *Effects on kidneys:* It decreases urinary volume.
4. *Effect on smooth muscles:* Serotonin causes contraction of smooth muscles of bronchioles, intestines, uterus, etc.
5. *Effect on gastrointestinal tract:* Serotonin increases peristalsis.

Metabolism and Excretion

Serotonin is oxidised by monoamine oxidase to 5-hydroxyindole acetic acid which is excreted in urine (Fig. 17.26).

A number of peptides described earlier as physiologically active peptides viz. angiotensin, bradykinin and met-enkephalin can also be considered as local hormones. **Nitric oxide**, besides having other functions, also acts as a local hormone.

Definition of hormones has broadened now. Several polypeptide growth factors which stimulate the growth of various target cells by acting through specific receptors may be considered as hormones. These include nerve growth factor (NGF), fibroblast growth factor (FGF), epidermal growth factor (EGF), platelet-derived growth factor (PDGF), etc. The cytokines which act on their target cells via specific receptors may also be regarded as hormones.

New compounds having hormone-like properties (candidate hormones) are being discovered with increasing frequency. Advances in molecular biology have made cloning, sequencing and characterisation of candidate protein hormones and their receptors easier. These

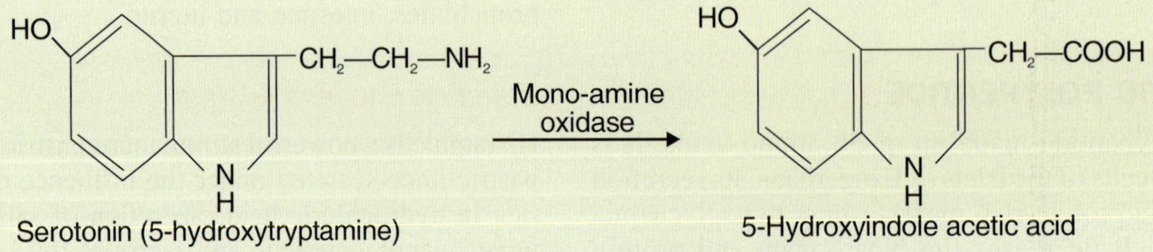

Fig. 17.26: Catabolism of serotonin

candidate hormones may become established as hormones in future. OB protein, the product of ob gene has become established as a hormone in mice. The analogous **leptin** protein, encoded by leptin gene, in human beings is more or less established as a hormone. It is secreted by adipocytes and decreases appetite byacting on hypothalamus.

EXERCISE

1. Describe the mechanism of action of protein hormones.

2. Describe the mechanism of action of steroid hormones. Explain the role of hormone response elements.

3. Write short notes on:
   a. Second messengers
   b. G-proteins
   c. Insulin receptor
   d. Nitric oxide
   e. Radio-immuno-assay
   f. ELISA
   g. Hypothalamic hormones
   h. ADH
   i. Hyperparathyroidism
   j. Serotonin
   k. Histamine
   l. Chorionicgonadotropin

4. Write 'true' or 'false':
   a. Hormone receptors have at least two domains.
   b. Receptors for protein hormones are intracellular.
   c. A hormone may have more than one type of receptors.
   d. A hormone may use more than one second messengers.
   e. A receptor may bind more than one hormones.
   f. G-protein is a tetramer having two α- and two β-subunits.
   g. G-proteins may be stimulatory or inhibitory.
   h. Displacement of GTP by GDP activates the G-protein.
   i. G-proteins carry the signal from receptor to the effector.
   j. Diacylglycerol activates protein kinase G.
   k. Insulin receptor possesses tyrosine kinase domain.
   l. Insulin-like growth factors mediate some of the effects of insulin.
   m. Pro-opiomelanocortin is the precursor of ACTH.
   n. Differential processing of pro-opiomelanocortin yields different peptides.
   o. Melatonin is synthesised from tryptophan.
   p. Metabolic effects of insulin are mediated by insulin receptor substrate-1.
   q. Blood-brain barrier is permeable to dopamine but not to epinephrine.
   r. Dihydrotestosterone is an inactive metabolite of testosterone.
   s. H_2 receptor blockers decrease the secretion of hydrochloric acid in gastric juice.
   t. Leptin, secreted by hypothalamus, increases appetite.

5. Fill in the blanks:
   a. Hormone receptors are chemically .... in nature.
   b. The .... subunit of G-proteins can bind GDP or GTP.
   c. Protein kinase A is activated by ....
   d. .... activates protein kinase G.
   e. Protein kinase C is activated by ....
   f. Tyrosine kinase domain is present in the .... subunit of insulin receptor.
   g. A decrease in the number of receptors is called ....
   h. .... is the second messenger for atrial natriuretic peptide.
   i. The second messenger for nitric oxide is ....
   j. Nitric oxide is synthesised from ....
   k. Phospholipase C hydrolyses phosphatidyl inositol-4,5-biphosphate into .... and ....
   l. Deficient secretion of .... causes diabetes insipidus.

m. Serotonin is synthesised from ....
n. A fasting plasma glucose above .... mg/dl on two occasions is diagnostic of diabetes mellitus.
o. Binding of epinephrine to .... receptors activates phospholipase C.
p. Urinary excretion of .... is increased in phaeochromocytoma.
q. Chorionic gonadotropin is secreted by ....
r. .... was the first hormone to be discovered.
s. Serotonin is degraded by the enzyme ....
t. .... is the only hormone which is a gas.

ANSWERS TO SHORT QUESTIONS

4. a. True
   c. True
   e. False
   g. True
   i. True
   k. True
   m. True
   o. True
   q. True
   s. True

   b. False
   d. True
   f. False
   h. False
   j. False
   l. False
   n. True
   p. False
   r. False
   t. False

5. a. Proteins
   c. cAMP
   e. Diacylglycerol
   g. Downregulation
   i. cGMP
   k. DAG, IP_3
   m. Tryptophan
   o. α_1-Adrenergic
   q. Placenta
   s. Mono-amine oxidase

   b. Alpha
   d. cGMP
   f. Beta
   h. cGMP
   j. Arginine
   l. ADH
   n. 126
   p. VMA
   r. Secretin
   t. Nitric oxide

18

Cancer: Proto-oncogenes, Oncogenes and Anti-oncogenes

Cancer is a disorder of **cell growth**. Normally, cell division is precisely regulated. As long as the regulatory mechanisms operate normally, the rate of cell division remains optimum. However, a disturbance in regulation leads to excessive cell division transforming normal cells into cancer cells. Apart from **uncontrolled cell division**, the cancer cells **invade** the neighbouring cells and tissues, and can **spread** to distant sites (metastasis). When a cancer cell divides, the daughter cells are also cancer cells. This shows that when a normal cell transforms into a cancer cell, some change occurs in its DNA which is transmitted to the daughter cells. The role of DNA in malignant transformation is also proved by transfection experiments. When DNA from a cancer cell is transferred into a normal cell, the recipient cell changes into a cancer cell.

Cancers of epithelial cells are known as **carcinomas,** and those of connective tissue are known as **sarcomas**. Both are also collectively known as malignant neoplasms or malignant tumours or malignant growths or malignancies.

Transformation of normal cells into cancer cells may be brought about by physical agents, chemical agents or biological agents.

Physical Agents

The physical agents that can cause cancer include ultraviolet rays, X-rays and γ-rays. These are also known to damage DNA. For example, ultraviolet rays cause the formation of pyrimidine dimers. X-rays and γ-rays generate free radicals, which can damage DNA.

Chemical Agents

Many mutagenic chemicals that damage DNA are also known to cause cancer. Such chemicals include benzpyrene, dimethylbenzanthracene, acetylamino-fluorene, dimethylnitrosamine, diethylnitrosamine, aflatoxin B, asbestos, beryllium, etc. Some of these can directly transform normal cells into cancer cells and are known as **carcinogens**. Some are not directly carcinogenic but can be converted into carcinogens in the body. These are known as **procar-**

cinogens. Conversion of a procarcinogen into a carcinogen usually involves microsomal hydroxylation of the compound.

Detection of Carcinogens

A number of new chemicals are introduced every year many of which may be carcinogenic. Their safety has to be established before their introduction in the market. Carcinogenicity testing in animals is expensive and time-consuming. A rapid and inexpensive test for detection of mutagenicity and potential carcinogenicity was devised by Ames, and is known as **Ames' assay**. In this test, a mutant tester strain of *Salmonella typhimurium* is used which has lost the ability to synthesise histidine due to a mutation. A culture of this tester strain is grown on agar gel in the **absence of histidine** in two petri dishes. The chemical being tested is added to one of the dishes. If the chemical is mutagenic (and hence potentially carcingenic), it will cause mutations in the tester strain. One of the mutations may restore the ability of the micro-organism to synthesise histidine. The dishes are compared after 48 hours. Very few colonies of bacteria will be seen in the dish without the mutagenic chemical while several colonies will be seen in the dish having the mutagenic chemical.

Since the bacteria lack the microsomal hydroxylase system which is required to convert procarcinogens into carcinogens, pre-incubation of the chemical with mammalian liver homogenate may be done to convert procarcinogens into carcinogens.

Biological Agents

Some DNA as well as RNA viruses can cause cancer in animals and human beings. Such viruses are known as **oncoviruses**. In this case also, the DNA of the infected cell is altered by the introduction of viral genes into the host cell genome.

ONCOGENES

Investigation of oncoviral genomes revealed the presence of oncogenes in these viruses. Rous sarcoma virus, which causes sarcoma in chickens, was the first oncovirus to be discovered. It was later found to possess an oncogene known as src gene. Other oncogenes found in viruses include ras, sis, myb, myc, abl, trk, fos, erb B, etc.

PROTO-ONCOGENES

Later on, some genes similar to viral oncogenes were discovered in healthy animals and human beings. These were named proto-oncogenes. It was suggested that conversion of proto-oncogenes into oncogenes transforms normal cells into cancer cells. Such a conversion may be brought about by radiations, mutagenic chemicals or viruses. Therefore, activation of proto-oncogenes is thought to be a critical event which pushes a normal cell into malignant transformation.

Functions of Proto-oncogenes

Since proto-oncogenes are present in normal cells, they must serve some purpose. Like all genes, they encode some proteins. These proteins are generally growth factors or receptors for growth factors or signal transducers that transmit growth signals from receptors to effectors. Growth factors are similar to protein hormones. They are secreted by some cells and may act on distant cells (endocrine), neighbouring cells (paracrine) or on the cells secreting the growth factor (autocrine). The target cells contain transmembrane receptors for growth factors. The cytoplasmic portion of the receptors may possess tyrosine kinase activity or may send signals to adenylate cyclase or phosphoinositidase (phospholipase C). A G-protein may also be involved in signal transduction. Binding of the growth factor to its receptor stimulates the cell to divide.

Growth factors discovered in human beings include platelet-derived growth factor (PDGF), epidermal growth factor (EGF), nerve growth factor (NGF), fibroblast growth factor (FGF), insulin-like growth factor-1 (IGF-1), insulin-like growth factor-2 (IGF-2), etc. When a proto-oncogene is activated to an oncogene, the encoded growth factor or receptor or transducer becomes abnormal either in quantity or in activity. This results in persistent stimulation of growth and the stimulated cell beings to divide uncontrollably. Some proto-oncogenes encode nuclear transcription factors that bind to DNA and regulate the expression of genes that affect cell growth. Some common proto-oncogenes and the proteins they encode are:

1. **Genes encoding growth factors:** sis gene encodes PDGF.
2. **Genes encoding receptors for growth factors:** erb B gene encodes the receptor for EGF, and trk gene encodes the receptor for NGF.
3. **Genes encoding signal transducers:** ras gene encodes a GDP/GTP binding protein.
4. **Genes encoding nuclear transcription factors:** fos gene encodes transcription factor, AP-1. myc gene encodes a DNA binding protein.

Activation of Proto-oncogenes to Oncogenes

Activation of proto-oncogenes to oncogenes may be brought about by incorporation of viral genome into the host cell genome. Even the viruses which do not have oncogenes can activate the proto-oncogenes. Physical and chemical agents can cause mutations which can result in abnormally high expression of proto-oncogenes or synthesis of abnormal products. Various mechanisms by which malignant transformation can occur are:

1. *Insertion of a Promoter*

When viral genome is incorporated into host cell genome, a viral promoter may be placed just upstream of a proto-oncogene. This can cause excessive expression of the proto-oncogene resulting in an abnormally high rate of cell growth.

2. *Insertion of an Enhancer*

Incorporation of viral genome into host cell genome may place a proto-oncogene under the control of a viral enhancer element. The enhancer element will cause increased expression of the normal proto-oncogene.

3. *Gene Amplification*

Multiple copies of a gene may be formed in the genome by gene amplification. Amplification of certain genes occurs during growing age, and ensures rapid growth. Amplification of some genes is seen in certain cancers. If a proto-oncogene is amplified, its product will be formed in large quantities leading to excessive cell growth.

4. *Chromosomal Translocation*

In some cancer cells, abnormal chromosomes are seen which result from translocation of a fragment of chromosome from one chromosome to another. Sometimes, the translocation is reciprocal, e.g. in **Burkitt's lymphoma**. In this B-cell cancer, reciprocal translocation occurs between chromosomes 8 and 14 as a result of which the myc gene of chromosome 8 migrates to chromosome 14, and is placed under the control of enhancer element of heavy (H) chain immunoglobulin gene. Therefore, the expression of myc gene is increased (Fig. 18.1).

5. *Deletion*

Deletion from a proto-oncogene can result in the synthesis of an abnormal protein. For example, erb B proto-oncogene encodes the **receptor for EGF**. The EGF receptor is a transmembrane polypeptide that possesses an EGF binding site on the extracellular side and a tyrosine kinase domain on the cytosolic side. Binding of EGF to two neighbouring receptors causes them to dimerise. This activates the tyrosine kinase domains of the dimer. Each receptor

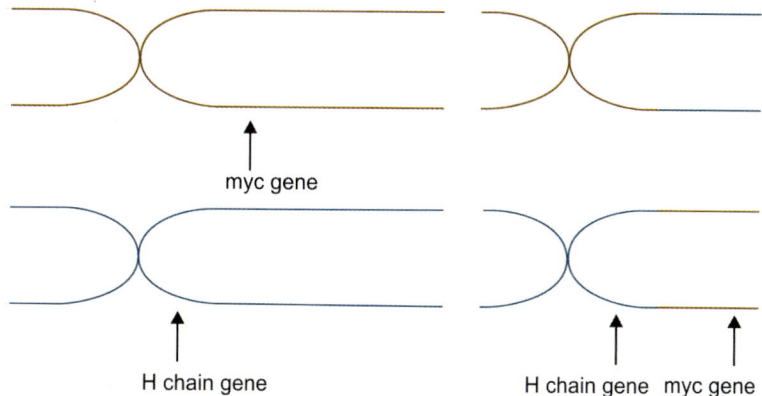

Fig.18.1: Chromosomal translocation in Burkitt's lymphoma. Expression of translocated myc gene is increased by the enhancer element of heavy (H) chain immunoglobulin gene

peptide phosphorylates the tyrosine residues of the other (Fig. 18.2).

The auto-phosphorylated tyrosine kinase domains phosphorylate the tyrosine residues of some target proteins. These proteins possess SH2 (src homology 2) domains which have an affinity for the auto-phosphorylated tyrosine kinase domain of the receptor. One such protein is growth factor receptor binding protein 2 (GRB 2). Phosphorylation of GRB 2 stimulates cell division by a cascade of reactions. (Fig. 18.3).

Deletion of a part of the erb B gene results in the synthesis of a **truncated receptor** which lacks the EGF binding site. The mutant receptor gets dimerised and auto-phosphorylated in the absence of EGF. Thus, growth signals are generated persistently even in the absence of EGF leading to unrestrained cell division.

6. *Point Mutation*

A single base substitution in a proto-oncogene may lead to the synthesis of an abnormal protein.

A gene implicated in several cancers is the **ras** proto-oncogene. It encodes a protein, **p21** which is a component of a long signal transduction pathway involving EGF and perhaps some other growth factors and hormones. p21 is analogous to G-proteins which act as signal transducers for many hormones. However, p21 is a monomer having a **GDP/GTP binding site.** When this site is occupied by GDP, p21 is inactive. Displacement of GDP by GTP makes p21 active. Active p21 sends signals to effectors that stimulate cell division and growth.

Like G-proteins, p21 possesses a **GTPase domain** which hydrolyses GTP into GDP and Pi. Conversion of GTP into GDP makes p21 inactive, terminating the growth

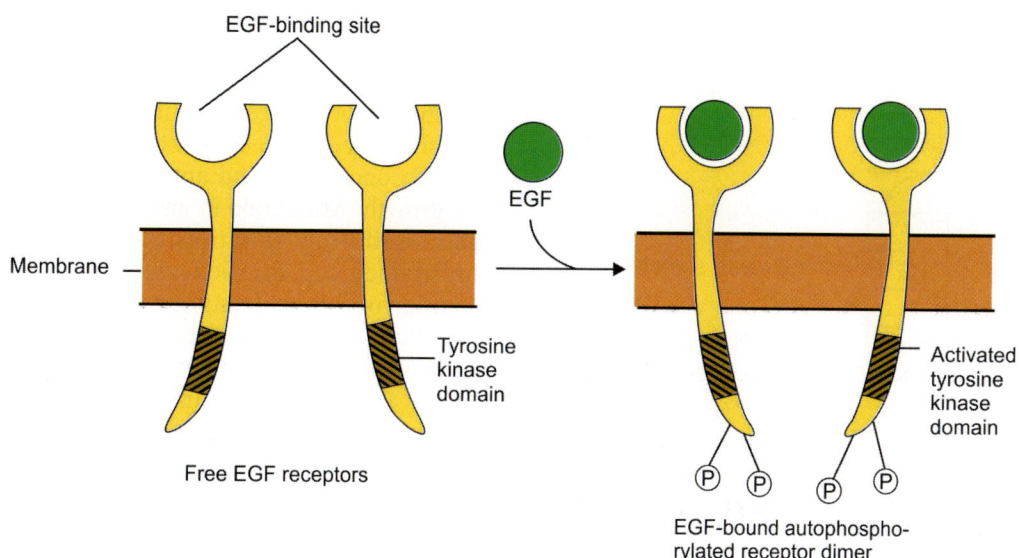

Fig.18.2: Binding of EGF to its receptors causes dimerisation of two receptors and activation of their tyrosine kinase domains. Each receptor molecule phosphorylates some tyrosine residues of the other. The auto-phosphorylated receptor phosphorylates the tyrosine residues of some target proteins generating growth signals

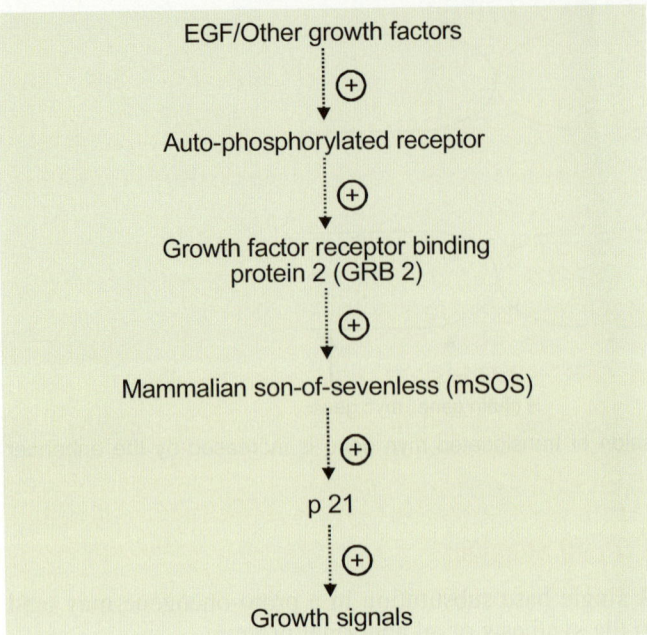

Fig. 18.3: A signal transduction cascade which activates p 21. Active p 21 sends growth signals to effectors that stimulate cell division

signals. However, another protein, **GTPase activating protein (GAP)** is required to switch on the GTPase activity of p21(Fig. 18.4).

Ras proto-oncogene is converted into an oncogene by a point mutation (GGC to GTC in codon 12). This results in the **substitution** of glycine by valine at position 12 in p21. This substitution **abolishes the GTPase activity** of p21 locking it permanently in its active state. Therefore, p21 sends growth signals persistently even in the absence of the growth factor resulting in excessive cell division.

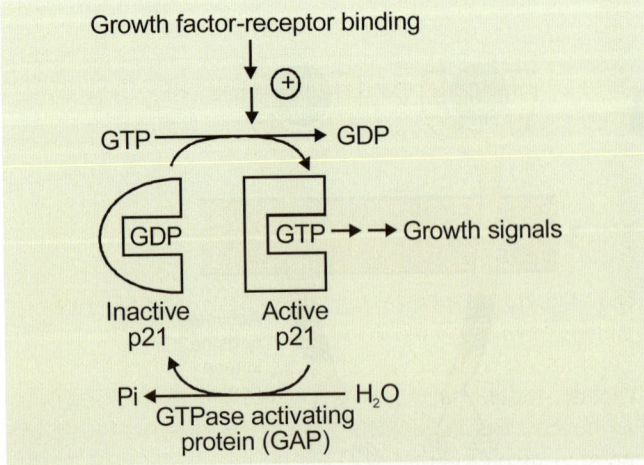

Fig. 18.4: Binding of the growth factor to its receptor starts a cascade of reactions that results in displacement GDP by GTP in p21 making it active. Active p21 sends growth signals. GTP is hydrolysed by the intrinsic GTPase activity of p21 which is switched on by GAP

Thus, activated proto-oncogenes can transform a healthy cell into a cancer cell either due to overexpression of genes resulting in excessive formation of the normal gene products or due to formation of abnormal gene products.

Oncoviruses transform infected cells by inserting their oncogene(s) into the DNA of the infected cells. The oncogenes are slightly altered versions of proto-oncogenes. Oncoviruses have most probably acquired these genes from animals (including man). When a virus infects an animal cell, the viral genome (or its DNA copy in case of retroviruses) is integrated into the host cell genome. When the viral genome breaks out of the host cell genome, it is not unusual for the virus to pick up some gene(s) from the host cell DNA. It is very likely that some viruses picked up proto-oncogenes from animal cells and, in time, these proto-oncogenes mutated and became oncogenes. When an oncovirus having an oncogene infects another host, the oncogene is incorporated in the DNA of the new host. The mutant oncogene is not subject to normal regulation or its protein product is abnormal. This leads to excessive growth of the host cell.

To differentiate between the proto-oncogenes normally present in animal and human cells, and the closely similar oncogenes present in viruses, letter 'c' is put before the names of cellular proto-oncogenes. Similarly, the letter 'v' is put before the names of viral oncogenes. Thus **c-ras** means the ras proto-oncogene present in animal cells, and **v-ras** means the ras oncogene present in viruses.

ANTI-ONCOGENES

Just as a number of growth-promoting proto-oncogenes are present in our genome, some genes having an opposite function are also present. These are known as anti-oncogenes or **tumour suppressor genes**. Anti-oncogenes were discovered much later than the oncogenes, and the information available about anti-oncogenes is much less than that about oncogenes. Anti-oncogenes encode proteins that **inhibit** cell division. A balance between the actions of proto-oncogenes and anti-oncogenes ensures optimal cell growth. Mutations in anti-oncogenes lead to **loss of their inhibitory function** tilting the balance towards unrestrained cell division. A major difference between proto-oncogenes and anti-oncogenes is that a mutation in one allele of a proto-oncogene is enough to alter its function while mutations in both the alleles are required to alter the function of an anti-oncogene. Thus, proto-oncogenes are dominant while anti-oncogenes are recessive. Some well investigated anti-oncogenes are:

1. p53 Gene

When p53 gene was discovered, it was believed to be an oncogene because its product, p53 protein, was found to be present in a number of cancers. p53 protein was presumed to be an oncoprotein because of its widespread occurrence in cancer cells. However, it was later discovered that healthy cells also had small concentrations of p53 which was slightly different from the p53 found in cancer cells. Comparison of these proteins showed that p53 present in healthy cells inhibits cell division while the p53 of cancer cells is a non-functional protein. Thus, it became evident that p53 gene is an anti-oncogene, and when it undergoes mutations, it forms an abnormal and non-functional protein which cannot restrain cell division. Unopposed action of activated proto-oncogenes can, then, cause malignant transformation.

p53 gene is expressed in nearly every cell. Its product, p53 protein plays a vital role in the cell cycle just before replication of DNA. It scans the DNA for signs of damage. If any damage is detected, it **arrests the cell cycle** in the G_1 phase to give time to DNA repair systems for repairing the damage. If the damage is repaired, it allows the cell cycle to proceed to the S phase. If the damage is not repaired, it pushes the cell into an alternate fate which is **apoptosis** (programmed cell death) so that the damaged DNA is not passed on to daughter cells. Thus, p53 acts as a watchdog to ensure that cells having damaged DNA do not divide and are eliminated.

Mutations in p53 gene have been seen in a number of cancers in a variety of tissues. Loss of inhibitory function of p53 protein is believed to play a key role in malignant transformation. **Inherited mutations** in p53 gene cause **Li-Fraumeni syndrome** in which a high incidence of a variety of cancers is seen in the affected families. The cancers develop at an early age.

2. RB 1 Gene

This is a tumour suppressor gene acting specifically in **retinoblasts**. It encodes a protein, p106. This protein can undergo reversible phosphorylation and dephosphorylation. The dephosphorylated form is the active form of the protein. The active protein binds to DNA and inhibits the expression of some growth-promoting genes. This inhibits cell division. Mutations in RB1 gene produce an abnormal p106 which cannot exercise its inhibitory control, and retinoblasts are transformed into cancer cells.

Like p53 gene, RB1 gene is a recessive gene. Therefore, mutations in both the alleles are required to produce an abnormal protein. Mutation in one allele may be inherited. If a mutation occurs in the second allele after birth, retinoblastoma will develop. This can occur in early childhood. If the mutation in the second allele occurs in a number of retinoblasts, multiple retinoblastomas will develop. The siblings having the mutant allele can also develop retinoblastomas. Sporadic retinoblastoma occurs in patients who have not inherited a mutant allele. In such persons, two mutations at the same locus are required for development of retinoblastoma. This is a rare occurrence. The tumour occurs at a later age and is solitary.

3. BRCA-1 Gene

BRCA-1 gene encodes a DNA repair protein. It is expressed mainly in mammary tissue. Mutations in both the alleles of BRCA-1 gene can cause breast cancer. Mutation in one allele may be inherited. Carriers of BRCA-1 mutation have 80–90% chance of developing breast cancer as only one more mutation in the second allele leads to loss of function and resultant malignant transformatilon. Ashkenazi Jews and inhabitants of Iceland have a high incidence of inherited BRCA-1 mutations.

4. BRCA-2 Gene

BRCA-2 gene encodes another DNA repair protein. It is expressed mainly in mammary tissue. Mutations in both the alleles can cause breast cancer. Again, mutation in one allele may be inherited. Carriers of BRCA-2 mutation have a higher risk of developing breast cancer than normal persons.

5. NF-1 Gene

NF (neurofibromin)-1 gene encodes GTPase activating protein (GAP). GAP is required to switch on the GTPase activity of p21. Mutations in NF-1 gene lead to the synthesis of a non-functional GAP. As a result, p21 remains persistently active causing malignant transformation. Mutations in NF-1 gene cause neurofibromatosis in which neurofibromas occur at multiple sites.

6. DCC Gene

A normal DCC gene prevents colon cancer. Absence of DCC (deleted in colon cancer) gene causes cancer of the colon.

7. p16 Gene

p16 gene encodes an inhibitor of cyclin D/CDK4 activity. This inhibition blocks the progression of cell cycle from G_1 phase to S phase giving time for DNA repair. Loss of function of p16 due to a mutation can cause malignant transformation. Mutations in p16 gene have been found in malignant melanoma and pancreatic cancers.

8. WT-1 Gene

WT-1 gene is specifically related to Wilm's tumour, a cancer of kidneys occuring in childhood. For long, WT-1 gene has been believed to be an anti-oncogene but some recent studies have shown expression of WT-1 gene in some cancers especially cancer of pancreas. This has created suspicion that WT-1 gene may, in fact, be a proto-oncogene.

To sum up, cancer may result from insertion of abnormal viral oncogenes, overexpression of normal proto-oncogenes, mutations in proto-oncogenes resulting in the synthesis of abnormal products or mutations in anti-oncogenes resulting in the synthesis of abnormal products that have lost their inhibitory control. Mutation in a single proto-oncogene or a single anti-oncogene is not enough to cause cancer. Usually, **a series of mutations** in proto-oncogenes as well as anti-oncogenes in the same cell is required to transform it into a cancer cell. As we grow older, we accumulate mutations. If the requisite combination of mutations occurs in some cell, it will cause malignant transformation. Accumulation of mutations is accelerated if we are exposed to DNA damaging agents or if the DNA repair systems are defective. A high incidence of cancers at a relatively early age is seen when the DNA repair systems are defective. A defect in the **nucleotide excision repair** system causes **xeroderma pigmentosum**. A defect in **mismatch repair** system causes **hereditary non-polyposis colon cancer.**

Malignant transformation changes the morphology and the metabolic profile of the cell. Morphological changes are used by the pathologist to diagnose cancer in a biopsy specimen. Metabolic changes are geared to ensure rapid growth of the cancer cells. Cancer cells appropriate nutrients and use them selfishly for their own growth. Synthesis of nucleotides, specially deoxyribonucleotides, DNA, RNA and proteins is increased. Glycolysis is increased. The cell begins to synthesise proteins that are normally synthesised in the undifferentiated embryonic and foetal stage. Some of these proteins can be used for diagnosis of cancer.

TUMOUR MARKERS

Tumour markers or cancer markers are proteins or others antigens synthesised specifically by cancer cells. Measurement of these compounds in plasma can be used to diagnose cancer. These include carcinoembryonic antigen (CEA), α-fetoprotein (AFP), prostate-specific antigen (PSA), carbohydrate antigen (CA) 15.3, CA 19.9, CA 125, CA 242, etc. Human chorionic gonadotropin (hCG) is raised specifically in choriocarcinoma. Rise in these tumour markers usually occurs when the disease is fairly advanced and is, therefore, not useful in early diagnosis of cancer. However, serial measurements of tumour markers are useful in monitoring the effectiveness of treatment and in early detection of recurrence.

EXERCISE

1. Describe the functions of proto-oncogenes. Explain the mechanisms by which proto-oncogenes can transform normal cells into cancer cells.

2. Write short notes on:
   a. Oncogenes   b. Tumour suppressor genes
   c. Ames' assay   d. Tumour markers

3. Write 'true' or 'false':
   a. Uncontrolled multiplication of cells is known as metastasis.
   b. Ultraviolet rays can cause the formation of pyrimidine dimers.
   c. Pro-carcinogens are converted into carcinogens usually by conjugation.
   d. Mutagenicity of chemicals can be detected by Ames' assay.
   e. Viruses causing cancer are known as oncoviruses.
   f. Oncoviruses possess proto-oncogenes.
   g. Many oncogenes are present in human DNA.
   h. Proteins encoded by proto-oncogenes function in growth of cells.
   i. p53 is a proto-oncogene.
   j. A series of mutations in proto-oncogenes and tumour suppressor genes is usually necessary to transform a healthy cell into a cancer cell.

4. Fill in the blanks:
   a. A tester strain of .... is used in Ames' assay.
   b. The tester strain of .... used in Ames' assay lacks the ability to synthesise ....
   c. GTPase activating protein is required to switch on the GTPase activity of ....
   d. Programmed cell death is known as ....
   e. RB1 is an anti-oncogene acting specifically in ....

ANSWERS TO SHORT QUESTIONS

3. a. False
   c. False
   e. True
   g. False
   i. False

   b. True
   d. True
   f. False
   h. True
   j. True

4. a. *S. typhimurium*
   c. p21
   e. Retinoblasts

   b. *S. typhimurium*, histidine
   d. Apoptosis

Immunochemistry

We are exposed to a vast variety of infectious agents, e.g. bacteria, viruses, parasites, etc. many of which are capable of causing serious, and even fatal, diseases. Micro-organisms that can cause disease are known as pathogens. To counter these invaders, nature has equipped us with a highly competent defense system. The defense system comprises **innate immunity** and **acquired (adaptive) immunity**.

The innate defense mechanisms include natural barriers which prevent the entry of infectious agents, specialised cells which engulf and destroy the invading micro-organisms and molecules which activate and aid the native defense mechanisms.

Skin and mucous membranes act as physical barriers against the entry of infectious agents. The secretions covering skin and mucous membranes contain chemical substances which make the environment inhospitable for infectious micro-organisms. If the invaders succeed in crossing these barriers and entering the body, they are attacked by **phagocytes**.

The principal phagocytes are **macrophages** and **polymorphonuclear leukocytes**. Macrophages are formed continuously from monocytes that leave the circulation and enter the tissues. They are present in most of the tissues, and are the first to challenge the pathogens that have entered the tissues. They have receptors that recognise some common structural patterns which are present on the surface of pathogens (lipopolysaccharides, peptido-glycans, lipoproteins, etc.) but not on self-cells. Macrophages ingest the pathogens in the form of vesicles known as phagosomes. Lysosomes fuse with phagosomes to form phagolysosomes. Lysosomal enzymes, then, hydrolyse the microbial biomolecules. Some other chemicals, e.g. nitric oxide, superoxide radicals, lactoferrin etc, also help in the destruction of pathogens.

An inflammatory response is also produced by the cytokines and chemokines released by the activated macrophages. The cytokines cause dilatation of local blood vessels and increase their permeability leading to release of plasma proteins and blood cells, e.g. neutrophils, into the infected area. Chemokines attract the neutrophils to the site of infection. Neutrophils further aid in phagocytosis. Complement proteins, acute phase proteins (C-reactive protein, mannose-binding protein, ceruloplasmin, α_1-antitrypsin, etc.), interferons and chemical mediators released by mast cells (histamine, chemotactic factors, platelet activating factor, leukotrienes, prostaglandins, thromboxanes, etc.) also play important roles in the fight against the infectious agents.

The innate defense mechanisms are non-specific in the sense that they operate against all microbial invaders irrespective of the antigens present on them. Another feature of the innate defense mechanisms is that repeated exposure to the same invader does not increase the efficacy or magnitude of the response.

In contrast to innate immunity, acquired (or adaptive) immunity acts specifically. Each cell or molecule responsible for acquired immunity recognises and acts against a specific foreign invader. The molecules recognised by the immune system are antigens. Repeated exposure to an antigen improves the immune response against it. Adaptive immunity is comprised of two arms:

1. Humoral Immunity

Humoral immunity operates through circulating **antibodies** which can recognise and act against specific extracellular antigens.

2. Cell-mediated Immunity

It operates through **activated lymphocytes** which act against antigens that have entered some self-cell and destroy the self-cell as well as the antigen.

ANTIGENS

Antigens are foreign chemicals that can evoke an immune response, humoral or cellular or both. We come in contact with a wide variety of foreign chemicals but all of them are not antigens. Antigens are generally foreign proteins or polysaccharides or synthetic compounds having high molecular weights. Their structure is complex with some recurring chemical group. They may enter as free molecules or as components of some cell, e.g. a bacterial cell. Only a small part of the antigen molecule, known as **epitope** or **antigenic determinant**, is recognised by the immune system. Some antigens have more than one epitope.

HAPTENS

Haptens are foreign compounds having low molecular weight which cannot evoke an immune response by themselves. But they can evoke an immune response when they are combined with some other large molecule. However, once an immune response develops, the free hapten can also be recognised by the immune system.

ROLE OF LYMPHOCYTES

Lymphocytes are the key cells of the immune system. These are formed in the bone marrow from stem cells, and differentiate into two types, **B lymphocytes** (B cells) and **T lymphocytes** (T cells). Both are processed before they reach the lymphoid tissue. B cells are processed in bone marrow and T cells in the thymus gland. B cells synthesise antibodies that provide humoral immunity, and T cells provide cell-mediated immunity. A given B cell or T cell can recognise only one particular antigen.

HUMORAL IMMUNITY

Antibodies are the molecules that provide humoral immunity. Chemically, antibodies are proteins belonging to the globulin fraction of plasma proteins. They are also known as immunoglobulins. Immunoglobulins are made up of two types of polypeptide chains, **light chains** and **heavy chains**. Lights chains are smaller (MW 23,000) than heavy chains (MW 50,000 to 70,000). The basic unit of an immunoglobulin molecule is made up of two heavy chains and two light chains. The two heavy chains are joined to each others by disulphide bonds. Each light chain is joined to a heavy chain by a disulphide bond (Fig. 19.1). The number and positions of disulphide bonds differ in different classes of immunoglobulins. Light chains are of two types: κ (kappa) and λ (lambda). A given immuno-globulin has either κ or λ light chains. Heavy chains are

of five types, α (alpha), δ (delta), ϵ (epsilon), γ (gamma) and μ (mu). A given immunoglobulin has only one type of heavy chains. Heavy chains are usually conjugated to some carbohydrates. The carbohydrate content is different in different types of heavy chains.

In a given type of light chain, the C-terminal half has an identical amino acid sequence. This portion of the chain is known as the **constant region** N-terminal halves of different light chains have different amino acid sequences. Therefore, the N-terminal half is known as the **variable region**. In the variable region of a light chain, there are three hypervariable regions in which the amino acid sequences are extremely variable. The heavy chains also possess constant regions and variable regions. In a given type of heavy chain, the C-terminal three-fourths has a constant amino acid sequence, and constitutes the constant region. The N-terminal quarter constitutes the variable region. There are three hypervariable regions in the variable region. The constant regions of light chains and heavy chains are denoted as C_L and C_H respectively. The variable regions of of light chains and heavy chains are denoted as V_L and V_H respectively (Fig.19.2). Immuno-globulins are usually depicted as Y-shaped molecules. The tip of each arm of the Y, made up of V_L and V_H regions constitutes an antigen-binding site. The antigen-binding sites on the two arms are identical. The stem of the Y, made up of C_H region, performs the effector function of the immunoglobulin.

However, the light and heavy chains are not linear. Like all polypeptide chains, they possess secondary and tertiary structures. Coiling and folding of the chains produce some distinctive domains in the molecule. The light chain has two domains V_L and C_L. The heavy chain usually has four domains, V_H, C_{H1}, C_{H2} and C_{H3}. Due to folding, the hypervariable regions of light chains and heavy chains come close to each other and constitute the **antigen-binding site**. The amino acid sequence in the hypervariable region of a given immunoglobulin molecule is unique. Therefore, the antigen-binding site has a unique conformation which is complementary to a particular antigen. The hypervariable regions are also known as **complementarity determining regions** (CDRs) as they

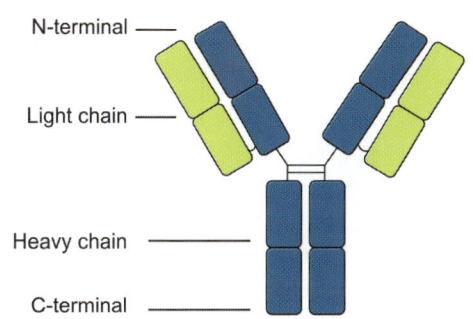

Fig. 19.1: Basic structure of an immunoglobulin

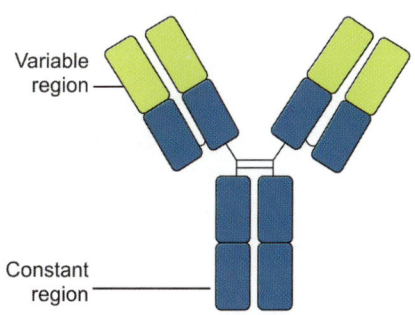

Fig. 19.2: Constant and variable regions of light and heavy chains of an immunoglobulin

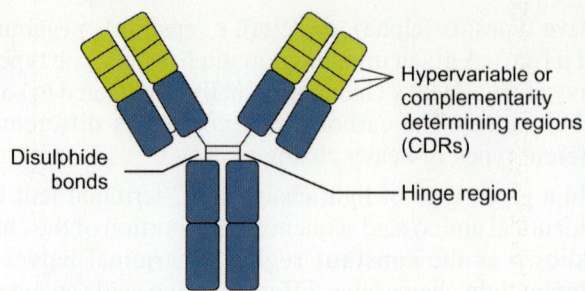

Fig. 19.3: Hypervariable regions in light and heavy chains

are responsible for the complementarity between the antibody and the antigen.

As mentioned earlier, only a small region of the antigen molecule, known as epitope or antigenic determinant, is recognised by the antibody. The portion of antibody molecule that contacts the epitope is known as paratope. The junctions between different domains of light chains and heavy chains have some flexibility, permitting movements between domains. The junction between C_{H1} and C_{H2} is more flexible, and is known as the hinge region where considerable movement is possible (Fig. 19.3).

Action of Papain

The antibody molecule can be cleaved in vitro by papain. Papain cleavage yields three fragments, two of which are identical (Fig. 19.4). The identical fragments are made up of paired V_L and V_H domains and paired C_L and C_{H1} domains. Since V_L and V_H domains possess the antigen-binding site, these fragments are capable of binding antigens, and are known as Fab fragments (*Fragment antigen binding*). The third fragment is made up of two paired C_{H2} domains and two paired C_{H3} domains. Since this fragment crystallises easily, it is known as Fc fragment (*Fragment crystallisable*). Treatment of antibodies with papain has thus shown that antigen-recognition is the function of variable regions of heavy chains and light chains.

Effector Functions of Antibodies

When an antibody finds an antigen having a complementary epitope, there is a non-covalent binding between the antibody and the antigen. The binding is reversible and invoves hydrogen bonds, electrostatic bonds, hydrophobic interactions and Van der Waals forces. Upon binding of antigen to the variable region of the antibody, the constant region performs the effector function. Antibody itself cannot destroy the antigen. It either prevents the antigen from exerting its noxious effects or recruits other effector cells and molecules that destroy the antigen. Important effector mechanisms by which the antibodies defend the organism are:

1. Neutralisation

Antibodies coat the antigens on the surface of the pathogens and prevent their entry into the host cells. Likewise, the toxins released by pathogens are coated by antibodies and their toxic effects are prevented.

2. Opsonisation

Antibodies coat the surface of the pathogens and facilitate phagocytosis by attracting phagocytes. Natural killer (NK) cells are also attracted by antibodies. NK cells cause antibody-dependant cell-mediated cytotoxicity (ADCC) which kills the pathogens. Both phagocytes and NK cells have receptors for the Fc regions of antibodies.

3. Complement Activation

Binding of antibodies to antigens on the surface of pathogens can activate the complement system which destroys the pathogens directly and/or facilitates their destruction by phagocytes.

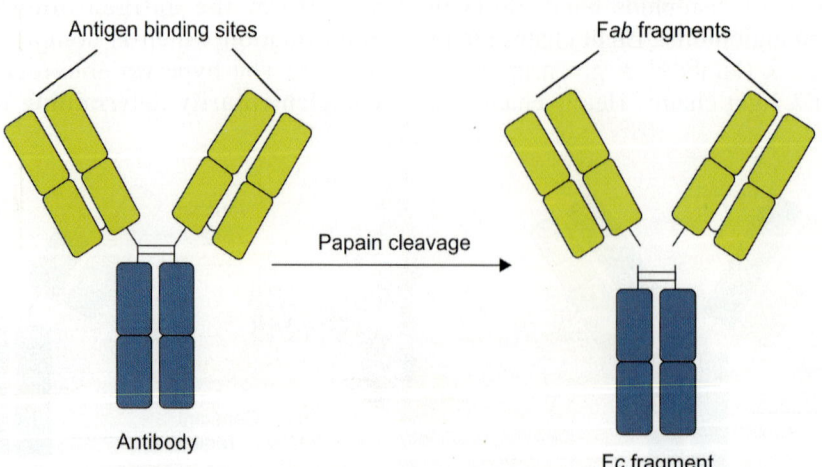

Fig. 19.4: Papain cleavage of antibody yields two F*ab* fragments and one F*c* fragment

Table 19.1: Classes of immunoglobulins

Immunoglobulin (Ig) class	Heavy chains	Light chains
IgA	α	κ or λ
IgD	δ	κ or λ
IgE	ε	κ or λ
IgG	γ	κ or λ
IgM	μ	κ or λ

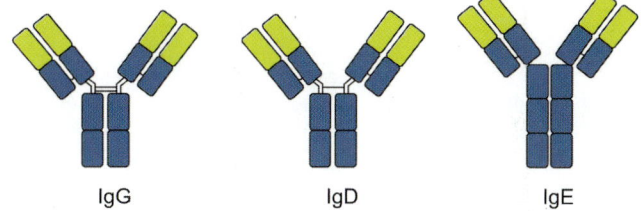

Fig. 19.5: Structures of IgG, IgD and IgE

Classification of Immunoglobulins

Immunoglobulins are classified on the basis of the heavy chains they possess into five classes (Table 19.1). In a given class, the heavy chains have a common amino acid sequence in the constant region. Since the effector function of the immunoglobulin depends upon the constant region of the heavy chains, different classes of immunoglobulins perform different effector functions.

Immunoglobulin G (IgG)

IgG is made up of two light chains and two heavy chains, and conforms to the general structure of immunoglobins (Fig. 19.5). It is the most abundant Ig in plasma and has the longest half-life. It can perform all the effector functions, e.g. neutralisation, opsonisation, complement activation, etc. It is the only class that can cross the placental barrier. During the first few weeks of life, the newborn is protected against pathogens by the maternal IgG antibodies received during intrauterine life. In human beings, IgG is further divided into four subclasses, IgG1, IgG2, IgG3 and IgG4, in the decreasing order of concentration in plasma.

Immunoglobulin A (IgA)

IgA is present in blood and exocrine secretions. IgA present in blood is a monomer, made up of two light chains and two heavy chains. It is of two types, IgA1 and IgA2. IgA1 is more abundant. IgA present in exocrine secretions (secretory IgA) is a dimer made up of four light chains and four heavy chains. It also possesses an additional J chain (MW 15000). Secretory IgA is synthesised beneath

the basolateral surface of epithelial cells. It binds to an Ig receptor on the basolateral surface of the epithelial cell and traverses the cell to reach its luminal surface. A part of the Ig receptor remains attached to the IgA dimer, and is known as the secretory component (SC). Secretory IgA is the only Ig present in exocrine secretions. It protects the epithelial cells against pathogens and their toxins, mainly by neutralisation. Secretory IgA present in breast milk enters the gut of the newborn and provides immunity against pathogens that enter the gastrointestinal tract (Fig. 19.6).

Immunoglobulin M (IgM)

IgM is the first immunoglobulin to be secreted upon entry of any antigen. It is the largest immunoglobulin. It is a pentamer made up of ten light chains and ten heavy chains. It also possesses a J chain. The heavy chains have five domains, and lack the hinge region (Fig. 19.7). IgM acts mainly by activating the complement system. It has weak neutralising and opsonising activity.

Immunoglobulin E (IgE)

IgE is quantitatively a minor immunoglobulin. It is a monomer made up of two light chains and two heavy chains. Its heavy chains have five domains and lack the hinge region. Most of the IgE is bound to mast cells and basophils. IgE antibodies are mainly antiparasitic. Upon binding of parasitic antigens to IgE, the mast cells release chemical mediators, e.g. histamine, leukotrienes, etc. that act on the parasite and also induce a localised inflammatory reaction. IgE also causes allergic reactions upon binding of innocuous antigens (allergens).

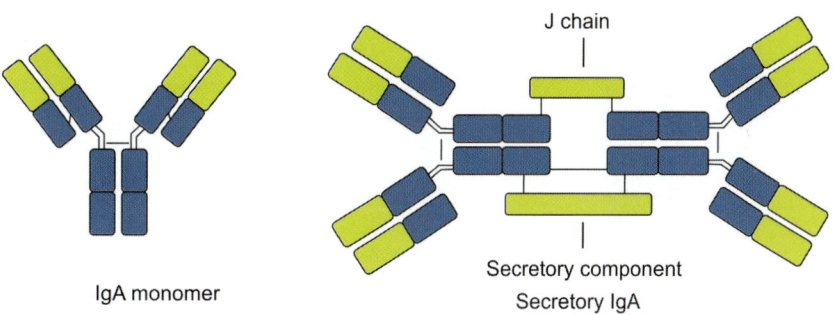

IgA monomer

J chain

Secretory component
Secretory IgA

Fig. 19.6: Structures of monomeric and secretory IgA

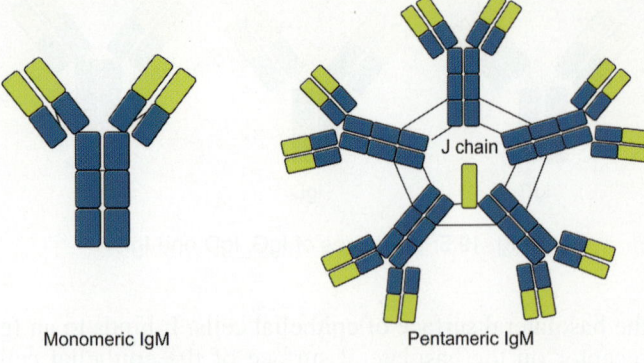

Monomeric IgM   Pentameric IgM

Fig. 19.7: Structures of monomeric and pentameric IgM

Immunoglobulin D (IgD)

IgD is a monomer having a structure similar to that of monomeric IgA. It is quantitatively a minor immunoglobulin having no known function.

Variants of the Basic Immunoglobulin Structure

1. Idiotypes

The variable region of an immunoglobulin molecule forms a typical three-dimensional structure (or cleft) which is complementary to the antigenic determinant of a particular antigen. This typical antigen-recognition structure consitutues an idiotype. Thus, we have a vast variety of immunoglobulin idiotypes, each recognising a particular antigen.

2. Isotypes

Immunoglobulins are divided into five classes, i.e. IgA, IgD, IgE, IgG and IgM. IgA is further subdivided into IgA1 and IgA2, and IgG into IgG1, IgG2, IgG3 and IgG4 subclasses. Each class and subclass is known as an isotype. Isotypic variations are due to differences in amino acid sequence in the constant region.

3. Allotypes

Mutations leading to substitution of one or two amino acids in the constant region give rise to immunoglobulin molecules of the same class or subclass differing slightly in the amino acid sequence in the constant region. These variants are known as allotypes. Such variants are found in a small proportion of the population, and are transmitted from parents to the progeny.

INSTRUCTION AND SELECTION THEORIES

Our immune system is capable of recognising practically every antigen. In early twentieth century, two contrasting theories were proposed to explain how antibodies capable of recognising a vast range of antigens could be formed. According to the instruction theory, upon first entry of an antigen in the body, the antigen acted as a template and an antibody complementary to the antigen was formed. Thus, the antigen instructed the synthesis of the antibody. The selection theory envisaged the presence of a wide range of pre-formed antibodies in small concentrations. Upon entry of an antigen in the body, the antigen would select an antibody having a complementary structure, and the production of this antibody would then increase.

To test the instruction theory, an antibody having a particular three-dimensional structure was unfolded by chemical means, and was allowed to re-fold in the presence of an unrelated antigen. If the antigen acted as a template, the re-folding should produce a conformation complementary to the antigen. However, this did not happen. The antibody re-folded to form its own original conformation. Moreover, our immune system was found to synthesise antibodies complementary to synthetic chemicals which it might never actually encounter. The instruction (template) theory was, therefore, discarded.

Selection (clonal selection) theory received acceptance as the evidence in its favour was found to be credible. It was found that each B lymphocyte is dedicated to form one particular antibody, a few molecules of which are

Class	Plasma level (mg/dl)	Half-life (days)	Active against	Special features
IgG	700–1,500	23	Bacteria and viruses	Can cross placenta and can activate complement system
IgA	60–500	5–6	Strongly antiviral and moderately antibacterial	Secretory IgA is present in exocrine secretions
IgM	40–200	5–6	Strongly antibacterial and moderately antiviral	Can activate complement system, first Ig to be formed upon entry of any antigen
IgE	0.01–0.1	2–3	Parasites	Mediates allergic reactions
IgD	0.3–40	2–3	Function unknown	

Table 19.2: Some important features of different classes of immunoglobulins

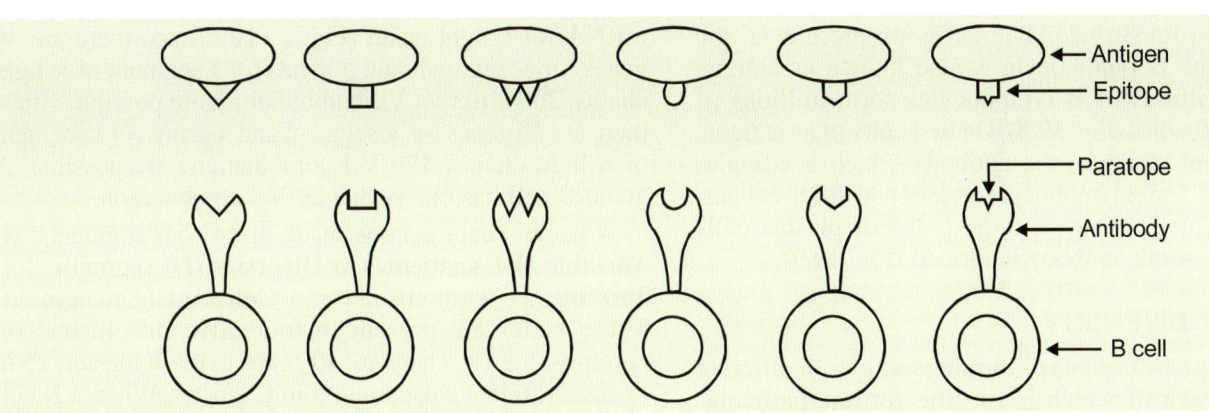

Fig. 19.8: Each B cell synthesises a particular antibody which is displayed on its surface. A wide range of antibodies recognising different antigens is present on the surface of different B cells

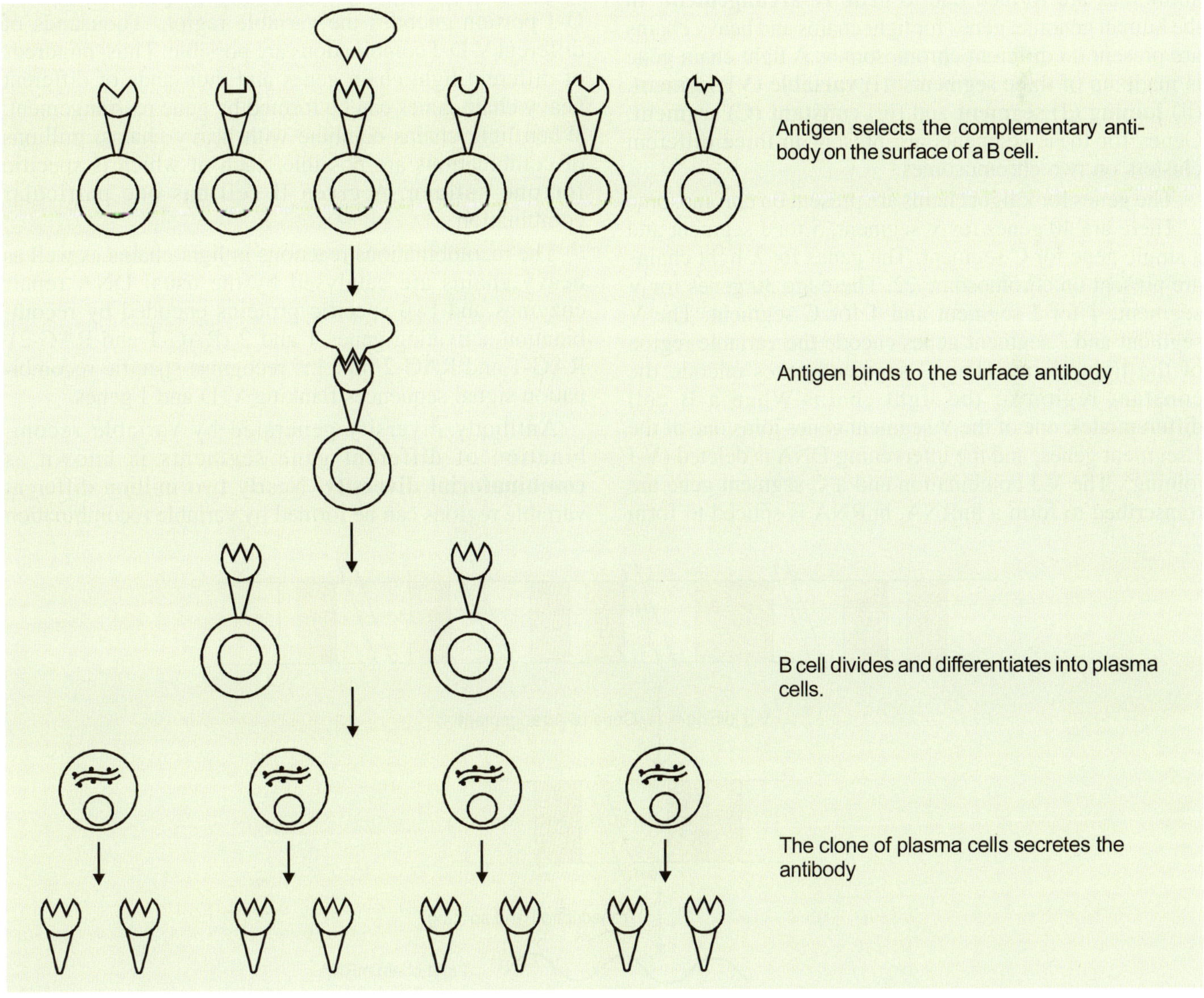

Antigen selects the complementary antibody on the surface of a B cell.

Antigen binds to the surface antibody

B cell divides and differentiates into plasma cells.

The clone of plasma cells secretes the antibody

Fig. 19.9: The antigen selects and binds to the complementary antibody on the surface of a B cell. The B cell divides and differentiates into plasma cells which secrete the antibody displayed on its surface. The antibody present on the surface of the B lymphocyte is also known as antigen receptor. Millions of B lymphocytes form millions of different antibodies (Fig. 19.8). On first entry of an antigen, it selects, and binds to, the antibody which is complementary to it. The B lymphocyte divides and differ-entiates into plasma cells. Thus, a large clone of plasma cells secreting the same antibody is formed (Fig. 19.9).

ANTIBODY DIVERSITY

Human beings are capable of forming millions of different antibodies each of which is specific for one particular antigen. Since antibodies are proteins, there should be millions of genes encoding different antibodies. However, the total number of genes in the human genome is only about 35,000 of which less than 200 are immunoglobulin genes. From this small number of genes, a huge variety of antibodies are formed due to **gene re-arrangement**. In the human genome, genes for light chains and heavy chains are present on different chromosomes. A light chain gene is made up of three segments: (i) **variable (V) segment**, (ii) **joining (J) segment** and (iii) **constant (C) segment**. Genes for these segments are present in three different clusters on two chromosomes.

The genes for κ light chains are present on chromosome 2. There are 40 genes for V segment, 5 for J segment and a single gene for C segment. The genes for λ light chains are present on chromosome 22. There are 30 genes for V segment, 4 for J segment and 4 for C segment. The V segment and J segment genes encode the variable region of the light chains. The C segment genes encode the constant region of the light chains. When a B cell differentiates, one of the V segment genes joins one of the J segment genes, and the intervening DNA is deleted (V-J joining). The V-J combination and a C segment gene are transcribed to form a hnRNA. hnRNA is spliced to form

mRNA for a light chain (Fig. 19.10). Since there are 40 genes for V segment and 5 genes for J segment of κ light chains, 200 different V-J combinations are possible. Since there are 30 genes for V segment and 4 genes for J segment of λ light chains, 120 V-J combinations are possible. A given B cell has one particular V-J combination.

A heavy chain gene is made up of four segments: (i) **Variable (V) segment**, (ii) **Diversity (D) segment**, (iii) **Joining (J) segment** and (iv) **Constant (C) segment**. These genes are present in four different clusters on chromosome 14. There are 40 genes in the V cluster, 25 in D cluster, 6 in J cluster and 9 in C cluster. When a B cell differentiates, one D segment gene joins one J segment gene, and the intervening DNA is deleted (D-J joining). One V segment gene joins D-J with deletion of intervening DNA (V-D-J joining). V-D-J combination and the first C segment gene (Cμ) are transcribed to form hnRNA. hnRNA is spliced to form heavy chain mRNA (Fig. 19.11). The V-D-J portion encodes the variable region. Thousands of different V-D-J combinations are possible. Thus, hundreds of different light chain genes and thousands of different heavy chain genes can be formed by gene rearrangement. When light chains combine with heavy chains, millions of combinations are possible, each of which is specific for one antigen. A given B cell has one particular combination.

The recombinations reactions in light chains as well as heavy chains are catalysed by the usual DNA repair enzymes and two specific proteins encoded by recombination-activating genes 1 and 2 (RAG-1 and RAG-2). RAG-1 and RAG-2 proteins recognise specific recombination signal sequences flanking V, D and J genes.

Antibody diversity generated by variable recombination of different gene segments is known as **combinatorial diversity**. Nearly two million different variable regions can be formed by variable recombination

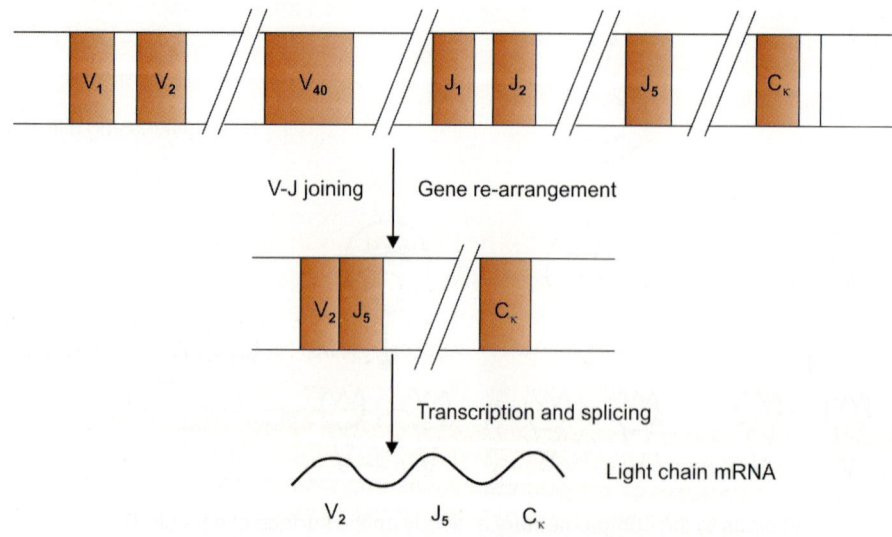

Fig. 19.10: Gene re-arrangement to form a light chain gene

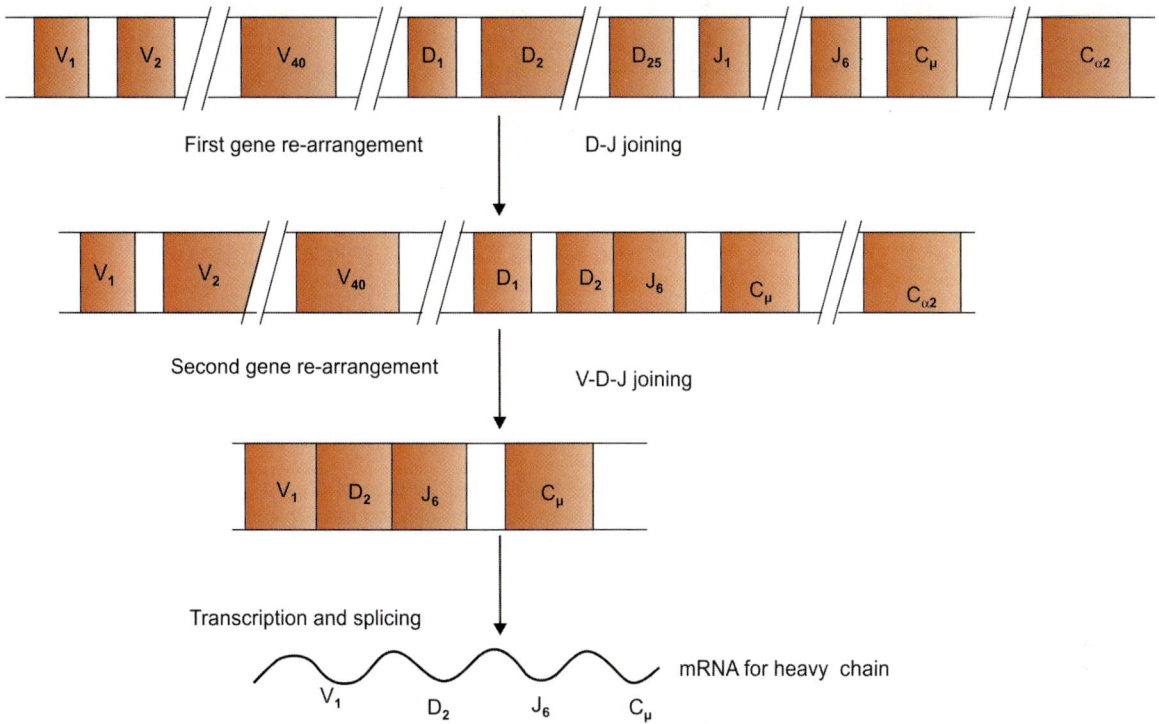

Fig. 19.11: Gene re-arrangement to form a heavy chain gene

of different segments and by variable combinations of light chains and heavy chains. Further diversity is generated by imprecise joining of different gene segments. At the time of joining, some nucleotides may be deleted by exonucleases and some nucleotides may be added by terminal deoxyribonucleotidyl transferase (TdT) leading to **junctional diversity**. A final source of diversity is **somatic hypermutation**. When a mature B cell encounters an antigen, a series of point mutations occur in the assembled variable region creating further diversity.

Like other genes, the Ig genes are preceded by a promoter. A regulator is present upstream of the promoter. An enhancer element is present downstream of the variable region (V-D-J). The first constant region gene is $C\mu$. Each constant region gene is preceded by a highly conserved short repetitive sequence known as switch sequence (Fig. 19.12). The promoter is weak but gene expression is increased by the enhancer element.

Class Switching

Different classes of immunoglobulins differ in their heavy chains and in their effector functions. Within a class, the heavy chains have a specific constant region. The genes

for the constant segment of heavy chains are present in a cluster. C_μ gene is at the 5'-end of the cluster. Each constant segment gene is preceded by a switch sequence which is a highly conserved short repetitive sequence. Once V-D-J joining has occurred, V-D-J is transcribed with C_μ which is the first constant segment gene at the 5'-end of the constant segment cluster. Therefore, IgM is the first immunoglobulin to be formed upon entry of an antigen. However, an immunoglobulin of a different class may be required to deal with the same antigen. For this, the V-D-J complex already formed is joined to a different constant segment gene downstream with deletion of the intervening DNA. Thus, an immunoglobulin of a different class but having the same antigen specificity is formed (Fig. 19.13). This is known as class (or isotype) switching. The switch sequences facilitate switching from one class to another. The lymphokines released by T cells also have a role in class switching.

PRIMARY RESPONSE

There are millions of B lymphocytes in circulation, each synthesising one particular immunoglobulin. Some immunoglobin molecules are present on the surface of each

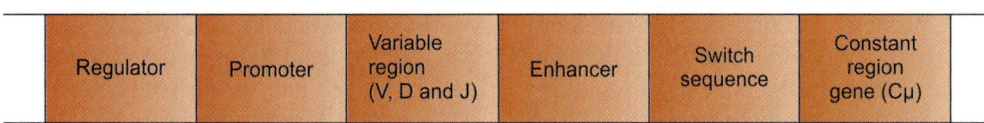

Fig. 19.12: A heavy chain gene with its regulator, promoter and enhancer

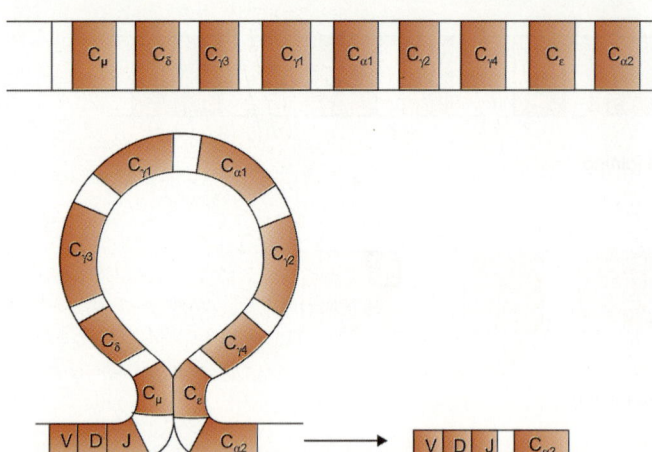

Fig. 19.13: Class switching. (a) Sequence of constant segment genes preceded by switch sequences; (b) Class switching from IgM to IgA2 with deletion of intervening DNA

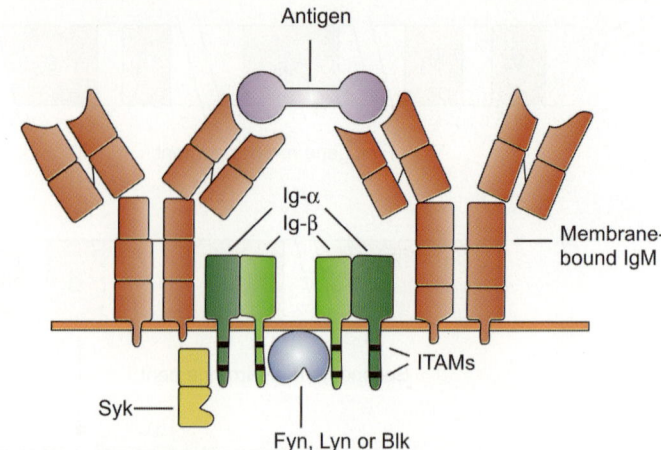

Fig. 19.14: Binding of an antigen to membrane-bond IgM on B cell causes oligomerisation of neighbouring IgM molecules that initiates differentiation of B cell into plasma cell

B lymphocyte. When an antigen enters the body for the first time, it will encounter some immunoglobulin molecule on the surface of some B lymphocyte having a complementary antigen-recognition site. The antigen binds to it. This binding stimulates the B lymphocyte to differentiate into a **plasma cell** and divide. The plasma cells secrete the immunoglobulin into plasma. This is termed as primary response. The primary response is weak and short-lived.

Differentiation of B lymphocytes into Plasma Cells

C_{H4} domain of the membrane-bound IgM is associated with two other transmembrane proteins – Ig-α and Ig-β. Cytoplasmic portions of Ig-α and Ig-β have two precisely spaced tyrosine residues that constitute an immunoreceptor tyrosine-based activation motif (ITAM). Binding of a specific antigen to the variable regions of membrane-bound immunoglobulins causes oligomerisation of neighbouring immunoglobulin molecules. This activates an intracellular tyrosine kinase, Lyn (and some other cytosolic tyrosine kinases, e.g. Fyn and Blk). Lyn phosphorylates the ITAMs of Ig-α and Ig-β. Phosphorylation of target proteins generates signals that stimulate the B cell to divide and differentiate into a plasma cell. The plasma cell synthesises the secreted form of immunoglobulin instead of the membrane-bound form. This change occurs due to alternative splicing of heavy chain hnRNA.

SECONDARY RESPONSE

The B cells which have encountered the antigen once are sensitised, and some of them are converted into **memory B cells** which retain the memory of the antigen. If the same antigen enters the body again, the memory B cells multiply rapidly, and are converted into antibody-secreting plasma cells. This is termed as secondary response. The secondary response is quick, strong and long-lasting. It ensures rapid and effective elimination of the antigen.

Immunisation

Active immunity against a variety of infectious diseases is induced by administration of a small dose of the antigen (**vaccine**) which will produce a primary response. The memory of the antigen is retained by the immune system. If the infectious agent enters the body naturally in future, a quick and strong secondary response will occur and the infectious agent will be destroyed. The vaccine may consist of:

1. **Killed micro-organisms** (typhoid vaccine, cholera vaccine, Salk's polio vaccine, etc),
2. **Live attenuated micro-organisms** (BCG vaccine, Sabin's polio vaccine, etc.),
3. **Toxoids** (tetanus toxoid, diphtheria toxoid, etc.) or
4. **Pure antigens** (recombinant hepatitis B vaccine).

Short-term passive immunity against an infection may be provided by administration of pre-formed antibodies. The antibodies may be obtained from animals or human beings or may be synthesised in the laboratory.

Production of Monoclonal Antibodies

Monoclonal antibodies are clones of each other. Monoclonal antibodies for diagnostic and therapeutic use can be produced in the laboratory by **hybridoma technology**, Hybridoma cells are hybrids of **B lymphocytes** and **myeloma cells**. Myeloma cells are antibody secreting malignant cells. To prepare monoclonal antibodies, a mouse is inoculated with a specific antigen. B lymphocytes are isolated from its spleen, and are fused with myeloma cells with the help of polyethylene glycol. All the cells may not fuse. The fused hybridoma cells are separated from unfused B lymphocytes and unfused myeloma cells by

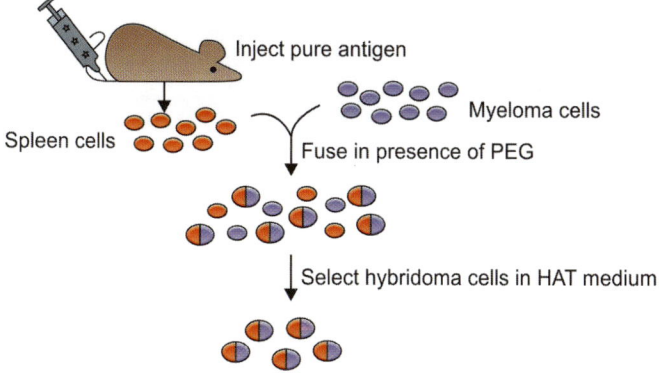

Fig. 19.15: Production of monoclonal antibodies

culturing them in HAT (Hypoxanthine-Aminopterin-Thymidine) medium (Fig. 19.15).

Unfused B lymphocytes do not survive long as they have a limited lifespan. Unfused myeloma cells can not survive because they are lacking in HGPRT and can not salvage hypoxanthine while de novo synthesis of purine nucleotides and thymidylate is blocked by aminopterin. Since hybridoma cells have acquired HGPRT from B lymphocytes, they can salvage hypoxanthine, and can grow in HAT medium. After sometime, only hybridoma cells will be left in the culture medium. These cells have acquired the property of immortality from myeloma cells and the property of secreting a particular antibody from B lymphocytes. Thus, an uninterrupted supply of a particular monoclonal antibody can be obtained from hybridoma cells (Fig. 19.16).

COMPLEMENT SYSTEM

The complement system consists of a group of proteins present in plasma which complements the actions of the immunoglobulins in dealing with the antigens. The members of this system include complement components C1-C9, factor B, factor D, etc. These proteins are inactive proenzymes which are converted into active enzymes by a cascade of reactions similar to the blood coagulation cascade. The cascade of reactions is triggered by the binding of some immunoglobulin molecules to antigen molecules present on the surface of a foreign cell, e.g. a microbial cell. The activated enzymes produce many effects, e.g. lysis of antigen-bearing cells, an inflammatory response at the site of microbial invasion, activation of phagocytes, basophils, mast cells, etc. There are two complement pathways–classic complement cascade and alternate complement pathway.

Classic Complement Cascade

The classic complement cascade proceeds through three stages – **recognition, activation** and **membrane attack**. The recognition unit is made up of complement components C1q, C1r and C1s. The activation unit comprises complement components C1, C2, C3 and C4. The membrane attack unit is made up of complement components C5, C6, C7, C8 and C9.

During the cascade of reactions, one complement component acts on the next, splitting a small peptide off and converting the inactive proenzyme into an enzyme. The small peptide released is denoted by the suffix 'a' and the larger fragment by the suffix 'b'. The enzymatically active fragment is denoted by a horizontal bar on it.

1. Recognition Phase

Recognition phase is initiated by binding of at least one IgM molecule or at least two IgG molecules to an antigen present on the surface of a foreign cell, e.g. a microbial cell. This attracts complement component C1 (made up of C1q, C1r and C1s) which binds to the constant region of the immunoglobulin (Fig. 19.17).

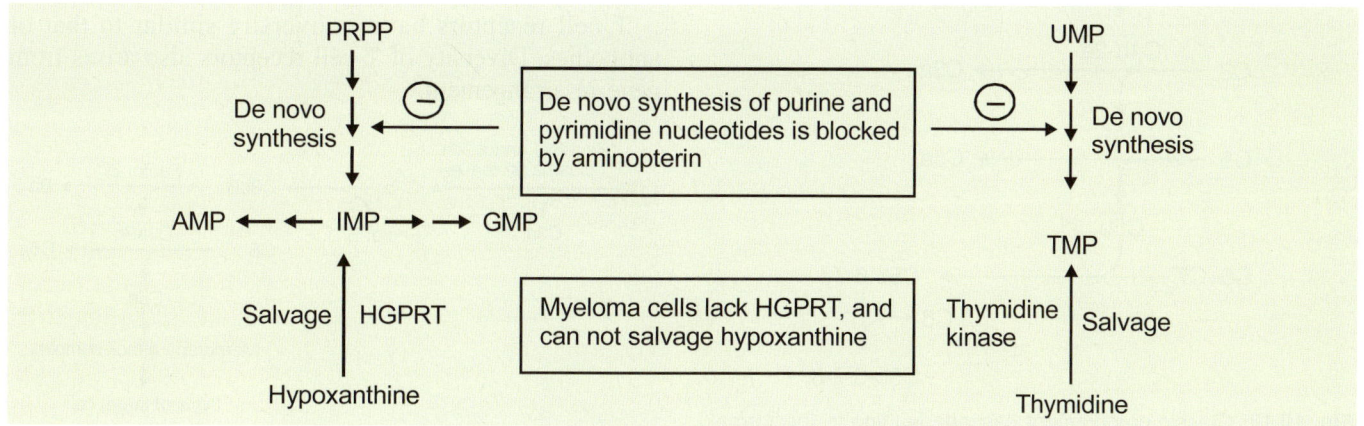

Fig. 19.16: Only hybridoma cells survive in HAT medium

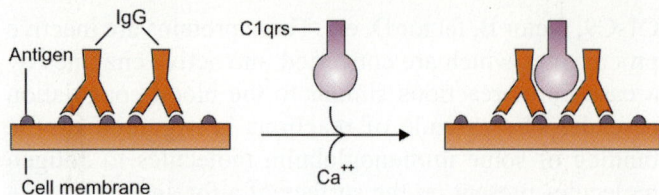

Fig. 19.17: Recognition unit of complement system (C1qrs) attaches to constant regions of two IgG molecules bound to surface antigen of a microbial cell

2. Activation Phase

Activated C1 ($\overline{C1qrs}$) acts on C4 splitting it into C4a and $\overline{C4b}$. Active $\overline{C4b}$ acts on C2 and splits it into $\overline{C2a}$ and C2b. $\overline{C4b}$ and $\overline{C2a}$ together act on C3 and split it into C3a and $\overline{C3b}$. This completes the activation phase. Active $\overline{C3b}$ initiates the next phase.

3. Membrane Attack Phase

$\overline{C3b}$ acts on C5 and splits it into C5a and $\overline{C5b}$. $\overline{C5b}$ activates and combines with C6 and C7. C8 binds to $\overline{C5b}$-6-7 to form the membrane attack unit which inserts in the cell membrane of the target microbial cell (Fig. 19.19).

Several molecules of C9 polymerise to form a trans-membrane annular structure (hole) through which the contents of the cell leak out leading to lysis of the target cell.

Although C3a and C5a released during the cascade are enzymatically inactive yet they play a role in dealing with microbial invasion. They induce an inflammatory response

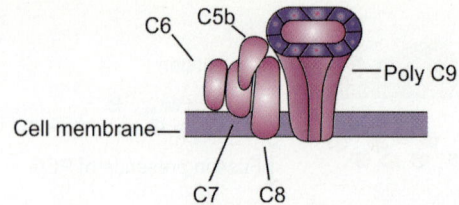

Fig. 19.19: Membrane attack complex inserted in the cell membrane of the target microbial cell

at the site of the microbial invasion which helps fight the invaders.

Alternate Complement Pathway

The alternate complement pathway does not involve antigen-antibody interaction and complement components C1, C2 and C4. In the presence of a bacterial endotoxin, C3 is slowly hydrolysed by some plasma protease or water into C3a and $\overline{C3b}$. Another protein, Factor B binds to $\overline{C3b}$ to form $\overline{C3bB}$. Factor D acts on $\overline{C3bB}$ and splits B into Ba and $\overline{Bb}$. $\overline{C3bBb}$, then, splits C5 into C5a and $\overline{C5b}$.

The rest of the pathway leading to the formation of membrane attack complex and lysis of the target cell is identical with the classic complement cascade.

CELL–MEDIATED IMMUNITY

Cell-mediated immunity is the function of T lymphocytes. T cells are of four types: (i) **cytotoxic** or **killer T cells**, (ii) **helper T cells**, (iii) **suppressor T cells** and (iv) **memory T cells**. Each T cell has transmembrane receptors on its surface that can recognise a specific antigen. The T cell receptor is a protein made up of an α chain and a β chain joined by a disulphide bond. Each chain has two extracellular domains, a transmembrane region and a short cytoplasmic tail. The α_1 and β_1 domains are similar to the variable regions of Ig light chains and heavy chains (V_L and V_H). The α_2 and β_2 domains are similar to the constant regions of Ig light chains and heavy chains (C_L and C_{H1}). The antigen-binding site or cleft is formed by the α_1 (or V_α) and β_1 (or V_β) domains (Fig. 19.21).

T cell receptors have a diversity similar to that of antibodies. Diversity of T cell receptors also arises from gene re-arrangement.

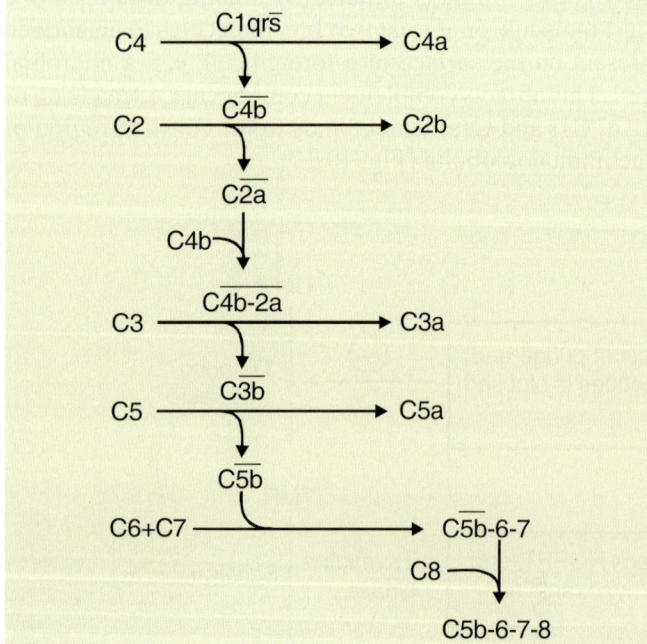

Fig. 19.18: Classic complement cascade leading to the formation of membrane attack unit

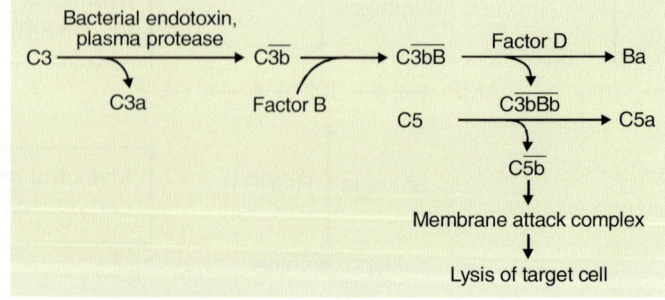

Fig. 19.20: Alternate complement pathway

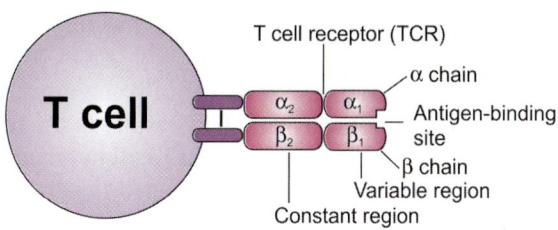

Fig. 19.21: T cell receptor

The gene for the variable region of a chain (V_α) is constructed from one of the 70 V segments and one of the 61 J segments. Thousands of different combinations are possible. The gene for the variable region of β chain (V_β) is constructed from one of the 52 V segments, one of the 2 D segments and one of the 13 J segments. Thousands of different combinations are possible. When an α chain combines with a β chain, millions of combinations are possible. A given T cell has one particular combination, and is specific for one particular antigen.

MHC Genes and Proteins

While T cell possesses receptors specific for an antigen, it cannot recognise the free antigen. The antigen must be attached to a cell, and it should be a self-cell. If a T cell is transferred from one person to another, it will not recognise the antigen. This means that the T cell not only recognises a foreign antigen but also recognises some molecule which are present on self-cells only. These self-molecules are proteins known as major histocompatibility complex (MHC). MHC proteins are present on the surface of all cells, and are unique to each individual. It is these MHC proteins which are responsible for rejection of transplanted organs as the immune system of the recipient recognises the MHC proteins of the donor as foreign antigens, and destroys the grafted organ unless strong immuno-suppressive drugs are used.

MHC Genes

The genes encoding MHC proteins are known as MHC genes, and can be divided into three classes. MHC class I

genes encode MHC I proteins. Foreign antigens combined with MHC I proteins are recognised by the receptors of cytotoxic T cells. MHC I proteins are present on the surface of all the cells. MHC class II genes encode MHC II proteins which are present on the surface of macrophages, B cells and follicular dendritic cells. Foreign antigens combined with MHC II proteins are recognised by the receptors of helper T cells. MHC class III genes encode proteins of the complement system and some other plasma proteins.

MHC Proteins

MHC proteins are transmembrane proteins. They have a peptide (antigen) binding cleft on their extracellular surface. They are synthesised on the endoplasmic reticulum. They pick up fragments of proteins formed by intracellular degradation of exogenous and endogenous proteins while on their way to the cell membrane. The fragments are bound firmly and displayed on the surface of the cell. If a T cell finds a foreign peptide bound to an MHC protein, cell-mediated immunity comes into operation. MHC class I proteins are made up of a large α subunit and a smaller β subunit (β_2-microglobulin). The α subunit has three extracellular domains (α_1, α_2 and α_3), a transmembrane region and a cytoplasmic tail. The α_1 and α_2 domains form the peptide binding cleft. They display fragments of proteins degraded by proteasome.

MHC class II proteins are made up of almost equal sized α and β subunits. Each subunit has two extracellular domains, a transmembrane region and a cytoplasmic tail. The α_1 and β_1 domains form the peptide binding cleft (Fig. 19.22). MHC class II proteins bind fragments of proteins degraded in intracellular vesicles called endosomes. These include proteins of pathogens that reside in endosomes and extracellular pathogens and proteins taken up by the cells by endocytosis. These proteins are degraded by cathepsins after fusion of the endosomes with lysosomes. Newly synthesised MHC class II proteins bind the peptide fragments, and travel to the cell membrane. MHC class II proteins get inserted in the cell membrane displaying the bound peptide on the surface of the cell.

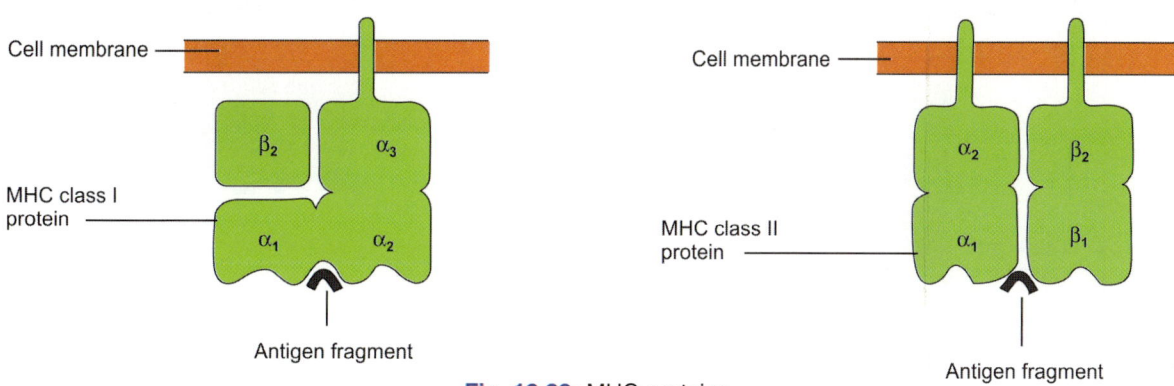

Fig. 19.22: MHC proteins

FUNCTION OF CYTOTOXIC (KILLER) T CELLS

Cytotoxic T cells destroy the infected self cells along with the pathogen present inside them. This prevents the spread of infection to healthy cells. Most viruses and several bacteria reside and replicate in the cytosol of the infected cells. Their proteins are degraded by proteasome. Peptide fragment are displayed on the surface of the cell by MHC class I proteins. The foreign peptide bound to a self MHC I protein is recognised by a particular cytotoxic T cell (Fig. 19.23).

The T cell receptor binds to the peptide: MHC I complex. A transmembrane protein, CD8 is also present in cytotoxic T cells, and acts as a co-receptor. CD8 is made up of an α and a β chain linked to each other by a disulphide bond. The extracelluar portion of CD8 binds to the $α_3$ domain of MHC class I protein. The cytoplasmic tail of CD8 is associated with Lck, a cytosolic tyrosine kinase. The cytoplasmic tail of T cell receptor is associated with six transmembrane polypeptides that constitute the CD3 complex. CD3 complex comprises a γ chain, a δ chain, two ε chains and two ξ chains. Their cytoplasmic portions have immunoreceptor tyrosine-based activation motifs (ITAMs). Upon binding of T cell receptor and CD8 to MHC I protein and antigen fragment, Lck becomes active. Active Lck phosphorylates the ITAMs of CD3 complex (Fig. 19.24).

Phosphorylated ITAMs act as a docking site for ZAP-70 (zeta associated protein of 70 kd). ZAP-70, then, phosphorylates the tyrosine residues of some other target proteins in the cytotoxic T cell. This results in the release of stored granules from the cytotoxic T cell targeted at the infected cell. The granules contain perforin, granzymes and granulysin.

Perforin inserts in the cell membrane of the infected cell. Several molecules of perforin polymerise to form transmembrane pores. Granzymes (serine proteases) hydrolyse the proteins of the infected cell as well as the proteins of the pathogen. Granulysin induces **apoptosis** of the infected cell. Apoptotic reactions fragment the DNA of the infected cell alongwith that of the pathogen. Thus the function of cytotoxic T cells is to destroy not only the pathogen but also the self-cells which have been infected by the pathogen so that the infection does not spread to healthy cells.

FUNCTION OF HELPER T CELLS

Helper T cells share the following common features with cytotoxic T cells:

1. Their T cell receptors are made up of α and β chains.
2. Cytoplasmic tail of T cell receptors is associated with similar CD3 complex having ITAMs.

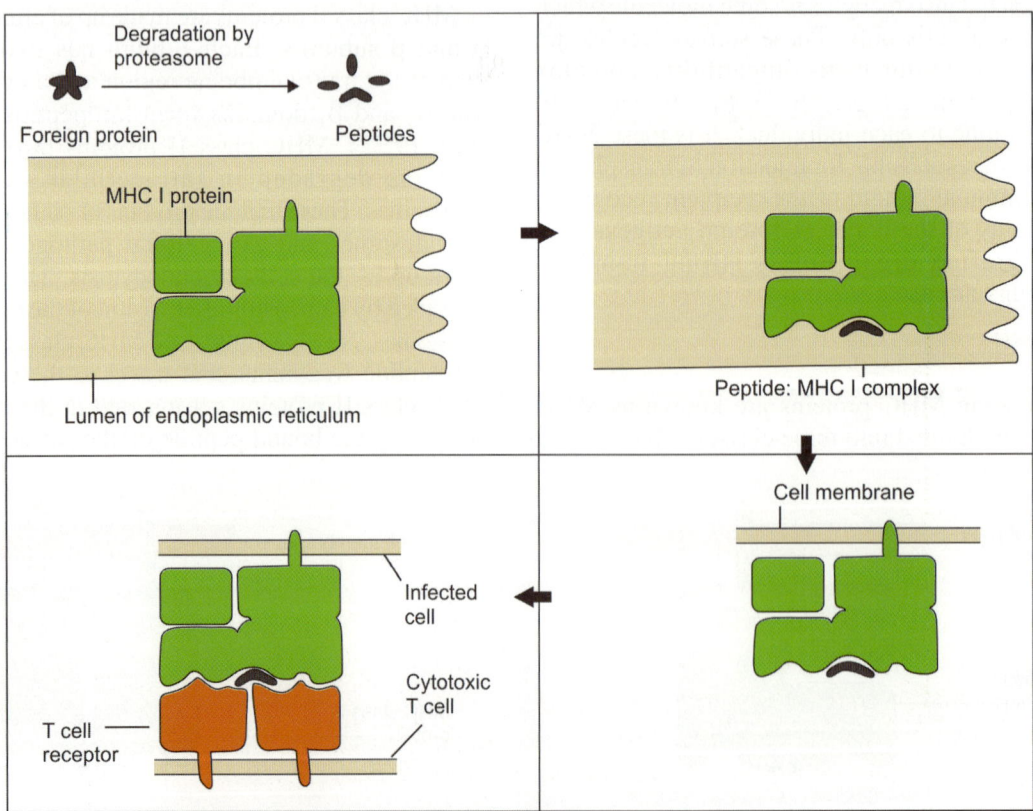

Fig. 19.23: An antigen enters a cell, and is broken up. A fragment attaches to MHC I protein. The MHC protein along with the bound antigen gets inserted in the cell membrane. T cell receptor of cytotoxic T cell binds to antigen fragment and MHC I protein

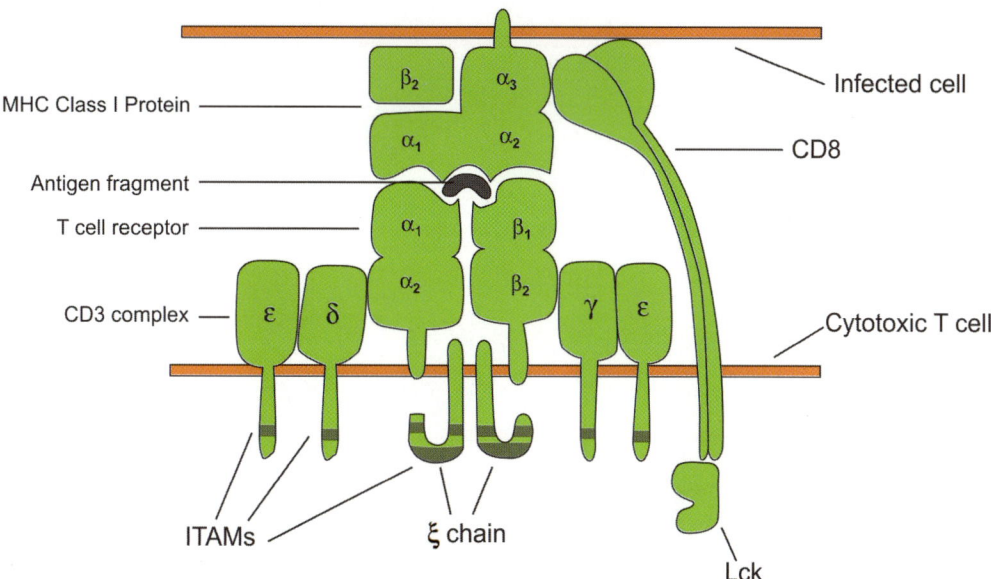

Fig. 19.24: Lck phosphorylates the ITAMs of CD3 complex. Phosphorylated ITAMs bind ZAP-70 which phosphorylates tyrosine residues of some target proteins which results in the release of stored granules from the cytotoxic T cell

3. They have co-receptors associated with Lck.
4. Intracellular signalling occurs by a cascade of phosphorylation reactions involving tyrosine residues.

Helper T cells differ from cytotoxic T cells in the following respects:
1. The co-receptor is CD4 made up of a single polypeptide chain folded into four extracellular domains – D1, D2, D3 and D4. The joint between D2 and D3 domains is flexible.
2. The T cell receptor recognises a foreign peptide bound to MHC class II protein.

MHC II proteins are present on macrophages, follicular dendritic cells and B lymphocytes. These cells are known as **antigen-presenting cells** (APCs). The T cell receptor of a helper T cell binds to a specific antigen fragment displayed by MHC class II protein on the surface of an APC. The D1 domain of CD4 binds to β_1 domain of the MHC II protein. This binding activates Lck. The active Lck phosphorylates ITAMs of CD3 complex (Fig. 19.25).

ZAP-70 binds to phosphorylated ITAMs and phosphorylates the tyrosine residues of some target proteins. This results in the release of cytokines (lymphokines) from the helper T cell.

Lymphokines

Lymphokines include:
1. Interleukins (ILs), e.g. IL-2, IL-3, Il-4, IL-5, IL-6, etc
2. Granulocyte colony stimulating factor (G-CSF)
3. Granulocyte-macrophage colony stimulating factor (GM-CSF)
4. Tumour necrosis factor (TNF)
5. Interferon-γ (IFNγ)

Actions of Lymphokines

IL-2 stimulates multiplication of helper T cells so that more helper T cells are available to mount an immune response. IL-3 stimulates the proliferation of bone marrow stem cells. IL-4 stimulates the proliferation of B cells, T cells and mast cells. IL-5 stimulates the growth of eosinophils. IL-10 stimulates the growth of mast cells, and increases the synthesis of MHC class II proteins in B lymphocytes. IFNγ activates macrophages and natural killer (NK) cells. TNF activates macrophages. GM-CSF stimulates the growth of granulocytes and macrophages, and also stimulates the differentiation of B cells and dendritic cells. Some lymphokines attract the phagocytic cells to the site of infection.

Thus, the release of lymphokines leads to:
1. Increase in the number of helper T cells themselves.
2. Increase in the number of cytotoxic T cells.
3. Increase in the number of B cells and plasma cells.
4. Increase in the number of antigen-presenting cells.
5. Increase in the number of phagocytic cells.
6. Activation of phagocytic cells.

In this way, both innate immunity and adaptive immunity are geared up to fight against the pathogen. The overall result of these actions is that an effective immune response is mounted to meet the challenge posed by the antigen/pathogen. Helper T cells respond to calls for help given by antigen-presenting cells in the form of an antigen fragment displayed on their surface. Helper T cells do not destroy the antigen themselves. They respond by activating all arms of the defence system and co-ordinating their actions so that the threat posed by the antigen is effectively met. Helper T cells are, therefore, described as the

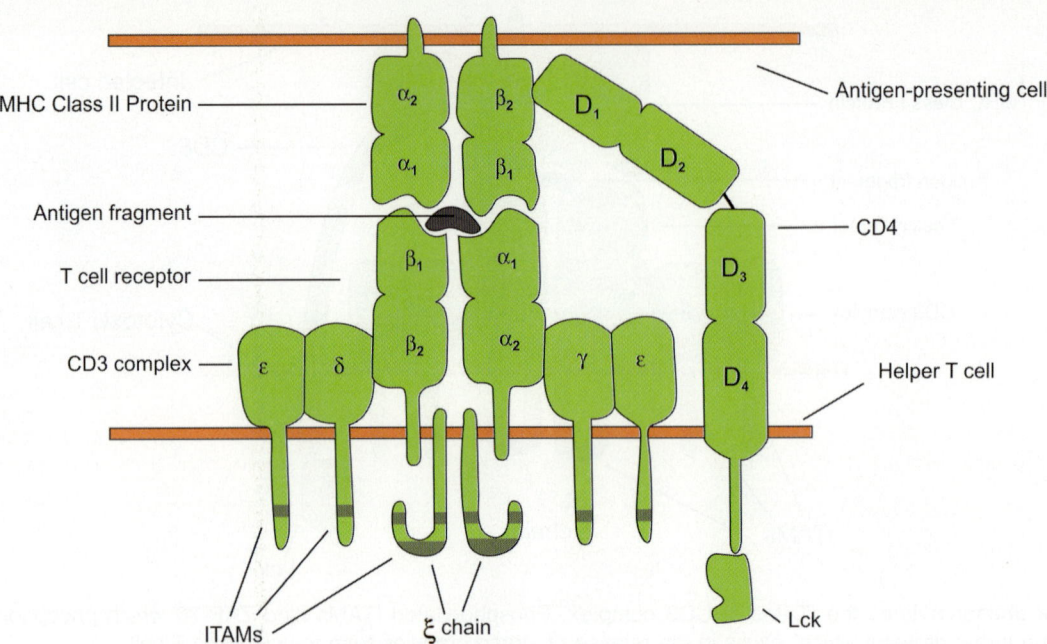

Fig. 19.25: An antigen enters a cell e.g. macrophage, and is broken up. A fragment of the antigen attaches to MHC II protein. MHC II protein along with the bound antigen gets inserted in the cell membrane. T cell receptor of helper T cell binds to the antigen fragment and MHC II protein. CD4 protein of helper T cell also binds to MHC II protein. Lck and CD3 complex are activated. This leads to the release of lymphokines from the helper T cells. The lymphokines activate all arms of the defence system

commanding officer of the defence force. If helper T cells are depleted or debilitated, the entire immune system is crippled.

FUNCTION OF SUPPRESSOR T CELLS

Suppressor T cells are also known as regulatory T cells. They play a regulatory role in the immune response. They suppress the activity of helper T cells and cytotoxic T cells, specially the former. This prevents a disproportionately high immune response.

FUNCTION OF MEMORY T CELLS

When a clone of T cells encounters an antigen for the first time, some of them counter the antigen by way of cell-mediated immunity but others retain the memory of the antigen and are preserved in the lymphoid tissue. These cells, known as memory T cells, can spread throughout the lymphoid tissue. When the same antigen is encountered again, the memory T cells are released into circulation, and an immune response is mounted quickly.

SELF AND NON-SELF

Many molecules having antigenic properties are present in our body also. While our immune system recognises and destroys foreign antigens, it does not act against self-antigens. Thus, our immune system is self-tolerant. This self-tolerance may partly be due to the action of suppressor T cells but there is a second, and more important mechanism.

As mentioned earlier, the newly formed lymphocytes are processed before reaching the lymphoid tissue. The processing occurs mostly in foetal life. The purpose of this processing is two-fold: (i) to allow only those lymphocytes to mature that are immunologically competent, and (ii) to eliminate those lymphocytes that can react with self-antigens.

Processing of T cells

Developing T cells express T cell receptor (TCR), CD4 and CD8. Some of the TCRs are incapable of recognising any self MHC protein, and such T cells would be functionally useless, if allowed to mature. Therefore, the developing T cells are first subjected to **positive selection**. If the TCR and CD8 bind to some MHC I protein, the cell is allowed to mature into a cytotoxic T cell, and expression of CD4 is suppressed. If the TCR and CD4 bind to some MHC II protein, the cell is allowed to mature into a helper T cell, and expression of CD8 is suppressed.

The positively selected cells are, then, subjected to **negative selection**. T cells that bind self-antigen: self-MHC complexes undergo apoptosis, and are eliminated.

Processing of B cells

Developing B cells that are capable of recognising self-antigens can have one of the following four fates:

1. Receptor Editing

Developing B cells that encounter multivalent self-antigens undergo further light chain gene rearrangement until the antigen receptor is so modified that it can not bind the self-antigen.

2. Clonal Deletion

If self-reactivity is not lost by receptor editing, the developing B cell undergoes apoptosis. Thus, the entire clone of self-reacting B cells is deleted.

3. Anergy

Developing B cells that encounter self-antigens of low valency become anergic. Their antigen receptor remains within the cell and signal transduction is impaired.

4. Immunological Ignorance

If the self-antigen is segregated in a compartment where B cells can not reach or if the self-antigen is present in insignificantly low concentration, the B cells capable of reacting with it will mature but will remain immuno-logically ignorant.

Thus, developing T cells and B cells are processed in such ways in foetal life that the cells capable of mounting an immune response against self-antigens are deleted or modified or incapacitated. This results in self-tolerance. However, self-tolerance is sometimes lost resulting in autoimmunity.

Autoimmune Diseases

If the immune system begins to react against a self-antigen, it results in an autoimmune disease. Autoimmune diseases can occur because:
1. Some self-molecules may combine with foreign antigens, for example microbial proteins, to form new antigens which are treated as foreign antigens by the immune system.
2. Some self-molecules having a close structural resemblance with foreign antigens may be targeted by the immune system.

Some diseases resulting from autoimmunity include Hashimoto's thyroiditis, myasthenia gravis, systemic lupus erythematosus, rheumatoid arthritis and some cases of diabetes mellitus, type1, male infertility and pernicious anaemia.

IMMUNODEFICIENCY

Immunodeficiency may be primary (inherited) or secondary (acquired). Impairment of immune system makes the patient unusually susceptible to infections. Inherited immunodeficiency diseases may affect humoral immunity or cell-mediated immunity or both.

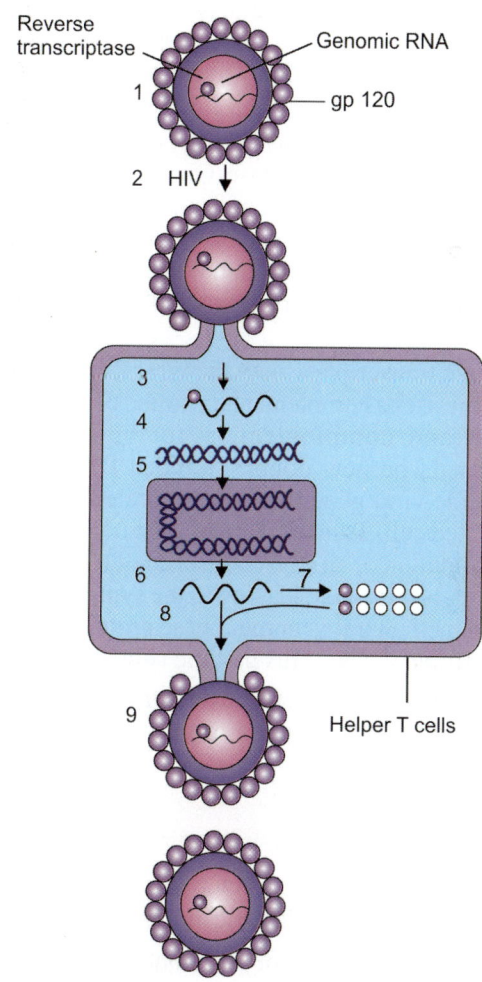

Fig. 19.27: Infection of a helper T (Th) cell by human immuno-deficiency virus (HIV). 1. HIV with its genomic RNA and reverse transcriptase (RT) in the interior and gp 120 on the surface. 2. Gp120 binds to CD4 of Th cell. Lipid bilayer of HIV fuses with the plasma membrane of Th cell. 3. Viral RNA and RT enter the cell. 4. RT synthesises a DNA copy of the HIV RNA. 5. DNA copy of the HIV genome is integrated in the DNA of Th cell. 6. Viral genome is transcribed. An RNA transcript of viral genome is formed. 7. Proteins encoded in the viral genome are synthesised. 8. Proteins surround the RNA. 9. Genomic RNA and proteins exit from the Th cell picking up a part of the lipid bilayer of Th cell on the way. 10. A new virus particle is formed

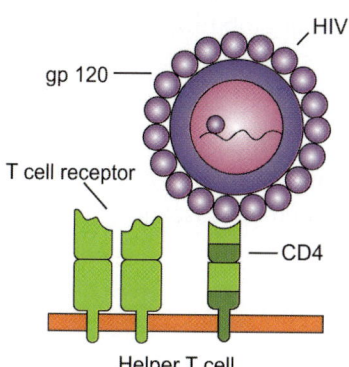

Fig. 19.26: Surface protein, gp 120 of HIV binds to CD4 of helper T cell

Congenital agammaglobulinaemia is an X-linked disease in which humoral immunity is impaired while cell-mediated immunity is normal. In DiGeorge syndrome, cell-mediated immunity is impaired as T cell processing doesn't occur due to lack of development of thymus. Inherited deficiency of purine nucleoside phosphorylase leads to impairment of cell-mediated immunity. Severe combined immuno-deficiency disease (SCID) can occur due to inherited deficiency of adenosine deaminase. Both humoral and cell-mediated immunity are severely impaired in SCID.

Acquired immunodeficiency of varying degrees may be caused by a variety of factors such as severe undernutrition, viral infections, immunosuppressive drugs, irradiation, etc. A particularly sinister form of such immunodeficiency is the **acquired immunodeficiency syndrome (AIDS)** caused by **human immunodeficiency virus (HIV)**.

HIV is a **retrovirus** having an RNA genome. It possesses reverse transcriptase. One of its surface proteins, gp 120 happens to have a conformation complementary to that of CD4. Due to this complementarity, HIV binds avidly to CD4 molecules present on the surface of helper T cells. The viral RNA and reverse transcriptase are injected into the helper T cell.

Reverse transcriptase uses the viral RNA as a template and synthesises a complementary strand of DNA. A second DNA strand complementary to the first strand is synthesised. The new double-stranded DNA, which is a copy of the viral genome, is incorporated in the DNA of the infected cell. Transcription of the viral genome results in the formation of an RNA transcript of the viral genome. This RNA is translated leading to the synthesis of proteins encoded by the viral genome. These proteins surround the RNA forming a new virus particle (Fig.19.27).

Multiple virus particles are formed due to repeated transcription and translation of the viral genome. When the number of virus particles becomes too large, the helper T cell ruptures, releasing the virus particles. The released virus particles infect other healthy helper T cells and destroy them. This ultimates leads to a severe depletion of helper T cells.

As seen earlier, helper T cells are the key cells of the immune system which activate different arms of the immune system and co-ordinate their actions. By killing and depleting helper T cells, HIV cripples the entire immune system. The patient becomes extremely susceptible to a variety of infections. These infections ultimately prove to be fatal.

ALLERGY

Allergy is described as a side effect of immunity. It is an altered immune response to an otherwise innocuous antigen. Antigens evoking an allergic response are called allergens. Allergens are small molecules present in pollens, dust mites, drugs, food, etc. Allergens bind to IgE (Reaginic antibody). IgE is normally present in minute concentration and protects against parasites.

Some persons have a relatively high level of IgE, influenced by genetic as well as environmental factors. High-affinity receptors present on mast cells bind IgE. Mast cells are present beneath mucosal cells and in connective tissue. When an allergen binds to IgE, the mast cells release their stored granules containing some chemical mediators. The chemical mediators include histamine, heparin, leukotrienes C4, D4 and E4, platelet activating factor, eosinophil chemotactic factor, etc.

These chemical mediators cause increase in capillary permeability, vasodilatation, itching, sneezing, broncho-spasm, etc depending upon the site where the allergic reaction has occurred. Allergic diseases include allergic dermatitis, allergic rhinitis, urticaria, bronchial asthma, drug allergies, food allergies, etc.

EXERCISE

1. Illustrate the general structure of an immunoglobulin with a labelled diagram. Mention the functions of individual parts. Describe the classification and functions of different classes of immunoglobulins.

2. Name different types of T lymphocytes and describe their functions.

3. Write short notes on:
   a. Haptens
   b. Clonal selection theory
   c. Basis of antibody diversity
   d. Class switching
   e. Monoclonal antibodies
   f. Classic complement cascade
   g. MHC proteins
   h. Helper T cells
   i. Cytotoxic T cells
   j. Autoimmunity
   k. Immunodeficiency
   l. AIDS

4. Write 'true' or 'false':
   a. The portion of antigen recognised by the antibody is known as paratope
   b. Haptens cannot evoke an immune response by themselves.

   c. Immunoglobulins are classified on the basis of their heavy chains.
   d. Antigen-binding site is present on the variable regions of heavy and light chains.
   e. IgM is present in plasma and exocrine secretions.
   f. IgG is the first immunoglobulin to be synthesised upon entry of an antigen in the body.
   g. The specific variable region of an immunoglobulin molecule constitutes an idiotype.
   h. IgG can cross the placental barrier.
   i. Antibodies are secreted by B lymphocytes.
   j. Diversity segment is present in light chain genes.
   k. MHC I proteins are present on the surface of all the cells.
   l. An antigen fragment, in conjunction with MHC I protein, is recognised by helper T cells.
   m. MHC proteins are unique to each individual.
   n. CD 8 protein is present in helper T cells.
   o. Cytotoxic T cells destroy self-cells infected by a foreign antigen.
   p. Human immunodeficiency virus infects helper T cells.
   q. Helper T cells are depleted in AIDS.
   r. Hybridoma cells are hybrids of T cells and myeloma cells.
   s. Monoclonal antibodies can be produced in hybridoma cells.
   t. Allergic response occurs on binding of an allergen to IgD.

5. Fill in the blanks:
   a. Epitope is present on .... molecules.
   b. Haptens are ....molecular weight compounds.
   c. Antibodies are secreted by .... cells.
   d. Antibody diversity arises from gene ....
   e. Secretory component is present in ....
   f. .... is the largest immunoglobulin.
   g. .... is the most abundant immunoglobulin in plasma.
   h. MHC .... proteins are present on the surface of macrophages, B cells and dendritic cells.
   i. Cytotoxic T cells release ...., granzyme and granulysin.
   j. Helper T cells release ....
   k. .... immunity does not improve on repeated exposure to the same antigen.
   l. CD 4 is a transmembrane protein present in .... cells.
   m. T cell receptors are made up of one .... and one .... chain.
   n. Antigen-presenting cells possess MHC .... protein.
   o. IL-2 stimulates the division of .... cells.
   p. Classic complement cascade is activated upon binding of .... or .... to an antigen present on the surface of a cell.
   q. Complement components are encoded by MHC class .... genes.
   r. .... response is quick, strong and long lasting.
   s. Hybridoma cells are cultured in .... medium.
   t. Hybridoma cells can be used to produce .... antibodies.

ANSWERS TO SHORT QUESTIONS

4. a. False   b. True
   c. True   d. True
   e. False   f. False
   g. True   h. True
   i. False   j. False
   k. True   l. False
   m. True   n. False
   o. True   p. True

q. True

s. True

5. a. Antigen

c. Plasma

e. IgA

g. IgG

i. Perforins

k. Innate

m. α, β

o. Helper T

q. III

s. HAT

r. False

t. False

b. Low

d. Re-arrangement

f. IgM

h. II

j. Lymphokines

l. Helper T

n. II

p. IgG, IgM

r. Secondary

t. Monoclonal

20

Prophyrins, Haemoglobin and Bilirubin

Porphyrins are formed by union of four pyrrole rings through methenyl bridges. The porphyrins usually contain a metal ion linked to the nitrogen atoms of the pyrrole rings. The biologically important porphyrins are usually conjugated proteins consisting of a metalloporphyrin linked to a protein. Some important compounds containing porphyrins are:

1. Haemoglobin

In haemoglobin, iron-porphyrin is linked with globin. Haemoglobin is a tetramer made up of four subunits. Each subunit contains a porphyrin nucleus, a ferrous ion and a polypeptide chain. Haemoglobin can reversibly combine with oxygen, and transports oxygen in the body.

2. Myoglobin

The structure of myoglobin is similar to that of haemoglobin with the difference that it is a monomer. It is present in muscles, and can reversibly combine with oxygen.

3. Cytochromes

Cytochromes contain iron-porphyrin conjugated to proteins. The iron-porphyrin portion is similar to that of haemoglobin. Cytochromes are components of respiratory chain in mitochondria, and transport electrons. Some cytochromes perform other functions as well, e.g. microsomal hydroxylation.

4. Catalase

This is an iron-porphyrin containing enzyme that is present mainly in animals. It acts on hydrogen peroxide.

5. Peroxidase

This is another iron-porphyrin containing enzyme that acts on hydrogen peroxide. It occurs mainly in plants.

6. Tryptophan Pyrrolase

This is an iron-porphyrin containing enzyme that acts on tryptophan.

CHEMISTRY

The structural units of porphyrins are pyrrole rings.

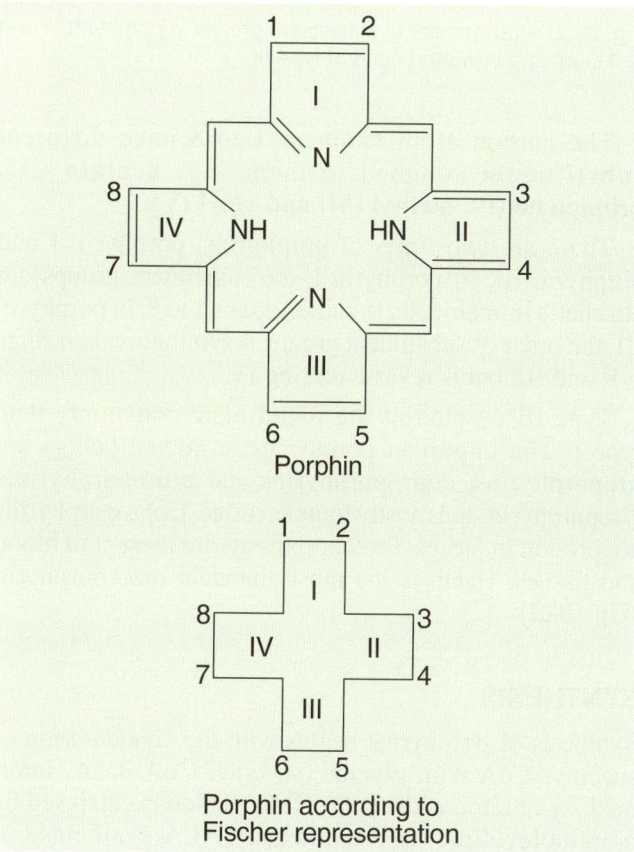

Four pyrrole rings combine to form the parent porphyrin, porphin. A simple representation of the porphin structure has been proposed by Fischer (Fig. 20.1).

Fig. 20.1: Porphin. The pyrrole rings are numbered I, II, III and IV. The arabic numerals show the positions of substituent groups

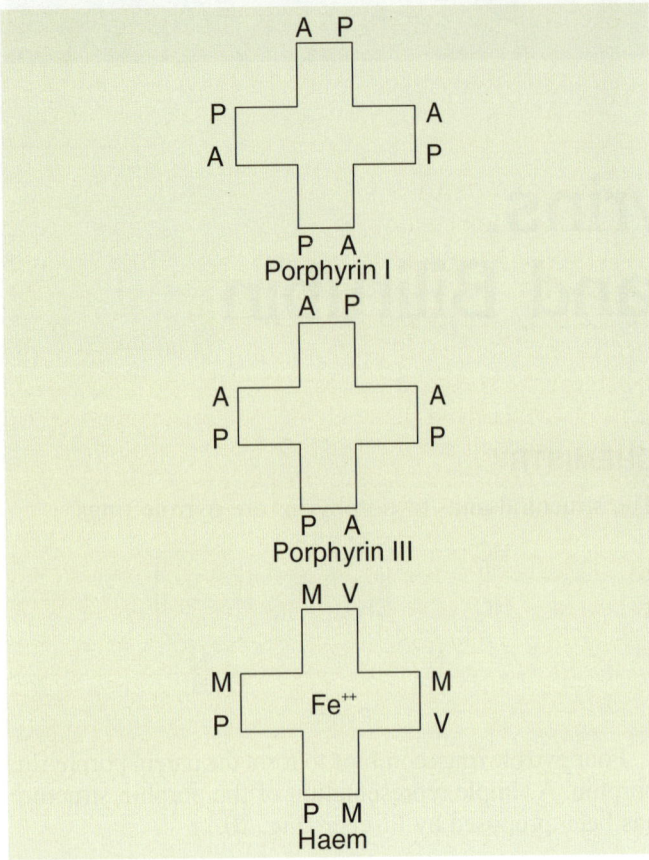

Fig. 20.2: Arrangement of substituent groups in porphyrins I and III. Haem is a protoporphyrin of type III

The carbon atom numbers 1 to 8 have different **substituents** attached to them, e.g. **acetate (A), propionate (P), methyl (M) and vinyl (V).**

There are two types of porphyrins, porphyrin I and porphyrin III. In porphyrin I, the substituent groups are attached symmetrically to carbon atoms 1 to 8. In porphyrin III, the order of substituent groups is symmetrical on rings I, II and III, but is reverse on ring IV.

Type III porphyrins are found more commonly than type I. The important porphyrins in human beings are uroporphyrins, coproporphyrins and protoporphyrins. Uroporphyrins are mostly found in urine. Coproporphyrins are present in faeces. Protoporphyrins are present in blood and tissues. Haem is the most abundant protoporphyrin (Fig. 20.2).

SYNTHESIS

Synthesis of porphyrins begins with the condensation of succinyl CoA with glycine (succinyl CoA is an intermediate of citric acid cycle). The reaction is catalysed by δ-aminolevulinic acid synthetase (ALA synthetase or AmLev synthetase). The product is α-amino-β-ketoadipic acid.

$$\begin{array}{c} CH_2-COOH \\ | \\ CH_2-C \sim S-CoA \\ \| \\ O \\ \text{Succinyl CoA} \end{array}$$

$$\begin{array}{c} CH_2-COOH \\ | \\ NH_2 \\ \text{Glycine} \\ CoA-SH \end{array} \Bigg\} \text{ALA synthetase}$$

$$\begin{array}{c} CH_2-COOH \\ | \\ CH_2-C-CH-COOH \\ \| \quad\quad | \\ O \quad\quad NH_2 \\ \text{α-Amino-β-ketoadipic acid} \end{array}$$

$$\text{Protoporphyrin III + Fe}^{++} \xrightarrow{\text{Haem synthetase}} \text{Haem}$$

α-Amino-β-ketoadipic acid is decarboxylated by ALA synthetase in the presence of pyridoxal phosphate (PLP) to form δ-aminolevulinic acid (ALA).

$$\begin{array}{c} CH_2-COOH \\ | \\ CH_2-C-CH-COOH \\ \| \quad\quad | \\ O \quad\quad NH_2 \\ \text{α-Amino-β-ketoadipic acid} \end{array}$$

$$\xrightarrow[CO_2]{\text{ALA synthetase, PLP}}$$

$$\begin{array}{c} CH_2-COOH \\ | \\ CH_2-C-CH_2-NH_2 \\ \| \\ O \\ \text{δ-Aminolevulinic acid} \end{array}$$

Two molecules of ALA are condensed by ALA dehydrase to form the first pyrrole compound, porphobilinogen.

$$\begin{array}{c} CH_2-COOH \\ | \\ CH_2-C-CH_2-NH_2 \\ \| \\ O \end{array}$$

$$\begin{array}{c} O=C-CH_2-NH_2 \\ | \\ CH_2-CH_2-COOH \\ \text{ALA} \end{array}$$

$$\xrightarrow[2H_2O]{\text{ALA dehydrase}}$$

$$\begin{array}{c} CH_2-COOH \\ | \\ C=C-CH_2-NH_2 \\ \diagup \quad\quad \diagdown \\ \quad\quad NH \\ \diagdown \quad\quad \diagup \\ C=C \\ | \quad\; H \\ CH_2-CH_2-COOH \\ \text{Porphobilinogen} \end{array}$$

Different porphyrins are formed from porphobilinogen. The exact reactions leading to the synthesis of porphyrins are not fully understood. Four porphobilinogen molecules react in the presence of uroporphyrinogen I synthetase to form hydroxymethylbilane. Hydroxymethylbilane spontaneously cyclises to form uroporphyrinogen I, or it can be enzymatically cyclised to uroporphyrinogen III by uroporphyrinogen I synthetase and uroporphyrinogen III cosynthetase. Coproporphyrinogens can be formed from uroporphyrinogens, and protoporphyrinogens from coproporphyrinogens (Fig. 20.3).

Protoporphyrin III is the most abundant and most important porphyrin. Haem is synthesised from protoporphyrin III in the presence of haem synthetase (ferrochelatase). Haem can combine with different polypeptides to form haemoglobin and other haemoproteins.

Regulation

The major purpose of porphyrin synthesis is to form **haem**. The regulatory enzyme in the pathway is **ALA synthetase**. The regulator is haem itself. Regulation occurs by **repression-derepression**. When haem is not being utilised, its concentration increases and it combines with an aporepressor to form the repressor. The repressor acts on the ALA synthetase gene and represses the synthesis of ALA synthetase. This decreases the synthesis of porphyrins. When haem begins to be utilised, its concentration decreases, and the synthesis of ALA synthetase is derepressed. The enzyme concentration increases and so does the porphyrin synthesis.

HAEMOGLOBIN

Haemoglobin (Hb) is the most abundant porphyrin-containing compound. It is a tetramer made up of four subunits. Each subunit contains a haem group and a polypeptide chain. The polypeptide chains are of five types viz. α, β, γ, δ and ε. The α chain is made up of 141 amino acids while other types have 146 amino acid residues each. Normal adult haemoglobin (HbA) is made up of four haem groups, two α chains and two β chains, and is represented as $\alpha_2\beta_2$. A small amount of HbA_2 is also found in adults which is $\alpha_2\delta_2$. Foetal haemoglobin (HbF) is $\alpha_2\gamma_2$. Embryonic haemoglobin is $\alpha_2\varepsilon_2$.

Each polypeptide chain is attached to the two **propionate** side chains of haem. The ferrous ion at the centre of each haem group has six electrons in its outermost orbit. Four of these link iron to the four nitrogen atoms of haem. The other two link iron to **two histidine residues** of the polypeptide chain. These are His_{58} and His_{87} in a chains, and His_{63} and His_{92} in β and other types of chains.

The distal iron-histidine bond is unstable and is broken when haemoglobin is exposed to high oxygen tension. This results in the formation of an iron-oxygen bond.

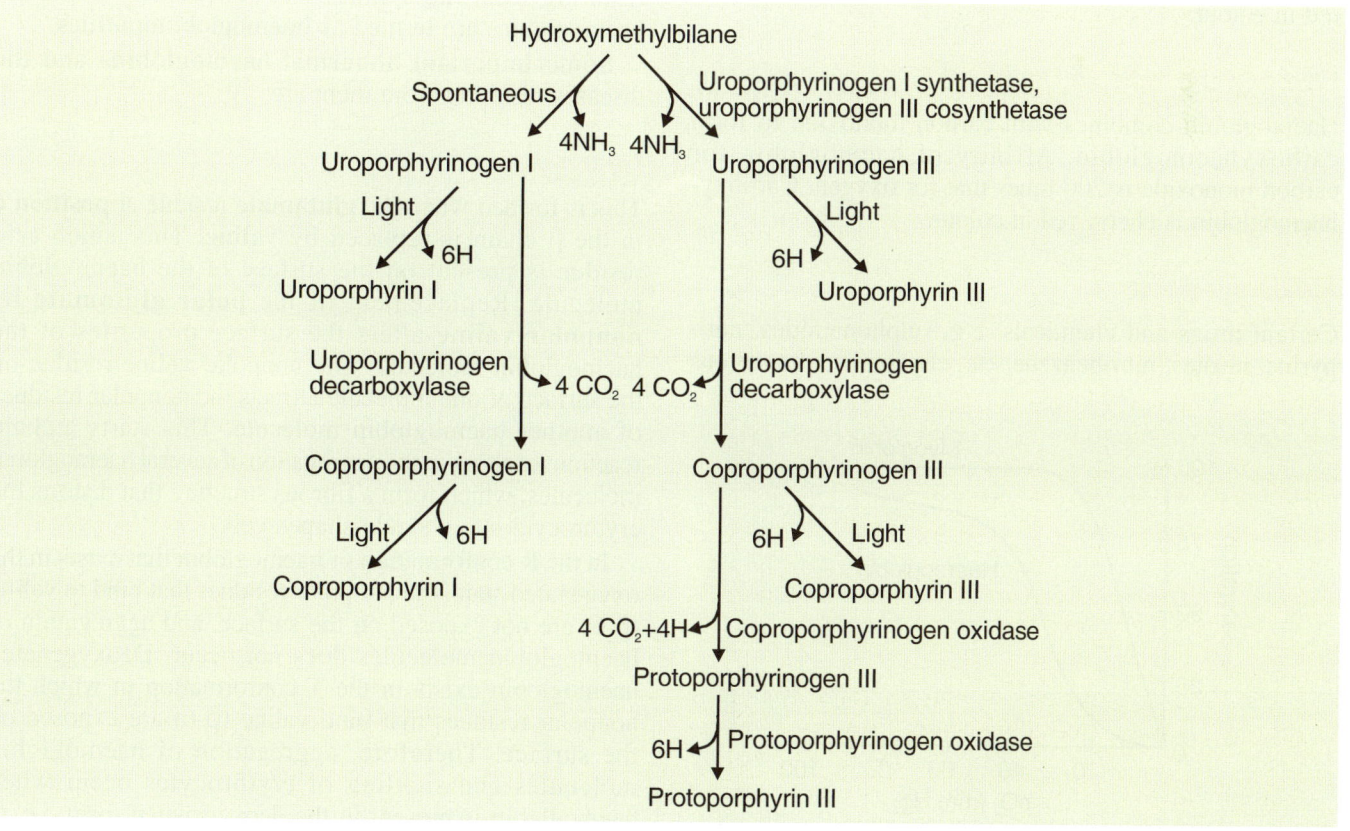

Fig. 20.3: Synthesis of different types of porphyrins from hydroxymethylbilane

The binding of oxygen to haemoglobin changes the conformation of haemoglobin. Two conformations have been described, T (taut) and R (relaxed). Deoxygenated Hb exists in T form which is stabilised by **2,3-biphospho-glycerate (2,3-BPG)** which is formed from 1,3-BPG (an intermediate in glycolytic pathway) when there is a deficiency of oxygen in the tissues. There is a central cavity in the haemoglobin molecule surrounded by the four polypeptide chains. 2,3-BPG enters this cavity and cross links the two β chains. When oxygen tension increases, 2,3-BPG is displaced and the T form changes into R form. During this transition, one pair of α and β subunits rotates by 15° relative to the other pair.

Each subunit of haemoglobin can bind one oxygen molecule. Since there are four subunits in a molecule of haemoglobin, one molecule can bind four oxygen molecules. Binding of one oxygen molecule to haemoglobin facilitates the binding of other oxygen molecules. This is known as **co-operative binding** and is responsible for the **sigmoidal** oxygen saturation/dissociation curve. This property is not shown by myoglobin which consists of a single monomeric unit. Oxygenated myoglobin releases oxygen only when oxygen tension is very low (Fig. 20.4).

Derivatives of Haemoglobin

Oxyhaemoglobin

This is the oxygenated form of haemoglobin and is bright red in colour.

Carboxyhaemoglobin

Haemoglobin combines with carbon monoxide to form carboxyhaemoglobin. Affinity of haemoglobin for carbon monoxide is 200 times that for oxygen. Carboxy-haemoglobin is cherry red in colour.

Methaemoglobin

Certain drugs and chemicals, e.g. sulphonamides, anti-pyrine, nitrites, nitrobenzene, etc. can oxidise the ferrous

iron of haemoglobin to ferric iron. Haemoglobin is converted into methaemoglobin, which is brownish red in colour. Methaemoglobin cannot combine with oxygen.

While haemoglobin cannot combine with cyanide, methaemoglobin can react with cyanide to form cyanmetha-emoglobin. This property is used in the treatment of **cyanide poisoning**. The patient is given sodium nitrite and sodium thiosulphate. The former converts haemoglobin into methaemoglobin which combines with cyanide to form non-toxic cyanmethaemoglobin. Sodium thiosulphate reacts with cyanide to form non-toxic sodium thiocyanate.

Sulphaemoglobin

Hydrogen sulphide and sulphonamides can convert haemoglobin into sulphaemoglobin which is dirty brown in colour, and cannot combine with oxygen.

Abnormal Haemoglobins

Several abnormal haemoglobins are formed due to mutations in the genes encoding polypeptide chains of haemoglobin. Often, a single amino acid is substituted. Hundreds of abnormal haemoglobins have been discovered, most of which are capable of normal or near-normal functioning. In some cases, when the amino acid substitution occurs in a critical region of the molecule, the functioning of haemoglobin is impaired. The diseases resulting from the synthesis of functionally abnormal haemoglobins are termed as **haemoglobinopathies**.

Some important abnormal haemoglobins and the diseases resulting from them are:

Haemoglobin S

This is formed when the **glutamate** residue at **position 6** in the β chain is replaced by **valine.** This amino acid residue is present on the surface of the haemoglobin molecule. Replacement of the **polar glutamate** by **nonpolar valine** alters the surface properties of the haemoglobin molecule. The nonpolar valine residue on the surface of one molecule attracts the nonpolar residues of another haemoglobin molecule. This starts a chain reaction resulting in the aggregation of several haemoglobin molecules, which form a fibrous structure that distorts the erythrocyte into a sickle-shaped cell.

In the R conformation of haemoglobin that exists in the oxygenated state, the nonpolar residues that bind to valine (β-6) are not exposed on the surface, and aggregation of haemoglobin molecules does not occur. Deoxygenated haemoglobin exists in the T conformation in which the nonpolar residues that bind valine (β-6) are exposed on the surface. Therefore, aggregation of haemoglobin molecules and sickling of erythrocytes occur when haemoglobin is present in the deoxygenated form, i.e. at low oxygen tension. Sickled erythrocytes are susceptible

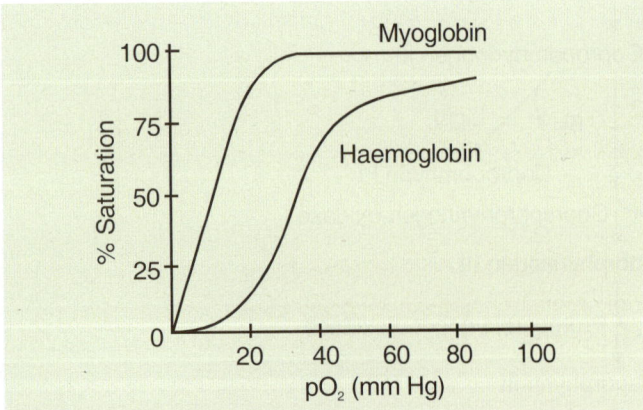

Fig. 20.4: Oxygen dissociation curve of haemoglobin and myoglobin

to premature destruction. Rapid destruction of erythrocytes causes haemolytic anaemia.

Inheritance of sickle cell anaemia is autosomal recessive. If the defect is inherited from one parent only, it results in **sickle cell trait** which doesn't cause any clinical abnormality. If the defect is inherited from both the parents, it results in **sickle cell disease** and severe haemolytic anaemia. Prenatal diagnosis can be made by **RFLP analysis** of foetal DNA (Chapter 16).

It has been shown that the presence of haemoglobin S gives some **protection against malaria**. The malarial parasite inhabiting erythrocytes gets killed when the erythrocytes are destroyed. Prevalence of haemoglobin S has been found to be higher in those areas where malaria is endemic.

Haemoglobin M

This is also known as haemoglobin Boston. It is formed when the histidine residue at position 58 in the α chain is replaced by tyrosine due to a point mutation. Bonding of phenol group of tyrosine with iron converts the ferrous form of iron into the ferric form (methaemoglobin) which cannot combine with oxygen.

Thalassaemia

This results from a decrease in, or lack of, synthesis of either α chains or β chains. Defective synthesis of α chains leads to **α-thalassaemia** and that of β chains leads to **β-thalassaemia.** A variety of genetic defects are known to cause thalassaemia, e.g. deletion of a part or whole of a gene, defective processing of the primary transcript, defective transport or translation of mRNA, premature termination, etc. Decreased synthesis or lack of synthesis of one type of chain leads to an overproduction of the unaffected chain resulting in the formation of a haemoglobin having only α chains or only β chains. When the defect is transmitted by only one parent, it results in **thalassaemia minor** which is symptomless. When the defect is transmitted by both the parents, it results in **thalassaemia major** which is associated with severe anaemia.

PORPHYRIAS

Porphyrias are a group of diseases in which large quantities of porphyrins or their precursors are excreted in urine. The abnormal excretion is due to a **defect in the synthetic pathway**. Absence or deficiency of an enzyme leads to accumulation of the intermediates proximal to the affected enzyme. The urine of the patients is normal in colour when fresh but becomes pink on exposure to light due to oxidation of porphyrinogens. Skin photosensitivity is often present. Early intermediates bind to nervous tissue, and produce neuropsychiatric abnormalities. Thus, a defect early in the pathway is more harmful than a defect in the later steps. Though the defective gene is present in all the tissues, the expression is usually confined to a particular tissue.

Depending upon the site of expression of the genetic defect, porphyrias may be divided into **hepatic porphyrias** and **erythropoietic porphyrias**. Hepatic porphyrias include acute intermittent porphyria, porphyria cutanea tarda, hereditary coproporphyria and variegate porphyria. Erythropoietic porphyrias include congenital erythro-poietic porphyria and protoporphyria. The enzymes deficient in these porphyrias are shown in Table 20.1. The clinical abnormalities are mainly neurovisceral in hepatic porphyrias and cutancous in crythropoictic porphyrias. However, some overlapping of signs and symptoms is not uncommon.

Hepatic Porphyrias

Acute attacks of abdominal pain, nausea and vomiting occur in hepatic porphyrias. Overactivity of the sympathetic nervous system produces tachycardia, tremors and hypertension. Psychiatric symptoms, e.g. anxiety, insomnia, disorientation and depression, are common. Motor neuropathy may cause progressive muscular weakness. Seizures can also occur. The biochemical basis of neurovisceral abnormalities is not known. In addition to the neurovisceral signs and symptoms, cutaneous photosensitivity of varying degrees is also present in hereditary coproporphyria, variegate porphyria and porphyria cutanea tarda.

Table 20.1: Inherited disorders of porphyrin synthesis			
	Mode of inheritance	*Affected enzyme*	*Site of expression*
Congenital erythropoietic porphyria	Autosomal recessive	Uroporphyrinogen III cosynthetase	Erythroid cells
Acute intermittent porphyria	Autosomal dominant	Uroporphyrinogen I synthetase	Liver cells
Porphyria cutanea tarda	Autosomal dominant	Uroporphyrinogen decarboxylase	Liver cells
Hereditary coproporphyria	Autosomal dominant	Coproporphyrinogen oxidase	Liver cells
Variegate porphyria	Autosomal dominant	Protoporphyrinogen oxidase	Liver cells
Protoporphyria	Autosomal dominant	Ferrochelatase (haem synthetase)	Erythroid and liver cells

Erythropoietic Porphyrias

Severe cutaneous photosensitivity from a very early age is the hallmark of erythropoietic porphyrias. Porphyrin precursors are present in skin, and damage the skin on exposure to sunlight. Multiple vesicles erupt on the skin. The skin is pigmented and fragile. Denuded areas on skin are prone to infections. Bones and teeth may be pigmented due to deposition of porphyrin precursors. Haemolysis may occur due to binding of porphyrin precursors to haemoglobin. In protoporphyria, liver damage also occurs in some patients.

While exposure to sunlight produces the cutaneous manifestations, the neurovisceral manifestations are precipitated by steroids, alcohol and a number of drugs, e.g. barbiturates, meprobamate, carbamazepine, mephenytoin, sulphonamides, griseofulvin, etc.

CATABOLISM

When the life-span of erythrocytes is over, they are broken down in the reticuloendothelial cells. Haem is removed from globin. The methenyl bridge between ring I and ring II is broken, releasing iron and converting haem into a green pigment, **biliverdin**. Biliverdin is reduced to yellow-coloured **bilirubin**, which is the major **bile pigment** in human beings. Biliverdin is formed from haem by microsomal haem oxygenase system, and bilirubin is formed from biliverdin by biliverdin reductase.

Bilirubin is released from reticuloendothelial cells into circulation. Since it is **insoluble in water**, it is transported in association with **albumin.** Albumin has two bilirubin-binding sites, a **high-affinity site** and a **low-affinity site**. Bilirubin is first bound to the high-affinity site. If the high-affinity sites on all the albumin molecules are saturated, excess bilirubin is bound to the low-affinity site. At a normal plasma albumin concentration, 20 to 25 mg of bilirubin can be bound to the high-affinity sites of the albumin molecules per 100 ml of plasma.

Water-insoluble bilirubin released from reticulo-endothelial cells is known as **unconjugated bilirubin**. It is taken up by liver cells from the circulating albumin with the help of a carrier-mediated **active transport** system. In hepatic parenchymal cells, bilirubin is conjugated with glucuronic acid to make it water-soluble. The conjugation reaction occurs in two steps. First, bilirubin reacts with UDP-glucuronic acid. UDP is released and bilirubin is converted into bilirubin monoglucuronide. The latter reacts with another molecule of UDP-glucuronic acid. UDP is releases and bilirubin monoglucuronide is converted into bilirubin diglucuronide. Both the reactions are catalysed by bilirubin UDP-glucuronyl transferase.

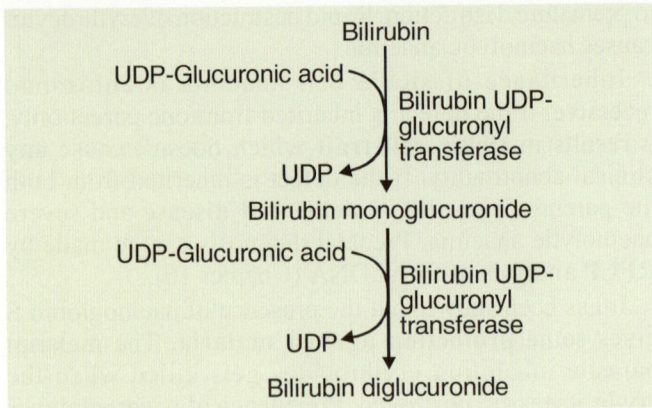

According to some authorities, the conversion of bilirubin monoglucuronide into bilirubin diglucuronide occurs by a trans-esterification reaction between two bilirubin monoglucuronide molecules, catalysed by bilirubin-glucuronide glucuronosyl transferase (dismutase):

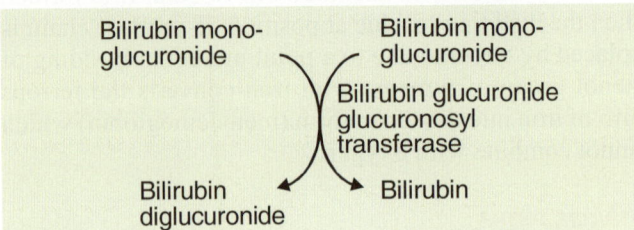

Bilirubin diglucuronide (**conjugated bilirubin**) is excreted into the intestine through bile. Excretion of conjugated bilirubin by hepatic cells into biliary canaliculi also takes place by an active transport mechanism. In the large intestine, bilirubin is freed from glucuronic acid, and is reduced to **urobilinogen** by the enzymes of intestinal bacteria. Most of the urobilinogen is excreted in the faeces. A small portion is reabsorbed into portal circulation, and is taken to liver which re-excretes most of it into the intestine (enterohepatic circulation of urobilinogen). A very small amount of urobilinogen enters the systemic circulation, and is excreted by the kidneys in urine.

JAUNDICE

Serum bilirubin concentration normally ranges from 0.2 to 1.0 mg/dl. This is total bilirubin, and includes conjugated as well as unconjugated bilirubin. The concentration of unconjugated bilirubin in serum varies from 0.1 to 0.6 mg/dl. This enters the circulation from the reticuloendothelial cells. The concentration of conjugated bilirubin in serum ranges from 0.1 to 0.4 mg/dl. This enters the circulation from liver after it has been conjugated. Conjugated bilirubin is also known as **direct reacting bilirubin** because, being water-soluble, it can directly react with Ehrlich's diazo reagent without the addition of an organic solvent. Unconjugated bilirubin is known as **indirect reacting bilirubin** because, being water-insoluble, it reacts with Ehrlich's diazo reagent only after addition of methanol or ethanol.

When serum bilirubin concentration rises above normal (**hyperbilirubinaemia**), bilirubin gets deposited in tissues which are stained **yellow**. This is known as **jaundice**. The yellow staining can be seen in skin and mucous membranes but is most clearly visible in the sclera. Jaundice can occur in a number of diseases. Depending upon the site of the disease, jaundice can be divided into three types:

1. Pre-hepatic Jaundice

This is also known as haemolytic jaundice. It is due to an increased rate of haemolysis. As the rate of breakdown of haemoglobin increases, bilirubin is formed in such large quantities that the capacity of the liver cells to take up, conjugate and excrete it is exceeded. The concentration of unconjugated bilirubin in serum rises and jaundice results. Since unconjugated bilirubin can not be excreted by the kidneys, urine does not contain bilirubin. As the rate of formation of bilirubin is increased, the rate of formation of urobilinogen is also increased, and urinary excretion of urobilinogen is raised.

A common cause of haemolytic jaundice is the "physiological jaundice of neonates". This occurs in some neonates between the third and tenth days of life. Erythrocytes formed during foetal life containing foetal haemoglobin are rapidly destroyed after birth. The rate of formation of bilirubin is increased. As the hepatic conjugating system is not fully developed in the first two weeks of life, unconjugated bilirubin accumulates in blood causing jaundice. This, however, is a transient and benign condition.

Haemolytic jaundice can occur in several other haemolytic diseases, the most serious of which is erythroblastosis foetalis or "haemolytic disease of the newborns". This occurs when an Rh-negative mother conceives an Rh-positive baby. The Rh-antigen can be transferred across the placenta from the foetus to the mother. The maternal system starts forming Rh-antibodies which can be transferred across the placenta to the foetus. The resulting Rh-incompatibility in the foetus causes severe haemolysis and unconjugated hyperbilirubinaemia. The baby is born with jaundice. If serum bilirubin (unconjugated) rises above **20–25 mg/dl**, the excess bilirubin is attached to the low-affinity site of albumin which is off-loaded in the central nervous system as the lipids of the nervous tissue can easily take up nonpolar bilirubin from the low-affinity site of albumin. In the central nervous system, bilirubin is attached to basal ganglia, hippocampus, cerebellum, medulla, etc. These tissues are stained yellow (**kernicterus**). Kernicterus is often fatal, and leaves behind permanent neurological damage if the patient survives.

2. Hepatic Jaundice

This is due to rapid destruction of liver cells as in viral hepatitis and on exposure to hepatotoxic drugs and chemicals. It is also known as **hepatocellular jaundice**. As the liver cells are destroyed, the capacity of the liver to take up, conjugate and excrete bilirubin is decreased. The concentration of unconjugated bilirubin in serum rises even though the rate of formation of bilirubin is normal.

In viral hepatitis, the surviving liver cells are inflamed and swollen, and compress the biliary canaliculi. This intraheptatic obstruction leads to regurgitation of conjugated bilirubin into systemic circulation. The concentration of conjugated bilirubin in serum is raised, and as it is water-soluble, it is excreted in urine. Thus, both unconjugated and conjugated bilirubin are raised in serum, and bilirubin is present in urine in viral hepatitis. Urinary urobilinogen is usually normal.

3. Post-hepatic Jaundice

This is also known as **obstructive jaundice** as it is caused by an obstruction to the flow of bile. The obstruction may be intrahepatic or extrahepatic. The commonest cause of biliary obstruction is the presence of gall stones in the biliary passage. The obstruction may also be due to compression of biliary channels by tumours, e.g. cancer of the head of pancreas. Rarely, atresia or stricture of biliary channels may cause obstruction.

As the flow of bile is obstructed, bilirubin which has been conjugated in the liver cells cannot be excreted into the intestine. Conjugated bilirubin is regurgitated into circulation. As it is water-soluble, it is excreted in urine. Since bilirubin cannot reach the intestine, formation of urobilinogen is stopped and urobilinogen is absent from urine. Therefore, the characteristic biochemical features of obstructive jaundice are a rise in the concentration of conjugated bilirubin in serum, presence of bilirubin in urine and absence of urobilinogen from urine.

Jaundice also occurs in the following inherited disorders of bilirubin metabolism:

Gilbert's Syndrome

This is a group of disorders in which the active transport system for hepatic uptake of circulating bilirubin is defective. The bilirubin UDP-glucuronyl transferase activity in liver cells is also sub-normal. The concentration of unconjugated biliburin is raised in serum. The inheritance is autosomal dominant.

Crigler-Najjar Syndrome

This is an autosomal recessive disorder. Two types have been recognised. In type I, hepatic bilirubin UDP-glucuronyl transferase activity is absent. Unconjugated bilirubin is greatly elevated in serum, kernicterus is common and the disease is often fatal. In type II, hepatic bilirubin UDP-glucuronyl transferase activity is decreased. Concentration of unconjugated bilirubin in serum is increased but it is not as high as in Crigler-Najjar syndrome, type I.

Lucey-Driscoll Syndrome

An inhibitor of bilirubin UDP-glucuronyl transferase, which is believed to be a progestational steroid, is present in the plasma of patients with Lucey-Driscoll syndrome. This causes unconjugated hyperbilirubinaemia.

Rotor's Syndrome

The active transport system, responsible for excretion of conjugated bilirubin in bile, is defective in Rotor's syndrome. This leads to conjugated hyperbilirubinaemia. The inheritance is autosomal recessive.

Dubin-Johnson Syndrome

The nature of the defect is similar to that in Rotor's syndrome. In addition, a black pigment, probably melanin, is deposited in liver. The concentration of conjugated bilirubin in plasma is raised. The inheritance is autosomal recessive.

EXERCISE

1. Describe haem synthesis and its regulation. Explain the difference between the oxygen dissociation curve of haemoglobin and myoglobin.

2. Describe the formation and excretion of bilirubin. Explain the changes in serum bilirubin in different types of jaundice.

3. Write short notes on:
   a. Methaemoglobin
   b. Haemoglobin S
   c. Thalassaemia
   d. Acute intermittent porphyria
   e. Kernicterus
   f. Crigler-Najjar syndrome
   g. Cyanmethaemoglobin

4. Write 'true' or 'false':
   a. Regulation of haem synthesis occurs by repression-derepression.
   b. Adult haemoglobin contains two alpha and two gamma chains.
   c. Oxygen dissociation curve of myoglobin is sigmoidal.
   d. Binding of oxygen to haemoglobin is co-operative.
   e. Cyanide can combine with methaemoglobin but not with haemoglobin.
   f. Haemoglobin S is formed due to substitution of glutamate by aspartate at position 6 in the β chain.
   g. Haemoglobin S has different surface properties as compared to normal haemoglobin.
   h. Haem synthetase is deficient in acute intermittent porphyria.
   i. Conjugated bilirubin is transported in circulation by albumin.
   j. An increase in serum bilirubin above 20-25 mg/dl can cause kernicterus.

5. Fill in the blanks:
   a. The regulatory enzyme for haem synthesis is ....
   b. An amino acid required for porphyrin synthesis is ....
   c. An intermediate of citric acid cycle required for porphyrin synthesis is ....
   d. Foetal haemoglobin contains two .... and two .... chains.
   e. Iron is present in the ....form in methaemoglobin.
   f. Urine turns ....in colour on exposure to atmosphere in porphyria.
   g. Haemoglobin is catabolised in .... cells.
   h. Albumin can bind ....molecules of bilirubin.
   i. Bilirubin is conjugated in ....
   j. .... bilirubin is soluble in water.
   k. Jaundice occurs due to a rise in the concentration of ....in plasma.
   l. .... bilirubin is raised in obstructive jaundice.
   m. Bilirubin is not present in urine in .... jaundice.
   n. Urobilinogen is not present in urine in .... jaundice.
   o. Concentration of .... bilirubin in serum is raised in Crigler-Najjar syndrome.

ANSWERS TO SHORT QUESTIONS

4. a. True
   c. False
   e. True
   g. True
   i. False

   b. False
   d. True
   f. False
   h. False
   j. True

5. a. ALA synthetase
   c. Succinyl CoA
   e. Ferric
   g. Reticuloendothelial
   i. Liver
   k. Bilirubin
   m. Haemolytic (pre-hepatic)
   o. Unconjugated.

   b. Glycine
   d. α, γ
   f. Pink
   h. Two
   j. Conjugated
   l. Conjugated
   n. Obstructive (post-hepatic)

21

Water-soluble Vitamins

Vitamins are a heterogeneous group of organic compounds which are essential for animals and human beings. They are required in very minute quantities. They do not provide energy but their dietary intake is essential as they perform biochemical functions **essential for normal health, growth and reproduction**. Deficiencies of vitamins produce specific diseases which can be prevented or cured by administration of the pure vitamins or intake of natural foods containing the concerned vitamins. Several deficiency diseases and, in some instances, their treatments were discovered long before the discovery of the vitamins themselves. Scurvy and beriberi are examples of diseases which could be cured by giving citrus fruits and rice polishings respectively even though the causes of these diseases were not known.

Since the chemical natures of vitamins were not known at the time of their discovery, they were named after the letters of the alphabet. These names have now been largely replaced by chemical names. Vitamins can be classified into two groups on the basis of their solubility:

Water-soluble Vitamins

These are soluble in water, and are not stored in the body. Their **excessive intake is wasteful** but does not cause any toxicity. The water-soluble vitamins essential for human beings are vitamins of the B-complex family (thiamin, riboflavin, niacin, pantothenic acid, pyridoxine, biotin, lipoic acid, folic acid and cobalamin) and vitamin C.

Fat-soluble Vitamins

These are soluble in fat but insoluble in water, and include vitamins A, D, E and K. They are present in food in association with dietary lipids. They can be stored in the body and their **excessive intake can be toxic**.

WATER-SOLUBLE VITAMINS

Since the water-soluble vitamins are not stored in the body to any appreciable extent, they have to be taken in the diet every day. Losses can occur during cooking as some of them are heat-labile. Some of the water-soluble vitamins

are **synthesised by intestinal bacteria**. If intestinal bacteria are destroyed, for example by **antibiotic therapy**, additional intake is required.

THIAMIN

Thiamin (vitamin B_1) is heat-stable in acidic medium but not in basic medium. It is oxidised by mild oxidising agents to thiochrome which is biologically inactive. Chemically, it is made up of a substituted pyrimidine linked through a methylene bridge to substituted thiazole (Fig. 21.1).

Functions

Thiamin forms a **coenzyme**, thiamin pyrophosphate (**TPP**) or thiamin diphosphate (**TDP**).

TPP is a coenzyme for **transketolase** (in HMP shunt) and **α-keto acid dehydrogenases,** e.g. pyruvate dehydrogenase, α-ketoglutarate dehydrogenase and branched-chain α-keto acid dehydrogenase. Impaired activity of α-keto acid dehydrogenases due to thiamin deficiency can limit the availability of energy.

Sources

Whole grain cereals, pulses, nuts, yeast, liver, kidney, heart and meat are good sources of thiamin. In **cereals,** thiamin is present mainly in the **outer layer of the grain**. Removal of the outer layer, e.g. by milling, causes considerable loss of thiamin.

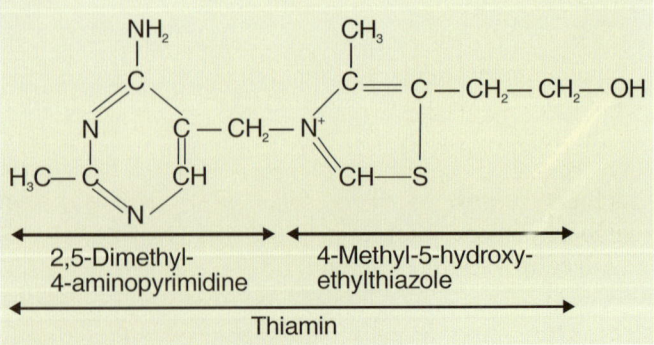

Fig. 21.1: Thiamin

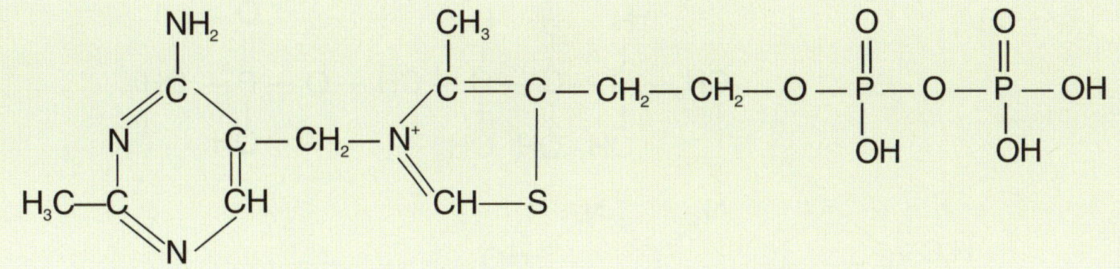

Fig. 21.2: Thiamin pyrophosphate (TPP) or thiamin diphosphate (TDP)

Requirement

The daily requirement of thiamin is 0.5 mg/1,000 kcal of energy or 1 to 1.5 mg/day in adults. The requirement increases in **alcoholics** and in **hypermetabolic states,** e.g. pregnancy, fever, hyperthyroidism, etc.

Deficiency

People consuming **polished rice** or **refined wheat flour** as their staple food are susceptible to thiamin deficiency due to removal of the outer layer of the grain. Parboiling of rice decreases the loss of thiamin. During parboiling, paddy is soaked in warm water for a few hours and, then, steam-dried. Thiamin percolates into the deeper part of the grain. Polishing of parboiled rice leads to a limited loss of thiamin. Alcoholics can develop deficiency as **alcohol impairs the absorption** of thiamin and its conversion into TPP.

Deficiency of thiamin causes beriberi which affects:

1. Central Nervous System

Thiamin deficiency causes peripheral neuritis involving sensory as well as motor nerves. Sensory involvement leads to hyperaesthesia, numbness, tingling and pain. Motor involvement leads to muscular weakness, sluggish reflexes, ataxia and paralysis.

2. Cardiovascular System

The heart muscle becomes weak resulting in congestive heart failure. This, in turn, causes oedema and ascites.

3. Gastrointestinal Tract

Involvement of gastrointestinal tract causes anorexia, dyspepsia and constipation.

Predominant involvement of central nervous system is known as **dry beriberi** as there is no collection of water in interstitial tissue in this condition. Predominant involvement of cardiovascular system is known as **wet beriberi** because of the occurrence of oedema. **Mixed beriberi** is more common in which different systems are involved in varying degrees.

Diagnosis of beriberi can be confirmed by some **laboratory investigations**. Concentration of pyruvic acid in blood is increased in beriberi. Thiamin concentration in erythrocytes is decreased. Urinary thiamin excretion after a test dose is decreased. In normal subjects, most of the test dose is promptly excreted in urine. Subjects deficient in thiamin retain most of the test dose in tissues and excrete less in urine. Measurement of transketolase activity in erythrocytes can confirm the diagnosis.

RIBOFLAVIN

Riboflavin (vitamin B_2) is heat-stable in neutral and acidic medium but not in basic medium. Its aqueous solution is unstable in sunlight and ultraviolet light. It can be readily reduced to leucoriboflavin. Chemically, riboflavin is 6,7-dimethyl-9-D-ribityl isoalloxazine (Fig. 21.3).

Functions

Riboflavin is a constituent of flavin mononucleotide (FMN) and flavin adenine dinucleotide (FAD). These two coenzymes can undergo reversible oxidation and reduction, and participate in a number of oxidation-reduction reactions. The riboflavin portion of FMN and FAD can reversibly combine with two hydrogen atoms.

FMN is a constituent of respiratory chain (electron transfer chain) and is a coenzyme for L-amino acid oxidase (Fig. 21.4).

FAD is a constitutent of respiratory chain, and is a coenzyme for several enzymes, e.g. D-amino acid oxidase, acyl CoA dehydrogenase, succinate dehydrogenase, glycerol-3-phosphate dehydrogenase, xanthine oxidase, sphingosine reductase, pyruvate dehydrogenase, α-ketoglutarate dehydrogenase, etc. It is also a constituent of the microsomal hydroxylase system (Fig. 21.5).

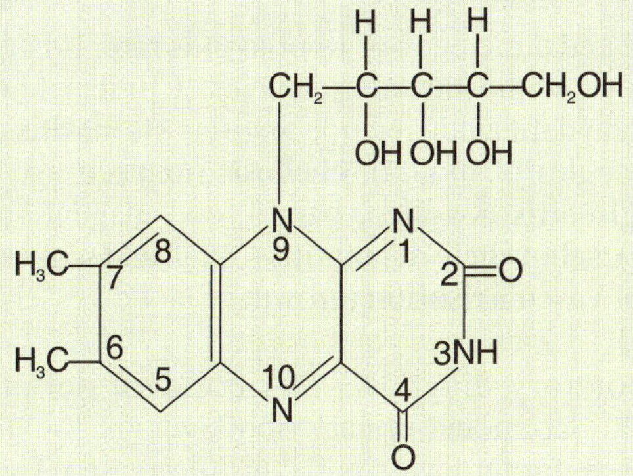

Fig. 21.3: Riboflavin

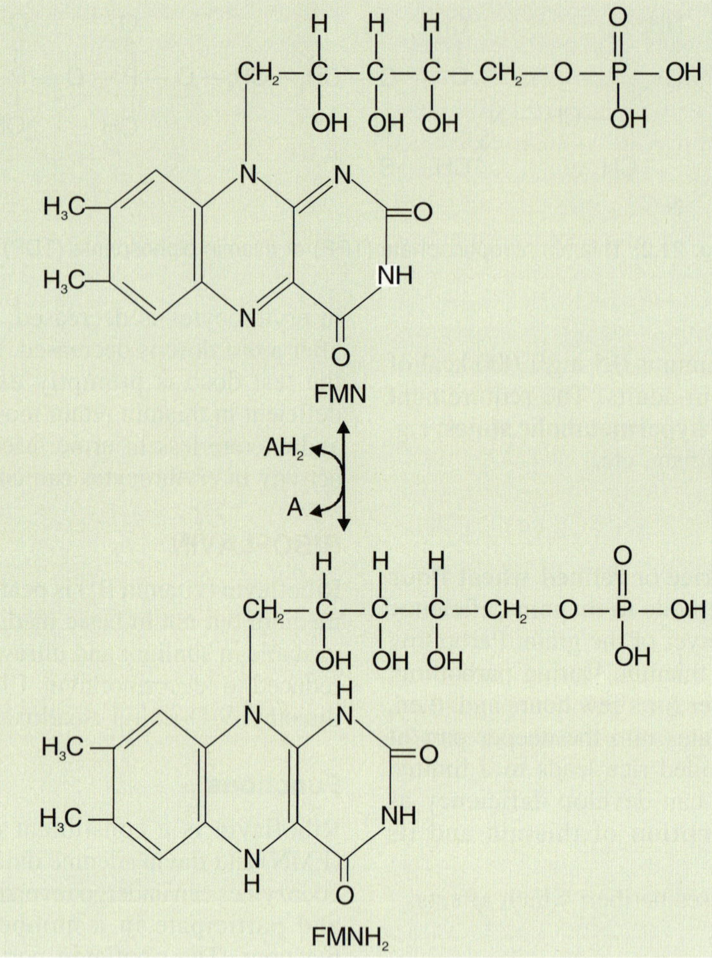

Fig. 21.4: Oxidised and reduced flavin mononucleotide (FMN).

Sources

Milk, eggs, liver, kidney, heart, yeast, germinating cereals and many vegetables are good sources of riboflavin.

Requirement

The daily requirement for riboflavin has been placed at 0.6 mg/1,000 kcal.

Deficiency

An isolated deficiency of riboflavin is rare. It is generally combined with other deficiencies. Clinical features of riboflavin deficiency include **angular stomatitis** (fissures at the angles of mouth), **cheilosis** (cracked and swollen lips), **glossitis** (swollen, painful and magenta-coloured tongue), **seborrheic dermatitis** (rough and scaly skin) and **corneal vascularisation** (growth of blood vessels into the cornea).

Laboratory diagnosis of riboflavin deficiency is difficult. Serum and urinary riboflavin are low in severe deficiency. Erythrocyte riboflavin is decreased. The urinary excretion of riboflavin after a test dose is decreased.

NIACIN

Niacin was known in the past as **anti-pellagra factor**, pellagra-preventing factor and vitamin B_3. It occurs in two forms, niacin (nicotinic acid) and niacinamide (nicotinamide). Both the forms are equally active. Niacin is converted into niacinamide in the body (Fig.21.6).

Niacin is a fairly stable vitamin. It is not destroyed by heat, light or oxidising agents.

Functions

Niacin performs its functions in the form of two coenzymes, nicotinamide adenine dinucleotide (**NAD**) and nicotinamide adenine dinucleotide phosphate (**NADP**) which can undergo reversible oxidation and reduction (Fig. 21.7).

Nicotinamide combines with ribose and phosphoric acid to form a nucleotide, which is linked with an adenine nucleotide to form NAD. An extra phosphate group is present in NADP (Fig. 21.8).

NAD and NADP act as coenzymes for several oxidoreductases in many metabolic pathways, e.g.

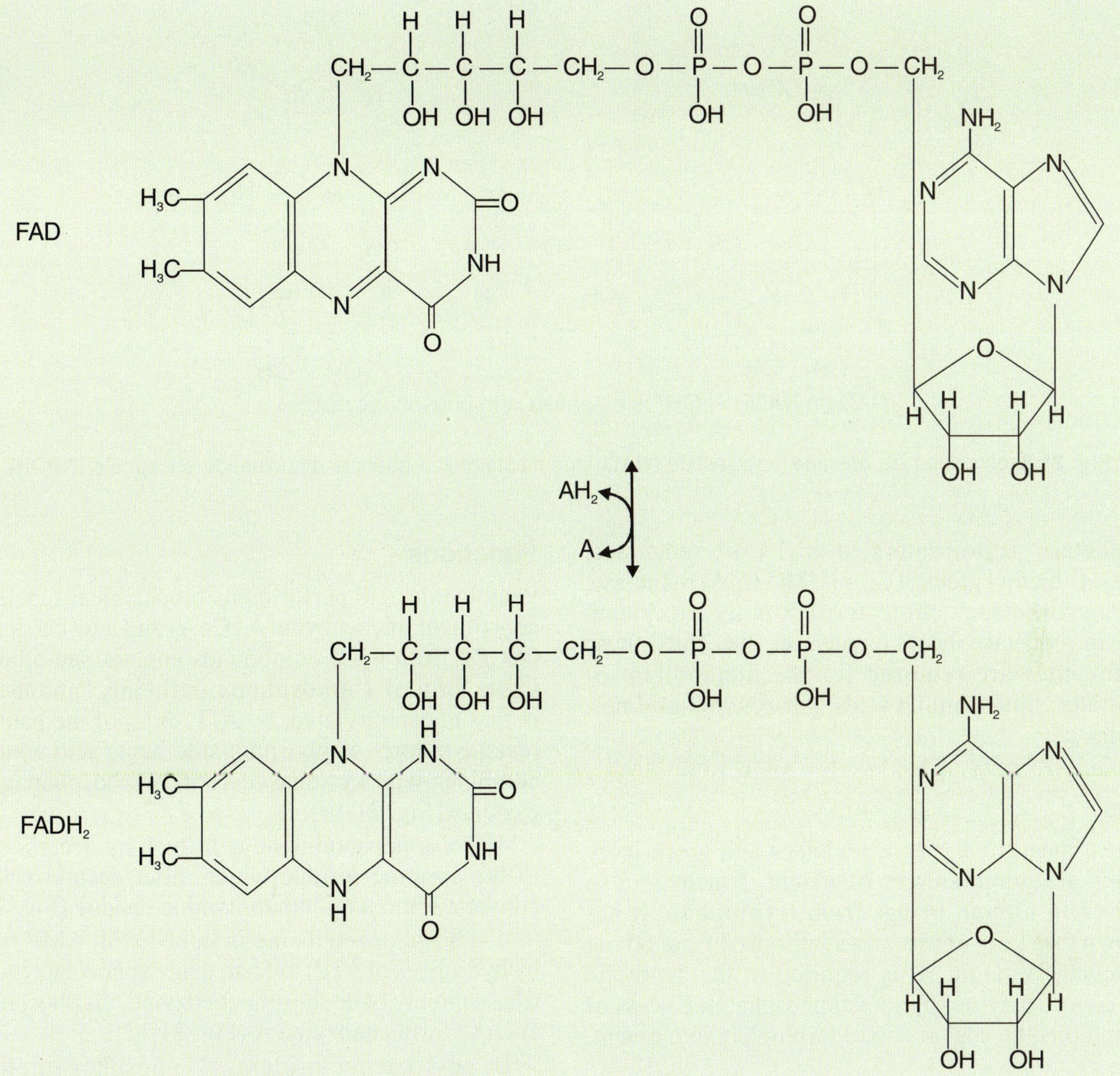

Fig. 21.5: Oxidised and reduced flavin adenine dinucleotide (FAD)

glycolysis, hexose monophosphate shunt, citric acid cycle, synthesis of fatty acids and steroids, oxidation of fatty acids, oxidative deamination of amino acids, etc. Generally, NAD acts as coenzyme in catabolic pathways and NADP in anabolic pathways. NAD is also a constituent of the respiratory chain. Some examples of enzymes which require NAD as a coenzyme are glyceraldehyde-3-phosphate dehydrogenase, lactate dehydrogenase, pyruvate dehydrogenase, isocitrate dehydrogenase, α-ketoglutarate dehydrogenase, malate dehydrogenase, β-hydroxyacyl CoA dehydrogenase, glutamate dehydrogenase, IMP dehydrogenase, etc. Examples of enzymes requiring NADP as a coenzyme include glucose-6-phosphate dehydrogenase, 6-phosphogluconate dehydrogenase, β-ketoacyl

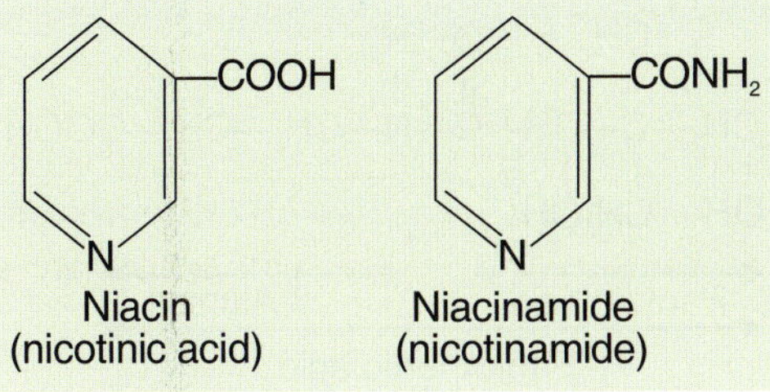

Fig. 21.6: Niacin and niacinamide

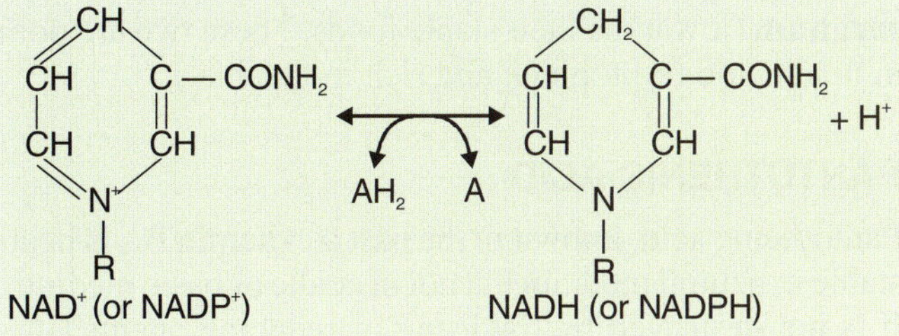

Fig. 21.7: Oxidised and reduced forms of NAD (or NADP)

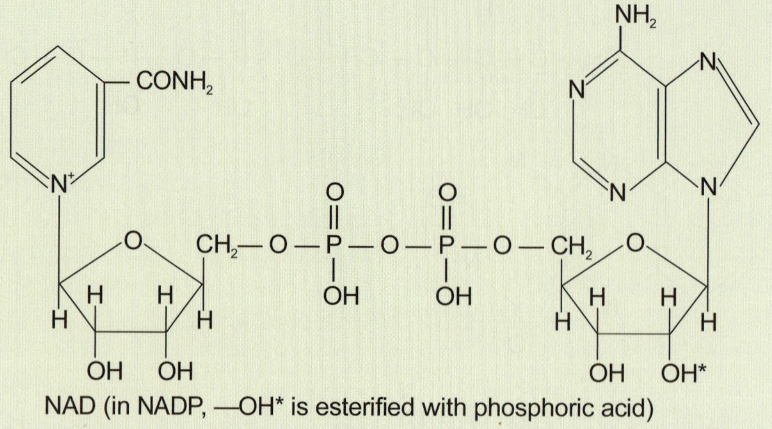

NAD (in NADP, —OH* is esterified with phosphoric acid)

Fig. 21.8: Nicotinamide adenine dinucleotide (NAD) and nicotinamide adenine dinucleotide phosphate (NADP)

CoA reductase, α,β-unsaturated acyl CoA reductase, β-hydroxy-β-methyl glutaryl CoA (HMG CoA) reductase, squalene synthetase, cholesterol 7-α-hydroxylase, thioredoxin reductase, haem oxygenase, etc. Thus, these two coenzymes are required for the metabolism of carbohydrates, lipids, amino acids, purines, pyrimidines, porphyrins, etc.

Sources

Milk, eggs, meat, liver, yeast, tomatoes and green leafy vegetables are good sources of niacin. Niacin is also **synthesised in human beings from tryptophan**. It has been shown that 1 mg of niacin is synthesised from 60 mg of tryptophan. Vitamin B_6 is required in the synthetic pathway as a coenzyme (pyridoxal phosphate). **Excess of leucine** inhibits the conversion of tryptophan into niacin.

Requirement

The daily requirement for niacin is 6.6 mg/1,000 kcal.

Deficiency

Deficiency of niacin causes **pellagra** which is characterised by stomatitis, glossitis, diarrhoea, dermatitis and dementia (mental degeneration). Dermatitis usually affects the exposed parts of the body. If untreated, the disease can be fatal.

Pellagra is common in people consuming **maize** and **sorghum** (jowar) as their staple foods. These two are poor in niacin and tryptophan, and rich in leucine.

PANTOTHENIC ACID

Pantothenic acid, known in the past as vitamin B_5, is heat-stable in neutral medium but not in acidic or basic medium. It is not destroyed by oxidising or reducing agents. It is made up of pantoic acid and β-alanine (Fig. 21.9).

Functions

Pantothenic acid performs its biochemical functions as a constituent of coenzyme A (**CoA**) and acyl carrier protein (**ACP**). Both these compounds contain pantothenic acid in the form of **4′-phosphopantetheine**. Pantothenic acid is first phosphorylated, by ATP, at C_4 of the pantoic acid residue to form 4′-phosphopantothenic acid which, then, combines with cysteine to form 4′-phosphopantothenyl cysteine (Fig. 21.10).

4′-Phosphopantetheine is formed by decarboxy-lation of the cysteine residue which, after decarboxylation, is converted into a thioethanolamine residue (Fig. 21.11).

4′-Phosphopantetheine is linked with AMP (provided by hydrolysis of ATP) to form dephosphocoenzyme A. The ribose moiety of dephosphocoenzyme A is phosphorylated at C_3 to form coenzyme A (Fig. 21.12).

In acyl carrier protein, 4′-phosphopantetheine is esterified with a serine residue of the protein. The –SH group of 4′-phosphopantetheine remains free.

A. *Role of Coenzyme A*

Coenzyme A is also represented as CoA-SH as its terminal **–SH group** binds various compounds. This coenzyme participates in a variety of reactions in the metabolism of carbohydrates, lipids and amino acids. Some examples of such reactions are:

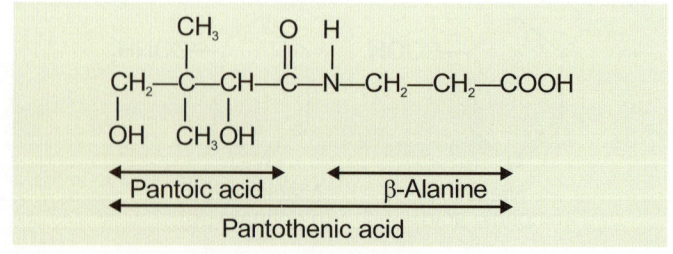

Fig. 21.9: Pantothenic acid

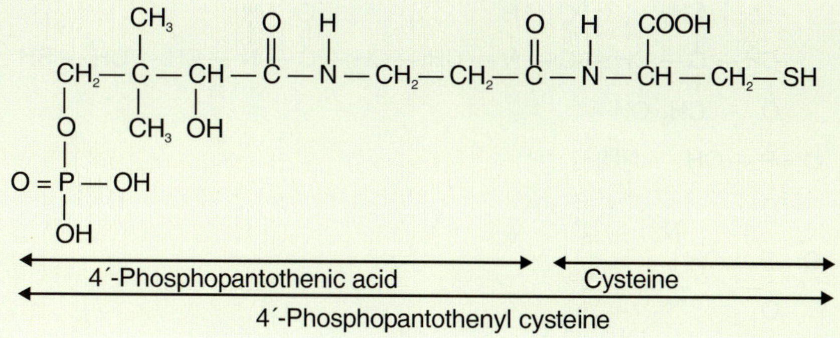

Fig. 21.10: 4´-Phosphopantothenyl cysteine

1. Oxidative Decarboxylation of α-keto Acids

A number of coenzymes are required in this reaction including CoA. The overall reaction is:

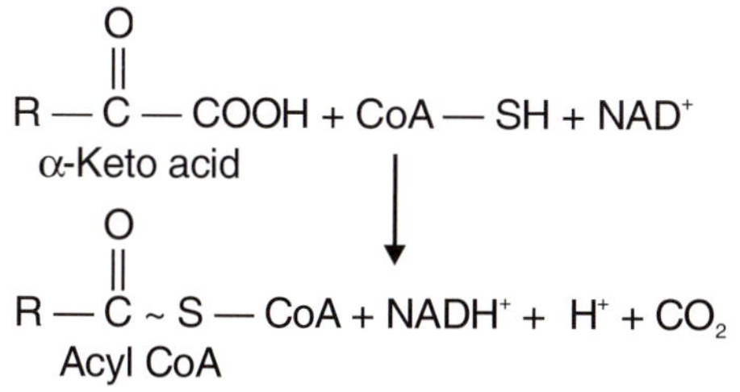

$$R - \overset{\overset{\displaystyle O}{\|}}{C} - COOH + CoA - SH + NAD^+$$
α-Keto acid

$$\downarrow$$

$$R - \overset{\overset{\displaystyle O}{\|}}{C} \sim S - CoA + NADH^+ + H^+ + CO_2$$
Acyl CoA

Pyruvate and α-ketoglutarate are converted into acetyl CoA and succinyl CoA respectively by this reaction.

2. Activation of Fatty Acids

Before fatty acids can take part in any reaction, they have to be converted into their CoA derivatives. This reaction, known as activation of fatty acids, is catalysed by acyl CoA synthetase (thiokinase).

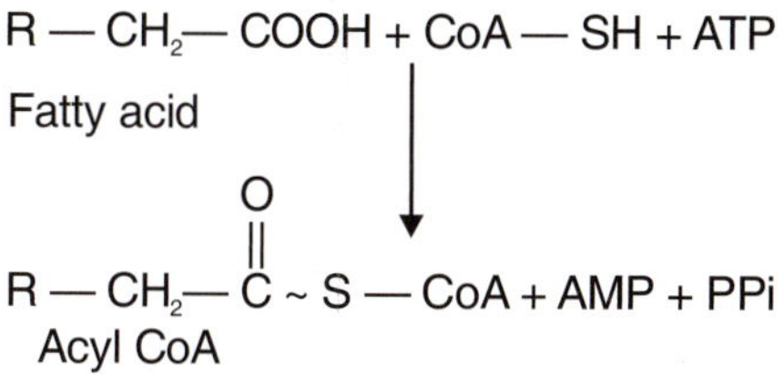

$$R - CH_2 - COOH + CoA - SH + ATP$$
Fatty acid

$$\downarrow$$

$$R - CH_2 - \overset{\overset{\displaystyle O}{\|}}{C} \sim S - CoA + AMP + PPi$$
Acyl CoA

3. Activation of Amino Acids

Some amino acids, e.g. leucine, isoleucine and valine, are converted into their CoA derivatives before they can be metabolised.

An important role of CoA is to provide active acetate (acetyl CoA) for various reactions, e.g. synthesis of fatty acids, cholesterol, ketone bodies, acetylcholine, etc. Active succinate (succinyl CoA) is required for haem synthesis and for gluconeogenesis from some amino acids.

B. Role of Acyl Carrier Protein

Acyl carrier protein is a constituent of the multienzyme complex which catalyses de novo synthesis of fatty acids.

Sources

Pantothenic acid is widely distributed in animal and plant foods. It is also synthesised by intestinal bacteria. Liver, kidney, meat, eggs, yeast, wheat, peas and sweet potatoes are good sources of pantothenic acid.

Requirement

The recommended daily intake is 10 mg though a smaller intake may be sufficient for infants and children.

Deficiency

Deficiency of pantothenic acid has not been reported in human beings. In animals, deficiency leads to loss of

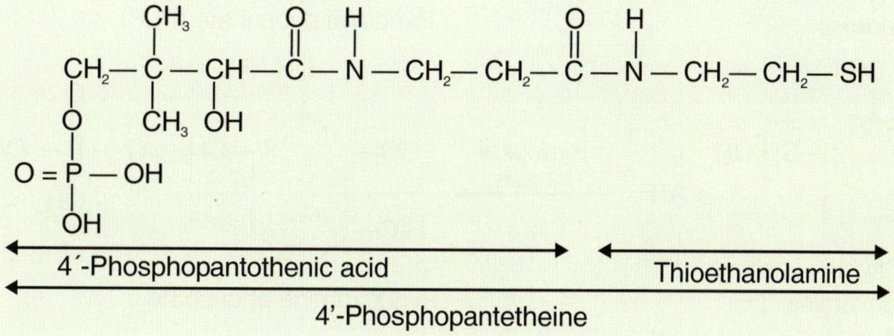

Fig. 21.11: 4´-Phosphopantetheine

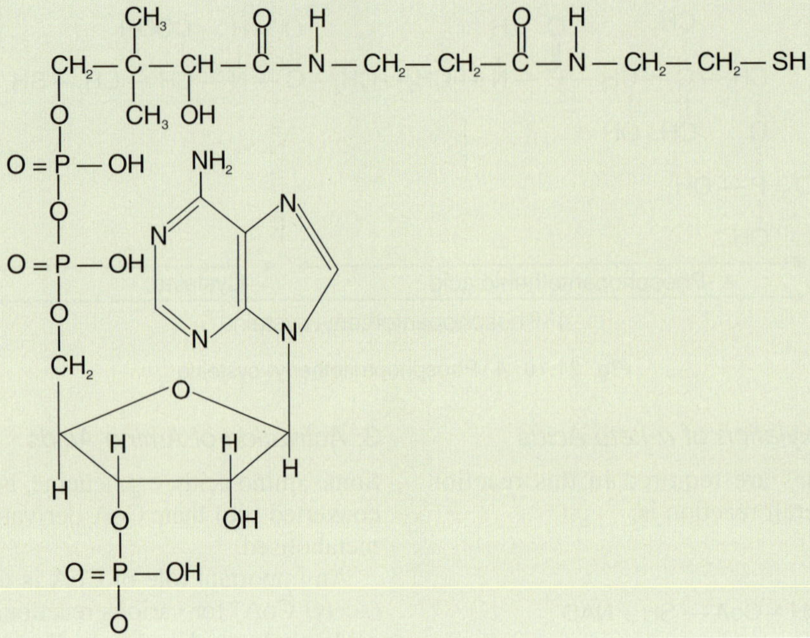

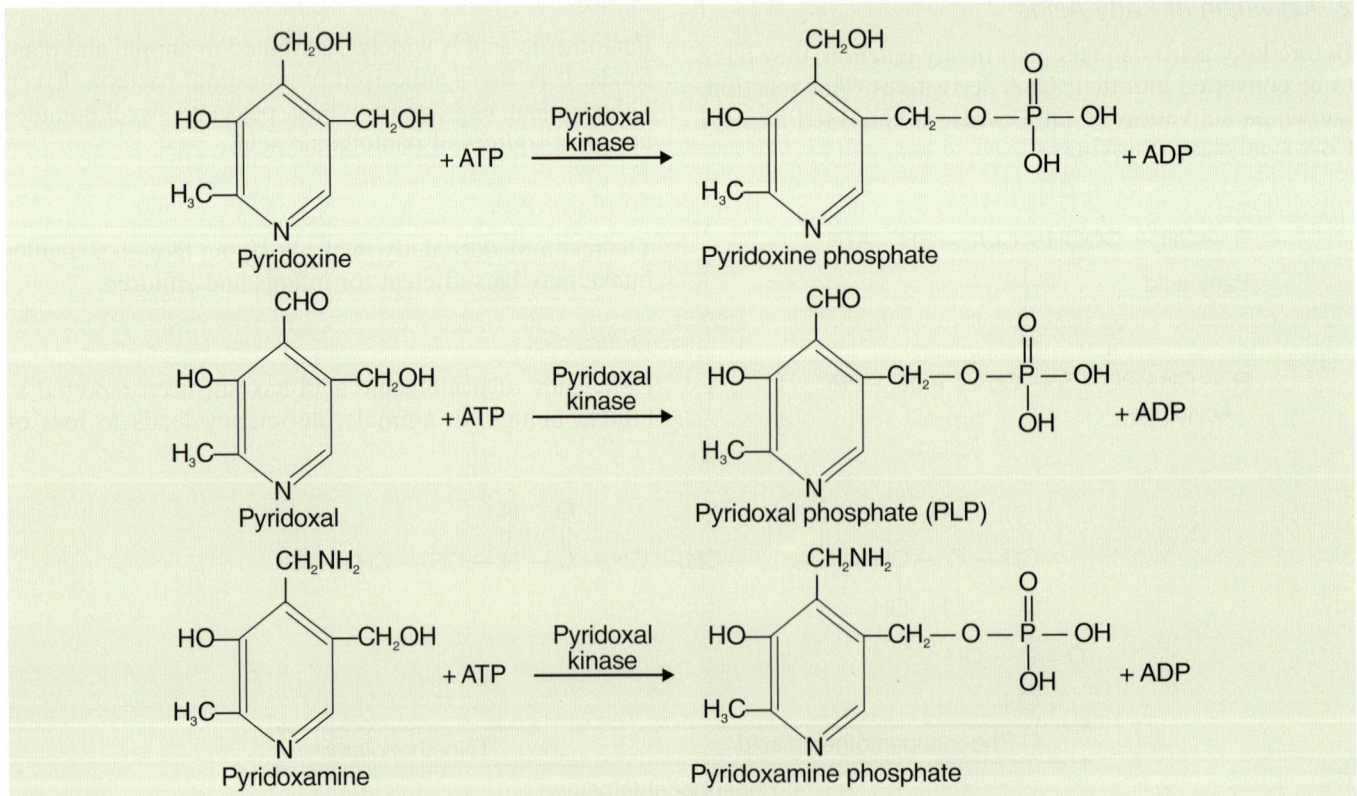

Fig. 21.12: Coenzyme A

weight, loss of hair, greying of hair, anaemia and necrosis of adrenal glands. Human deficiency can be produced experimentally, which causes neurological and gastro-intestinal disturbances.

PYRIDOXINE

Pyridoxine was known in the past as vitamin B_6. Vitamin B_6 consists of three closely related pyridine derivatives, pyridoxine, pyridoxal and pyridoxamine (Fig. 21.13). All the three are equally active as vitamins.

Fig. 21.13: Three forms of vitamin B_6 and their respective phosphates

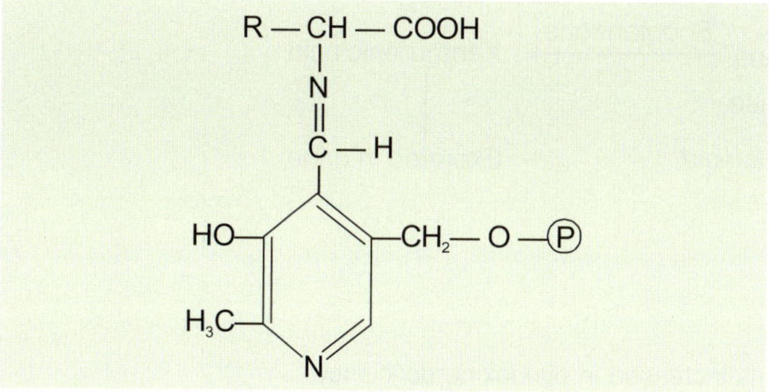

Fig. 21.14: Schiff base

Functions

Pyridoxine, pyridoxal and pyridoxamine are phosphorylated by ATP in the presence of pyridoxal kinase to form pyridoxine phosphate, pyridoxal phosphate and pyridoxamine phosphate respectively. The three are interconvertible.

Pyridoxal phosphate and pyridoxamine phosphate serve as coenzymes, mainly in the metabolism of amino acids. Pyridoxal phosphate (PLP) can form a Schiff base with an α-amino acid. The union occurs between the α-amino group of the amino acid and the aldehyde group of pyridoxal phosphate. The amino acid, thus bound, can undergo various reactions (Fig. 21.14).

Vitamin B_6 coenzymes participate in the following reactions:

1. Transamination

Such reactions are catalysed by specific transaminases. The amino group of an amino acid is transferred to an α-keto acid forming a new amino acid and a new α-keto acid. PLP acts as a carrier of the amino group (Fig. 21.15).

Transamination reactions are important for the formation of new amino acids, and also in the catabolism of amino acids.

2. Deamination

PLP acts as a coenzyme for serine deaminase and threonine deaminase.

3. Decarboxylation

PLP is a coenzyme for decarboxylases acting on glutamate, arginine, tyrosine, etc.

4. Transulphuration

PLP is a coenzyme for cystathionine synthetase and cystathionine γ-lyase which transfer sulphur from homocysteine to serine forming cysteine.

5. Desulphydration

PLP is a coenzyme for cysteine desulphydrase which removes the –SH group from cysteine.

6. Tryptophan Metabolism

One of the intermediates in the catabolism of tryptophan is 3-hydroxykynurenine which is converted into 3-hydroxyanthranilic acid by kynureninase, a PLP-dependent enzyme. When PLP is not available, 3-hydroxyanthranilic acid is not formed, and 3-hydroxykynurenine is spontaneously converted into an alternate metabolite, xanthurenic acid which is excreted in urine. Urinary excretion of xanthurenic acid can serve as an indicator of pyridoxine deficiency (Fig. 21.16).

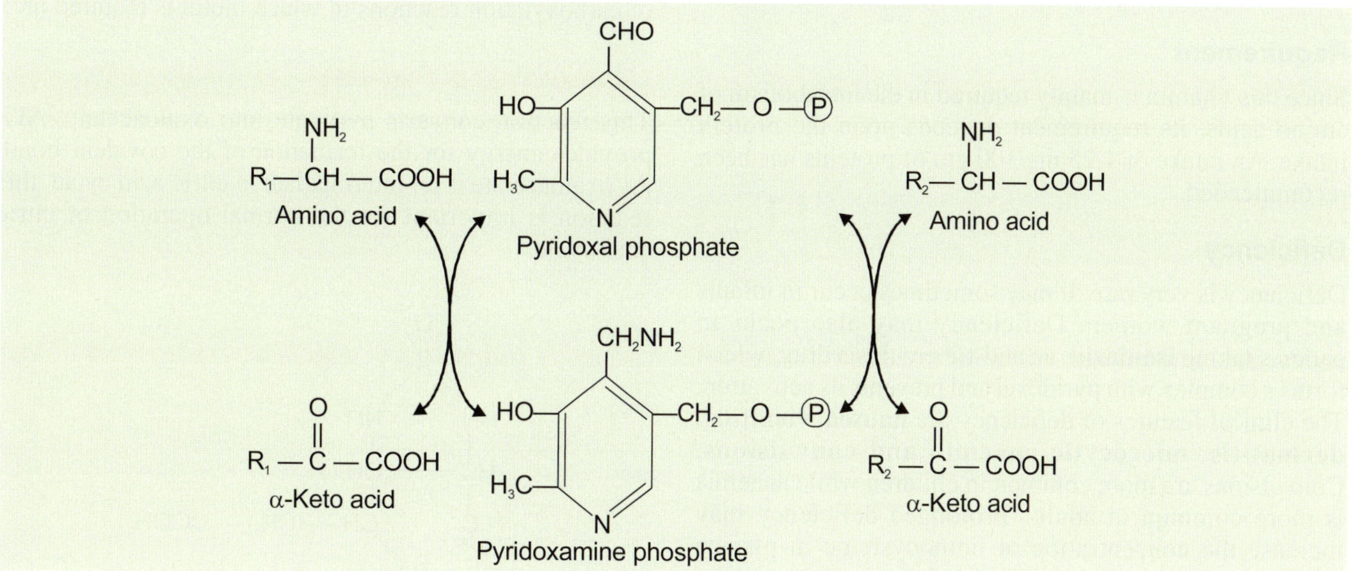

Fig. 21.15: Role of pyridoxal phosphate in transamination

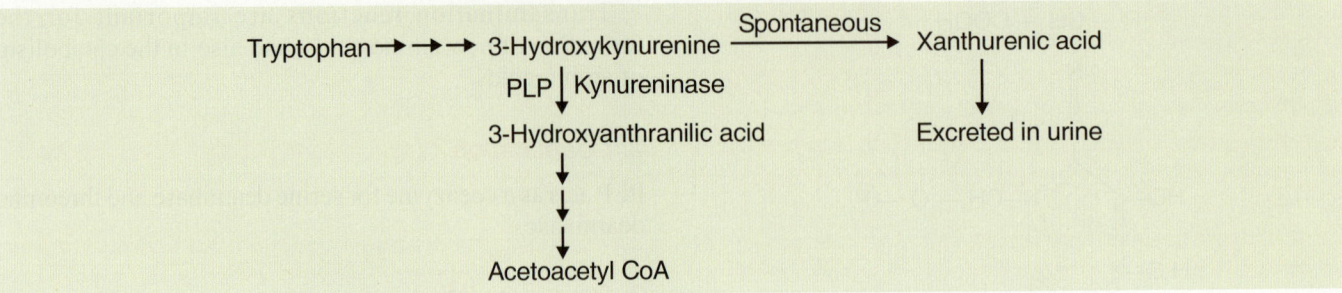

Fig. 21.16: Excretion of xanthurenic acid is increased in pyridoxine deficiency

7. Synthesis of Haem

One of the enzymes involved in the synthesis of haem is δ-aminolevulinic acid synthetase which requires PLP as a coenzyme.

8. Cellular uptake of Amino Acids

Cellular uptake of L-amino acids is an active process which requires the participation of PLP.

9. Formation of γ-amino Butyric Acid

Gamma-amino butyric acid (GABA) acts as a neuro-transmitter in brain. It is formed by the action of glutamate decarboxylase on glutamate. PLP is required as a coenzyme in this reaction.

10. Glycogenolysis

PLP is a coenzyme for **phosphorylase** which catalyses glycogen breakdown.

Sources

Liver, eggs, milk, yeast, wheat, corn and green leafy vegetables are excellent sources of the vitamin. Another source is bacterial synthesis in the intestine.

Requirement

Since this vitamin is mainly required in the metabolism of amino acids, its requirement depends upon the protein intake. An intake of 1.25 mg/100 gm of proteins has been recommended.

Deficiency

Deficiency is very rare. It may sometimes occur in infants and pregnant women. Deficiency may also occur in patients taking **isoniazid**, an anti-tuberculosis drug, which forms a complex with pyridoxal and prevents its activation. The clinical features of deficiency are **nausea, vomiting, dermatitis, microcytic anaemia and convulsions**. Convulsions are more common in children while anaemia is more common in adults. Prolonged deficiency may increase the concentration of homocysteine in plasma **(hyperhomocysteinaemia)** which increases the risk of cardiovascular diseases.

Laboratory diagnosis of pyridoxine deficiency can be confirmed by measuring the excretion of xanthurenic acid in urine after giving a test dose of tryptophan. The **urinary excretion of xanthurenic acid** is increased in pyridoxine deficiency.

BIOTIN

Biotin is also known as **anti-egg white injury factor**. When raw egg white is fed to rats, they develop certain symptoms which are relieved by biotin. It has been shown that raw egg white contains a protein, **avidin**, which forms a complex with biotin preventing its intestinal absorption. This leads to a deficiency of biotin. Avidin is inactivated by heat. Therefore, cooked eggs do not hamper absorption of biotin.

Biotin is heat-stable. It is a heterocyclic, sulphur-containing, monocarboxylic acid (Fig. 21.17).

Functions

Biotin is a coenzyme for carboxylases and is, therefore, also known as **co-carboxylase**. The carboxyl group of biotin forms a bond with the epsilon-amino group of a lysine residue in the apoenzyme molecule. In this way, biotin becomes an integral part of the holoenzyme. Some examples of carboxylation reactions in which biotin is required are:

Carboxylation of Pyruvate

This reaction converts pyruvate into oxaloacetate. ATP provides energy for the formation of the covalent bond. As oxaloacetate is an intermediate in citric acid cycle, this reaction is important for the normal operation of citric acid cycle.

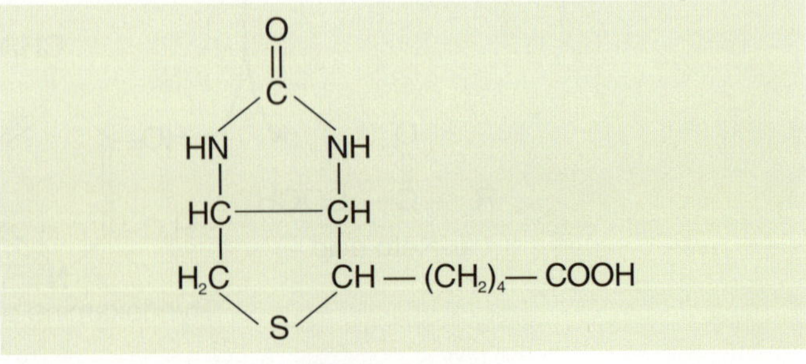

Fig. 21.17: Biotin

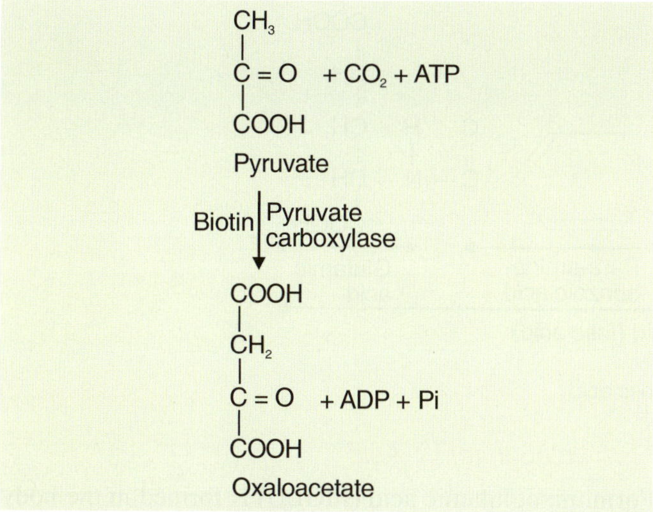

$$
\begin{array}{c}
CH_3 \\
| \\
C = O \quad + CO_2 + ATP \\
| \\
COOH \\
Pyruvate
\end{array}
$$

$$
\xrightarrow[\text{carboxylase}]{\text{Biotin} \mid \text{Pyruvate}}
$$

$$
\begin{array}{c}
COOH \\
| \\
CH_2 \\
| \\
C = O \quad + ADP + Pi \\
| \\
COOH \\
Oxaloacetate
\end{array}
$$

Carboxylation of Acetyl CoA

This reaction converts acetyl CoA into malonyl CoA. ATP provides the energy. This reaction is important for fatty acid synthesis.

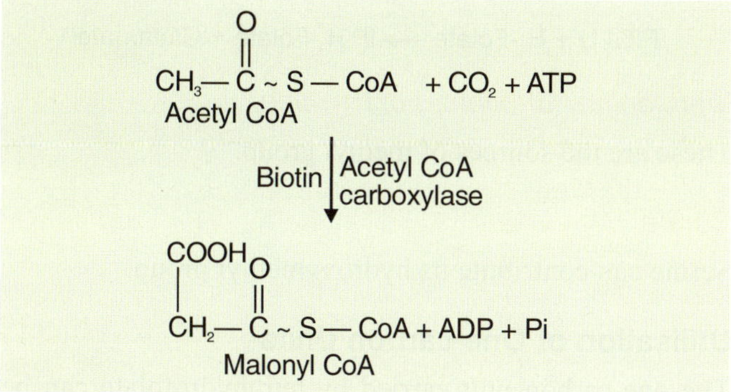

$$
\begin{array}{c}
\quad\quad O \\
\quad\quad \| \\
CH_3 - C \sim S - CoA \quad + CO_2 + ATP \\
Acetyl\ CoA
\end{array}
$$

$$
\xrightarrow[\text{carboxylase}]{\text{Biotin} \mid \text{Acetyl CoA}}
$$

$$
\begin{array}{c}
COOH\ \ O \\
| \quad\ \| \\
CH_2 - C \sim S - CoA + ADP + Pi \\
Malonyl\ CoA
\end{array}
$$

Carboxylation of Propionyl CoA

Propionyl CoA is carboxylated to D-methylmalonyl CoA. This is one of the reactions in the gluconeogenic pathway for conversion of propionate into glucose.

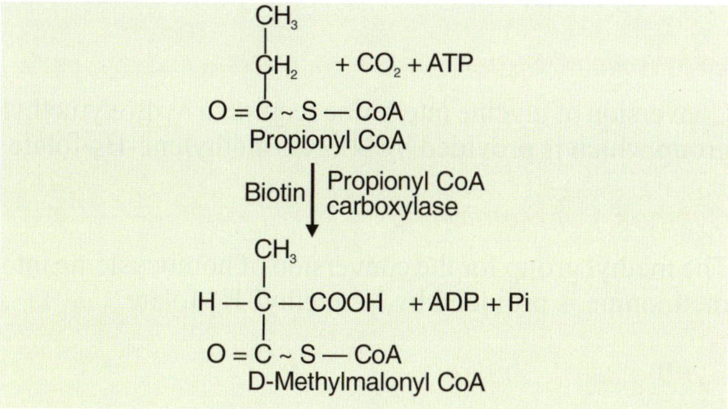

$$
\begin{array}{c}
CH_3 \\
| \\
CH_2 \quad + CO_2 + ATP \\
| \\
O = C \sim S - CoA \\
Propionyl\ CoA
\end{array}
$$

$$
\xrightarrow[\text{carboxylase}]{\text{Biotin} \mid \text{Propionyl CoA}}
$$

$$
\begin{array}{c}
CH_3 \\
| \\
H - C - COOH \quad + ADP + Pi \\
| \\
O = C \sim S - CoA \\
D\text{-Methylmalonyl CoA}
\end{array}
$$

Sources

Bacterial synthesis in the intestine provides ample amounts of biotin. Dietary sources include egg yolk, liver, kidney, yeast, peas, tomatoes, cauliflower, etc.

Requirement

Biotin requirement is not known with certainty as the intestinal bacteria meet most of the requirement. The daily intake has been estimated to be 100 to 300 mg.

Deficiency

Deficiency of biotin is unknown in human beings as sufficient vitamin is provided by intestinal bacteria, and the vitamin is widely distributed in both animal and plant foods. Deficiency may occur in animals when they are fed raw egg white. It is clinically characterised by retarded growth, loss of weight, dermatitis, loss of hair, muscular inco-ordination and paralysis.

LIPOIC ACID

Lipoic acid is a sulphur-containing fatty acid. It is also known as thioctic acid or 6,8-dithio-octanoic acid. It can exist in a reduced form and an oxidised form (Fig. 21.18).

Functions

Lipoic acid acts as a coenzyme in some oxidation-reduction reactions because of its ability to undergo reversible oxidation and reduction. It is required as a coenzyme in the **oxidative decarboxylation of α-keto acids** such as pyruvate and α-ketoglutarate.

Sources

Lipoic acid is widely distributed in foodstuffs. The quantities required by human beings are easily obtained from an ordinary diet.

Requirement

The exact requirement for lipoic acid is not known. The vitamin is probably required in very minute quantities.

Deficiency

Deficiency of lipoic acid has not been reported in human beings. Attempts to induce lipoic acid deficiency in higher animals have also been unsuccessful.

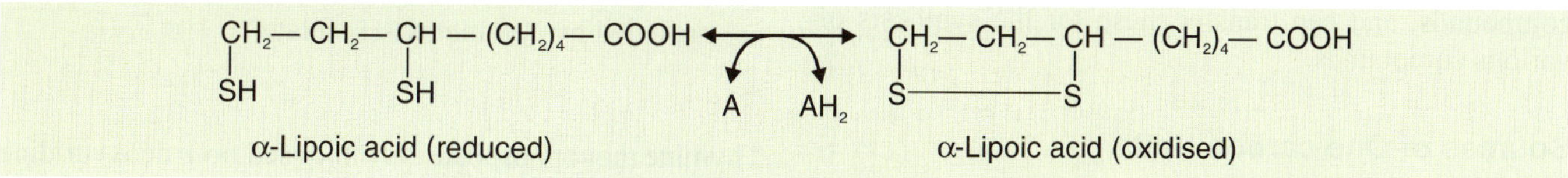

$$
\begin{array}{c}
CH_2 - CH_2 - CH - (CH_2)_4 - COOH \\
| \qquad\qquad | \\
SH \qquad\quad SH
\end{array}
\xrightleftharpoons[A \quad AH_2]{}
\begin{array}{c}
CH_2 - CH_2 - CH - (CH_2)_4 - COOH \\
| \qquad\qquad | \\
S \overline{\qquad\qquad} S
\end{array}
$$

α-Lipoic acid (reduced) α-Lipoic acid (oxidised)

Fig. 21.18: Reduced and oxidised forms of lipoic acid

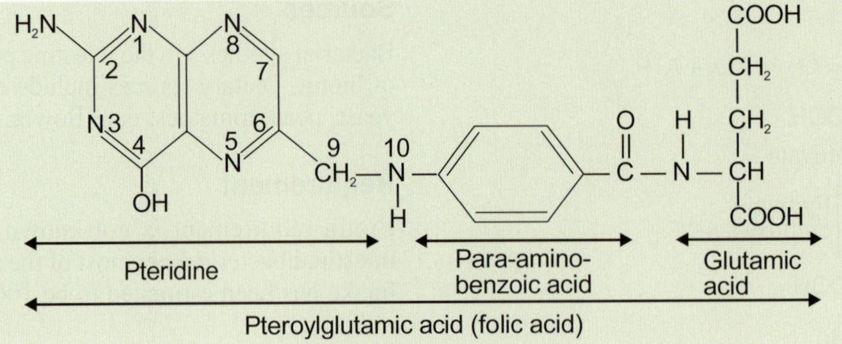

Fig. 21.19: Folic acid

FOLIC ACID

Folic acid is also known as folacin or pteroylglutamic acid. It is made up of pteridine, para-aminobenzoic acid and glutamic acid (Fig. 21.19).

Folic acid is found in foodstuffs as pteroylmonoglutamate, pteroyltriglutamate and pteroylheptaglutamate. The last two are converted into pteroylmonoglutamate in the intestinal mucosa. Folic acid is heat-stable in neutral medium.

Functions

Folic acid forms a coenzyme, **tetrahydrofolate**. Folic acid is first reduced to 7,8-dihydrofolate (H_2-folate or FH_2) and then to 5,6,7,8-tetrahydrofolate (**H_4-folate or FH_4**) by dihydrofolate reductase.

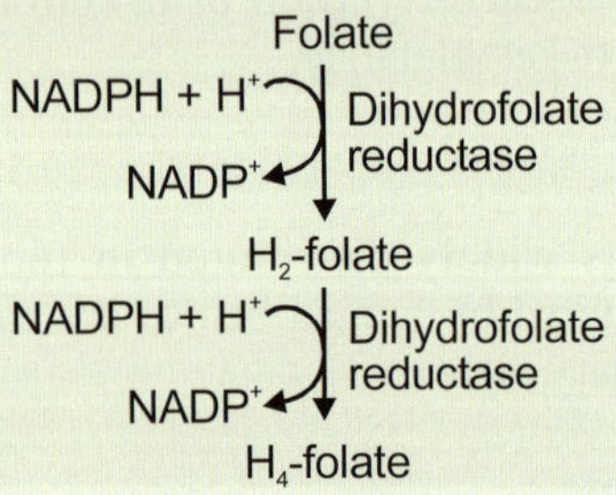

Amethopterin and aminopterin are competitive inhibitors of dihydrofolate reductase, and act as **folic acid antagonists**.

H_4-Folate is a carrier of **one-carbon units,** e.g. formyl (–CHO), formate (–HCOO=), methyl (–CH_3), methylene (=CH_2), methenyl (=CH) or formimino (–CH = NH) groups. The one-carbon unit may be attached to N^5 or N^{10} of H_4-folate.

H_4-Folate can receive one-carbon units from various compounds, and can transfer these for the synthesis of various compounds.

Sources of One-carbon Units

Tetrahydrofolate may receive one-carbon units from:

Formiminoglutamic Acid

Formiminoglutamic acid (FIGLU) is formed in the body from histidine.

$$\text{Histidine} \longrightarrow \text{Urocanic acid} \longrightarrow \longrightarrow \text{Figlu}$$

FIGLU can transfer its formimino group to tetrahydrofolate.

$$\text{FIGLU} + H_4\text{-Folate} \longrightarrow fi^5\text{-}H_4\text{-Folate} + \text{Glutamate}$$

Methionine, Choline and Thymine

These are the sources of methyl group.

Serine

Serine can contribute its hydroxymethyl group.

Utilisation of One-carbon Units

The one-carbon unit carried by tetrahydrofolate can be utilised in the following reactions:

Synthesis of Purines

The carbon atoms two and eight of purines are contributed by f^{10}-H_4-folate.

Synthesis of Serine

Conversion of glycine into serine requires a hydroxymethyl group which is provided by N^5, N^{10}-methylene-H_4-folate.

Synthesis of Methionine

The methyl group for the conversion of homocysteine into methionine is provided by N^5-methyl-H_4-folate.

Synthesis of Choline

The methyl groups for the synthesis of choline from serine are provided by N^{10}-methyl-H_4-folate.

Synthesis of Thymine

Thymine monophosphate is synthesised from deoxyuridine monophosphate. The methyl group for this conversion is

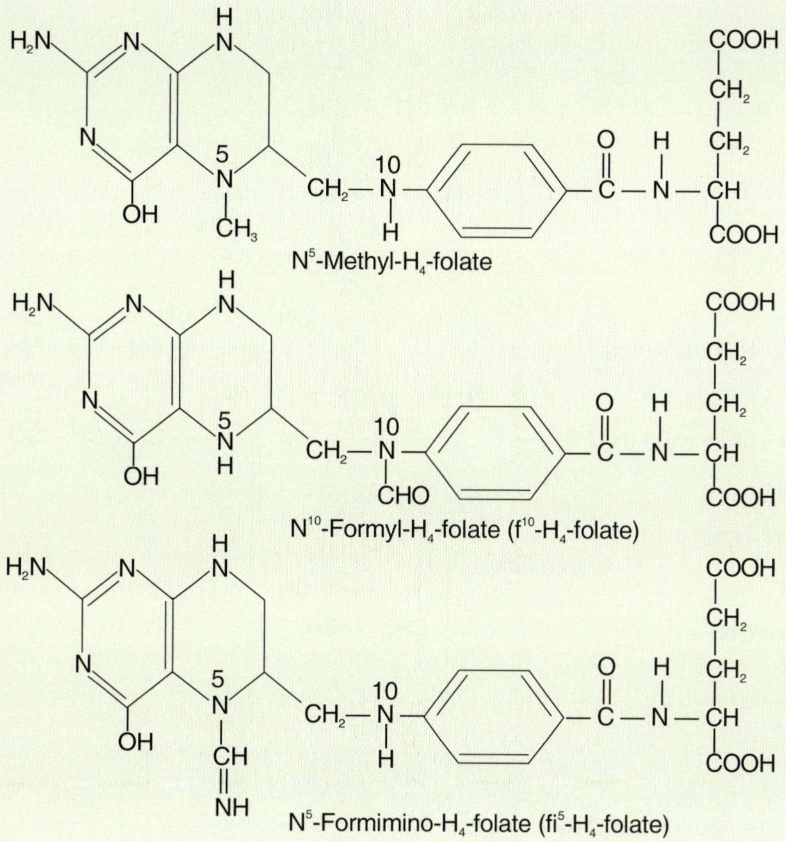

Fig. 21.20: One-carbon units attached to H_4-folate (tetrahydrofolate) at N^5 and N^{10}

provided by N^5, N^{10}-methylene-H_4-folate, which is converted into H_2-folate. H_2-Folate has to be reduced to H_4-folate so that it can continue to function as a coenzyme.

Synthesis of n-formylmethionine

n-Formylmethionine is required to initiate protein synthesis in prokaryotes. The formyl unit of f^{10}-H_4-folate is transferred to methionine which converts it into n-formylmethionine.

Sources

Folic acid is obtained from green leafy vegetables, yeast, liver, kidney, meat, fish, milk, etc. Intestinal bacteria also synthesise folic acid.

Requirement

Infants and children	: 100 µg/day
Adult men and women	: 100 µg/day
Pregnant women	: 300 µg/day
Lactating women	: 150 µg/day

Deficiency

As folic acid is required for the synthesis of purines and thymine, its deficiency impairs the synthesis of nucleic acids. This leads to growth failure and megaloblastic anaemia. Leukopenia can also occur.

Laboratory diagnosis of deficiency can be made by giving a test dose of histidine and measuring the **urinary excretion of figlu** which is increased in subjects deficient in folic acid.

COBALAMIN (VITAMIN B$_{12}$)

Cyanocobalamin was the first B_{12} vitamin isolated from liver in 1948. Vitamin B_{12} activity was later found in several compounds in which the cyanide group is replaced by a hydroxyl group (hydroxycobalamin), a methyl group (methylcobalamin), a nitro group (nitrocobalamin) or a chloride group (chlorocobalamin).Molecular formula of vitamin B_{12} is $C_{63}H_{88}O_{14}N_{14}PCo$. It has four pyrrole rings with a cobalt atom at the centre (corrin ring). The cobalt atom forms co-ordination bonds with the nitrogen atoms of four pyrrole rings, a cyanide group and 5,6-dimethyl-benzimidazole which, in turn, is linked with ribose-3-phosphate. The phosphate group of ribose-3-phosphate is linked with the pyrrole ring D (IV) through aminopropanol.

Vitamin B_{12} is fairly heat-stable. It is also known as the **extrinsic factor of Castle** or **anti-pernicious anaemia factor** as its deficiency causes pernicious anaemia.

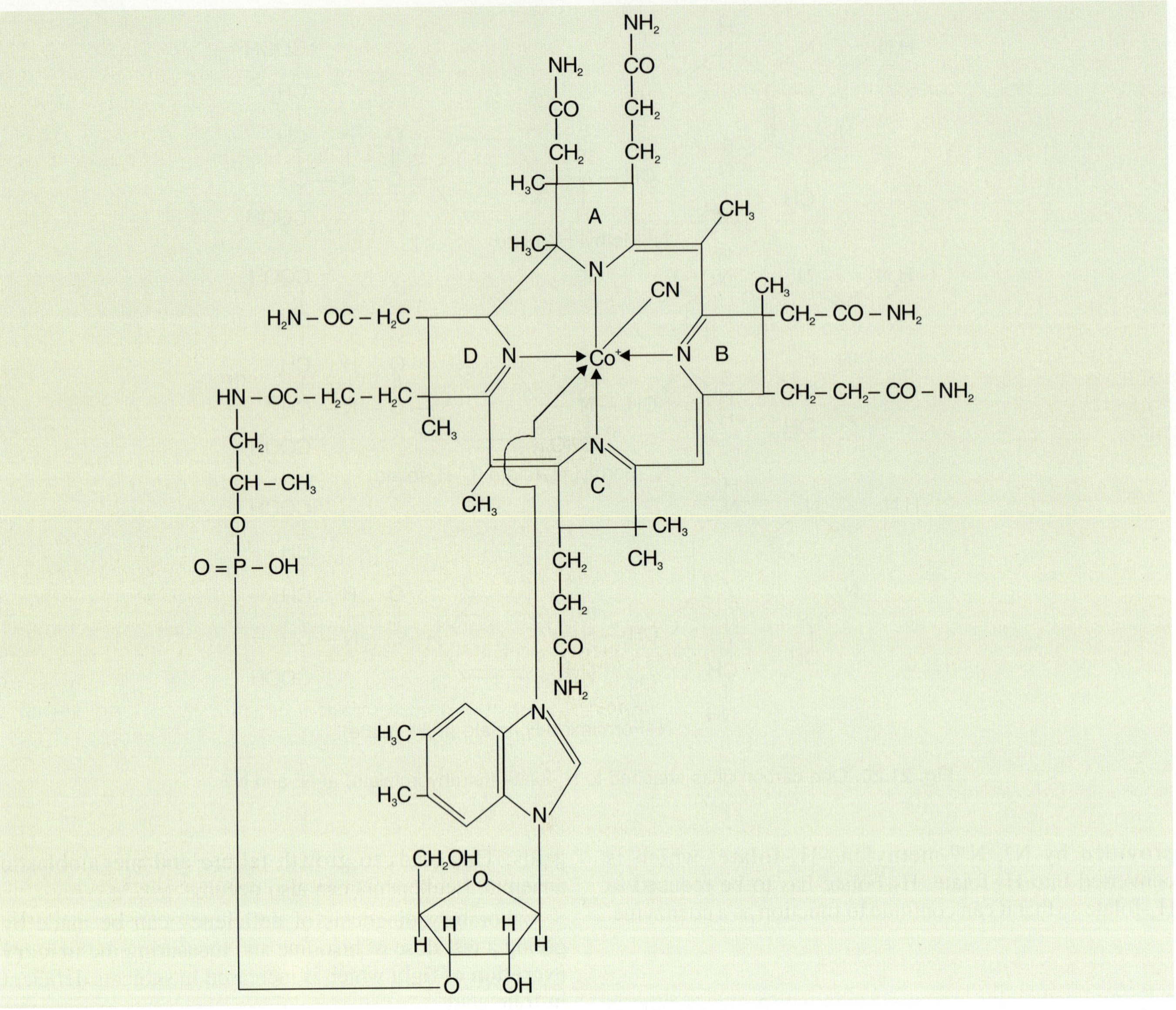

Fig. 21.21: Cyanocobalamin

Functions

Vitamin B_{12} forms coenzymes known as cobamides. Cobamides are formed by replacement of the cyanide group of vitamin B_{12} by 5′-deoxyadenosine. There are three **cobamides** which differ from each other in the benzimidazole portion. These are:

5,6-Dimethylbenzimidazole cobamide: 5,6-Dimethylbenzimidazole is present as such as in vitamin B_{12}.

Benzimidazole cobamide: Benzimidazole is present instead of 5,6-dimethylbenzimidazole.

Adenyl cobamide: Adenine replaces 5,6-dimethylbenzimidazole.

Besides these three, methylcobalamin is active as a coenzyme as such. The cobamides function as coenzymes in the following reactions:

1. Transfer of One-carbon Units

Apart from H_4-folate, cobamides are also involved in the transfer of one-carbon units. The two act in concert. An example of one such reaction is the synthesis of methionine from homocysteine.

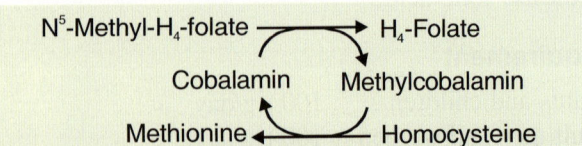

H_4-Folate is returned to the folate pool so that it can again participate in various one-carbon transfer reactions. Thus, cobamides help in one-carbon transfer reactions by sharing a part of the load on H_4-folate.

If there is a deficiency of cobalamin, methyltetrahydrofolate cannot transfer its methyl group to cobalamin. Most of the folate is trapped as methyltetrahydrofolate. This leads to a functional deficiency of folate as folate is not available to carry other one-carbon units. This is known as **folate trap**. Replenishment of cobalamin or large doses of folic acid can overcome the folate trap.

2. Formation of Succinyl CoA

Cobamides act as a coenzyme in the conversion of methylmalonyl CoA into succinyl CoA. Methylmalonyl CoA is formed directly from valine and via propionyl CoA from isoleucine, methionine and fatty acids having an odd number of carbon atoms. Succinyl CoA may be converted into glucose or oxidised in citric acid cycle.

$$
\begin{array}{c}
CH_3 \\
| \\
HOOC - C - H \\
| \\
C \sim S - CoA \\
\| \\
O \\
\text{L-Methylmalonyl CoA}
\end{array}
$$

Cobamide | Methylmalonyl CoA isomerase

$$
\begin{array}{c}
CH_2 - COOH \\
| \\
CH_2 - C \sim S - CoA \\
\| \\
O \\
\text{Succinyl CoA}
\end{array}
$$

In vitamin B_{12} deficiency, methylmalonic acid is excreted in large amounts in urine (**methylmalonic aciduria**). Rarely, methylmalonic aciduria may be caused by an inherited defect in methylmalonyl CoA isomerase.

Absorption, Transport and Storage

The ingested vitamin B_{12} is released by gastric hydrochloric acid. Most of the vitamin binds to R-protein secreted in gastric juice and saliva. Gastric parietal cells also secrete intrisic factor (IF), a glycoprotein of 45 kd which can bind vitamin B_{12}. However, at low pH, the affinity of vitamin B_{12} for R-protein is much higher than that for IF. Therefore, most of the vitamin binds to R-protein in stomach. In the duodenum, R-protein is hydrolysed, and vitamin B_{12} is bound to IF. One IF molecule binds one molecule of vitamin B_{12}. A specific receptor on ileal mucosa binds the IF:vitamin B_{12} complex. The vitamin is taken up by the mucosal cells and is transferred to plasma. Most of the vitamin is bound to transcobalamin II in plasma. The circulating transco-balamin II:vitamin B_{12} complex is taken up by cells with the help of a specific receptor. Transcobalamin II is hydrolysed in the cell by lysosomal enzymes. A significant amount of vitamin B_{12} is stored in the body, principally in liver. Most of the vitamin is bound to transcobalamin I in liver.

Sources

Vitamin B_{12} cannot be synthesised by any plant or animal. It is synthesised only by some bacteria. Animals acquire it through bacterial synthesis in their intestines. Liver, kidney, meat, eggs, milk and cheese are good sources of vitamin B_{12}. Bacteria present in the human intestine also synthesise vitamin B_{12}.

Requirement

Infants and children	: 0.3 to 0.5 µg/day
Adult men and women	: 1 µg/day
Pregnant and lactating women	: 1.5 µg/day

Deficiency

Deficiency of vitamin B_{12} can occur due to deficient intake (**nutritional deficiency**) or due to impaired absorption. Absorption is impaired when IF is absent due to atrophy of gastric mucosa or after gastrectomy. The condition arising from absence of IF is known as **pernicious anaemia**. Clinical features of deficiency may take long to develop as the hepatic stores of vitamin B_{12} can last a considerable length of time. **Nutritional deficiency** causes **megaloblastic anaemia**. An additional feature in pernicious anaemia due to absence of IF is **sub-acute combined degeneration** of lateral and posterior columns of spinal cord leading to sensory as well as motor disturbances.

ASCORBIC ACID

Ascorbic acid (vitamin C) prevents a specific deficiency disease, **scurvy**. Therefore, it is also known as **antiscorbutic factor**. It is very heat-labile, specially in basic medium. Chemically, its structure resembles that of hexoses. It can exist as L- and D- isomers. Only the **L-isomer** possesses vitamin activity. It can be readily oxidised to dehydro-ascorbic acid. Both L-ascorbic acid and L-dehydroascorbic acid possess equal vitamin activity (Fig. 21.22).

Vitamin C is synthesised by all plants and animals except guinea pigs and primates which lack **L-gulono-lactone oxidase**, the enzyme that converts L-gulonolactone into L-ascorbic acid.

Functions

1. Vitamin C is required for the formation and main-tenance of intercellular cement substance.
2. Since it can undergo reversible oxidation and reduction, it takes part in some oxidation-reduction reactions. There is considerable evidence in support of the role of vitamin C in the oxidation of phenylalanine and tyrosine.
3. It is required for post-translational hydroxylation of proline and lysine residues, and is, therefore, essential for the **conversion of procollagen into collagen** which

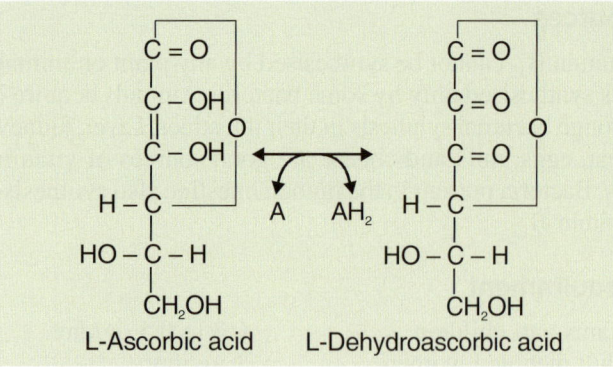

Fig. 21.22: Reduced and oxidised forms of vitamin C

is rich in hydroxyproline and hydroxylysine. Through collagen synthesis, it plays a role in the formation of matrix of bones, cartilages, dentine and connective tissue.

4. By converting ferric ions into ferrous ions, it helps in the absorption of iron.

5. It is required for the formation of bile acids from cholesterol.

6. It acts as an **anti-oxidant**. It inhibits the formation of nitrosamines during digestion. Nitrosamines are powerful carcinogens.

7. Adrenal gland is rich in ascorbic acid. Its ascorbic acid content decreases rapidly in stressful conditions. This suggests that ascorbic acid may play a role in the synthesis of adrenocortical steroid hormones.

Tissue Distribution

Total amount of ascorbic acid in an adult is 2 to 3 gm. It is distributed in all tissues and body fluids. It is present in high concentrations in the glands. The highest concentration is found in the adrenal glands, followed by the pituitary gland, thymus and corpus luteum. Leukocytes are also rich in ascorbic acid. The concentration in plasma is 0.5 to 1.5 mg/dl. The vitamin begins to appear in urine when the plasma level exceeds 1 mg/dl.

Sources

Citrus fruits, e.g. amla, lemon and orange, are very rich in vitamin C. Guava, tomatoes, green leafy vegetables and germinating pulses are also good sources. Potatoes are a fair source. Since considerable losses of vitamin C can occur during cooking, some raw fruits and salads should be included in the daily diet.

Requirement

Vitamin C is required in much larger quantities than any other vitamin. The Indian requirements, as recommended by Indian Council of Medical Research, are:

Infants and children	: 30–50 mg/day
Adult men and women	: 60 mg/day
Pregnant and lactating women	: 80 mg/day

Deficiency

Deficiency of vitamin C produces scurvy. A full-blown picture of scurvy is rare these days but isolated signs and symptoms of vitamin C deficiency are still seen which include:

1. The gums become swollen and spongy, and bleed easily on slight pressure. This may be one of the early signs of vitamin C deficiency.

2. Loosening of teeth.

3. The capillaries rupture easily due to increased fragility. Small haemorrhagic spots (petechial haemorrhages) are seen in the skin.

4. Anaemia can occur due to repeated haemorrhages and impaired absorption of iron.

5. Retardation of skeletal growth.

6. Easy fracturability of bones.

7. Delayed union of fractures.

8. Delayed healing of wounds.

9. Hypercholesterolaemia can occur due to decreased conversion of cholesterol into bile acids.

Laboratory diagnosis of deficiency can be made by **ascorbic acid saturation test**. After a test dose of ascorbic acid, urinary excretion of ascorbic acid is low in subjects deficient in the vitamin.

EXERCISE

1. Describe the functions, sources and requirement of folic acid. What are the clinical features of folic acid deficiency? Explain the biochemical basis of use of folic acid antagonists as anti-cancer drugs.

2. Describe the functions, sources and requirement of ascorbic acid. Explain the clinical features and laboratory diagnosis of ascorbic acid deficiency.

3. Write short notes on:
   a. Beriberi
   b. Pellagra
   c. Functions of pyridoxine
   d. Cobamides
   e. Scurvy
   f. Folic acid antagonists

4. Write 'true' or 'false':
   a. Thiamin pyrophosphate is coenzyme for transaldolase.
   b. Thiamin requirement is greater in alcoholics.
   c. Wet beriberi is accompanied by oedema.
   d. Polished rice is poor in thiamin.
   e. Peripheral neuropathy occurs in riboflavin deficiency.
   f. Coenzymes formed from riboflavin are FMN and FAD.
   g. Niacin can be synthesised in human beings from threonine.
   h. Niacin deficiency causes pellagra.
   i. Pellagra is common is people consuming refined wheat floor as their staple food.
   j. Pantothenic acid is used to form CoA and acyl carrier protein.
   k. Pyridoxal phosphate is required mainly in the metabolism of amino acids.
   l. Carboxyl group of an amino acid reacts with the phosphate group of pyridoxal phosphate to form a Schiff base.
   m. Pyridoxal phosphate is a coenzyme for phosphorylase.
   n. Isoniazid therapy can cause pyridoxine deficiency.
   o. Biotin deficiency may be caused by consumption of raw egg white.
   p. Lipoic acid acts as a coenzyme in oxidative deamination.
   q. Amethopterin prevents regeneration of tetrahydrofolate.
   r. Folic acid deficiency causes microcytic anaemia.
   s. Vitamin B_{12} is the intrinsic factor of Castle.
   t. Citrus fruits are rich in vitamin C.

5. Fill in the blanks:
   a. .... is the coenzyme for transketolase.
   b. Deficiency of thiamin causes ....
   c. Predominant involvement of nervous system causes .... beriberi.
   d. FAD contains .... phosphate, ribose and adenine.
   e. One mg of niacin can be synthesised from .... mg of ....
   f. ....is common in people consuming maize as their staple food.
   g. .... is a coenzyme for transaminases.
   h. Urinary excretion of .... is increased in pyridoxine deficiency.
   i. .... is a coenzyme for carboxylases.
   j. A protein, ... present in raw egg white, prevents the absorption of biotin.
   k. TPP, FAD, NAD, CoA and lipoic acid are required in .... of α-keto acids.
   l. Tetrahydrofolate is a carrier of .... units.
   m. Amethopterin is a .... antagonist.
   n. Folic acid deficiency causes .... anaemia.
   o. Urinary excretion of .... is increased in folic acid deficiency.
   p. .... is the extrinsic factor of Castle.
   q. .... are the coenzymes formed from vitamin B_{12}.
   r. Absence of intrinsic factor causes .... anaemia.

s. .... deficiency causes scurvy.

t. Vitamin C is required for .... of proline and lysine residues of collagen.

ANSWERS TO SHORT QUESTIONS

4. a. False
   b. True
   c. True
   d. True
   e. False
   f. True
   g. False
   h. True
   i. False
   j. True
   k. True
   l. False
   m. True
   n. True
   o. True
   p. False
   q. True
   r. False
   s. False
   t. True

5. a. TPP
   b. Beriberi
   c. Dry
   d. Riboflavin
   e. 60, tryptophan
   f. Pellagra
   g. PLP
   h. Xanthurenic acid
   i. Biotin
   j. Avidin
   k. Oxidative decarboxylation
   l. One-carbon
   m. Folic acid
   n. Megaloblastic
   o. FIGLU
   p. Vitamin B_{12}
   q. Cobamides
   r. Pernicious
   s. Vitamin C
   t. Hydroxylation

22

Fat-soluble Vitamins

VITAMIN A

Vitamin A is found only in animals though its precursors are found in a variety of plants. It occurs in three forms, **retinol** (alcohol form), **retinal** (aldehyde form) and **retinoic acid** (acid form). Chemically, each form contains a β-ionone ring attached to a polyene chain (Fig. 22.1). All the double bonds in the polyene chain have a *trans*-configuration in naturally occurring vitamin A (all-*trans*-vitamin A).

Retinol may be esterified with a fatty acid or phosphoric acid. The storage form of vitamin A is generally retinyl palmitate. Some of the functions of vitamin A are performed by retinyl phosphate. Vitamin A can be formed in our body from its precursors (**provitamins A**). The precursors are **carotenes** (or carotenoids) which are

naturally occurring pigments found in most yellow and green fruits and vegetables. α-Carotene, β-carotene and γ-carotene are important precursors of vitamin A. Of these, **β-carotene** is the most important. One molecule of β-carotene can be converted into two molecules of retinal.

A molecule of β-carotene contains two β-ionone rings connected by an 18-carbon polyene chain. β-Carotene is cleaved in the middle by β-carotene dioxygenase and molecular oxygen to form two molecules of retinal. Bile salts facilitate the reaction.

α-Carotene and γ-carotene contain only one β-ionone ring, and can form only one retinal molecule each. Retinal is reduced to retinol by retinaldehyde (retinine) reductase. Some retinal is spontaneously oxidised to retinoic acid. While retinal and retinol are interconvertible, retinoic acid cannot be converted back into retinal (Fig. 22.2).

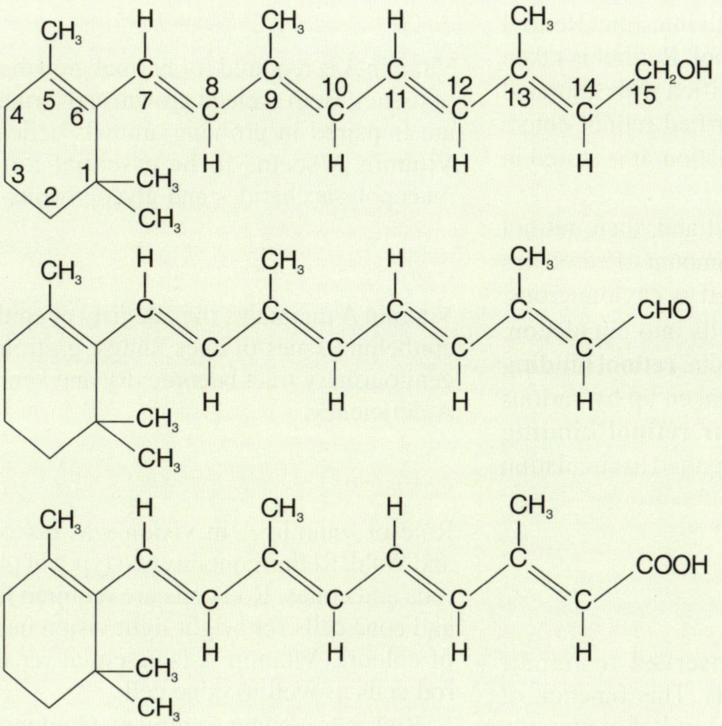

Fig. 22.1 Retinol, retinal and retinoic acid

335

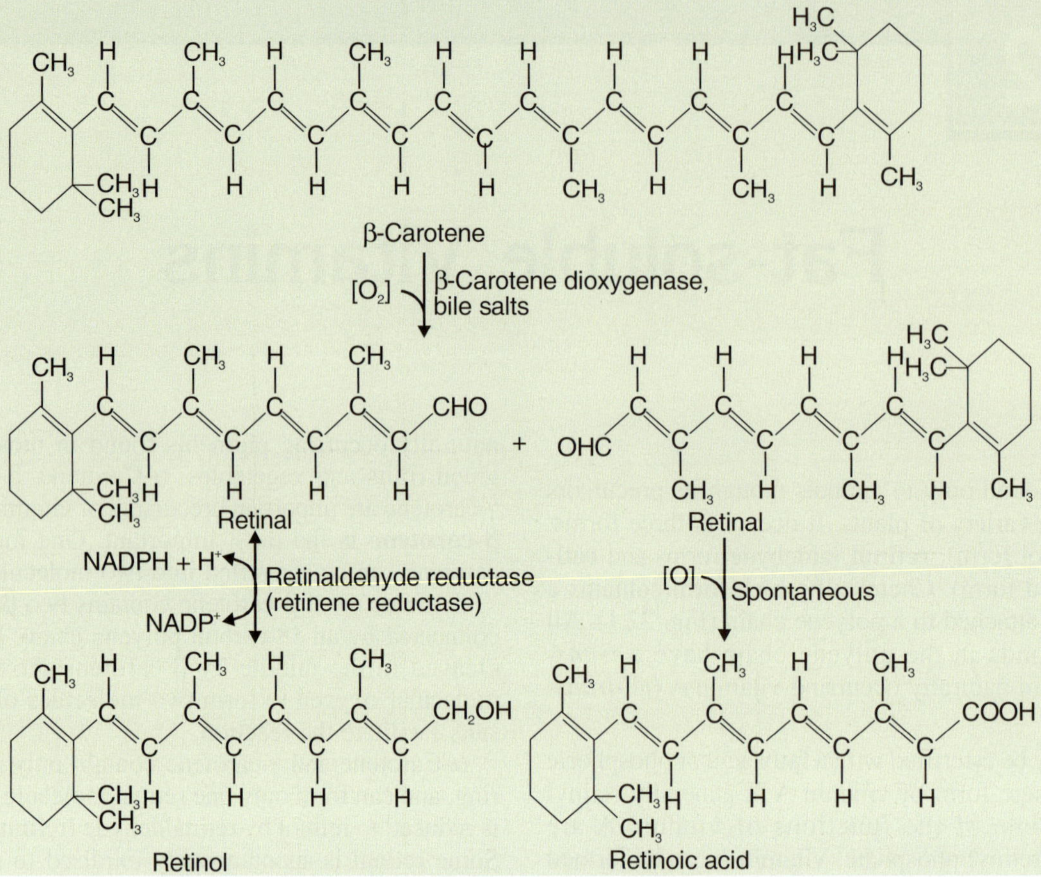

Fig. 22.2: Conversion of β-carotene into retinal, and of retinal into retinol and retinoic acid

Vitamin A is absorbed from the small intestine. Retinyl esters are hydrolysed to form free retinol. Retinol is taken up by the mucosal cells. It is is re-esterified with saturated fatty acids in the mucosal cells. Esterified retinol enters the lacteals and reaches liver via circulation. It is stored in the hepatic lipocytes.

Conversion of carotenes into retinal and, then, retinol occurs in the small intestine. A small amount of carotenes may be absorbed as such and transported by chylomicrons.

Retinol is released from hepatic cells into circulation. It is transported in blood by an α_1-globulin, **retinol binding protein (RBP)**. Circulating retinol is taken up by various cells in which it is bound to **cellular retinol binding protein (CRBP)**. Retinoic acid is transported in circulation in association with albumin.

Functions

1. Reproduction

Vitamin A deficiency has been observed to impair reproductive function in some animals. This function of vitamin A is probably mediated by control of expression of certain genes by retinol bound to CRBP.

2. Growth and Differentiation

Vitamin A is required for normal growth and differentiation of tissues. Both skeletal growth and formation of soft tissues are impaired in growing animals deficient in vitamin A. Vitamin A seems to be essential for the synthesis of mucopolysaccharides and glycoproteins in various tissues.

3. Integrity of Epithelial Tissues

Vitamin A maintains the integrity of epithelial tissues. The epithelial tissues of eyes, lungs, gastrointestinal tract and genitourinary tract become dry and keratinised in vitamin A deficiency.

4. Vision

Role of vitamin A in vision was discovered by Morton and Wald. Retina contains two types of photoreceptor cells, rods and cones. Rod cells are required for dimlight vision and cone cells for bright light vision including perception of colours. Vitamin A is essential for the functioning of rod cells as well as cone cells.

Rod cells contain a pigment, **rhodopsin** (visual purple). Rhodopsin is a conjugated protein made up of opsin

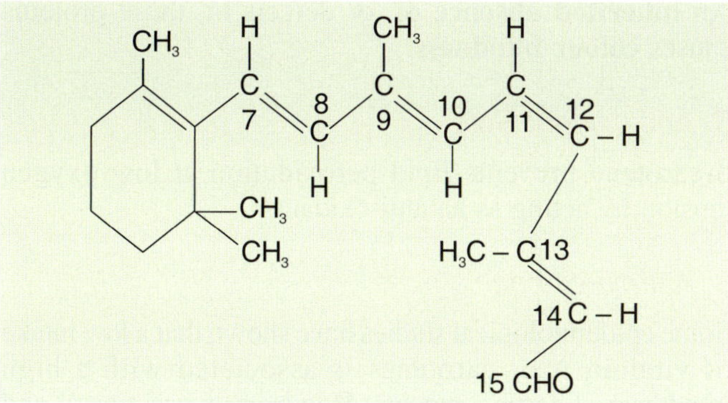

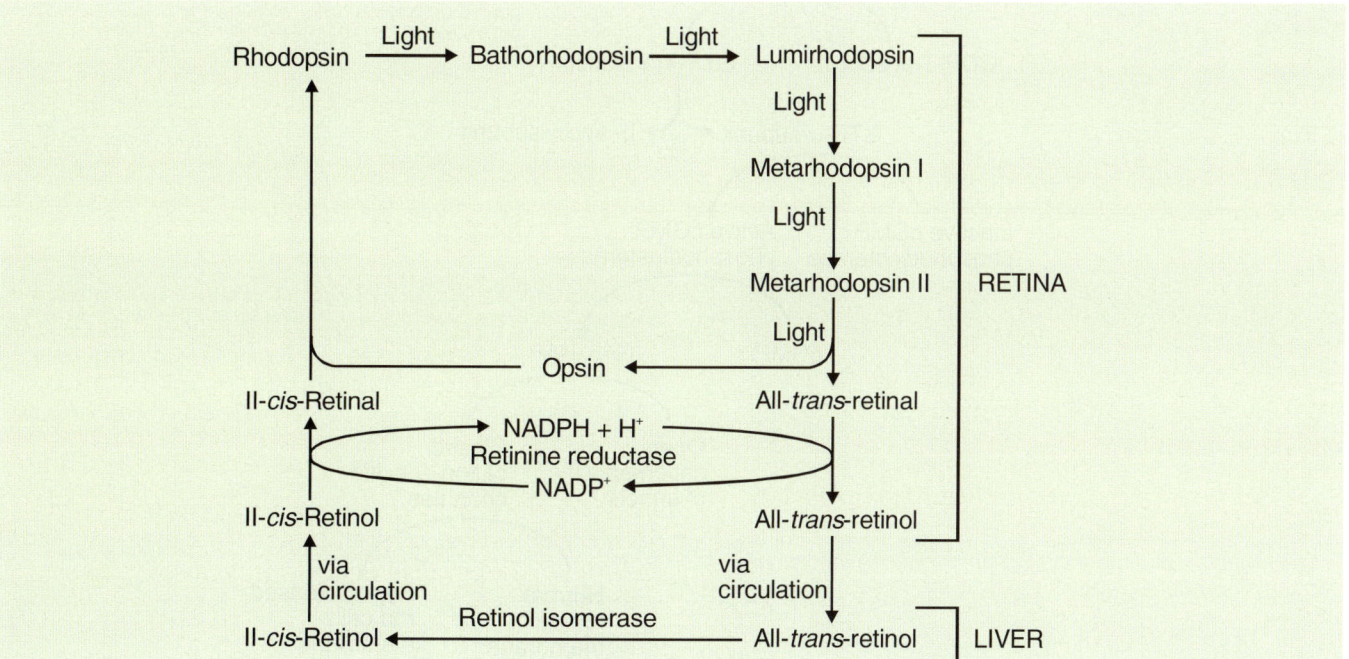

Fig. 22.3: 11-*cis*-Retinal

(a protein) and **11-cis-retinal,** an isomer of all-*trans*-retinal (Fig. 22.3).

The aldehyde group of 11-*cis*-retinal is bonded with the epsilon-amino group of a lysine residue of opsin by Schiff base linkage. Rhodopsin molecules are present in large numbers in rod cells.

When light strikes rod cells, 11-*cis*-retinal is converted into all-*trans*-retinal. Conformation of all-*trans*-retinal is such that it can not bind with opsin. Therefore, opsin and all-*trans*-retinal dissociate. A number of transient intermediates are formed before dissociation of opsin and all-*trans*-retinal.

When a person moves from dimlight into bright light, all the rhodopsin molecules are rapidly dissociated. When he moves back into dimlight, he is unable to see until rhodopsin is re-formed. For this, all-*trans*-retinal has to be isomerised to 11-*cis*-retinal. The enzyme system for the isomerisation reaction is present only in liver. Therefore, all-*trans*-retinal is reduced to all-*trans*-retinol in retina, and is released into circulation. It is taken up by liver, and is converted into 11-*cis*-retinol which is released into circulation. Retina takes up the circulating 11-*cis*-retinol and oxidises it to 11-*cis*-retinal. The latter combines with opsin to form rhodospin. This sequence of reactions is known as **visual cycle** (Fig. 22.4).

The time taken for regeneration of rhodospin is known as the **dark adaptation time** which depends upon the vitamin A content of liver. When liver contains adequate stores of vitamin A, the dark adaptation time is short. In vitamin A deficiency, dark adaptation time is prolonged.

Mechanism of Vision

Rhodopsin is a transmembrane protein. When photons strike it, they cause a conformational change in the rhodopsin molecule as a result of which it is activated (photo-excited). The photo-excited form is probably metarhodopsin II. Another membrane-bound protein, **transducin** is present in close vicinity of rhodopsin. Transducin belongs to the family of G-proteins, and is made up of three subunits, α-subunit, β-subunit and γ-subunit. The α-subunit has a site for GDP or GTP. Normally, this site is occupied by GDP. Photo-excited rhodopsin causes displacement of GDP by GTP. The α-subunit containing GTP dissociates from the β- and γ-subunits, and activates another membrane-bound protein, cGMP phosphodiesterase. The active enzyme converts cGMP into G-5'-MP as a result of which the concentration of cGMP in the rod cell rapidly decreases. This causes

Fig. 22.4: Visual cycle

hyperpolarisation of the rod cell membrane. The rod cell membrane contains a number of cation-specific channels which are normally kept open by cGMP leading to continuous influx of sodium ions into the rod cell. The decrease in cGMP concentration leads to **closure of cation-specific channels,** accumulation of sodium ions outside the rod cell and the consequent hyperpolarisation of the membrane (Fig. 22.5). The nerve impulse generated as a result of hyperpolarisation is transmitted to appropriate areas of brain (visual cortex).

The α-subunit of transducin possesses intrinsic GTPase activity. Therefore, GTP bound to the α-subunit is slowly hydrolysed into GDP. When GTP is converted into GDP, the α-subunit reassociates with the β- and γ-subunits forming transducin containing GDP. cGMP phosphodiesterase becomes inactive again, and the whole chain of events is terminated.

Vitamin A is also required for bright light vision. The cone cells of retina contain three conjugated proteins, **porphyrinopsin, iodopsin** and **cyanopsin**. These are sensitive to red, green and blue light respectively. The prosthetic group is 11-*cis*-retinal in each of these but the protein part is different. These proteins become photo-excited on exposure to light of specific colour. A nerve impulse is, then, generated in much the same way as in rod cells. A given cone cell contains only one of these three proteins, and can perceive only one particular colour.

An **inherited absence** of, or defects in, these proteins causes **colour blindness**.

5. *Anti-oxidant Role*

β-carotene prevents lipid peroxidation at low oxygen tension by acting as an anti-oxidant.

6. *Anti-carcinogenic Role*

Some epidemiological studies have shown that a low intake of vitamin A or carotenes is associated with a high incidence of certain cancers. However, experimental and clinical confirmation of this finding is yet to be obtained.

Since retinol and retinal are interconvertible and can also be converted into retinoic acid, they can perform all the functions of vitamin A. Retinoic acid can support growth and differentiation, and can maintain epithelia but cannot perform other functions of vitamin A. 13-*cis*-Retinoic acid, a synthetic compound, is more active than naturally occurring retinoic acid.

Sources

Preformed vitamin A is present only in animal foods, e.g. fish liver oils, liver, eggs, milk, butter, cream, cheese, etc. Provitamins A are found in green leafy vegetables, e.g. spinach, coriander leaves, mustard leaves, cabbage, lettuce, etc. and in red and yellow vegetables and fruits, e.g. carrot,

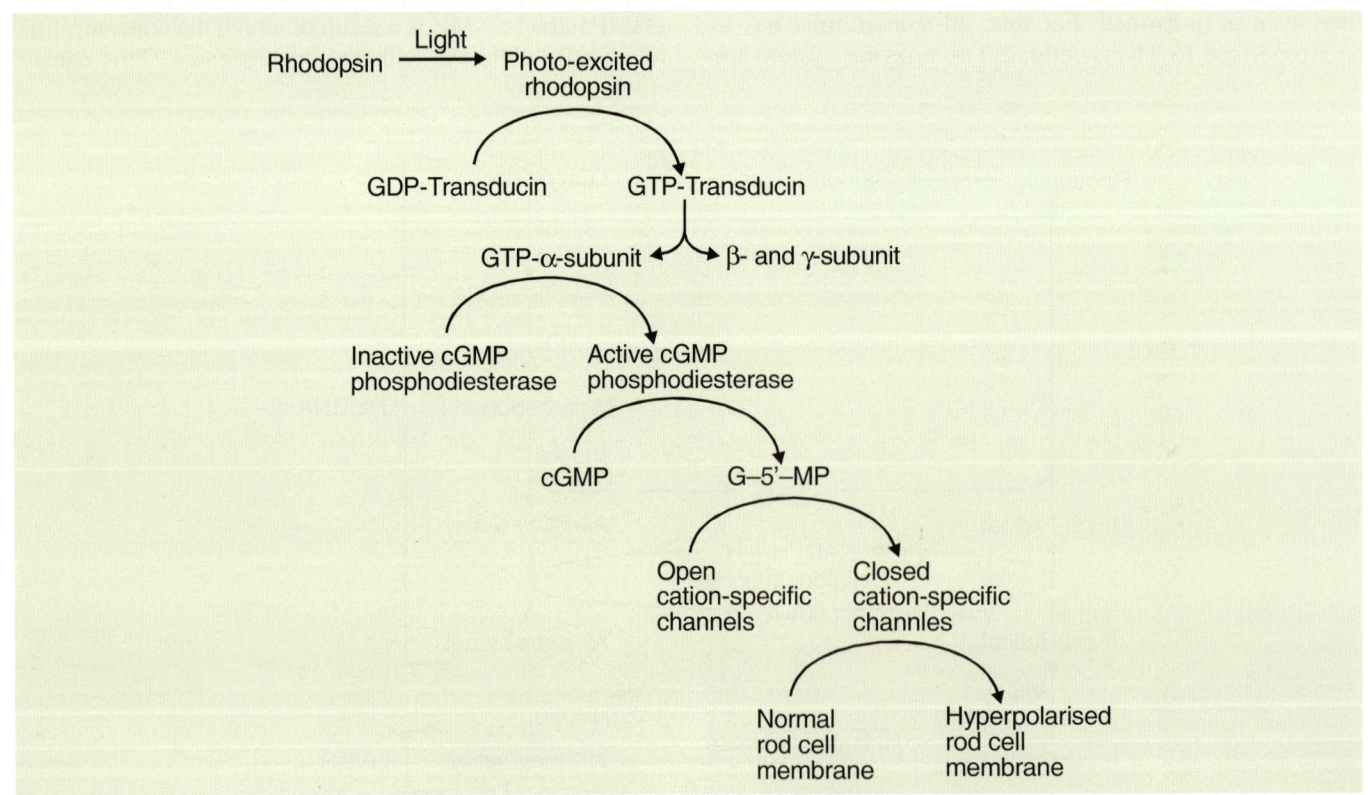

Fig. 22.5: Cascade of events converting light energy into a nerve impulse in a rod cell

tomato, mango, papaya, plums, etc. Maize and soyabean are also fair sources of provitamins A.

Requirement

Since vitamin A is present in food in many different forms which differ in their vitamin A activity, it is not possible to express the requirement for vitamin A in terms of its actual weight. For instance, if we take equal amounts of retinol, β-carotene and α- or γ-carotene, their vitamin A activities would be different. To overcome this difficulty, relative vitamin A activities of different compounds were compared in rats, and were expressed in terms of international units (IU). One IU is the activity present in 0.3 μg of retinol, 0.344 μg of retinyl acetate or 0.6 μg of β-carotene. Daily requirements were expressed in IU for a long period. Subsequently, it was found that intestinal absorption and utilisation of carotenes were much less efficient in human beings than in rats. Therefore, vitamin A activities were converted into retinol equivalents (RE). One RE is the activity present in 1 μg of retinol, 6 μg of β-carotene or 12 μg of other carotenes. The daily requirement of vitamin A, in terms of IU and RE, is given in Table 22.1.

Deficiency

A deficiency of vitamin A can arise from inadequate intake, inadequate absorption or inadequate conversion of carotenes into vitamin A. Zinc deficiency may impair the mobilisation of vitamin A from liver. The clinical manifestations of deficiency are:

1. Xerophthalmia

The lacrimal glands become keratinised, and stop secreting lacrimal fluid. The eyes become dry. Bitot's spots (small, opaque spots) may appear on cornea.

2. Keratomalacia

The cornea is softened, and is finally destroyed.

3. Nyctalopia

Initially, dark adaptation time is prolonged which may be **the earliest indication** of deficiency. Finally, the ability to see in dimlight is completely lost which is known as night blindness or nyctalopia.

4. Blindness

In severe and prolonged deficiency, there is total loss of vision due to functional and structural changes in the eyes.

5. Follicular Hyperkeratosis

There is hyperkeratinisation of skin especially around hair follicles.

6. Susceptibility to Infections

Susceptibility to infections may be increased due to epithelial damage.

Toxicity

Hypervitaminosis A may occur if large doses of vitamin A, usually in **pharmacological form**, are taken over **long periods**. It is characterised by rough skin, hair loss, anorexia, weight loss, headache, vertigo, irritability, hyperaesthesia, hepatosplenomegaly, liver damage, etc.

VITAMIN D

Vitamin D is also known as **anti-rachitic factor** or anti-rachitic vitamin as it prevents a deficiency disease, **rickets** (rachitis).

Of the several compounds possessing vitamin D activity, the most important are vitamin D_2 (**ergocalciferol**) and vitamin D_3 (**cholecalciferol**). These are formed from provitamin D_2 (**ergosterol**) and provitamin D_3 (**7-dehydrocholesterol**) respectively on exposure to **ultraviolet light** (Fig. 22.6).

Ergosterol occurs in plants e.g. ergot and yeast. 7-Dehydrocholesterol occurs in animals. It is formed from cholesterol. 7-Dehydrocholesterol present in skin is converted into cholecalciferol on exposure to sunlight. Cholecalciferol is synthesised in human beings also.

Functions

1. Vitamin D increases the intestinal absorption of calcium. The absorption of phosphorus is also increased secondarily.
2. Vitamin D increases the renal tubular absorption of calcium, and decreases that of phosphorus.
3. Vitamin D is required for mineralisation of bones. Bone formation is a continuous and dynamic process. Calcium salts are continuously deposited into and resorbed from bones by osteoblasts and osteoclasts respectively. In growing age, deposition exceeds resorption leading to skeletal growth. In adult life, deposition and resorption are finely balanced leading to remodeling of bones. Vitamin D is required for bone growth as well as remodeling.

Table 22.1: Requirement of vitamin A

	IU/day	RE/day
Infants	1,500–2,000	400
Children	2,000–4,000	400–700
Adult men	5,000	1,000
Adult women	4,000	800
Pregnant women	5,000	1,000
Lactating women	6,000	1,200

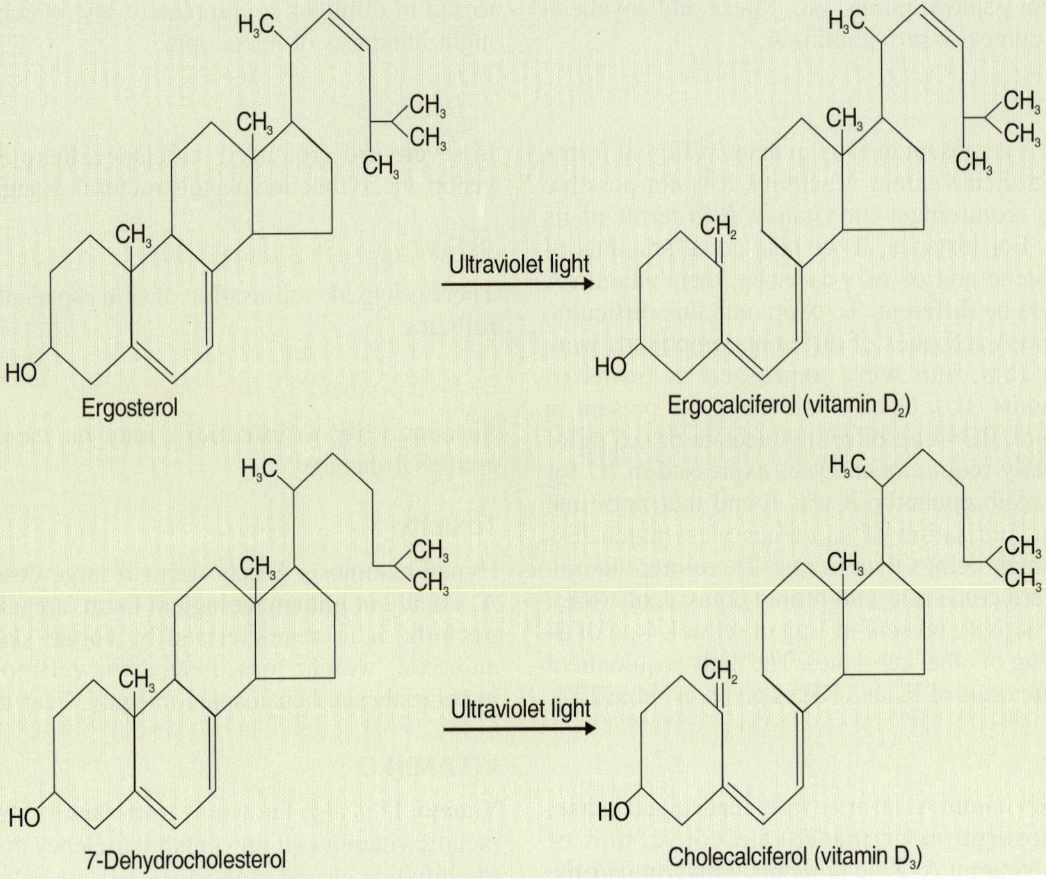

Fig. 22.6: Synthesis of vitamins D₂ and D₃ from their precursors

Thus, the main functions of vitamin D are to regulate the metabolism of calcium and the mineralisation of bones. However, these functions are not performed by vitamin D itself. Vitamin D is first hydroxylated at C_{25} to form 25-hydroxycholecalciferol in the liver. 25-Hydroxycholecalciferol is further hydroxylated at C_1 in the kidneys to form **1,25-dihydroxycholecalciferol (1,25-DHCC or calcitriol)**. 1,25-DHCC is the metabolically active form of vitamin D. 1,25-DHCC acts as a **hormone** and, therefore, vitamin D may be regarded as a prohormone. The mechanism of action of 1,25-DHCC is similar to that of steroid and thyroid hormones. It binds to its intracellular **receptors** in the target cells. The hormone-receptor complex binds to a hormone response element in DNA and increases the transcription and translation of certain genes.

In the intestinal mucosa, 1,25-DHCC induces the synthesis of calcium-binding protein, Ca^{++}-dependent ATPase and alkaline phosphatase. These proteins are responsible for the active absorption of calcium. Vitamin D acts in concert with **parathormone**. Parathormone activates the renal hydroxylase which converts 25-hydroxycholecalciferol into 1,25-DHCC. Increased absorption of calcium leads to a rise in plasma calcium, which inhibits parathormone secretion (Fig. 22.7).

Sources

Plant foods are poor sources of vitamin D. Though ergocalciferol is present in some plants, its intestinal absorption is poor. Cholecalciferol is the major dietary form of vitamin D. Fish liver oils are very rich in cholecalciferol. Eggs, butter and cheese are fairly good sources. An important source of vitamin D is its **endogenous synthesis** in the skin. Where sunshine is good and people are adequately exposed to sunlight, enough vitamin D is synthesised in the body to meet the daily requirement.

Requirement

Due to differences in the anti-rachitic activity of different compounds possessing vitamin D activity, the requirement is expressed in international units (IU). One IU is the activity present in 0.025 µg of cholecalciferol. The requirement is 400 IU/day in infants, children, and pregnant and lactating women. The adult requirement is 200 IU/day.

Deficiency

Deficiency can occur due to inadequate intake, inadequate absorption or inadequate exposure to sunlight. Two distinct

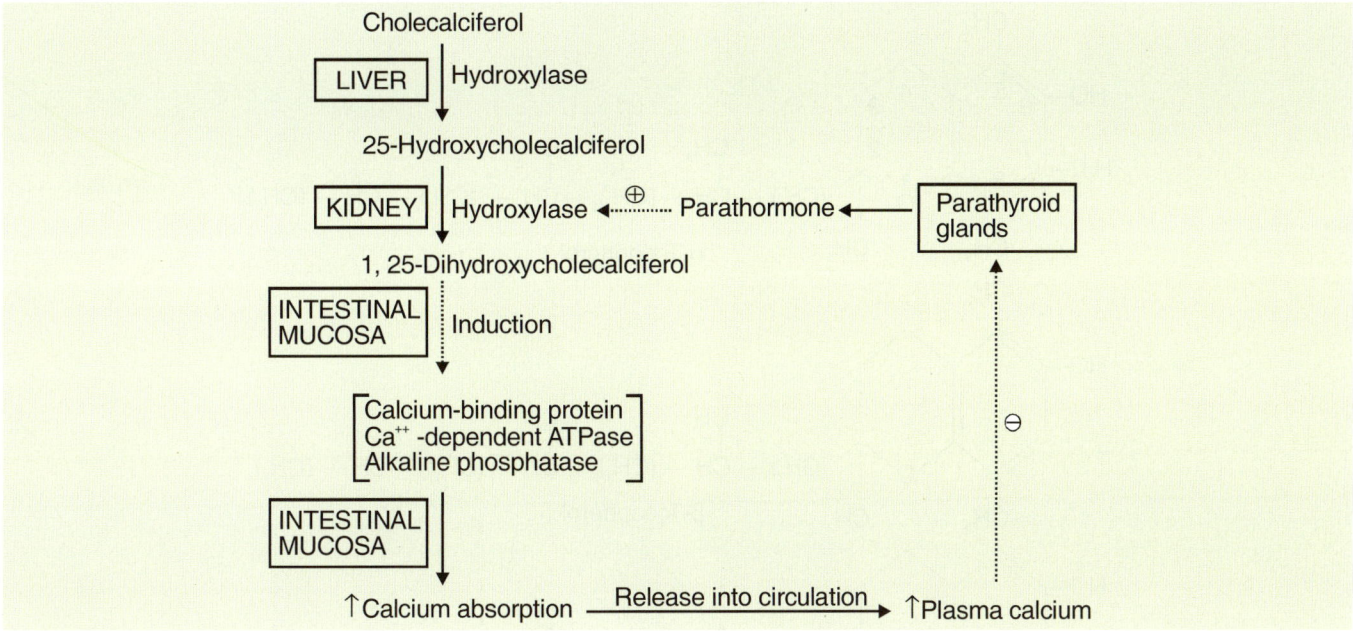

Cholecalciferol
LIVER | Hydroxylase
25-Hydroxycholecalciferol
KIDNEY | Hydroxylase ← ⊕ ⋯ Parathormone ← Parathyroid glands
1, 25-Dihydroxycholecalciferol
INTESTINAL MUCOSA | Induction
[Calcium-binding protein
Ca⁺⁺-dependent ATPase
Alkaline phosphatase]
INTESTINAL MUCOSA
↑Calcium absorption —— Release into circulation → ↑Plasma calcium
⊖

Fig. 22.7: Role of cholecalciferol and parathormone in calcium absorption and regulation of plasma calcium concentration

syndromes arise from deficiency of vitamin D, **rickets** in childhood and **osteomalacia** in adult life.

Rickets

The most susceptible periods for development of rickets are infancy and puberty when skeletal growth occurs rapidly. Deficiency of vitamin D causes deficient mineralisation of bones and overgrowth of epiphyses. This results in some typical skeletal deformities such as:
1. Delayed closure of fontanelles and bossing of skull.
2. *Craniotabes:* The skull bones are soft.
3. *Pigeon chest:* The anteroposterior diameter of chest is increased.
4. *Rickety rosary:* The costochondral junctions of ribs are enlarged, and appear to the beaded. This series of beads on the chest gives the appearance of a rosary worn around the neck.
5. *Vertebral deformities:* Kyphosis, lordosis or scoliosis may occur due to forward, backward or lateral bending of vertebral column.
6. *Pelvic deformities:* The size of the pelvic outlet may be decreased.
7. *Bowlegs and knock knees:* The leg bones may become curved under the weight of the body (bowlegs) and the two knees may touch each other while standing erect (knock knees).
8. *Enlarged wrists and knees:* Wrists and knees may be enlarged due to overgrowth of epiphyses of the long bones.

Apart from the skeletal deformities, some changes in serum and urine chemistry are also seen. Serum calcium and inorganic phosphorus are decreased. Serum alkaline phosphatase is increased. Hypocalcaemia increases the secretion of parathormone. Urinary excretion of calcium is decreased, and that of phosphorus is increased by parathormone.

Osteomalacia

Pregnant and lactating women are particularly prone to osteomalacia. Matrix of the bones is normal but demineralisation occurs to varying extents. Aches and pains may occur in bones and susceptibility to fractures is increased. Changes in serum and urine chemistry are similar to those in rickets.

Toxicity

Prolonged intake of large doses of vitamin D in pharmacological form may cause hypervitaminosis D. Serum calcium is raised. Hypercalcaemia may cause loss of appetite, polydipsia, polyuria, constipation, muscular weakness, etc. Calcification may occur in soft tissues, e.g. arteries, bronchi, muscles, kidneys, etc. Stones may be formed in the kidneys.

VITAMIN E

Vitamin E is sometimes described as anti-sterility vitamin. However, its anti-sterility function is seen only in some animals and not in human beings. Vitamin E activity is present in several **tocopherols**, the most important being α-, β-, γ- and δ- tocopherol (Fig. 22.8).

α-Tocopherol is the most abundant tocopherol in foodstuffs, and is taken as the standard. The official reference standard is synthetic DL-α-tocopherol acetate.

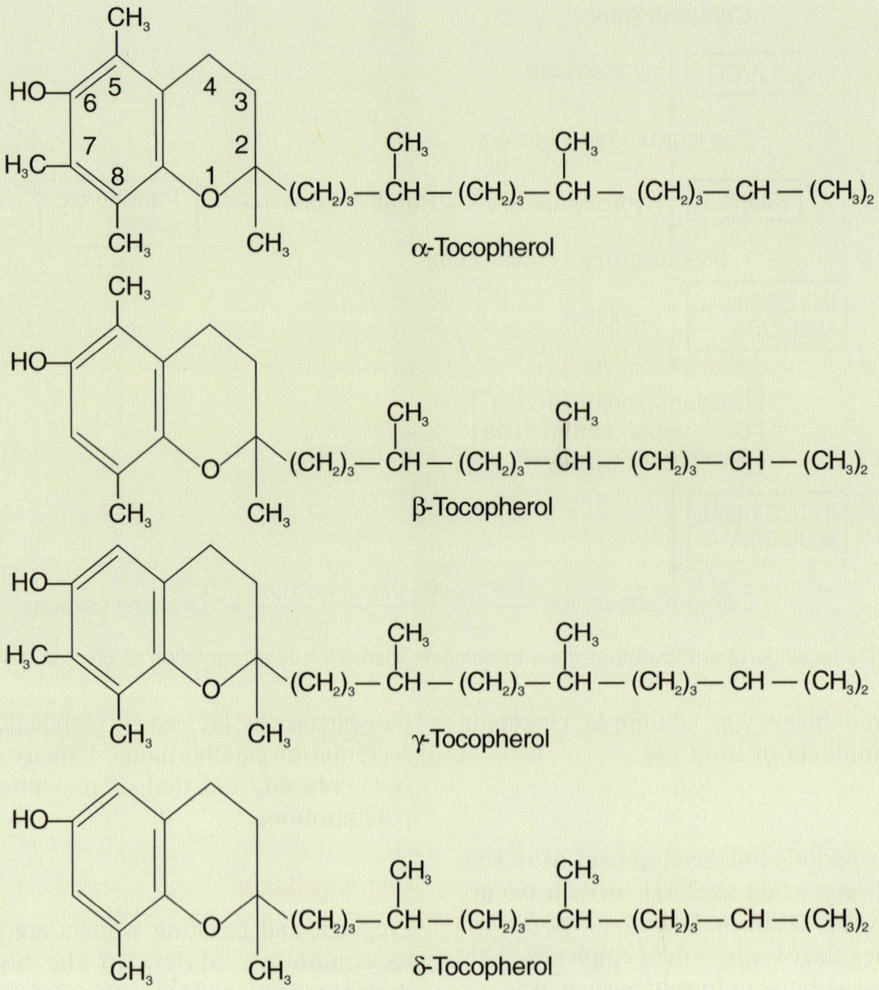

Fig. 22.8: Various forms of vitamin E

The vitamin E activity present in 1 mg of this compound is described as one international unit (IU). The vitamin E activity of 1 mg of naturally-occurring D-α-tocopherol is 1.5 IU. The vitamin E activities of other tocopherols are much lower.

Functions

The most important function of vitamin E in human beings is to act as an **anti-oxidant**. Vitamin E is readily oxidisable, and prevents the oxidation of other, less oxidisable compounds. It prevents the oxidation of other antioxidants, e.g. carotenes, vitamin A and vitamin C. It prevents peroxidation of unsaturated fatty acids, and protects the tissues against the harmful effects of lipid peroxides. It protects the RBC membrane from oxidants, and makes the RBCs resistant to haemolysis. It protects the pulmonary tissue from atmospheric oxidants.

Sources

Vegetable oils, e.g. wheat germ oil, rice bran oil, corn oil, soya bean oil, cottonseed oil, etc. are very rich in vitamin E. Other good sources are green leafy vegetables, nuts, legumes, milk, eggs and meat.

Requirement

Infants   : 4–5 IU/day
Children   : 7-12 IU/day
Adult men   : 15 IU/day
Adult women   : 12 IU/day
Pregnant and lactating women   : 15 IU/day

The requirement of vitamin E is related to the intake of polyunsaturated fatty acids (PUFA). It has been suggested that an intake of 0.8 mg of D-α-tocopherol (or 1.2 IU of vitamin E) per gm of PUFA in diet will prevent vitamin E deficiency.

Deficiency

Deficiency of vitamin E is uncommon because of its widespread distribution in foods. Moreover, the foods which are rich in PUFA, e.g. vegetable oils, are also rich in vitamin E. Deficiency may occur in severely

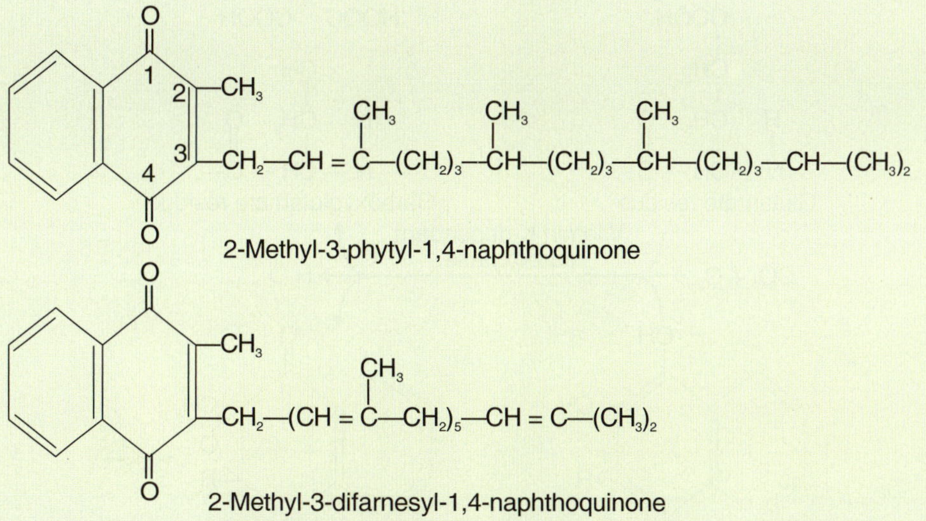

2-Methyl-3-phytyl-1,4-naphthoquinone

2-Methyl-3-difarnesyl-1,4-naphthoquinone

Fig. 22.9: Naturally-occurring forms of vitamin K

undernourished children and in premature infants fed on artificial milk not containing vitamin E. The clinical manifestations of deficiency are oedema, haemolytic anaemia and thrombocytosis.

VITAMIN K

Vitamin K activity is present in many compounds having a 2-methyl-1,4-naphthoquinone nucleus. Two naturally-occurring compounds having this nucleus are 2-methyl-3-phytyl-1,4-naphthoquinone (**phylloquinone** or **vitamin K_1**) and 2-methyl-3-difarnesyl-1,4-naphthoquinone (**menaquinone** or **vitamin K_2**). The former occurs in plants and the latter in bacteria (Fig. 22.9).

Some synthetic compounds having vitamin K activity have also been prepared. These include menadione, sodium menadiol diphosphate and menadione sodium bisulphite (Fig. 22.10). These three are water-soluble.

Functions

Vitamin K is essential for normal **coagulation of blood**. Concentrations of several coagulation factors in plasma are decreased in vitamin K deficiency. These include prothrombin (Factor II), proconvertin (Factor VII), Christmas factor (Factor IX) and Stuart-Prower Factor (Factor X). All these coagulation factors are chemically proteins, and vitamin K is required for post-translational modification of these proteins, which is necessary for their activation.

Prothrombin is synthesised in liver in the form of an inactive precursor, pre-prothrombin. Hydroquinone (reduced) form of vitamin K is required for **carboxylation of glutamate residues** of pre-prothrombin as a result of which pre-prothrombin is converted into prothrombin. During this reaction, hydroquinone form of vitamin K is converted into 2,3-epoxide form. Hydroquinone form is

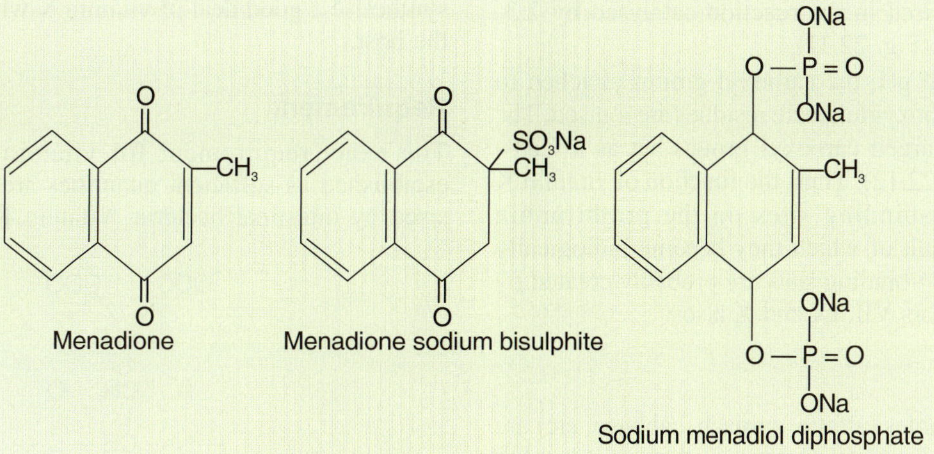

Menadione

Menadione sodium bisulphite

Sodium menadiol diphosphate

Fig. 22.10: Synthetic forms of vitamin K

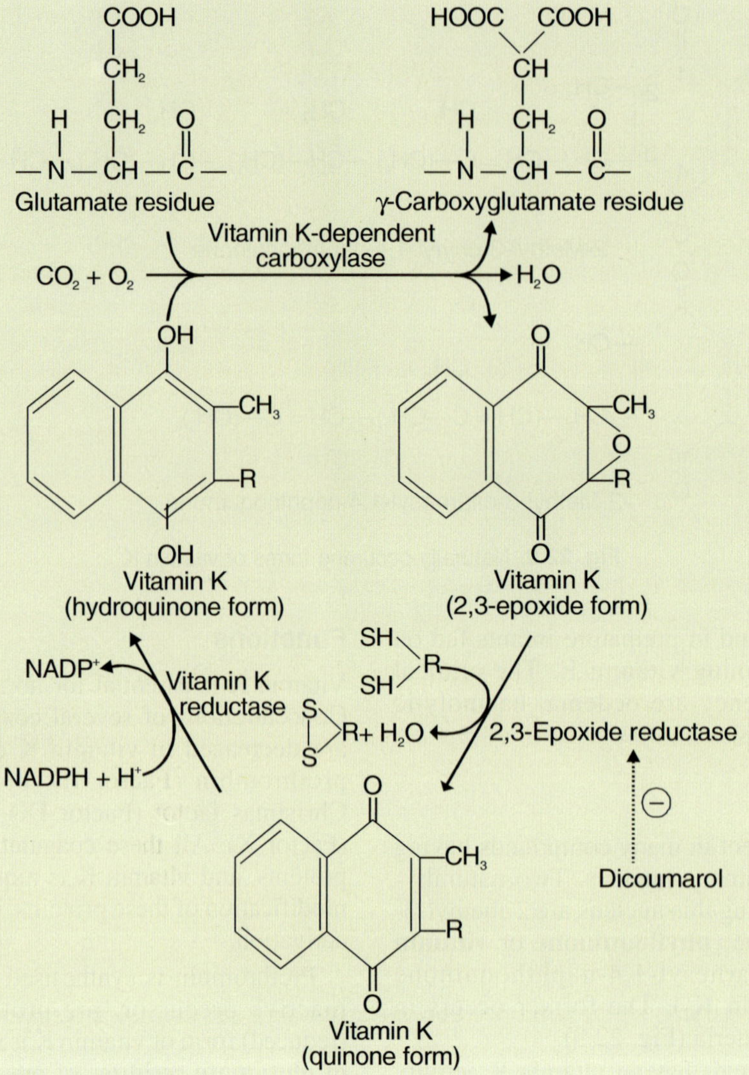

Fig. 22.11: γ-Carboxylation of glutamate residues and regeneration of hydroquinone form of vitamin K (dicumarol, an anticoagulant, disrupts the cycle by inhibiting 2,3-epoxide reductase)

regenerated via quinone form by 2,3-epoxide reductase and vitamin K reductase. An as yet unidentified sulphydryl compound is required in the reaction catalysed by 2,3-epoxide reductase (Fig. 22.11).

At physiological pH, the carboxyl groups attached to the γ-carbon of carboxyglutamate residues are ionised. The two negatively charged carboxyl groups act as a **Ca⁺⁺-binding site** (Fig. 22.12). Thus, the function of vitamin K is to create Ca⁺⁺-binding sites on the prothrombin molecules as a result of which they become biologically active. Similar Ca⁺⁺-binding sites are probably created by vitamin K on Factors VII, IX and X also.

Sources

Green leafy vegetables (alfalfa, spinach, cabbage, etc) are rich in vitamin K. Cauliflower and peas are also good sources. Liver is a fair source. Small amounts are present in milk and eggs also. A very important source is bacterial synthesis in the intestine. The intestinal bacteria synthesise a good deal of vitamin K which is available to the host.

Requirement

The exact requirement for vitamin K has not been established as sufficient quantities are normally synthesised by intestinal bacteria. Vitamin K supplements are

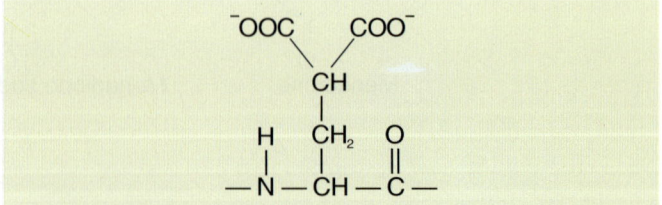

Fig. 22.12: Ionised γ-carboxyglutamate residue

required only when the intestinal bacteria are destroyed, e.g. by antibiotic therapy or when fat absorption is impaired, e.g. in sprue, coeliac disease, obstructive jaundice, etc. The normal daily requirement is probably less than 0.1 mg.

Deficiency

Deficiency of vitamin K leads to a disturbance in the normal mechanism of coagulation of blood. Even a slight injury causes prolonged **bleeding** in a subject deficient in vitamin K. Diagnosis can be made by measuring **prothrombin time** which is prolonged in vitamin K deficiency. Prothrombin time may also be prolonged in patients with liver damage due to inability of the liver to synthesise prothrombin. These two conditions can be distinguished by parenteral administration of vitamin K. Prothrombin time returns to normal in subjects deficient in vitamin K but not in patients with liver damage.

EXERCISE

1. Describe the functions of vitamin A. What are the clinical features of vitamin A deficiency and toxicity?

2. Describe the biochemical role of anti-oxidant vitamins.

3. Write short notes on:
   a. Visual cycle
   b. Calcitriol
   c. Functions of vitamin E
   d. Functions of vitamin K
   e. Rickets

4. Write 'true' or 'false':
   a. Vitamin A can be formed from carotenes.
   b. Retinal and retinol are interconvertible.
   c. Retinoic acid is an inactive metabolite of retinal.
   d. One molecule of retinal is formed from one molecule of β-carotene.
   e. Anti-oxidant activity is present in β-carotene.
   f. On exposure to light, all-*trans*-retinal is converted into 11-*cis*-retinal.
   g. 7-Dehydrocholesterol is the precursor of ergocalciferol.
   h. 25-Hydroxylation of cholecalciferol occurs in liver.
   i. 1,25-Dihydroxycholecalciferol is the active metabolite of cholecalciferol.
   j. Serum calcium is decreased and serum inorganic phosphorus is increased in rickets.
   k. Vitamin E acts as an anti-oxidant.
   l. Vitamin E prevents sterility in human beings.
   m. Vitamin K can be synthesised by intestinal bacteria.
   n. Prothrombin time is decreased in vitamin K deficiency.
   o. Vitamin K is required for post-translational modification of prothrombin.

5. Fill in the blanks:
   a. Retinal is converted into .... spontaneously.
   b. .... transports retinol in circulation.
   c. Rhodopsin is made up of .... and opsin.
   d. When light falls on .... cells, rhodopsin dissociates into .... and opsin.
   e. Dark adaptation time is prolonged in .... deficiency.
   f. One retinol equivalent is the activity present in one .... of retinol.
   g. .... is the precursor of cholecalciferol.
   h. .... is the immediate precursor of calcitriol.
   i. .... induces the synthesis of calcium-binding protein.
   j. Bowlegs and knock-knees can occur in ....
   k. The activity present in .... of cholecalciferol is known as one international unit of vitamin D.
   l. Serum calcium is ....in hypervitaminosis D.
   m. Vitamin ....prevents peroxidation of unsaturated fatty acids.
   n. Menadione is soluble in ....
   o. Vitamin K creates .... binding sites on prothrombin molecules by γ-carboxyation of .... residues.

ANSWERS TO SHORT QUESTIONS

4. a. True
   c. False
   e. True
   g. False
   i. True
   k. True
   m. True
   o. True

   b. True
   d. False
   f. False
   h. True
   j. False
   l. False
   n. False

5. a. Retinoic acid
   c. 11-*cis*-retinal
   e. Vitamin A
   g. 7-Dehydrocholesterol
   i. Calcitriol
   k. 0.25 µg
   m. E
   o. Ca++, glutamate

   b. Retinol binding protein
   d. Rod, all-*trans*-retinal
   f. µg
   h. 25-Hydroxycholecalciferol
   j. Rickets
   l. Increased
   n. Water

Minerals

Of the large number of minerals present in nature, only a few are essential for human beings. Some of these are required in relatively large quantities, and are known as **principal elements** or **macronutrients**. These include calcium, phosphorus, magnesium, sodium, potassium, chlorine and sulphur. Some minerals are required in minute quantities, and are known as **trace elements** or **micronutrients**. These include iron, iodine, copper, zinc, cobalt, manganese, molybdenum, chromium, selenium and fluorine.

CALCIUM

Calcium is the most abundant mineral in human beings. It is used mainly to form bones and teeth but performs some other functions as well.

Distribution

Total calcium in an average adult is about 1,000 gm of which nearly 99% is present in bones and teeth. The rest (about 10 gm) is distributed in various tissues and body fluids. Muscles and nerves have relatively more calcium than other tissues.

Calcium is present in bones mainly in the form of calcium phosphate. Small amounts of carbonate, hydroxide, fluoride, citrate and other salts of calcium are also present. Calcium phosphate is first deposited in an amorphous form which is later converted into crystalline form. The crystalline form is known as **hydroxyapatite**, and its rough composition is $Ca_{10}(PO_4)_6(OH)_2$. The crystals are rod-shaped. There is a continuous exchange of calcium between bones and extracellular fluid.

Concentration of calcium in intracellular and extracellular fluids is delicately regulated. The concentration of calcium in plasma (or serum) is 9 to 11 mg/dl (4.5 to 5.5 mEq/L). About 50% of this is bound to proteins, and can not diffuse through capillaries (protein-bound or non-diffusible calcium). About 5% is associated with organic anions, e.g. citrate, and is diffusible. The remaining 45% is free **ionised calcium**, and is freely diffusible. Almost all the physiological functions of calcium are performed by ionised calcium.

Functions

1. Formation of Bones and Teeth

As mentioned earlier, the major function of calcium is to form bones and teeth. Calcium phosphate is deposited in bones the around collagen fibres in the zone of ossification in an amorphous form. The amorphous form changes later into hydroxyapatite crystals. Osteoblasts mineralise the bones and osteoclasts remove calcium phosphate from the bones.

During growing age, osteoblastic activity is more than the osteoclastic activity leading to skeletal growth. In adults, the activities are balanced leading to a continuous remodelling of the bones.

2. Excitability and Conductivity of Nerves

Excitability of nerves depends upon a number of cations including Ca^{++}. A raised plasma calcium level decreases, and a lowered plasma calcium level increases the excitability of nerves. Transmission of impulses across synapses occurs due to release of neurotransmitters which requires calcium ions.

Neurotransmitters are present in the cell inside synaptic vesicles. There are two pools of synaptic vesicles, reserve pool and releasable pool. In the reserve pool, a synaptic vesicle is bound to actin filaments through a protein, synapsin I (dephosphorylated). Release of Ca^{++} activates **calmodulin (CaM) kinase II** which phosphorylates **synapsin I**. This leads to dissociation of the synaptic vesicle from actin filaments. Synaptic vesicle moves to releasable pool from where it releases the neurotransmitter molecules by exocytosis (Fig. 23.1).

3. Neuromuscular Transmission

Neuromuscular transmission occurs through release of acetylcholine from the motor endplate which requires the presence of calcium ions.

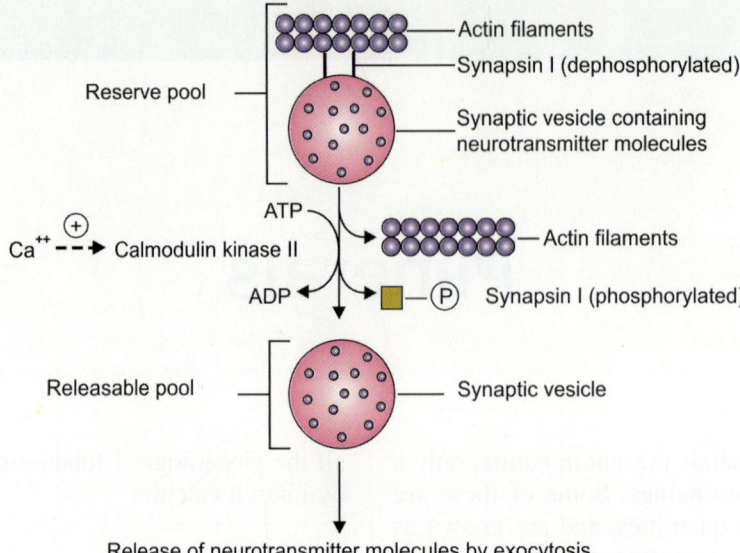

Fig. 23.1: Role of Ca⁺⁺ in the release of neurotransmitters

4. Excitability and Contractility of Myocardium

The rhythmic generation of impulses in heart and contraction of heart muscle also require calcium ions. An increase in the concentration of ionised calcium increases cardiac contractility and vice versa.

5. Coagulation of Blood

Ionised calcium is one of the coagulation factors. Coagulation of blood occurs by a cascade of reactions. Calcium ions are required in most of these reactions. Many of the anticoagulants which are used to prevent in vitro coagulation of blood, e.g. oxalate, citrate, EDTA, etc. act by binding calcium ions.

6. Action of Hormones

Ionised calcium acts as a **second messenger** for some hormones. Moreover, secretion of hormones which are stored in granular form requires the presence of Ca⁺⁺.

Absorption

Absorption of calcium occurs by an active uptake system in the upper part of small intestine. Normally, 10 to 20% of the dietary calcium is absorbed. The absorption is affected by the following factors:

1. pH

A relatively low pH increases the solubility of calcium salts and favours calcium absorption.

2. Calcium: Phosphorus Ratio

Since calcium and phosphorus are absorbed together, they must be present in the diet in a proper ratio. The ideal ratio is 1:1 but absorption can occur satisfactorily as long as the ratio lies between 1:2 and 2:1.

3. Proteins

Presence of proteins and amino acids in the food together with calcium facilitates the absorption of calcium.

4. Vitamin D and Parathormone

Vitamin D and parathormone play an important role in the metabolism of calcium. Cholecalciferol is converted into its active metabolite, 1,25-dihydroxycholecalciferol (1,25-DHCC or calcitriol) with the help of parathormone as described in Chapter 22. 1,25-Dihydroxychole-calciferol induces the synthesis of **calcium-binding protein**, **calcium-dependent ATPase** and **alkaline phosphatase** in the intestinal mucosa. These are required for the active absorption of calcium.

As calcium is absorbed, plasma calcium level rises. When plasma calcium rises above the normal range, it causes feedback inhibition of parathormone secretion. This switches off the series of reactions responsible for raising the plasma calcium level. Thus, vitamin D and parathormone act in concert to regulate calcium absorption and the plasma calcium level.

Requirement

Infants	: 400–600 mg/day
Children	: 800 mg/day
Adolescents	: 1200 mg/day
Adults	: 800 mg/day
Pregnant and lactating women	: 1200 mg/day

Dietary Sources

Milk, cheese, eggs, figs, nuts, beans, lentils, cabbage and cauliflower are good sources of calcium.

Abnormal Serum Calcium Levels

Serum calcium level may rise or fall in some pathological conditions. A rise in serum calcium level (hypercalcaemia) occurs in hyperparathyroidism, hypervitaminosis D, bone cancer, multiple myeloma, leukaemia, polycythaemia, milk alkali syndrome, sarcoidosis, idiopathic infantile hypercalcaemia, etc.

A decrease in serum calcium level (hypocalcaemia) is seen in hypoparathyroidism, rickets, osteomalacia, steatorrhoea, chronic renal failure, nephrotic syndrome, etc.

If serum calcium level remains elevated over a long period, calcium may get deposited in soft tissues such as kidneys, liver, arteries, etc. A sudden decrease in serum calcium may cause **tetany** (involuntary contraction of skeletal muscles).

PHOSPHORUS

Distribution

Next to calcium, phosphorus is the most abundant mineral in human beings. About 700 gm of phosphorus is present in the body of an average adult. Nearly 80% of it is present in bones and teeth. The remainder is distributed all over the body. Nerves and muscles are particularly rich in phosphorus. Phosphorus is mainly an intracellular mineral. Serum inorganic phosphorus level is 2.5 to 4.0 mg/dl in adults and 4 to 7 mg/dl in children. The product of serum calcium concentration (mg/dl) and serum inorganic phosphorus concentration (mg/dl) remains nearly constant at 40 in adults and 50 in children.

Functions

1. *Formation of Bones and Teeth*

As mentioned earlier, calcium phosphate is the principal salt in bones and teeth. Formation of bones and teeth is one of the major functions of phosphorus.

2. *Formation of High-energy Compounds*

Phosphorus is a constituent of most of the high-energy compounds in our body, e.g. ATP, creatine phosphate, phosphoenol pyruvate, etc.

3. *Role in Metabolism*

Phosphorus is a constituent of many coenzymes, e.g. FMN, FAD, NAD, NADP, thiamin pyrophosphate, pyridoxal phosphate and coenzyme A. Phosphorus plays an important role in metabolic reactions in the form of these coenzymes. Moreover, phosphorus plays a unique role in the metabolism of carbohydrates. Carbohydrates have to be phosphorylated before they can enter any metabolic pathway.

4. *Formation of Nucleic Acids*

Phosphorus is required for the formation of nucleotides which, in turn, form nucleic acids.

5. *Formation of Membranes*

Phosphorus participates in the formation of biomembranes in the form of phospholipids.

6. *Formation of Nervous Tissue*

Phosphorus also takes part in the formation of nervous tissue in the form of phospholipids.

7. *Maintenance of pH*

Inorganic phosphorus exists as HPO_4^{--} and $H_2PO_4^-$ which constitute a buffer pair and help in the maintenance of pH. Phosphate buffer is more abundant in intracellular fluid.

Absorption

Phosphorus is absorbed from the small intestine along with calcium. If calcium absorption is normal, so will be that of phosphorus.

Requirement

Infants	: 250–400 mg/day
Children	: 800 mg/day
Adolescents	: 1200 mg/day
Adults	: 800 mg/day
Pregnant and lactating women	: 1200 mg/day

Dietary Sources

Phosphorus is widely distributed in foodstuffs. If calorie and protein intakes are sufficient, a dietary deficiency of phosphorus is unlikely to occur. Milk, cheese, eggs, meat, nuts and beans are particularly good sources of phosphorus.

Abnormal Serum Phosphorus Levels

A rise in serum inorganic phosphorus level (hyper-phosphataemia) occurs in hypoparathyroidism, acromegaly, diabetes mellitus, hypervitaminosis D, chronic renal failure, etc.

A low serum inorganic phosphorus level (hypophos-phataemia) is seen in rickets, osteomalacia, hyperparathyroidism, steatorrhoea, Fanconi syndrome and familial hypophosphataemic rickets (renal rickets or vitamin D-resistant rickets). The last is an inherited disorder (X-linked dominant) in which renal tubular reabsorption of phosphate is greatly decreased. A transient decrease in serum inorganic phosphorus occurs following insulin injections.

MAGNESIUM

Distribution

The total magnesium in an average adult is about 20 gm. Bones contain about 70%, and the remainder is present in other tissues and body fluids, e.g. muscles, blood, CSF, etc. Serum magnesium level is 2 to 3 mg/dl. Concentration of magnesium in the intracellular compartment is higher than that in the extracellular compartment.

Functions

1. Excitability of Nerves

Together with some other cations, magnesium ions also affect the excitability of nerves. A low magnesium level increases the excitability, and a high magnesium level decreases the excitability.

2. Cofactor for Enzymes

Magnesium is a cofactor for all the enzymes requiring ATP as a second substrate as ATP participates in biochemical reactions as Mg^{++}- ATP complex. These include enzymes involved in the metabolism of carbohydrates, lipids, amino acids, purines and pyrimidines, e.g. hexokinase, phosphofructokinase, thiokinase, mevalonate kinase, squalene synthetase, glutamine synthetase, carbamoyl phosphate synthetase, PRPP synthetase, etc. Some other enzymes requiring Mg^{++} as a cofactor are enolase, glucose-6-phosphate dehydrogenase, transketolase, etc.

Absorption

Magnesium is absorbed from the small intestine. The extent of absorption depends on the magnesium content of the diet and is independent of the requirement. On an average diet, about half of the ingested magnesium is absorbed. The absorption may increase on a low-magnesium diet, and may fall on a high-magnesium diet. The regulation of magnesium balance is the function of kidneys. Aldosterone plays a role in the renal regulation. A high aldosterone level decreases the tubular reabsorption of magnesium.

Requirement

Infants	: 60–70 mg/day
Children	: 150–250 mg/day
Adult men	: 350 mg/day
Adult women	: 300 mg/day
Pregnant and lactating women	: 450 mg/day

Dietary Sources

Nuts, beans, wheat, milk, eggs, orange and spinach are good sources of magnesium. Almond is particularly rich in magnesium.

Abnormal Serum Magnesium Levels

Serum magnesium level is decreased (hypomagnesaemia) in chronic alcoholism, chronic diarrhoea, hyperparathyroidism and aldosteronism. A high serum magnesium level (hypermagnesaemia) is commonly seen in renal failure.

SODIUM

Distribution

Total amount of sodium in an average adult is about 60 gm. About 20 gm is present in bones. The rest is distributed in other tissues. Sodium is the major cation of the **extracellular fluids**. Plasma sodium level is 310 to 340 mg/dl or 136 to 145 mEq/L. Other extracellular fluids are also rich in sodium. The intracellular fluid contains only about 10 mEq/L.

Functions

1. Maintenance of Osmotic Pressure

Being the major cation of extracellular fluids, sodium plays on important role in maintaining the osmotic pressure of body fluids, and guards against excessive water loss. It should be remembered that osmotic pressure depends upon the number of solute particles and not on their size. And sodium ions outnumber all the other solute particles in extracellular fluids.

2. Maintenance of pH

In the form of sodium bicarbonate, it is a component of the bicarbonate-carbonic acid buffer which is a major buffer of the extracellular fluids. Renal excretion of hydrogen ions in exchange for sodium ions is also important in maintaining the pH of body fluids.

3. Nerve Excitability and Conduction

Maintenance of normal excitability of nerves and conduction of nerve impulses are also important functions of sodium. Cations and anions are so distributed across the cell membrane of nerve fibres that the exterior of the membrane is slightly electropositive in relation to the interior. This potential difference is known as the resting potential. When a stimulus is applied to the nerve, the stimulated area immediately becomes permeable to sodium ions which move into the interior of the nerve fibre. The interior becomes electropositive in relation to the exterior. Thus, a nerve impulse is generated. Transmission of the nerve impulse also occurs due to influx of sodium ions along the entire length of the nerve fibre.

4. Active Transport

Several compounds enter the cells against their concentration gradient by active absorption. **Sodium pump**, which ejects sodium ions from the interior of the cell to the exterior, is linked with the active absorption of glucose, galactose and some amino acids.

Absorption

Sodium enters gastrointestinal tract through ingested food and through digestive secretions. The latter is a far more abundant source as compared to dietary intake. Almost all the sodium is absorbed from the gastrointestinal tract. The absorption occurs from the entire length of the small and large intestines. As the concentration of sodium in intestinal lumen is far greater than that inside the mucosal cells, sodium diffuses from the lumen into the cells. The intracellular sodium is actively transported into blood by the sodium pump. This keeps the intracellular concentration of sodium in the mucosal cells at a low level so that more sodium can diffuse from the intestinal lumen into the mucosal cells.

Requirement

There has been considerable controversy about the daily requirement of sodium. The requirement depends upon daily loss of sodium from the body which depends upon climate. In a tropical country like India, a daily intake of 4 to 6 gm of elemental sodium or 10 to 15 gm of sodium chloride is sufficient to maintain sodium balance. In recent years, a direct relationship between excessive sodium intake and prevalence of **hypertension** has been shown. As far as sodium nutrition is concerned, the problem is really one of preventing excessive intake rather than one of guarding against a dietary deficiency.

Dietary Sources

Table salt (sodium chloride) is one of the chief sources of sodium in our daily diet. Baking powder (sodium bicarbonate) can also contribute significant amounts. Meat, fish, fowl, eggs, milk, cheese and cereals are rich in sodium. Carrot, radish, cauliflower, spinach, turnip, legumes and nuts are also good sources of sodium.

Abnormal Serum Sodium Levels

Sodium metabolism is controlled by adrenocortical hormones. Mineralocorticoids, such as aldosterone, are the most potent in this regard followed by glucocorticoids and sex hormones. These hormones cause retention of sodium and loss of potassium from the body. Therefore, abnormal serum sodium levels are to be expected in adrenocortical disorders. Excessive loss of sodium in gastrointestinal secretions and urine can also affect the serum sodium level.

Hyponatraemia (low serum sodium) occurs in adrenocortical insufficiency, severe diarrhoea, chronic renal disease, excessive sweating, etc. Hyponatraemia may also occur due to dilution of plasma when dehydrated patients are rehydrated with salt-free fluids.

Hypernatraemia (high serum sodium) occurs in adrenocortical hyperactivity, prolonged steroid therapy and dehydration. In dehydration, hypernatraemia occurs due to haemoconcentration.

POTASSIUM

Distribution

Total amount of potassium in an average adult is about 140 gm. Potassium is the chief cation of the **intracellular compartment**, and is present in all cells. The potassium content of intracellular fluid is about 140 mEq/L while that of extra-cellular fluid is only about 5 mEq/L. Serum potassium level is 3.5 to 5 mEq/L.

Functions

1. Maintenance of Osmotic Pressure

Potassium is involved in the maintenance of osmotic pressure within the cells in the same way as sodium does in extracellular compartment. Nearly half the osmolarity of intracellular fluid is due to potassium.

2. Maintenance of pH

Potassium, in the form of KH_2PO_4 and K_2HPO_4, helps to maintain the pH of intracellular fluid.

3. Nerve Excitability and Conduction

Together with sodium, potassium plays a role in maintaining the normal excitability of nerves and in the conduction of nerve impulses. It also affects the excitability and contractility of muscles, particularly heart muscles. Marked alterations in serum potassium level often cause serious abnormalities in the functioning of the heart.

4. Cofactor for Enzymes

Potassium functions as a cofactor for some enzymes, e.g. pyruvate kinase.

5. Active Transport

Along with sodium, potassium is also involved in active transport . The sodium pump, involved in active transport of glucose, galactose, amino acids, etc. is really a sodium-potassium pump as it causes energy-dependent efflux of sodium and influx of potassium.

Absorption

Potassium absorption occurs down the concentration gradient from small intestine as well as large intestine.

Requirement

The exact potassium requirement is not known with certainty. A daily intake of 4 gm is sufficient to maintain potassium balance.

Dietary Sources

Potassium is very widely distributed in foodstuffs. Meat, fish, fowl, cereals, vegetables, apricots, peaches, oranges and pineapples are rich is potassium.

Abnormal Serum Potassium Levels

Hypokalaemia (low serum potassium) occurs in adreno-cortical hyperactivity, prolonged steroid therapy, diarrhoea, wasting diseases, metabolic alkalosis, familial periodic paralysis and after insulin injection. Hypokalaemia may also be caused by prolonged use of thiazide diuretics which promote urinary excretion of potassium. It may also occur when a dehydrated patient is rehydrated with potassium-free fluids. Hypokalaemia causes irritability, muscular weakness, tachycardia, cardiac dilatation and ultimately cardiac arrest. Characteristic **electrocardiographic changes,** e.g. flattened or inverted T waves and depressed ST segment, may be more valuable in the diagnosis of potassium deficit than the serum potassium level.

Hyperkalaemia (high serum potassium) is seen in adrenocortical insufficiency, renal failure, dehydration, etc. Indiscriminate intravenous potassium therapy may also cause hyperkalaemia. Hyperkalaemia causes mental confusion, numbness and tingling, muscular weakness and paralysis, bradycardia, peripheral circulatory failure and cardiac arrest. Electrocardiographic changes are also characteristic and include lengthening of P-R interval, widening of QRS complex and elevation of T waves. Finally, the P wave disappears altogether.

CHLORINE

Distribution

The total amount of chlorine in an average adult is about 80 gm. Chlorine, in the form of chloride ions, is the chief anion of extracellular compartment. Normal serum chloride level is 100 to 106 mEq/L (355 to 375 mg/dl). The chloride content of cerebrospinal fluid is 120 to 130 mEq/L. The interstitial fluid contains about 110 mEq/L. The intracellular fluid contains only about 4 mEq/L.

Functions

1. Maintenance of Osmotic Pressure

Alongside sodium, chloride ions play an important role in maintaining the osmotic pressure of extracellular fluids as they are present in a high concentration in extracellular fluids.

2. Maintenance of pH

Chloride ions help in maintaining the pH of blood by the mechanism of chloride shift.

3. Formation of Hydrochloric Acid

Hydrochloric acid is an important constituent of gastric juice. Chloride ions are necessary for its formation.

Absorption

Chloride ions are absorbed passively down the concentration gradient in the upper portion of the small intestine. In distal ileum and colon, they are absorbed in exchange for bicarbonate ions.

Requirement

Chloride is commonly present in food as sodium chloride. Therefore, sodium and chloride intakes are parallel. If daily requirement of sodium is met, so will be that of chloride.

Dietary Sources

Table salt is the most abundant source of chloride in our daily diet. Foods that provide sodium also provide chloride, e.g. meat, fish, fowl, eggs, milk, cheese, cereals, etc.

Abnormal Serum Chloride Levels

With a few exceptions, changes in serum chloride level are parallel to those in serum sodium level. Serum chloride level is raised (hyperchloraemia) in dehydration, respiratory alkalosis, metabolic acidosis (e.g. renal failure and diarrhoea) and adrenocortical hyperactivity.

Serum chloride level is lowered (hypochloraemia) in severe vomiting, prolonged gastric suction, respiratory acidosis, metabolic alkalosis and Addison's disease.

SULPHUR

Distribution

About 100 gm of sulphur is present in an average adult. Inorganic sulphur, in the form of sulphate ions, is present in very small amounts. Organic sulphur is the predominant form of sulphur in the body. It is present in most proteins in the form of **sulphur-containing amino acids**, cysteine and methionine.

Functions

1. Sulphur is a component of most of the proteins in the form of cysteine and methionine. The sulphydryl (–SH) groups of cysteine residues not only stabilise the structure of proteins by forming disulphide bonds but

are also essential for the biological activity of many proteins, particularly the enzymes.

2. Several mucopolysaccharides, e.g. heparin, chondroitin sulphate and keratan sulphate, contain sulphur.

3. Sulphur is a constituent of many vitamins, e.g. thiamin, biotin, lipoic acid, etc. Active form of pantothenic acid, i.e. coenzyme A and acyl carrier protein, also contain sulphur.

4. Detoxification of many harmful substances is done in the liver by conjugating them with sulphate.

Absorption

Sulphur is absorbed from the intestine mainly in the form of sulphur-containing amino acids. Absorption of inorganic sulphate is very poor.

For sulphation of various compounds, e.g. muco-polysaccharides, cerbrosides, etc sulphur is converted into its active form, phosphoadenosine phosphosulphate (PAPS; active sulphate) which acts as a donor of the sulphate group.

Requirement

The daily excretion of sulphur is about 5 gm in average adults. Most of it is derived from proteins. If protein intake is adequate, it will provide sufficient sulphur as well.

Dietary Sources

As mentioned earlier, inorganic sulphate is very poorly absorbed from the intestine. It is the sulphur of the proteins that meets our sulphur requirements. Therefore, protein-rich foods, e.g. eggs, milk, cheese, meat, fish, nuts and legumes, are the main sources of sulphur in our daily diet.

IRON

Distribution

Total amount of iron in an adult human being is 3.5 to 4.5 gm. Blood and blood-forming organs are the largest reservoirs of iron in our body. But small amounts of iron are present in nearly every tissue. Important iron-containing compounds are haemoglobin, myoglobin, ferritin, haemosiderin, transferrin, cytochromes and iron-containing enzymes. About 70% of the body iron is present in haemoglobin and 5% in myoglobin. Ferritin and haemosiderin, which are storage forms of iron, contain about 20% of the body iron. Transferrin, which is an iron carrier protein present in plasma, contains 0.1% of the body iron. The remaining iron is present in cytochromes and enzymes. Structure and functions of haemoglobin, myoglobin and cytochromes have been described earlier. Important features of other iron-containing compounds are described as follows:

Ferritin

Ferritin is present in liver, spleen, bone marrow, brain, kidneys, intestine, placenta, etc. It is one of the **storage** forms of iron. The protein portion is known as apoferritin. Apoferritin combines with iron to form ferritin.

The first step in the synthesis of ferritin is the formation of apoferritin induced by the entry of ferrous iron in the cell. This is followed by oxidation of ferrous iron to the ferric form. Ferric iron forms ferric hydrophosphate micelles, which enter the protein shell to form ferritin.

Apoferritin is made up of 24 identical subunits, each having a molecular weight of 22,000 to 24,000. The subunits are arranged at the vertices of a pentagonal dodecahedron with a hollow space in the centre. Ferric hydrophosphate micelles are present in this space. When fully saturated, a molecule of ferritin contains 5,000 atoms of iron, and has a molecular weight of 900,000.

Haemosiderin

Haemosiderin is a granular iron-rich protein. It is insoluble in water unlike ferritin. The exact structure of haemosiderin is not known. It has been shown that iron is first stored in the body in the form of ferritin. As the iron stores increase, the older ferritin molecules are aggregated to form haemosiderin. Some of the protein is degraded in this process. Therefore, the percentage of iron in haemosiderin is higher as compared to that in ferritin. Normally, about two thirds of the stored iron is in the form of ferritin and one third in the form of haemosiderin.

Transferrin

Transferrin is a **carrier protein** which transports iron in circulation. Free iron is toxic, and has a tendency to precipitate. These problems are overcome by combining iron with transferrin. Transferrin is a β_1-globulin with a molecular weight of about 90,000. It is made up of two non-identical subunits. One molecule of transferrin can transport two ferric atoms.

Transferrin carries iron to and from various tissues through circulation. There are specific receptors for transferrin on the cell membranes of the cells requiring iron, e.g. red cell precursors. Transferrin-iron complex attaches to these receptors. This attachment produces a conformational change in the transferrin molecule as a result of which the iron is released. The free transferrin molecules are then displaced from the cell membrane by molecules carrying iron.

The concentration of transferrin in plasma is 200 to 400 mg/dl. This amount of transferrin is capable of carrying 250 to 400 mg of iron per dl of plasma. This is known as the **total iron binding capacity** of plasma. Normal plasma iron level is 50 to 175 µg/dl which means that the iron binding capacity of plasma is only about 30% saturated in healthy subjects.

Iron-containing Enzymes

Several enzymes require iron for their catalytic activity. In some cases, iron forms an integral part of the enzyme molecules. In others, presence of iron is required for the catalytic activity of the enzymes. The iron-containing enzymes are mostly concerned with biological oxidations. Examples of such enzymes are catalase, peroxidase, aconitase, succinate dehydrogenase, xanthine oxidase, etc.

Functions

1. Transport of Oxygen

The most important function of iron is to transport oxygen in the body in the form of **haemoglobin**. A similar function is performed in muscles by **myoglobin**.

2. Oxidative Reactions

As a component of the various **oxidoreductase enzymes** mentioned earlier, iron plays a role in a number of oxidative reactions.

3. Tissue Respiration

As a component of **cytochromes** in the respiratory chain, iron is involved in tissue respiration. It is the iron component of the cytochromes that accepts and donates electrons.

Iron Balance

Iron status depends upon the relative rates of iron absorption and iron excretion. Iron absorption is important not only from the nutritional point of view but also because this is the major mechanism for maintaining normal iron balance. Iron metabolism is said to occur within a **closed system** in the body, i.e. there is little exchange of iron between man and his environment. The iron present in the body is continuously reutilised. Only a minute amount of iron is lost everyday from the body in the form of exfoliated cells. The faecal iron loss in 0.4 to 0.5 mg a day. The urinary iron loss is about 0.1 mg a day. About 0.2 to 0.3 mg of iron is lost daily from the skin alongwith the exfoliated cells. Thus, the **total iron loss** is just under one mg a day.

In **premenopausal women**, there are two additional routes of iron loss. About 20 to 25 mg of iron is lost with **menstrual blood** in each cycle. This is equivalent to a daily loss of 0.7 to 0.8 mg of iron. During **pregnancy**, there is no menstrual loss but the expectant mother has to provide iron to the **foetus**. This amounts to about 0.6 mg a day in the first trimester, about 2.8 mg a day in the second trimester, and about 4 mg a day in the third trimester of pregnancy.

The iron losses are balanced by intestinal absorption of iron. The intestinal absorption is affected by body iron stores, erythropoietic activity, degree of saturation of plasma transferrin, the amount of dietary iron, valency of ingested iron (Fe^{++} or Fe^{+++}) and presence of other substances in the food. Absorption is more when body iron stores are low, erythropoietic activity is increased, saturation of plasma transferrin is low and iron is ingested in ferrous form. Presence of ascorbic acid, succinic acid, histidine and cysteine in the food increases iron absorption. Phytates and phosphates retard iron absorption.

Iron can be absorbed from all segments of the small intestine but presence and normal functioning of stomach are also essential. Patients with **achlorhydria** and those who have undergone **gastrectomy** absorb less iron as compared to normal persons. Gastric enzymes and hydrochloric acid release iron from iron-containing compounds and reduce ferric iron to the ferrous form.

The exact mechanism of iron absorption is still imperfectly understood. It is believed that ferritin content of mucosal cells of the intestine regulates the absorption of iron. These cells are formed in the crypts of Leiberkuhn. They gradually reach the tip of the villi and are shed off into the intestinal lumen. Their average life-span is three days. The function of ferritin in these cells is to block the absorption of iron. Those cells which are formed during a period of iron overload are rich in ferritin. These cells will absorb little iron during their life-span. Moreover, when these are shed off, their iron content will also be lost in faeces. Conversely, the cells formed during a period of iron deficiency are poor in ferritin. These cells absorb more iron and transfer it into the plasma.

Requirement

Though the actual requirement of iron is very small, much larger amounts have to be provided in diet because only a small proportion of the dietary iron is normally absorbed. The daily requirement in different age groups is as follows:

Infants	: 6–10 mg/day
Children	: 10 mg/day
Adolescents	: 12 mg/day
Adult men and post-menopausal women	: 10 mg/day
Premenopausal and lactating women	: 15 mg/day
Pregnant women	: 30 mg/day

Dietary Sources

Liver, heart, kidney, spleen, meat, fish and eggs are good sources of iron. The vegetable sources include whole wheat, figs, dates, nuts, beans, spinach, molasses, etc. A much greater proportion of iron can be absorbed from animal foods than from vegetable foods. On a mixed diet, healthy subjects absorb 5 to 10% of the dietary iron.

Iron Deficiency

Iron deficiency is widespread both in poor and in affluent countries. Iron deficiency is the commonest cause of anaemia throughout the world. Deficiency can be caused by **inadequate intake** of iron especially when the requirement is high, e.g. in infancy, adolescence and pregnancy. **Malabsorption** resulting from steatorrhoea, coeliac disease, gastrectomy, etc can also cause iron deficiency. Persistent **blood loss**, e.g. from genital tract, gastrointestinal tract, hookworm infestation, etc. can also result in iron deficiency.

When iron deficiency develops, the earliest change is a depletion of body iron stores. Other changes follow progressively. Plasma transferrin saturation is decreased. Plasma iron is decreased. A **microcytic, hypochromic anaemia** develops. Poikilocytosis becomes evident. Hemoglobin level falls. Severe and prolonged deficiency leads to tissue changes, e.g. koilonychia, angular stomatitis, glossitis, pharyngeal and oesophageal webs, atrophic gastritis, partial villus atrophy, etc.

Iron Overload

Iron overload is much less common than iron deficiency. Two types of iron overload syndromes are known. When excessive iron is deposited in reticuloendothelial cells without tissue damage, it is known as **haemosiderosis**. This occurs when excessive amounts of iron enter the body through the parenteral route. Repeated blood transfusions given to patients with thalassaemia and sideroblastic anaemia may lead to deposition of iron in reticuloendothelial cells.

When excess iron enters the body through the alimentary route, it gets deposited in parenchymal cells and causes tissue damage. This condition is known as **haemochromatosis**. It may be primary or secondary. Primary (genetic) haemochromatosis is far more common. The gene responsible for this and the protein encoded by it have not been identified. The genetic defect leads to excessive intestinal absorption of iron. Excess iron is deposited in liver, heart, pancreas and other endocrine glands, skin, etc. Hepatomegaly, cardiomegaly, congestive heart failure, hypogonadism, diabetes mellitus and bronze-coloured pigmentation of skin are the usual clinical abnormalities. The condition is also known as **bronzed diabetes**.

Serum iron, ferritin and per cent saturation of iron-binding capacity are increased in haemochromatosis. Phlebotomy and iron-chelating agents, e.g. desferrioxamine are used to remove excess iron.

Secondary haemochromatosis may occur in alcoholic liver disease in which iron deposition is usually confined to hepatic tissue. South African Bantus are known to develop haemochromatosis due to excessive ingestion of iron present in an alcoholic beverage brewed in iron vessels.

IODINE

Distribution

Iodine is present in small amounts in human beings. The total amount of iodine in the body of an average adult is 45–50 mg. About 10 to 15 mg of iodine is present in the thyroid gland. Muscles contain about 25 mg. About 5 mg is present in skin, 3 mg in the skeleton and 2 mg in liver.

Functions

The only known function of iodine is in the synthesis of thyroid hormones. The thyroid gland actively takes up iodide ions from plasma, oxidises them to iodine, and incorporates iodine into tyrosine residues of thyroglobulin to form mono-iodo-tyrosine (MIT) and di-iodo-tyrosine (DIT). Two DIT residues combine to form thyroxine (T_4), and one MIT and one DIT residue combine to form tri-iodo-thyronine (T_3).

Absorption

Iodine is absorbed from all parts of the alimentary tract, particularly from the small intestine. Iodine and iodate are converted into iodide prior to absorption. Other mucous membranes and skin can also absorb iodine.

The iodide absorbed from the alimentary tract and elsewhere enters the circulation. About one third of the circulating iodide is taken up by the thyroid gland. The remainder is excreted, mainly by the kidneys. Small amounts of iodide are excreted in saliva, bile, milk, sweat and expired air.

Plasma iodine level is 4 to 10 µg/dl. Only 10% of it is present in the form of inorganic iodide. Organic iodine is present mostly in the form of thyroid hormones bound to proteins (protein bound iodine).

Requirement

Infants	:	40–50 µg/day
Children	:	70–120 µg/day
Adults	:	150 µg/day

Dietary Sources

Iodine is present in water and soil. Foods, both animal and plant, obtain iodine from water and soil. Iodine content of foodstuffs depends upon the **iodine content of water and soil**. Sea water is rich in iodine. Therefore, sea foods, e.g. fish, oysters, lobsters, etc. are the best sources of iodine. As we go away from the sea, the iodine content of water and soil, and hence of the foodstuffs, decreases.

Iodine Deficiency

Iodine deficiency is common in certain areas of the world. These areas constitute the so-called **goitre belt**. Sub-Himalayan region of India is a part of this belt as the iodine content of soil and water is poor in this region. A high prevalence of non-toxic goitre (endemic goitre) is seen in this region. The thyroid gland becomes hypertrophic in order to produce enough hormones from the available iodine. A severe deficiency can produce hypothyroidism. Endemic goitre can be prevented by providing iodised table salt in the goitre belt. **Iodised salt** is prepared by mixing potassium iodate with common salt in the proportion of 1:10,000 to 20,000. Injection of iodised poppyseed oil has also been successfully used in some countries. One dose is sufficient for 2 to 4 years.

COPPER

Distribution

About 60 to 100 mg of copper is present in the body of an average adult. Relatively large amounts of copper are present in muscles (30 to 50 mg), bones (12 to 20 mg) and liver (9 to 15 mg). Plasma copper level is 100 to 200 mg/dl. Nearly 90% of the plasma copper is tightly bound to a copper-containing protein, **ceruloplasmin** which is synthesised in the liver. Rest of the plasma copper is loosely attached to **albumin**. Albumin is the major carrier of copper as it can easily release copper. Many tissues contain minute amounts of copper in the form of copper-containing enzymes.

Functions

Copper performs its physiological functions in the form of copper-containing enzymes. These include cytochrome oxidase, superoxide dismutase, monoamine oxidase, tyrosinase, dopamine hydroxylase, etc. Ceruloplasmin also functions as ferroxidase which oxidises ferrous iron to the ferric form.

Copper is also essential for synthesis of haemoglobin, formation of bones and maintenance of myelin sheath of nerves.

Absorption

About one third of the dietary copper is normally absorbed, mainly from small intestine. **Copper-binding P-type ATPase**, an enzyme present in intestinal mucosa (and many other cells) transfers copper into portal circulation. Albumin carries it to liver. A different copper-binding P-type ATPase present in liver is required for incorporation of copper into ceruloplasmin, and its excretion in bile.

Daily Requirement

Adults require about 2.5 mg of copper daily. Infants and children require about 0.05 mg/kg of body weight.

Dietary Sources

Liver, kidney, meat, nuts, legumes and raisins are good source of copper.

Disorders of Copper Metabolism

Wilson's disease (hepatolenticular degeneration) is an autosomal recessive disease in which the synthesis of ceruloplasmin is impaired. Large amounts of copper are deposited in liver, basal ganglia and around cornea. Serum copper and ceruloplasmin levels are low. Urinary excretion of copper is increased. Recent work has shown that **copper-binding P-type ATPase is congenitally deficient in liver** in this disease. This impairs the **incorporation of copper into apoceruloplasmin** and its biliary excretion leading to **copper toxicity**. Another inherited disorder of copper metabolism is **Menkes disease** which is an X-linked recessive disease. In this disease, copper-binding P-type ATPase is deficient in intestinal mucosa and most other tissues except liver. Copper accumulates in intestinal mucosa but can not be released into circulation. This leads to a **deficiency of copper** in tissues. The deficiency causes cerebral degeneration, hypochromic microcytic anaemia and steely or kinky hair.

Copper may also be involved in the aetiology of Indian childhood cirrhosis in which excessive deposition of copper has been shown in liver. It has been suggested that excess copper enters the body when milk boiled in copper or brass utensils is fed to infants.

Serum copper and ceruloplasmin levels are elevated in pregnancy, infections, leukaemia, collagen diseases, myocardial infarction, cirrhosis of liver and after administration of oestrogen or oral contraceptives.

ZINC

Distribution

The total amount of zinc in an average adult is 1.3 to 2.1 gm. Its tissue distribution is very wide. Prostate, liver, kidneys, muscles, heart, skin, bones and teeth are particularly rich in zinc. Plasma zinc level is 50 to 150 µg/dl. Blood cells, erythrocytes and leukocytes, have a higher concentration of zinc than plasma.

Functions

1. Zinc is essential for normal **growth** and **sexual development**. It is required for the synthesis of nucleic acids, which is essential for cell division and growth.

2. In the form of zinc fingers, it is a constituent of some proteins which regulate transcription.

3. Many **enzymes** require zinc for their catalytic activity. These include carbonic anhydrase, carboxypeptidase, lactate dehydrogenase, malate dehydrogenase, glutamate dehydrogenase, alcohol dehydrogenase, alkaline phosphatase, etc.

4. Zinc is present in the β-cells of the islets of Langerhans. It is probably required for the **storage and release of insulin**.

Absorption

Zinc is absorbed from the small intestine. Copper, cadmium and calcium interfere with the absorption of zinc. Phytates also retard zinc absorption by forming an insoluble complex with zinc.

Requirement

Infants	:	5 mg/day
Children	:	10 mg/day
Adult men	:	15 mg/day
Adult women	:	12 mg/day
Pregnant women	:	15 mg/day
Lactating women	:	20 mg/day

Dietary Sources

Zinc is widely distributed in foodstuffs. Liver, kidney, meat, fish, eggs, milk, yeast and whole grain cereals are good sources of zinc.

Zinc Deficiency

A dietary deficiency of zinc may occur in vegetarians taking refined wheat flour as their staple diet. It can also occur in **acrodermatitis enteropathica**. It causes retardation of growth, dwarfism, delayed puberty and hypogonadism. A milder deficiency may cause poor wound healing and impaired perception of taste.

COBALT

About one mg of cobalt is present in the body of an average adult. It is chiefly distributed in liver, kidneys and bones. It is present almost entirely as a constituent of vitamin B_{12}.

Inorganic cobalt is not known to perform any biological function in human beings. It functions solely as a component of vitamin B_{12}. It must be provided in the diet as vitamin B_{12}. Inorganic cobalt is not absorbed from the alimentary tract. Injected cobalt is rapidly excreted in urine.

MANGANESE

About 12 to 20 mg of manganese is present in an average adult. Liver, pancreas and kidneys contain relatively more manganese than other tissues. Manganese is present mainly in the mitochondria and nuclei of the cells.

Manganese is absorbed from the small intestine. Less than 5% of the ingested manganese is normally absorbed.

Manganese is required for the formation of the matrix of bones and cartilages, for normal reproduction and for the normal functioning of the central nervous system. It gives stability to the structure of nucleic acids. A number of enzymes require manganese as a cofactor, e.g. superoxide dismutase, arginase, acetylcholine esterase, RNA polymerase, carboxylases, and glycosyl transferases involved in the synthesis of mucopolysaccharides and glycoproteins.

The daily manganese requirement is believed to be 2 to 5 mg. Whole-grain cereals, legumes, nuts, green vegetables and fruits are good sources of manganese.

MOLYBDENUM

Molybdenum is present in very small amounts in the human body, principally in liver and kidneys. It is a component of xanthine oxidase, aldehyde oxidase and sulphite oxidase. Sulphite oxidase converts sulphite and sulphur dioxide into sulphate.

The exact requirement for molybdenum is unknown. An average diet provides 75 to 100 µg of molybdenum a day. Molybdenum deficiency is unknown in human beings. Excessive intake of molybdenum may cause copper deficiency.

CHROMIUM

The total amount of chromium in the body of an average adult is about 6 mg. It is widely distributed in the body. Chromium is a constituent of glucose tolerance factor (GTF) which binds to insulin and potentiates its actions. A relationship between chromium deficiency and glucose intolerance has been shown which can be corrected by chromium supplementation.

The absorption of chromium is less than 1%. Stainless steel utensils contain chromium which can also be absorbed. Chromium requirement is about 0.2 mg/day. Excess chromium can be toxic.

SELENIUM

Selenium is present in human body in minute amounts. About 6 mg of selenium is present in the body of an average adult. It is widely distributed in the body. Renal cortices, liver, muscles, pancreas, pituitary and skin contain selenium in relatively large amounts.

The role of selenium in the nutrition of animals has been known for sometime. It is involved in normal growth, reproductive functions and prevention of hepatic necrosis and muscle dystrophy in several animal species. Its exact role in human beings is still being investigated. It may be involved in the synthesis of coenzyme Q. It is also believed to play a role in immune reactions. It is a component of some proteins in the form of selenocysteine. The most definitive role of selenium, discovered so far, is in the **prevention of peroxidation of lipids** and other compounds. Hydrogen peroxide, formed in the tissues by the action of aerobic dehydrogenases and superoxide dismutase, is a toxic compound. It is detoxified by reduced glutathione.

$$2\ G - SH + H_2O_2 \longrightarrow GS - SG + 2\ H_2O$$
Reduced glutathione   Oxidised glutathione

The above reaction is catalysed by **glutathione peroxidase**. Selenium is a constituent of this enzyme. Glutathione peroxidase can also detoxify the fatty acid hydroperoxides (ROOH) that have already been formed by the action of hydrogen peroxide on fatty acids.

$$2\ G-SH + R-OOH \longrightarrow$$
$$\text{Fatty acid}$$
$$\text{hydroperoxide}$$
$$GS-SG + R-OH + H_2O$$
$$\text{Alcohol}$$

Thus, selenium acts as an **anti-oxidant**, and protects the tissues against the potentially toxic effects of hydrogen peroxide. Vitamin E also does the same but by a different mechanism.

The daily requirement for selenium is about 70 µg in adult man and 55 µg in adult women.

FLUORINE

About 2.6 gm of fluorine is normally present in the human body. More than 95% of it is present in **bones** and **teeth**. Fluorine is ingested in the form of fluorides. It is readily absorbed from the intestine, and enters the extracellular fluids.

Fluoride makes the bones resistant to **osteoporosis** in later life. It makes the teeth resistant to **dental caries**.

Certain bacteria, which are normal inhabitants of the oral cavity, act upon dietary carbohydrates and convert them into lactic acid. Lactic acid corrodes the enamel of the teeth and produces cavities (dental caries). Fluoride hardens the enamel of the teeth, and makes it resistant to attack by lactic acid.

Drinking water is the main source of fluoride. Seafood, cheese and tea may provide small amounts but other foods are generally poor in fluoride. The **fluoride intake** generally depends upon the **fluoride content of water**. In a tropical country like India, where water intake is relatively high, a fluoride content of 0.5 to 0.8 parts per million (ppm) in water will provide sufficient fluoride. If the fluoride content is less than this, dental caries may become a public health problem. In such areas, fluoride must be added to the drinking water (fluoridation) to raise its fluoride concentration to 0.5 to 0.8 ppm.

Fluoride is potentially toxic. If the fluoride content of water exceeds 1.2 ppm (or the daily fluoride intake exceeds 3 mg), it may cause fluorosis. In mild cases, only the teeth are affected (**dental fluorosis**). The teeth become mottled and corroded.

In severe cases, the bones are also affected (**skeletal fluorosis**). The bones of the vertebral column, pelvis and limbs become deformed. Tendons and ligaments are calcified. Fluorosis generally occurs in certain geographical areas where the fluoride content of water is high.

EXERCISE

1. Describe the maintenance of calcium homeostasis, and functions of calcium.

2. Write short notes on:
   a. Iron deficiency
   b. Haemochromatosis
   c. Wilson's disease
   d. Menkes disease
   e. Selenium
   f. Fluorosis

3. Write 'true' or 'false':
   a. About 45% of serum calcium is ionised.
   b. Proteins hamper the intestinal absorption of calcium.
   c. A sudden decrease in serum calcium causes tetany.
   d. Serum inorganic phosphorus is lower in children than in adults.
   e. Magnesium is required in all reactions involving ATP.
   f. Sodium is the major cation of intracellular fluid.
   g. Hypokalaemia and hyperkalaemia cause characteristic ECG changes.
   h. Iron is transported in circulation by ferritin.
   i. Iron loss is about 10 mg/day in adult men.
   j. Bronzed diabetes occurs due to copper overload.
   k. Consumption of iodised salt is recommended in hypertension.
   l. Hair becomes kinky and steely in Wilson's disease.
   m. Acrodermatitis enteropathica can cause zinc deficiency.
   n. Selenium is a constituent of glutathione reductase.
   o. Fluorosis increases the incidence of dental caries.

4. Fill in the blanks:
   a. .... is the most abundant mineral in human beings.
   b. A high plasma calcium level causes feedback inhibition of .... secretion.
   c. Renal tubular reabsorption of .... is greatly decreased in vitamin D-resistant rickets.
   d. Excessive sodium intake increases the prevalence of ....
   e. Aldosterone .... the urinary excretion of potassium.
   f. Chloride is the chief anion in .... fluid.
   g. Apoferritin is made up of .... identical subunits.
   h. .... transports iron in circulation.
   i. Iodine is required for the synthesis of ....
   j. .... is the major carrier of copper in circulation.
   k. Ceruloplasmin possesses .... activity.
   l. A severe deficiency of .... occurs in Menkes' disease.
   m. .... is a trace element present in glucose tolerance factor.
   n. Selenium acts as an ....
   o. Fluorosis can affect .... and ....

ANSWERS TO SHORT QUESTIONS

3. a. True
   c. True
   e. True
   g. True
   i. False
   k. False
   m. True
   o. False

   b. False
   d. False
   f. False
   h. False
   j. False
   l. False
   n. False

4. a. Calcium
   c. Phosphate
   e. Increases
   g. 24
   i. Thyroid hormones
   k. Ferroxidase
   m. Chromium
   o. Teeth, bones®

   b. Parathormone
   d. Hypertension
   f. Extracellular
   h. Transferrin
   j. Albumin
   l. Copper
   n. Anti-oxidant

24

Water Balance

Water is the most abundant component of our body. It accounts for nearly 70 percent of the total body weight in an adult male and 60 percent in an adult female. In obese individuals, the proportion of water is relatively less. Water bathes all cells, is present in all cells, is the solvent for all ions and molecules, and is the medium in which all biochemical reactions occur. Water has been chosen as the universal solvent for all living organisms. Some properties of water which make it an ideal medium for body fluids are:

1. Solvent Power

Water is an efficient and suitable solvent for most of the solutes present in our body. Some compounds which do not dissolve readily in water can form colloidal solutions.

2. Dielectric Constant

Water has a high dielectric constant because of which a large number of oppositely charged particles can co-exist in water.

3. Specific Heat

Water has a very high specific heat which means that a large amount of heat is required to raise the temperature of water. This ensures that the body temperature is not raised appreciably when thermal energy is released in the body during oxidation of carbohydrates, lipids and proteins.

4. Latent Heat of Evaporation

Water has a high latent heat of evaporation relative to other liquids. A large amount of thermal energy has to be spent for evaporation of water. When water evaporates from skin and lungs, a large amount of heat is lost, and a rise in body temperature is prevented. This is important for maintaining body temperature.

DISTRIBUTION OF WATER

In an average adult man weighing 70 kg, nearly 50 litres of water is present. About 70 percent of total body water or 35 litres is present in intracellular compartment. This is known as intracellular fluid (ICF). The remaining 30 percent, i.e. 15 litres is extracellular fluid (ECF). The ECF is further distributed in the following sub-compartments:

1. Plasma

About 3 litres of water is present as plasma in the vascular compartment.

2. Interstitial Fluid

About 7 litres of water is present in tissues in between the cells.

3. Transcellular Fluid

About 1 litre of water is present in cavities, e.g. cerebrospinal fluid, pleural fluid, pericardial fluid, peritoneal fluid, etc.

4. Unexchangeable Fluid

About 4 litres of water is present in bones, cartilages, dense connective tissue etc which does not exchange easily with other compartments.

OSMOLALITY

Osmolality is the **concentration of solutes or particles** in a fluid, expressed in **milliosmol (mosm) per kg**. The distribution of water in different compartments is determined by the osmolality of the compartment. The major osmotically active solutes in body fluids are:

a. **Electrolytes,** e.g. Na^+, K^+, Cl^-, HCO_3^-, phosphate, etc. and

b. **Proteins**.

The average concentrations of these solutes in important compartments are shown in Table 24.1.

Effective osmolality (or **tonicity**) of a compartment is determined by the solutes restricted to that compartment. The selective distribution of ions in intracellular and extracellular compartments is maintained by specific ion

Table 24.1: Concentrations of osmotically active substances (mEq/L) in major body fluids

	Intracellular fluid	Interstitial fluid	Plasma
CATIONS			
Na⁺	10	137	142
K⁺	160	5	5
Mg⁺⁺	24	3	3
Ca⁺⁺	6	5	5
Total	200	150	155
ANIONS			
Cl⁻	5	113	100
HCO₃⁻	5	27	27
Sulphate	15	1	1
Inorganic phosphate	25	2	2
Organic phosphates	70	–	–
Organic anions	15	5	5
Proteins	65	2	20
Total	200	150	155

channels and ion pumps. In fact, a lot of energy has to be spent daily for maintaining the differential distribution of ions in the intracellular and extracellular compartments. Potassium is present in a very high concentration in the intracellular fluid while very little potassium is present in extracellular fluid. Sodium is present in a very high concentration in the extracellular fluids but in a very low concentration in the intracellular fluid. This differential distribution is maintained by Na⁺, K⁺-exchanging ATPase. Proteins are present in a fairly high concentration in intracellular fluid, in a smaller but significant concentration in plasma and in a negligible concentration in interstitial fluid. Chloride and bicarbonate are the major anions in extracellular fluids while the major anions in intracellular fluid are phosphates and proteins.

Sodium and its associated anions determine the effective osmolality of the extracellular fluid. Potassium and its associated anions determine the effective osmolality of the intracellular fluid. The specific distribution of ions and molecules, and their concentrations, in the intracellular fluid are vital for the functioning of the cells, and are zealously maintained. Therefore, changes in osmolality of intracellular fluid are usually due to movement of water in and out of cells rather than the movement of solutes. For instance, hyperosmolality of extracellular fluid will draw water out of cells into the extracellular compartment, and hypoosmolality of extracellular fluid will drive water

out of the extracellular compartment into the intracellular compartment. Shrinkage or swelling of cells due to a shift of water out of or into the cells can seriously affect the functioning of cells.

Osmolality of **plasma** is 275 to 290 mosmol/kg. A 0.9 percent solution of sodium chloride (saline) or a 5 percent solution of glucose (dextrose) in water has the same osmolality (or tonicity) as that of plasma, and is said to be isosmotic or isotonic. Osmotic pressure exerted by proteins is called **oncotic pressure** (or colloid osmotic pressure). The normal oncotic pressure of plasma is about 25 mm of Hg. If there is a decrease in the concentration of proteins in plasma, e.g. due to proteinuria, oncotic pressure of plasma decreases. Water forced out of capillaries at the arterial end due to greater hydrostatic pressure can not re-enter at the venous end if the oncotic pressure becomes less than the hydrostatic pressure. This will result in oedema.

WATER INTAKE AND OUTPUT

Water balance of the body depends upon the relative intake and output of water. Water is taken in as drinking water and in the form of food and beverages. Some water is also formed in the body during metabolic reactions due to oxidation of hydrogen atoms removed from carbohydrates, lipids and amino acids. In a temperate climate, intake of drinking water averages about 1.5 litres/day, water in the form of food and beverages about 1 litre/day and metabolic water about 0.3 litre/day. Thus, the total intake is about 2.8 litres/day.

Water is lost from the body in the form of urine (about 1.5 litres/day), faeces (about 0.1 litre/day), water vapour in expired air (about 0.4 litre/day) and water lost through skin in the form of sweat (about 0.8 litre/day). Thus, the total output is also about 2.8 litres/day. In hot climates, sweat loss is much more which is compensated by increased intake of drinking water. If it is not compensated, urine output will decrease. However, urine output can not decrease below a certain level. Normally, about 600 milliosmol solutes have to be excreted by the kidneys everyday. Minimum water required to dissolve 600 milliosmol solutes is 500 ml. A decrease in urine output below 500 ml/day (oliguria) will decrease the excretion of metabolic waste.

Regulation of Water Balance

Water balance is regulated by antidiuretic hormone (ADH) of posterior pituitary and the thirst centre located in the hypothalamus. These two receive signals about the osmolality of plasma from **osmoreceptors** located in the hypothalamus. Osmoreceptors can perceive a change of even 1 to 2 percent in the osmolality of plasma. If there is an increase in the osmolality of plasma,

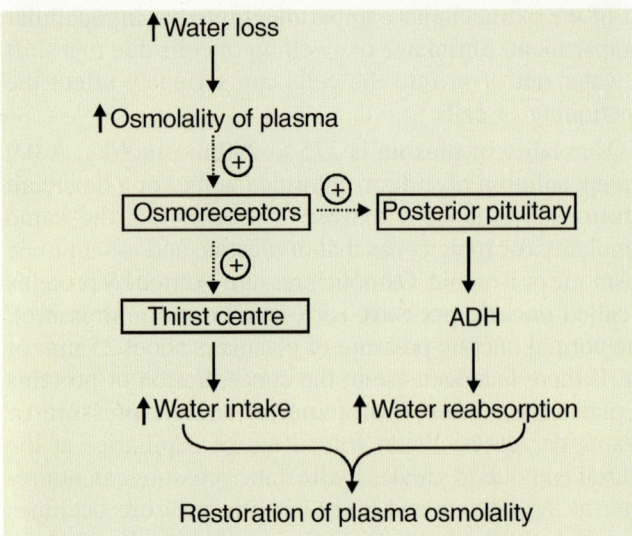

Fig. 24.1: Restoration of plasma osmolality following water loss

a. **Posterior pituitary** secretes ADH which decreases urine output, and

b. **Thirst centre** is stimulated which increases water intake.

The resulting increase in water content of plasma restores its osmolality (Fig. 24.1). ADH secretion begins when the osmolality of plasma reaches about 285 mosmol/kg. Thirst centre is stimulated when the osmolality of plasma reaches about 295 mosmol/kg.

When blood circulates through the kidneys, about 125 ml of glomerular filtrate is formed every minute or about 180 litres every day. When the filtrate passes through the tubules, a large amount of solutes is absorbed by the cells of proximal convoluted tubules and loop of Henle. A corresponding amount of water is also reabsorbed due to the osmotic effect of the solutes. This is known as **obligatory reabsorption** of water, and amounts to 85% of the glomerular filtrate or about 153 litres per day.

The cells of the distal convoluted tubules and collecting ducts, specially the latter, are not permeable to water in the absence of ADH. Binding of ADH to specific receptors (V_2 receptors) on the cell membrane of these cells activates adenylate cyclase. This increases the intracellular concentration of cAMP, which activates protein kinase A. Protein kinase A phosphorylates some cytosolic proteins which translocate water channels (aquaporins) from cytosol into the cell membrane. Water moves into the cell through the water channels (Fig. 24.2).

Thus, the reabsorption of water in distal convoluted tubules and collecting ducts is regulated by ADH, and is proportional to the concentration of ADH in plasma. The ADH-regulated reabsorption is known as **facultative reabsorption** of water. Normally, this is about 25.5 litres per day. The remaining 1.5 litres of water is excreted in the form of urine every day. The facultative reabsorption can be adjusted to maintain the water balance of the body.

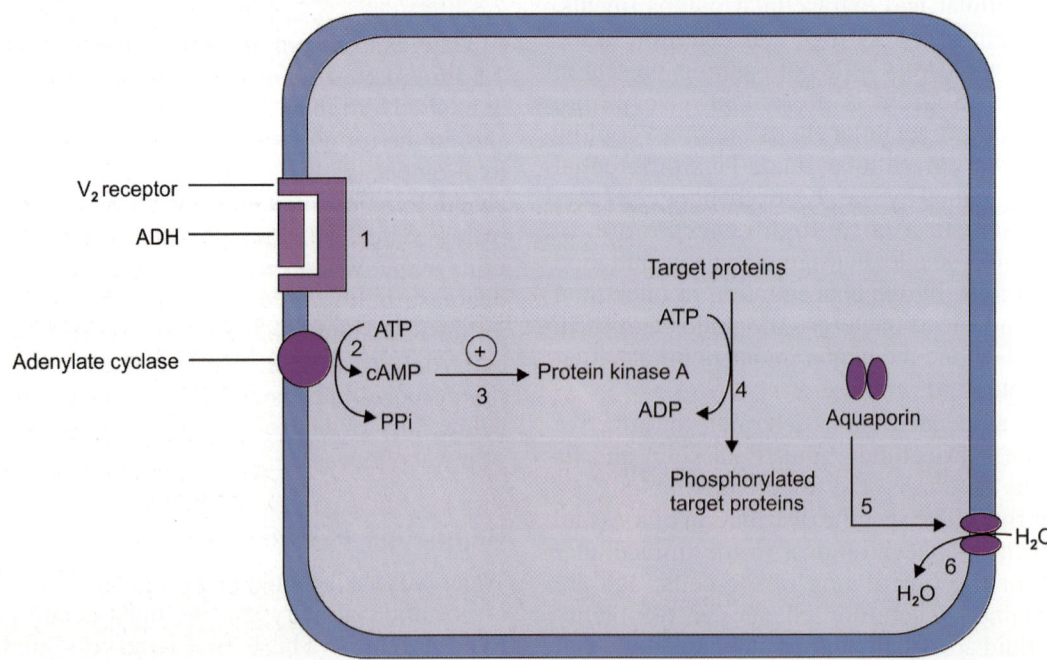

Fig. 24.2: Facultative reabsorption of water under the influence of antidiuretic hormone (ADH) in distal convoluted tubules and collecting ducts. 1. ADH binds to V_2 receptor. 2. Adenylate cyclase is activated, and forms cAMP. 3. Protein kinase A is activated. 4. Protein kinase A phosphorylates some target proteins. 5. Phosphorylated target proteins insert water channels (aquaporins) in the cell membrane. 6. Water moves into the cell through aquaporins.

Dehydration

Dehydration can result from diminished intake of water or from excessive loss of water. The latter is a far more common cause of dehydration. Excessive water loss can occur due to excessive sweating, vomiting, diarrhoea, haemorrhage, burns, etc. In uncontrolled diabetes mellitus resulting in glycosuria, urinary water output increases to dissolve the glucose being excreted in urine. Urinary water loss may also be increased in renal diseases in which the kidneys fail to reabsorb water, e.g. chronic glomerulonephritis. Severe water loss can occur in diabetes insipidus resulting from decreased secretion of ADH (central diabetes insipidus) or decreased responsiveness of target cells to ADH (nephrogenic diabetes insipidus). Dehydration can be corrected by administration of fluids either orally or intravenously. The composition of the fluid administered should be similar to that of the fluid lost.

Water Intoxication

Excessive retention of water in the body can occur in acute renal failure when the kidneys fail to excrete water. Sometimes, it can result from overadministration of intravenous fluids. Hypersecretion of ADH is a rare cause of water retention. Apart from the treatment of the primary cause, diureties may be used to increase the output of urine.

Diuretics

Most of the diuretics act by inhibiting the reabsorption of some solutes. Water is lost in urine to dissolve the extra solutes. The following are some commonly used diuretics:

1. *Acetazolamide:* This is a competitive inhibitor of carbonic anhydrase. It decreases the formation of carbonic acid in the proximal convoluted tubules. Normally, carbonic acid dissociates into H^+ and HCO_3. H^+ is secreted into tubular fluid in exchange for Na^+. By disrupting this exchange, acetazolamide increases the urinary excretion of Na^+. Extra water is excreted to dissolve Na^+. Excessive use of acetazolamide can cause acidosis due to decreased excretion of H^+.

2. *Spironolactone:* This is a structural analogue of **aldosterone.** It binds to aldosterone receptors, and prevents the action of aldosterone on the distal convoluted tubules. This decreases the reabsorption of sodium and chloride. Water excretion is increased due to the osmotic effect of sodium and chloride.

3. *Thiazides:* They inhibit sodium reabsorption in the distal convoluted tubules. They also increase K^+ loss.

4. *Furosemide:* Furosemide decreases the reabsorption of sodium and chloride in the loop of Henle. Therefore, it is known as a **loop diuretic**. It is a potassium-sparing diuretic as it does not cause potassium loss.

5. *Ethacrynic acid:* Action of ethacrynic acid is very similar to that of furosemide. This is also a potassium-sparing loop diuretic.

6. *Mannitol:* Mannitol is an osmotic diuretic. It is filtered by the glomeruli but is not reabsorbed by the tubules. Extra water is lost in urine to dissolve mannitol.

ECF CONTRACTION AND EXPANSION

Dehydration described above is never due to a pure water loss. The fluids lost from the body contain electrolytes also. The loss usually occurs from the extracellular compartment as the intracellular fluid is tightly protected. Therefore, dehydration results in a decrease in ECF volume (ECF contraction). ECF contraction can secondarily affect ICF volume. Depending upon the osmolality of the fluid lost, ECF contraction can be isotonic, hypotonic or hypertonic.

Retention of water causes an increase in the volume of ECF (ECF expansion). This again can be isotonic, hypotonic or hypertonic. The nature of the fluid lost in different types of ECF contraction and the fluid retained in different types of ECF expansion alongwith some representative causes thereof are summarised in Table 24.2.

Table 24.2: The nature of the fluid lost or retained in different types of ECF contraction and expansion, and some representative causes of these disturbances

		ECF contraction		ECF expansion
ISOTONIC	1.	Isotonic fluid is lost from the body.	1.	Isotonic fluid accumulates in Interstitial tissue.
	2.	It can occur in diarrhoea due to loss of isotonic secretions and in intestinal obstruction due to collection of secretions in the gut.	2.	It can occur due to oedema caused by hypertension, congestive heart failure, nephrotic syndrome, cirrhosis of liver, etc.
HYPOTONIC	1.	Hypertonic fluid is lost from the body.	1.	More water is retained than solutes.
	2.	It can occur in Addison's disease due to excessive loss of sodium and chloride in urine.	2.	It can occur in acute glomerulonephritis due to decreased glomerular filtration.
HYPERTONIC	1.	Hypotonic fluid is lost from the body.	1.	Retention of solutes is more than that of water.
	2.	It can occur in fevers and heat exposure due to excessive sweating or insensible perspiration.	2.	It can occur in primary aldosteronism and Cushing's disease due to excessive retention of sodium and chloride.

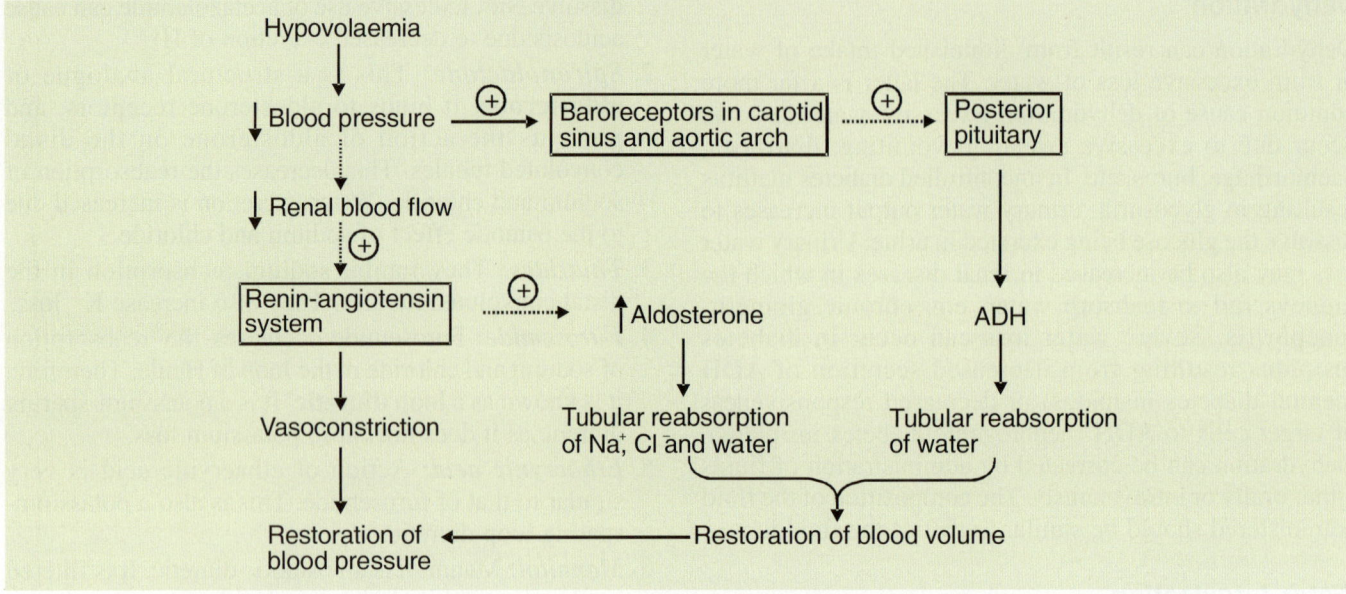

Fig. 24.3: Role of renin-angiotensin system, aldosterone and ADH in correction of hypovolaemia.

Isotonic contraction or expansion of ECF will not affect the ICF. But if the ECF becomes hypotonic or hypertonic, secondary changes will occur in the ICF.

Hypovolaemia

ECF contraction is clinically manifested commonly as a decrease in blood volume (hypovolaemia). Sudden and excessive loss of fluids from the body can cause life-threatening hypovolaemia. But hypovolaemia is not always due to loss of fluids. It can occur when the total body water is normal, or even increased, due to shifting (redistribution) of water from the vascular compartment into interstitial tissue.

A decrease in blood volume decreases the blood pressure. Restoration of blood volume and blood pressure requires the actions of renin-angiotensin system, aldosterone and ADH (Fig. 24.3).

The compensatory mechanisms may be unable to correct hypovolaemia if it is too severe and if the pathological condition causing hypovolaemia persists. Pathological conditions causing hypovolaemia may do so by:

A. Fluid Loss

This can be caused by renal or extra-renal sodium and water loss.

1. *Renal sodium and water loss*: This can occur in chronic renal diseases, diabetes mellitus, Addison's disease, diabetes insipidus, etc. It can also be caused by excessive use of diuretics.
2. *Extra-renal sodium and water loss*: This can occur in fevers, heat exposure, vomiting, diarrhoea, intestinal obstruction, burns, haemorrhage, etc.

B. Redistribution of Water

A shift of water from the vascular compartment into interstitial tissue (oedema) can cause hypovolaemia. Oedema can occur due to a decrease in oncotic pressure of plasma or due to an increase in capillary permeability. Common causes of oedema include congestive heart failure, nephrotic syndrome, cirrhosis of liver, etc.

Like ECF contraction, hypovolaemia can also be **isotonic** (e.g. in diarrhoea, intestinal obstruction, etc), **hypotonic** (e.g. in chronic renal disease, excessive use of thiazide diuretics, Addison's disease, congestive heart failure, nephrotic syndrome, cirrhosis of liver, etc.) or **hypertonic** (e.g. in fevers, heat exposure, severe burns, etc.).

Treatment of hypovolaemia should comprise treatment of the primary cause and correction of fluid balance. In hypovolaemia due to shifting of water from the vascular compartment, correction of the imbalance requires salt restriction and diuretics. In hypovolaemia due to sodium and water loss, correction of the imbalance requires oral or intravenous administration of fluids. In mild cases, oral rehydration is preferable. In severe cases, intravenous fluids are required. In isotonic (normonatraemic) hypovolaemia, isotonic (0.9%) saline should be given. In hypotonic (hyponatraemic) hypovolaemia, hypertonic (3%) saline is preferable. In hypertonic (hypernatraemic) hypovolaemia, hypotonic (0.45%) saline or 5% GDW (glucose in distilled water) is preferable. While giving intravenous fluids, a watch should be kept on serum potassium and care should be taken not to overhydrate the patient. Many of the pathological conditions causing hypovolaemia may cause disturbances in acid-base balance as well, which should be corrected together with the correction of fluid imbalance.

EXERCISE

1. Write short notes on:
   a. Facultative reabsorption
   b. Diuretics
   c. ECF contraction
   d. ECF expansion

2. Write 'true' or 'false':
   a. About 30% of total body water is present in the intracellular compartment
   b. Osmolality of body fluids is expressed in milliosmol per litre.
   c. Effective osmolality of a compartment is determined by the solutes restricted to that compartment.
   d. A 0.9% solution of sodium chloride is isotonic with plasma.
   e. Oncotic pressure is exerted by electrolytes.
   f. ADH binds to V_1 receptors on the cells of distal convoluated tubules.
   g. Acetazolamide is an aldosterone antagonist.
   h. Spironolactone inhibits carbonic anhydrase.
   i. Hypotonic contraction of ECF can occur in Addison's disease.
   j. Nephrogenic diabetes insipidus is due to decreased responsiveness of target cells to ADH.

3. Fill in the blanks:
   a. Sodium and its associated anions determine the effective osmolality of .... fluid.
   b. Osmolality of plasma is 275–290 ....
   c. Osmotic pressure exerted by .... is called oncotic pressure.
   d. The normal average oncotic pressure of plasma is about 25 ....
   e. .... is the second messenger for ADH in renal tubular cells.
   f. ADH regulates the .... reabsorption of water.
   g. ADH causes insertion of .... in the cell membrane of cells of distal convoluted tubules and collecting ducts.
   h. .... is an inhibitor of carbonic anhydrase.
   i. .... blocks aldosterone receptors in distal convoluted tubules.
   j. Furosemide and ethacrynic acid act on the ....

ANSWERS TO SHORT QUESTIONS

2. a. False
   b. False
   c. True
   d. True
   e. False
   f. False
   g. False
   h. False
   i. True
   j. True

3. a. Extracellular
   b. Milliosmol/kg
   c. Proteins
   d. mm of Hg
   e. cAMP
   f. Facultative
   g. Aquaporins
   h. Acetazolamide
   i. Spironolactone
   j. Loop of Henle

Acid-base Balance

For normal functioning of the body, pH of body fluids has to be maintained within a narrow range. Acids and bases are constantly formed during metabolic reactions, and can also enter from outside. In some pathological conditions, there may be abnormal losses of acids or bases from the body. To meet these challenges, elaborate mechanisms have evolved to maintain the acid-base balance of the body fluids.

ACIDS AND BASES

Acids and bases are defined according to whether they donate or accept hydrogen ions, i.e. protons. An acid is a proton (H^+) donor. A base is a proton (H^+) acceptor.

H_2CO_3	$\rightleftharpoons$	H^+	+	HCO_3^-
HNO_3	$\rightleftharpoons$	H^+	+	NO_3^-
H_3PO_4	$\rightleftharpoons$	H^+	+	$H_2PO_4^-$
$H_2PO_4^-$	$\rightleftharpoons$	H^+	+	HPO_4^{--}
Acid		Proton		Base

An alkali releases hydroxyl ions, e.g. NaOH and KOH.

STRENGTH OF ACIDS

Acids, for example hydrochloric acid and carbonic acid, dissociate into their component ions:

HCl	$\rightleftharpoons$	H^+	+	Cl^-
H_2CO_3	$\rightleftharpoons$	H^+	+	HCO_3^-

However, different acids do not dissociate to the same extent. In a solution containing hydrochloric acid, the acid is almost completely dissociated and, therefore, the hydrogen ion concentration is very high. In a solution containing carbonic acid, majority of carbonic acid molecules are undissociated and, therefore, the hydrogen ion concentration is low.

An acid which dissociates to a greater extent will be a stronger acid as compared to the one that dissociates to a lesser extent. Mineral acids are strong acids. Organic acids are generally weak acids.

pH Scale

Hydrogen ion concentrations present in biological fluids are extremely low. The pH scale was devised by Sorensen in 1909 to express the minute hydrogen ion concentrations conveniently. pH represents the negative log of the hydrogen ion concentration (mol/litre).

$$pH = -\log [H^+]$$

Water dissociates into hydrogen ions and hydroxyl ions, and its ion product (K_w) is:

$$K_w = [H^+][OH^-] = 10^{-14}$$

Since pure water yields equal number of hydrogen and hydroxyl ions, the concentration of hydrogen ions as well as hydroxyl ions in pure water is 10^{-7} mol/litre. Therefore, the pH of water is:

$$\text{pH of water} = -\log [H^+] = -\log 10^{-7} = -(-7) = 7$$

If the pH of a solution is less than 7, its hydrogen ion concentration would be more than that of water and the solution would be acidic. If the pH is more than 7, the hydrogen ion concentration would be less than that of water, and the solution would be basic. If the pH is exactly 7.0, the solution would be neutral. The normal pH of arterial blood is 7.35 to 7.45 (average 7.4) which means that the reaction of blood is slightly basic.

The reaction of a fluid can also be described in terms of its actual hydrogen ion concentration. Since the hydrogen ion concentrations in plasma and other body fluids are very low, these are expressed in nanomol/litre.

$$1 \text{ mol/litre} = 10^9 \text{ nanomol/litre}$$

At pH 7.4, the hydrogen ion concentration is 40 nanomol/litre. It is preferable to describe changes in the reaction of body fluids in nanomol/litre as the pH scale is not linear. For example, the hydrogen ion concentration at pH 7.5 is 31 nanomol/litre and at pH 7.6, it is 25 nanomol/litre. Therefore, an increase in pH from 7.4 to 7.5 represents a decrease of 9 nanomol/litre in hydrogen ion concentration whereas an increase in pH from 7.5 to 7.6 represents a decrease of only 6 nanomol/litre. However, due to prolonged usage, the pH scale has come to stay.

Regulation of pH Body Fluids

For normal physiological functioning, pH of blood and other body fluids has to be maintained within a narrow range. Departures from the normal range can cause serious consequences. Conformation of proteins is extremely sensitive to changes in pH. Changes in conformation of enzymes resulting from derangement of pH can impair the functioning of metabolic machinery. Therefore, mechanisms are required for maintaining the pH of body fluids within the normal range. There are three principal mechanisms for regulation of pH:

Chemical Buffers

These can instantly neutralise the acids and bases which are produced in the body or which enter from outside.

Respiratory Mechanism

This mechanism regulates the elimination of carbonic acid which is a major end product of metabolism in the form of carbon dioxide. Respiratory buffering occurs within minutes or hours.

Renal Mechanism

The kidneys help in the regulation of pH by eliminating excess acids or bases in urine. The renal regulation is very thorough but not very prompt. Renal buffering occurs over a period of hours or days.

CHEMICAL BUFFERS

A buffer is a chemical substance or system which, when present in a solution, prevents or resists a change in pH on addition of an acid or a base. A buffer is usually made up of a weak acid and its alkali salt. The pH of a buffer can be calculated from Henderson-Hasselbalch equation:

$$pH = pK_a + \log \frac{[Salt]}{[Acid]}$$

pK_a is the negative log of the dissociation constant (K_a) of the acid component of the buffer. Since pK_a is constant, the pH depends upon the ratio of the salt component and the acid component. The major buffers in body fluids are the following:

1. Bicarbonate-carbonic Acid Buffer

This is quantitatively the major buffer of extracellular fluids specially plasma. Carbonic acid is formed from carbon dioxide and water, and is in equilibrium with dissolved carbon dioxide. Carbonic acid dissociates to form the second component of the buffer, i.e. bicarbonate. Since sodium is the major cation of extracellular fluids, bicarbonate forms sodium bicarbonate. pK_a of carbonic acid (in equilibrium with dissolved CO_2) is 6.1. Average concentrations of bicarbonate and carbonic acid in plasma are 27 mEq/L and 1.35 mEq/L respectively. Therefore, the pH would be:

$$pH = pK_a + \log \frac{[HCO_3^-]}{[H_2CO_3]}$$
or $$pH = 6.1 + \log \frac{27}{1.35}$$
or $$pH = 6.1 + \log 20$$
or $$pH = 6.1 + 1.3 = 7.4$$

As long as the ratio of bicarbonate:carbonic acid is 20:1, the pH would be maintained at 7.4. A buffer is most effective near its pK_a. pK_a of carbonic acid is rather distant from 7.4 yet bicarbonate-carbonic acid is an important buffer in plasma because it is present in high concentration.

The salt component of the buffer can convert strong acids into weak acids:

$$HCl + NaHCO_3 \rightarrow H_2CO_3 + NaCl$$

Since H_2CO_3 is a much weaker acid than HCl, the change in pH would be minimal. The acid component of the buffer can convert strong bases into weak bases:

$$NaOH + H_2CO_3 \rightarrow NaHCO_3 + H_2O$$

Since $NaHCO_3$ is a much weaker base than NaOH, the change in pH would be minimal. Thus, the buffer resists a change in pH on addition of acids as well as bases.

Measuring pCO_2 is easier than measuring H_2CO_3. Concentration of H_2CO_3 can be calculated by multiplying pCO_2 by a constant. The constant depends upon the solvent and the temperature. For plasma at 37°C, the constant is 0.0301 or approximately 0.03. Therefore, in the equation for calculating pH, $[H_2CO_3]$ can be replaced by $pCO_2 \times 0.03$.

2. Phosphate Buffer

Concentration of inorganic phosphate in extracellular fluids is rather low yet it is an important buffer as its pK_a is closer to 7.4. Phosphate ions are present in two forms, dihydrogen phosphate ($H_2PO_4^-$) and monohydrogen phosphate (HPO_4^{--}). $H_2PO_4^-$ is a weak acid as it can donate a proton, and HPO_4^{--} is a base as it can accept a proton. In extracellular fluids, these exist as NaH_2PO_4 and Na_2HPO_4, and constitute a buffer. Na_2HPO_4 can neutralise acids and NaH_2PO_4 can neutralise bases:

$$HCl + Na_2HPO_4 \rightarrow NaCl + NaH_2PO_4$$
$$NaOH + NaH_2PO_4 \rightarrow H_2O + Na_2HPO_4$$

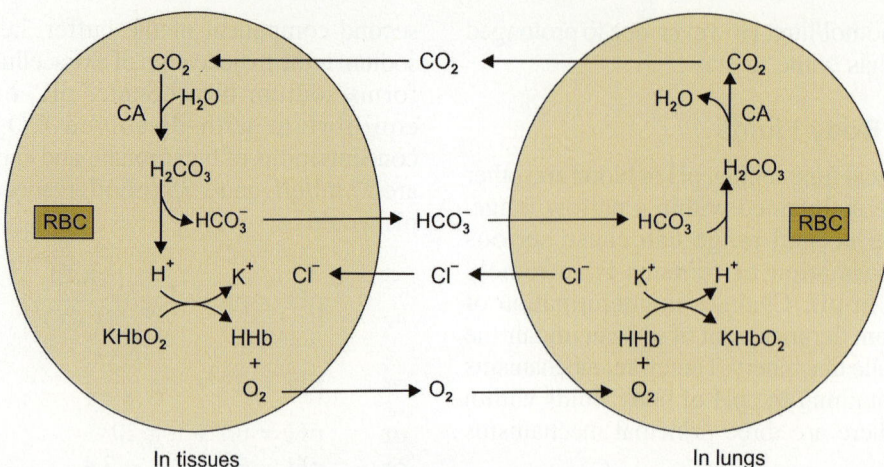

Fig. 25.1: In tissues, carbon dioxide enters RBCs, and is converted into carbonic acid by carbonic anhydrase (CA). Carbonic acid dissociates into hydrogen ions and bicarbonate ions. Hydrogen ion combine with haemoglobin (Hb), and bicarbonate ions are released into plasma in exchange for chloride ions. In lungs, these processes are reversed

In the first reaction, a strong acid is converted into a weak acid. In the second reaction, a strong base is converted into a weak base. Thus, the change in pH on addition of an acid or a base would be minimal.

The pH of a fluid containing phosphate buffer depends upon pK_a of HPO_4^{--} which is 6.8, and the ratio of HPO_4^{--} to HPO_4^{--} which is 4:1 in plasma. Therefore, the pH of plasma will be maintained at:

$$pH = pK_a + \log \frac{\left[HPO_4^{--} \right]}{\left[H_2PO_4^- \right]}$$

or $pH = 6.8 + \log 4$

or $pH = 6.8 + 0.6 = 7.4$

3. Proteins

Proteins act as buffers because of their amphoteric nature. In acidic medium, they act as bases and neutralise acids. In basic medium, they act as acids and neutralise bases. The amino acid residues having pK_a close to 7.4 are the most effective in buffering. Among different amino acids, pK_a of histidine is the closest to 7.4.

Proteins are present in high concentrations in intracellular fluid and in a significant concentration in plasma. But other extracellular fluids have a low protein content. Hence, the buffering action of proteins is exerted mainly in the intracellular fluid and plasma.

4. Haemoglobin

Haemoglobin is important not only for transporting oxygen and carbon dioxide but in this process, it also acts as a buffer. It buffers the large amount of carbonic acid which is formed from carbon dioxide produced in various metabolic reactions. In fact, haemoglobin is responsible for 60% of the buffering capacity of blood. The large

number of histidine residues in haemoglobin make it an effective buffer.

RESPIRATORY REGULATION

Haemoglobin transports a large amount of carbon dioxide to the lungs without any change in the pH of blood. The lungs regulate the elimination of carbon dioxide. Respiratory centre in the medulla is sensitive to pCO_2, pH and pO_2 of the blood. The chemoreceptors located in the aortic arch and carotid sinus transmit information about changes in pCO_2, pH and pO_2 to the respiratory centre which, accordingly, regulates the rate and depth of respiration.

Increased pCO_2 is the most important stimulant of the respiratory centre. A rise in pCO_2 stimulates the respiratory centre which increases the rate and depth of respiration. This increases the elimination of CO_2, and a decrease in pH resulting from accumulation of CO_2 (and carbonic acid) is prevented. Changes in pH also affect the respiratory centre. A fall in pH stimulates the respiratory centre leading to hyperventilation and increased elimination of CO_2. Changes in pO_2 affect the respiratory centre only to a limited extent. However, marked anoxaemia can stimulate respiratory centre (for example, at high altitudes) resulting in hyperventilation.

Thus, the respiratory mechanism tends to restore the ratio of bicarbonate:carbonic acid in blood by altering the concentration of carbonic acid (and dissolved CO_2) if bicarbonate concentration has changed due to any metabolic factor (e.g. decrease in bicarbonate in ketosis).

RENAL REGULATION

During the course of normal metabolism, the body produces a large amount of acids. The kidneys prevent a change in pH by excreting hydrogen ions in urine and returning

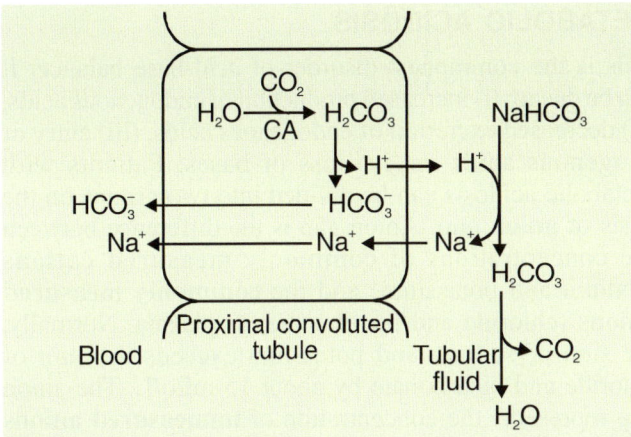

Fig. 25.2: Sodium and bicarbonate ions filtered in glomeruli are returned to blood by cells of proximal convoluted tubules

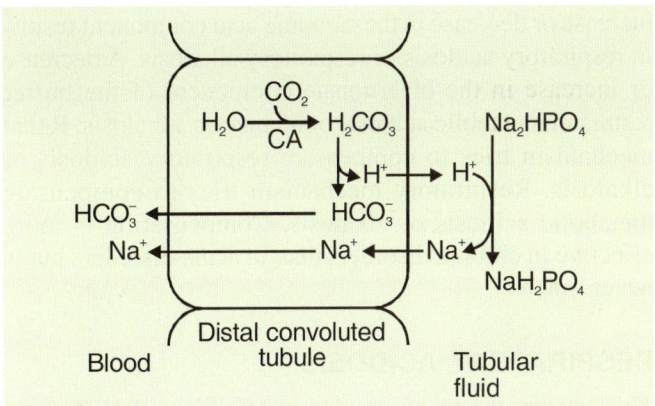

Fig. 25.3: Acidification of monohydrogen phosphate

bicarbonate to blood. Therefore, the pH of urine is usually acidic whereas the pH of blood and glomerular filtrate is slightly basic. The renal regulation operates in three major ways:

1. Reabsorption of Bicarbonate

On an average diet, about 40 mEq of acid is produced everyday as sulphate, phosphate and organic acids. If these acids are not excreted, the pH of blood will become acidic. More than 4,000 mEq of bicarbonate is filtered by glomeruli and enters the tubular lumen everyday. If this bicarbonate is lost in urine, it will be a major drain on alkali reserve and will deplete the main chemical buffer of plasma. However, tubular reabsorption (reclamation) of bicarbonate prevents this loss.

Bicarbonate is present in glomerular filtrate alongwith the cation sodium as sodium bicarbonate. Carbonic anhydrase (CA) present in the tubular cells convents water and carbon dioxide into carbonic acid which dissociates into hydrogen ion and bicarbonate ion. The tubular cell actively secretes the hydrogen ion into tubular lumen in exchange for sodium ion. The sodium ion entering the tubular cell from the lumen and the bicarbonate ion produced in the tubular cell diffuse into capillaries. The hydrogen ion secreted into the tubular lumen combines with bicarbonate to from carbonic acid which is converted into carbon dioxide and water by carbonic anhydrase bound to luminal surface of the tubular cells (Fig. 25.2).

2. Acidification of Monohydrogen Phosphate

After all the bicarbonate has been reabsorbed, hydrogen ion secretion proceeds against Na_2HPO_4 in the distal convoluted tubules. Na_2HPO_4 is converted into NaH_2PO_4 by the hydrogen ions secreted by the tubular cells, and sodium ions are reabsorbed in exchange for hydrogen ions.The sodium ions entering the tubular cells and bicarbonate ions produced from carbonic acid diffuse into

capillaries (Fig. 25.3). As a result of conversion of Na_2HPO_4 into NaH_2PO_4 in the lumen, the tubular fluid is acidified. The acidity due to NaH_2PO_4 is known as titratable acidity.

3. Secretion of Ammonia

Reabsorption of sodium ions also occurs against ammonium ions in distal convoluted tubules. Ammonia is formed by deamination of amino acids, particularly glutamine in the tubular cells. Ammonia combines with a hydrogen ion to form an ammonium ion. Ammonium ions are secreted into tubular fluid, and sodium ions are reabsorbed in exchange for ammonium ions (Fig. 25.4).

Renal regulation can respond to changes in the acid-base balance of blood. If production of acids increases, the kidneys cause greater acidification of urine and vice versa. Any deficiency in chemical and respiratory buffering is corrected by the kidneys. The renal response is slow but very thorough.

DISORDERS OF ACID-BASE BALANCE

When regulatory mechanisms fail to maintain the pH, acidosis or alkalosis results. Disorders occur when the bicarbonate: carbonic acid ratio deviates from 20:1. An

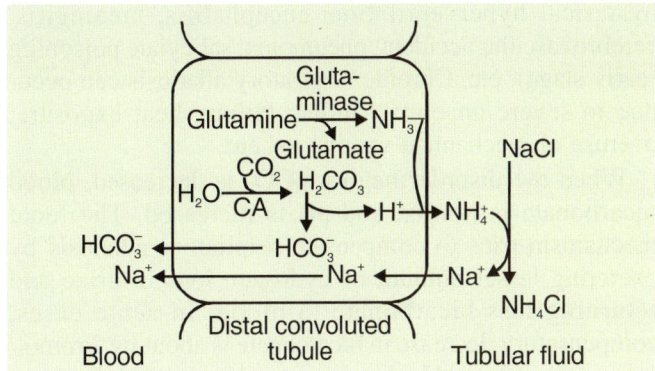

Fig. 25.4: Ammonium ion secretion against sodium ions in distal convoluted tubules

increase or decrease in the carbonic acid component results in respiratory acidosis or respiratory alkalosis. A decrease or increase in the bicarbonate component of the buffer results in metabolic acidosis or metabolic alkalosis. Renal mechanism tries to compensate respiratory acidosis or alkalosis. Respiratory mechanism tries to compensate metabolic acidosis or alkalosis. Compensation is more effective in chronic disorders than in acute disorders but is never 100%.

RESPIRATORY ACIDOSIS

This occurs due to accumulation of carbon dioxide (and carbonic acid) in the body due to hypoventilation resulting in decreased elimination of carbon dioxide or due to inspiring air having high carbon dioxide content.

Acute respiratory acidosis can occur due to collapse of lungs, pneumothorax, haemothorax, head injury depressing respiratory centre or due to overdose of opiates, general anaesthetics, alcohol or sedatives that depress the respiratory centre.

Chronic respiratory acidosis may occur in bronchial asthma, emphysema, bronchiectasis, chronic bronchitis, myopathies, myasthenia, intracranial tumours, etc.

When respiratory acidosis begins, pCO_2 is elevated, blood bicarbonate is normal and pH is decreased. The renal mechanism tries to compensate respiratory acidosis by excreting more hydrogen ions in urine and returning more bicarbonate to blood. In acute cases, bicarbonate increases by 1 mmol/L for every 10 mm Hg rise in pCO_2 as a compensatory measure. In chronic cases, bicarbonate increases by 4 mmol/L for every 10 mm Hg rise in pCO_2.

RESPIRATORY ALKALOSIS

This is the least common type of acid-base disorder. It results from a decrease in carbon dioxide (and carbonic acid) content of blood. The decrease is due to hyperventilation leading to excessive elimination of carbon dioxide from the lungs. Acute respiratory alkalosis can occur due to hysterical hyperventilation, encephalitis, meningitis, cerebrovascular accident, pneumonia, salicylate poisoning (early stage), etc. Chronic respiratory alkalosis can occur due to severe anaemia, cardiac failure, heat exposure, overuse of mechanical ventilators, etc.

When the disorder begins, pCO_2 is decreased, blood bicarbonate is normal and pH is increased. The renal mechanism tries to compensate respiratory alkalosis by excreting lesser amount of hydrogen ions in urine and returning less bicarbonate to blood. In acute cases, compensatory decrease in bicarconate is about by 2 mmol/L for every 10 mm Hg decrease in pCO_2. In chronic cases, bicarbonate decreases by 4 mmol/L for every 10 mm Hg decrease in pCO_2.

METABOLIC ACIDOSIS

This is the commonest disorder of acid-base balance. It can be due to: (i) increased production of endogenous acids, (ii) decreased excretion of endogenous acids, (iii) entry of exogenous acids or (iv) loss of bases. Patients with metabolic acidosis can be divided into two groups on the basis of **anion gap**. Anion gap is the difference between the concentrations of **commonly measured cations** (sodium and potassium) and the **commonly measured anions** (chloride and bicarbonate) in plasma. Normally, the sum of sodium and potassium exceeds the sum of chloride and bicarbonate by about 15 mEq/L. The anion gap represents the concentration of **unmeasured anions** in plasma, e.g. pyruvate, phosphate, sulphate, anionic proteins, etc.

$$\text{Anion gap} = [Na^+ + K^+] - [Cl^- + HCO_3^-]$$

1. Metabolic Acidosis with Normal Anion Gap

In these patients, plasma bicarbonate is low but the anion gap is normal due to a reciprocal increase in chloride. Hence, this condition is also known as **hyperchloraemic metabolic acidosis**. The causes are diarrhoea, gastrointestinal fistula, intestinal obstruction, renal tubular acidosis, administration of ammonium chloride, carbonic anhydrase inhibitors, etc. Respiratory compensation occurs by way of hyperventilation. pCO_2 decreases by 1.25 mm Hg for every 1 mmol/L decrease in bicarbonate.

2. Metabolic Acidosis with Increased Anion Gap

These patients have low blood bicarbonate and normal chloride. Anion gap is increased due to the presence of some abnormal and unmeasured anions. The causes include diabetic ketoacidosis, ketoacidosis of starvation, alcoholic ketoacidosis (sudden withdrawal), uraemia, lactic acidosis, salicylate intoxication (in later stages), intoxication with methanol, ethylene glycol, paraldehyde, formic acid, oxalic acid, boric acid, etc.

The respiratory mechanism compensates the acidosis by increasing the rate and depth of respiration so that pCO_2 decreases and the bicarbonate:carbonic acid ratio returns to the normal. pCO_2 decreases by 1.25 mm Hg for every 1 mmol/L decrease in bicarbonate.

METABOLIC ALKALOSIS

This can occur from loss of acids or excess of bases. The common causes are loss of HCl due to severe vomiting or prolonged gastric aspiration, excessive use of antacids, potassium loss, etc.

In the beginning, blood pH is high, bicarbonate is high, chloride is reciprocally low and pCO_2 is normal. The respiratory mechanism compensates metabolic alkalosis by decreasing the rate and depth of respiration so that more carbon dioxide is retained and the bicarbonate:carbonic acid ratio is brought to the normal.

pCO$_2$ increases by 0.75 mm of Hg for every 1mmol/L increase in bicarbonate.

MIXED ACID-BASE DISORDERS

Some patients may have two or more diseases simultaneously which may produce independent but concomitant disturbances in acid-base balance. For example, a diabetic with renal complications or an independent renal disease may develop metabolic acidosis due to ketosis as well as due to renal disease. The two together may result in severe acidosis, especially because renal compensation will not occur. Or a diabetic with simultaneous lung disease may develop metabolic acidosis as well as respiratory acidosis. The expected respiratory compensation will not occur in such a case. Alcoholic acidosis may be complicated by metabolic alkalosis if vomiting occurs. In gastroenteritis, vomiting may produce metabolic alkalosis and diarrhoea may produce metabolic acidosis.

A mixed acid-base disturbance may be present in salicylate intoxication when respiratory alkalosis has not abated and metabolic acidosis has set in. Very careful clinical examination and laboratory investigations are required in such patients.

EXERCISE

1. Describe the different mechanisms by which the pH of body fluids is maintained.

2. Write short notes on:
   a. Blood buffers
   b. Respiratory acidosis
   c. Anion gap
   d. Metabolic acidosis

3. Write 'true' or 'false':
   a. A bicarbonate: carbonic acid ratio of 20:1 would maintain the pH at 7.4.
   b. Respiratory acidosis occurs due to loss of bicarbonate.
   c. Anion gap is the difference in the plasma concentrations of (sodium + potassium) and (chloride + bicarbonate).
   d. Anion gap is normal in diabetic ketoacidosis.
   e. Metabolic alkalosis can occur in diarrhoea.

4. Fill in the blanks:
   a. Haemoglobin is responsible for ....% of the buffering capacity of blood.
   b. Retention of .... would cause respiratory acidosis.
   c. Anion gap represents the concentration of .... anions in plasma.
   d. Anion gap is .... in hyperchloraemic metabolic acidosis.
   e. Metabolic .... can occur in severe vomiting.

ANSWERS TO SHORT QUESTIONS

3. a. True
   c. True
   e. False
   b. False
   d. False

4. a. 60
   c. Unmeasured
   e. Alkalosis
   b. Carbon dioxide
   d. Normal

Nutrition and Diet

One of the major functions of food is to provide energy for various biological activities. The daily energy intake should be sufficient to meet the energy requirement of an individual. The conventional unit of energy is **calorie**. The thermal energy required to raise the temperature of 1 gm of water by 1°C is known as 1 calorie (cal or small calorie). In human physiology, energy is generally expressed in terms of **kilocalories** (Calorie, large calorie or kcal). One kcal is equal to 1,000 cal.

In the international system of units, the unit of energy has now been changed to **joule** (J). One joule is the energy required to move a mass of one kg by one metre distance by a force of one newton. One calorie equals 4.184 (or roughly 4.2) joules. Therefore,

1 kcal   =   4.2 kJ
1,000 kcal   =   4.2 MJ (megajoule)
240 kcal   =   1.0 MJ

However, kcal is still widely used as a unit of energy.

CALORIFIC VALUE OF FOODS

The three major classes of energy-yielding nutrients are carbohydrates, lipids and proteins. Energy value of carbohydrates, lipids and proteins can be measured by a **bomb calorimeter**. A weighed amount of the substance is burned in the burning chamber of bomb calorimeter by an electrically heated platinum wire in the presence of oxygen. The heat evolved is absorbed by a fixed quantity of water which surrounds the burning chamber. The rise in temperature of water is measured by a thermometer. The heat evolved by complete burning of one gm of the substance is calculated, and is known as its calorific value. The calorific values of different classes of compounds as determined by bomb calorimetry are:

Carbohydrates :   4.1 kcal/gm
Lipids   :   9.3 kcal/gm
Proteins   :   5.4 kcal/gm

However, when these compounds are oxidised in the body, their calorific values are not the same as measured by bomb calorimetry.

Carbohydrates and lipids liberate slightly less energy in the body as their digestion and absorption is not 100 percent. A major difference is seen in case of proteins. In a bomb calorimeter, the proteins are completely oxidised. But in the human body, the end product of protein catabolism is urea which still contains some energy. However, this energy is not available.

Therefore, the calorific value of proteins in the body is significantly less. The calorific values of carbohydrates, lipids and proteins in the body are:

Carbohydrates :   4 kcal/gm
Lipids   :   9 kcal/gm
Proteins   :   4 kcal/gm

Alcohol (ethanol) is another energy-rich compound, and its calorific value is 7 kcal/gm.

ENERGY EXPENDITURE OF A PERSON

The energy actually spent by a living person can be measured by **direct calorimetry** or **indirect calorimetry**. In direct calorimetry, the subject is kept in an insulated chamber surrounded by water. The rise in temperature of water is measured over a period of some hours. From this, the energy produced per hour or per minute can be calculated.

In indirect calorimetry, the energy production is measured from the volume of oxygen consumed and carbon dioxide eliminated by a person over a fixed period. The ratio of the volume of CO_2 expired and O_2 inspired is known as the **respiratory quotient (RQ)**. The RQ of carbohydrates, lipids and proteins is different.

RQ of Carbohydrates

RQ of carbohydrates is nearly one. For example, complete oxidation of one molecule of glucose requires six molecules of oxygen and produces six molecules of carbon dioxide.

$$C_6H_{12}O_6 + 6\,O_2 \longrightarrow 6\,CO_2 + 6\,H_2O$$

$$\therefore \quad RQ = \frac{6}{6} = 1$$

RQ of Lipids

Lipids contain less oxygen in their molecules than carbohydrates. Therefore, they require more oxygen for their oxidation. For example, complete oxidation of one molecule of stearic acid requires 26 molecules of oxygen, and produces 18 molecules of carbon dioxide.

$$C_{17}H_{35}COOH + 26 O_2 \longrightarrow 18 CO_2 + 18 H_2O$$

$$\therefore \quad RQ = \frac{18}{26} = 0.7$$

RQ of Proteins

Molecular formulae of proteins are quite variable because of differences in their amino acid compositions. Therefore, different proteins differ in their RQ. The average RQ of proteins is about 0.8.

On a mixed diet, the RQ is about 0.85. At an RQ of 0.85, every litre of oxygen consumed by an individual represents an energy production of 4.825 kcal. In this way, the total energy spent by an individual over a given period can be calculated from the volume of oxygen consumed by him and the volume of carbon dioxide eliminated.

ENERGY REQUIREMENT

Energy requirement of an individual is equal to his energy expenditure. Ideally, the energy requirement should be calculated from the energy expenditure of individuals. But this is not practicable. Recommendations have to be made for a whole community regarding energy requirement. Factors which have to be considered while calculating energy requirement are:
a. Basal metabolic rate (BMR),
b. Specific dynamic action (SDA) of food,
c. Physical activity, and
d. Provision for growth.

Basal Metabolic Rate

The total energy spent or heat produced by a subject in basal condition, i.e. complete physical and mental rest, is known as basal metabolic rate. BMR is expressed in kcal/hour/square metre of body surface area. This energy is spent for maintaining vital physiological activities e.g. circulation, respiration, peristalsis, maintenance of body temperature etc. These activities are going on even when one is at rest or asleep. And a certain amount of energy is required to sustain these functions which is known as the BMR. A provision has to be made for BMR while calculating the energy requirements.

Measurement of BMR

The measurement is made after a 12-hour period of rest and fasting. The subject should be recumbent but awake during the measurement. The environmental temperature should be comfortable and not above the body temperature.

BMR is usually measured by Benedict-Roth apparatus. The subject comfortably breathes into the mouthpiece of the apparatus. The oxygen consumed over a 6-minute period is measured and corrected to NTP (normal temperature and pressure). This is multiplied by 10 to get the hourly oxygen consumption. Assuming an RQ of 0.85, each litre of oxygen consumed is supposed to produce 4.825 kcal of energy. The energy produced per hour is divided by the body surface area of the subject to get the BMR.

Body surface area of the subject can be calculated by:
1. Du Bois formula, which is:

$$A = H^{0.725} \times W^{0.425} \times 71.84/10,000$$

where A is body surface area in square metres, H is height in cm and W is weight in kg.

2. Nomograms which directly relate the height and weight of a subject with his body surface area.

The BMR is high in childhood and gradually decreases until old age. The average BMR of adult men is 40 kcal/hour/square metre while the average BMR of adult women is 36 kcal/hour/square metre.

BMR can be affected by a number of physiological and pathological conditions. The BMR is higher in males, in young age, in colder climate and in non-vegetarians. BMR is increased in pregnancy, hyperthyroidism, fevers, severe anaemia, polycythaemia, etc. It is decreased in starvation, hypothyroidism, adrenal insufficiency, etc.

Specific Dynamic Action

Consumption of food increases the energy production in the body, even in the basal state. This is due to SDA or **thermogenic effect** of food. After consumption of food, some energy is spent by the body for digestion, absorption, transport, metabolism and interconversion of carbohydrates, lipids and proteins. The energy spent by the body to metabolise food is known as the SDA of the food. Proteins have the highest SDA. When 25 gm protein is ingested, about 30 kcal are spent in metabolising it. The energy value of 25 gm of protein is 100 kcal but 30 kcal have to be spent to gain this energy. So, the net gain of energy from 25 gm of protein will be 70 kcal only. Thus, the SDA of proteins is about 30 percent. SDA of lipids is about 13 percent and of carbohydrates about 5 percent.

When different foodstuffs are taken together, the SDA is less than the sums of SDA of individual foodstuffs. Carbohydrates and lipids lower the SDA. Lipids cause a greater lowering of SDA than carbohydrates. A mixed diet containing proteins, lipids and carbohydrates has an SDA of about 10 percent. This means that if a mixed diet having a calculated energy value of 3,000 kcal is taken in a day, the net energy gain would be 2,700 kcal only because 300 kcal would be spent on account of SDA to metabolise the foodstuffs. Therefore, an additional provision of 10 percent has to be made for SDA while calculating the energy requirement of a person.

Physical Activity

Physical activity involves muscular work. This increases the energy expenditure above the basal level. Therefore, an extra provision has to be made for physical activity. The increment depends upon the type of physical activity and its duration. In general, physical activity can be divided into three types depending upon one's occupation, **sedentary, moderate work** and **heavy work**.

Men, sitting at rest, spend about 100 kcal/hour. While standing, the energy expenditure rises to about 110 kcal/hour. Average energy expenditure of office workers is about 110 kcal/hour. During moderate work, e.g. tailoring, laundering, carpentry, wall painting, dish washing etc, the energy expenditure is about 150 kcal/hour. During heavy work, e.g. masonry, farming, blacksmithy, rickshaw-pulling, etc. the energy expenditure goes up to about 280 kcal/hour. During swimming, running, weight training, etc. the energy expenditure is still higher.

Women, sitting at rest, spend about 70 kcal/hour. During standing, the energy expenditure goes upto 80 kcal/hour. During sedentary work, e.g. household work or office work, the energy expenditure is about 90 kcal/hour. During moderate work, the energy expenditure of women is about 125 kcal/hour, and during heavy work, about 210 kcal/hour.

Provision for Growth

During infancy and childhood, an extra provision has to be made for growth because nutrients are also used for formation of tissues. An extra provision has also to be made in pregnancy to meet the requirements of the growing foetus. During lactation, an extra allowance is to be made which should be equivalent to the energy value of milk secreted by the nursing mother.

RECOMMENDED ENERGY INTAKE

The daily energy requirement of an individual can be calculated from his/her BMR, SDA, physical activity pattern, the hours spent in sleep, at rest and in occupational work, and growth requirements, if any. The requirements differ from country to country. Indian requirements have been recommended by Indian Council of Medical Research (ICMR). These requirements are for a reference man or woman of the community. Necessary adjustments are made for any deviation from the reference standard.

An Indian reference man is between 20 and 39 years of age and has a body weight of 60 kg. He sleeps for eight hours daily. He spends eight hours a day in light occupational work. He spends six hours a day sitting at rest, reading, writing, etc. and two hours a day doing household work, walking, recreational exercise, etc.

An Indian reference woman is between 20 and 39 years, and weighs 50 kg. She spends eights hours in bed and eight hours in household work or light occupational work. She spends six hours a day sitting at rest, reading, writing, etc and two hours a day in walking, light recreational exercise, etc.

We can now calculate the energy requirement of the reference man, a moderately active man and a very active man (Table 26.1).

Similarly, we can calculate the daily energy requirement of a reference woman, a moderately active woman and a very active woman (Table 26.2).

Based on such calculations, ICMR (1980) has recommended energy allowances (safe energy intake) for Indian males and females of different age groups (Table 26.3).

Table 26.1: Calculation of energy requirement of men

Activity	Hours	Sedentary Kcal/hr	Sedentary Kcal (total)	Moderately active Kcal/hr	Moderately active Kcal (total)	Very active Kcal/hr	Very active Kcal (total)
Sleep	8	65	520	65	520	65	520
Sitting	6	100	600	100	600	100	600
Standing	2	110	220	110	220	110	220
Occupational work	8	110	880	150	1200	280	2240
Total			2220		2540		3580
SDA (10%)			222		254		358
Grand total			2442		2794		3938
Rounded off			2400		2800		3900

Table 26.2: Calculation of energy requirement of women

Activity	Hours	Sedentary		Moderately active		Very active	
		Kcal/hr	Kcal (total)	Kcal/hr	Kcal (total)	Kcal/hr	Kcal (total)
Sleep	8	55	440	55	440	55	440
Sitting	6	70	420	70	420	70	420
Standing	2	80	160	80	160	80	160
Occupational work	8	90	720	125	1000	210	1680
Total			1740		2020		2700
SDA (10%)			174		202		270
Grand total			1914		2222		2970
Rounded off			1900		2200		3000

DIET

The energy requirements discussed earlier are provided by food. The foodstuffs consumed daily constitute diet. However, provision of energy is not the sole function of diet. The diet must meet all the metabolic requirements of an individual. The essential components of diet are:

1. Proteins,
2. Lipids,
3. Carbohydrates,
4. Vitamins,
5. Minerals, and
6. Water.

The first three constitute the **proximate principles** of diet, and will be discussed here. The roles of vitamins, minerals and water have been discussed earlier.

PROTEINS

Proteins are required mainly for formation of tissues. Even adults require proteins for replacement of worn out tissues. When proteins are taken in excess, they can be used as a source of energy also, either directly or after their conversion into carbohydrates and lipids. When energy is not available in the form of carbohydrates and lipids, tissues proteins may be broken down and used as a source of energy.

While considering the nutritional role of proteins, we have to take into account their quality as well as quantity.

Quality of Proteins

All the dietary proteins are not of equal nutritional quality. The nutritional quality of proteins is usually assessed on the basis of the following:

1. Essential Amino Acid Content

Eight amino acids are considered to be essential for human beings as these are not synthesised in the human body.

These are valine, leucine, isoleucine, threonine, methionine, lysine, phenylalanine and tryptophan. Two amino acids, arginine and histidine, are considered to be semi-essential because their endogenous synthesis is not sufficient to meet the requirements of infants and children. The other amino acids can be synthesised in the body in adequate quantities. Cysteine can meet the requirement of methionine to some extent but not completely. Similarly, tyrosine can partially meet the requirement of phenylalanine.

Table 26.3: Recommended energy allowance, kcal/day (ICMR, 1980)

Infants (up to 6 months)	120/kg of body weight
Infants (7–12 months)	100/kg of body weight
Children (1–3 years)	1200
Children (4–6 years)	1500
Children (7–9 years)	1800
Children (10–12 years)	2100
Boys (13–15 years)	2500
Girls (13–15 years)	2300
Boys (16–19 years)	3000
Girls (16–19 years)	2200
Men (sedentary work)	2400
Women (sedentary work)	1900
Men (moderate work)	2800
Women (moderate work)	2200
Men (heavy work)	3900
Women (heavy work)	3000
Pregnancy	+ 300
Lactation (first 6 months)	+ 500
Lactation (second 6 months)	+ 400

A good protein should contain all the essential amino acids. Deficiency of even a single amino acid can impair the synthesis of proteins. Animal proteins contain all the essential amino acids. Vegetable proteins are usually deficient in one or more essential amino acids. The essential amino acid which is deficient in a protein is known as its **limiting amino acid**. Lysine and threonine are the limiting amino acids in cereals. Methionine is the limiting amino acid in pulses. Groundnut is poor in lysine, threonine and methionine. Maize is poor in lysine, methionine and tryptophan. Soya bean is somewhat deficient in methionine. Thus, animal proteins are superior to vegetable proteins in terms of essential amino acid content.

2. Digestibility Coefficient (DC)

This is the percentage of ingested protein which is absorbed into the blood stream after digestion in the gastrointestinal tract.

3. Biological Value (BV)

This is the percentage of ingested protein (or nitrogen) retained in the body after digestion and absorption.

4. Net Protein Utilisation (NPU)

This is a measure of utilisation of dietary proteins for protein synthesis in the body. It depends upon digestibility coefficient and biological value.

$$NPU = \frac{DC \times BV}{100}$$

5. Protein Efficiency Ratio (PER)

This is the gain in body weight (gm) per gm of protein ingested.

Protein content, DC, BV, NPU and PER of some common sources of proteins are given in Table 26.4.

Thus, the major animal sources of proteins (egg, milk, meat and fish) are superior to vegetable sources (cereals, pulses, nuts and beans) in terms of digestibility, absorption and utilisation in the body. Therefore, animal proteins are considered to be first class proteins or **proteins of high biological value** while vegetable proteins are described as second class proteins or proteins of **low biological value**. It is recommended that at least half of the protein requirement should be met from animal proteins.

However, animal foods are beyond the reach of large sections of population in developing countries. For example, per capita consumption of animal proteins in India is 6 gm/day while it is 60 to 65 gm/day in developed countries.

Since it is not always possible to increase the consumption of animal proteins, measures should be taken

Table 26.4: Protein content, digestibility coefficient (DC), biological value (BV), net protein utilisation (NPU) and protein efficiency ratio (PER) of some protein-rich foods

	Protein content (%)	DC	BV	NPU	PER
Egg (hen's)	13.3	98	98	96	3.8
Milk (cow's)	3.5	95	85	81	2.0
Meat	20	96	82	79	2.8
Fish	22	96	80	77	1.7
Wheat	12	85	60	51	1.3
Rice	7	93	70	65	1.7
Maize	11	85	50	43	1.0
Bengal gram	23	84	62	52	1.1
Black gram	24	82	55	45	1.0
Green gram	24	85	58	49	0.8
Red gram	22	83	56	46	0.8
Groundnut	27	92	54	50	1.7
Soya bean	40	86	64	55	0.9

to improve the quality of vegetable proteins. The drawback of vegetable proteins is the absence or deficiency of one or more essential amino acids. This can be made good by two methods:

1. Mutual Supplementation

An essential amino acid deficient in one vegetable food may be present in another vegetable food. If these two foods are taken together, all the essential amino acids can be obtained. This is known as mutual supplementation. The following combinations can significantly improve nutritional quality of vegetable proteins.

   i. Wheat + groundnuts
   ii. Wheat + pulses
  iii. Rice + pulses
   iv. Rice + groundnuts
   v. Wheat + soya bean
   vi. Bengal gram + sesame
 vii. Cereals + legumes + leafy vegetables

2. Fortification with Amino Acids

The limiting amino acid can be added to a food. This is known as fortificatio. For example, wheat flour can be fortified with its limiting amino acid, lysine. The limiting amino acids in most of the vegetable proteins are lysine, methionine, threonine and tryptophan. Lysine and methionine are being manufactured on commercial scale at economic prices, and can be used for fortification of vegetable foods. It has been shown that fortification of vegetable foods with their limiting amino acids leads to a significant improvement in their protein efficiency ratio (Table 26.5).

Table 26.5: Protein efficiency ratio (PER) of some common vegetable foods before and after fortification with limiting amino acids

Food	PER
Wheat	1.3
Wheat + lysine	2.4
Rice	1.7
Rice + lysine + threonine	2.0
Maize	1.0
Maize + lysine + methionine + tryptophan	2.2
Soya bean	0.9
Soya bean + methionine	3.2
Groundnut	1.7
Groundnut + lysine + threonine + methionine + tryptophan	2.9

Table 26.6: Recommended protein intake (ICMR, 1981)

	Daily protein intake	
	gm/kg of body weight	total (gm)
Up to 3 months	2.3	
4–9 months	1.8	
10–12 months	1.5	
1–3 years	1.8	22
4–6 years	1.6	29
7–9 years	1.35	36
10–12 years (boys)	1.24	43
13–15 years (boys)	1.10	52
16–18 years (boys)	0.94	53
Adult men (60 kg)	1.0	60
10–12 years (girls)	1.17	43
13–15 years (girls)	0.95	43
16–18 years (girls)	0.88	44
Adult women (50 kg) *	1.0	50

* An extra intake of 14 gm/day is recommended in the last six months of pregnancy, and 25 gm/day during the first six months of lactation.

Protein Requirement

Protein requirement is more in growing age than in adults. Protein requirement is also increased in pregnancy and lactation. ICMR has recommended the protein requirements of Indian subjects on the basis of body weight (Table 26.6).

LIPIDS

Lipids are commonly known as fats and oils. Fats are solid at room temperature while oils are liquid at room temperature. Fats and oils are really triglycerides. These are the major lipids present in food. Smaller amounts of other lipids, e.g. phospholipids, glycolipids, cholesterol, etc. may also be present in foods. Except for polyunsaturated fatty acids (PUFA), all the lipids can be synthesised in the body. For this reason, PUFA are also known as **essential fatty acids (EFA)**. Thus, one major role of dietary lipids is to provide essential fatty acids. Some other functions are as follows.

1. They act as carriers of fat-soluble vitamins.
2. They are a concentrated source of energy, and spare proteins from being used as a source of energy.
3. They make the food palatable.

Therefore, a certain amount of lipids must be present in the diet. The quantity and chemical nature of dietary lipids should be such that our requirement of essential fatty acids can be met but atherosclerosis is not promoted. Excessive intake of triglycerides, cholesterol and saturated fatty acids promotes atherosclerosis by raising the concentration of cholesterol in serum. PUFA have an opposite effect.

Therefore, the lipid content and composition of diet should be determined keeping the following points in mind.

1. The total lipid intake should be just enough to meet the requirements.

2. Cholesterol intake should be cut down to the minimum, preferably below 300 mg/day.
3. PUFA should replace saturated fatty acids to the extent possible.

ICMR (1981) has recommended that lipid intake should be such that it provides 20 percent of the total energy requirement. The essential fatty acids should provide at least 3 percent of the total energy in adults, and 5 to 6 percent in infants, children, and pregnant and lactating women.

Lipids may be present in food as **visible fat** or **invisible fat**. Vegetable oils, hydrogenated vegetable oils, butter, ghee, etc. which are pure lipids, are known as visible fat. The lipids present in milk, meat, fish, cereals, pulses, vegetables, etc constitute invisible fat. According to ICMR (1981), half of the total lipid intake should be in the form of invisible fat. The content of invisible fat in some common dietary sources of lipids is shown in Table 26.7. Among these, animal foods are richer in saturated fatty acids while vegetable foods are richer in PUFA. The percentage of saturated, monounsaturated and polyunsaturated fatty acids in oils and fats (visible fat) in shown in Table 26.8.

The PUFA essential for human beings are linoleic acid, α-linolenic acid and arachidonic acid. Most of the PUFA present in oils and fats is linoleic acid. Among vegetable oils, the only good source of α-linolenic acid is soya bean oil. α-Linolenic acid is also present in green leafy

Table 26.7: Lipid content (%) of some common foods

Food	Lipid	Food	Lipid
Egg (hen's)	11	Wheat	1.0
Fish	10	Rice	0.5
Meat	13.3	Maize	3.5
Milk (cow's)	3.8	Pulses	5
Milk (buffalo's)	7.5	Groundnut	40
Cheese	31	Soya bean	20

Table 26.9: Cholesterol content (mg/100 gm) of some common foods

Food	Cholesterol	Food	Cholesterol
Egg	550	Milk, whole	11
Liver	300	Milk, skimmed	5
Meat	65	Butter	250
Fish	70	Cheese	100

vegetables. The requirement for α-linolenic acid is very small. Arachidonic acid requirement is even smaller which is easily obtained from invisible fat.

Hydrogenated vegetable oils have become a popular cooking medium in poor strata because of their better keeping quality. During hydrogenation, unsaturated fatty acids are converted into saturated fatty acids. Thus, the EFA content is decreased. The *cis* double bonds may also be converted into *trans* double bonds. Therefore, natural vegetable oils should be preferred over hydrogenated oils.

Some of the disadvantages of vegetable oils can be removed by the use of refined oils. Vegetable oils are refined by treating them with steam, alkalis, etc. In this process, free fatty acids and substances responsible for bad odour, taste and rancidity, are removed. However, refined oils are more expensive than natural oils.

The cholesterol content of food is also important. Cholesterol is present only in animal foods. Cholesterol content of some common foods is given in Table 26.9.

CARBOHYDRATES

No carbohydrate is really essential for human beings as all the carbohydrates can be synthesised in the human body. However, carbohydrates form a major component of diet because they are a relatively **cheap source of energy**. Carbohydrates are present in food generally in three forms.

Starch

Starch is the most abundant carbohydrate in food. It is present in cereals, pulses, roots, tubers, etc.

Sugars

These include monosaccharides, e.g. glucose, fructose and galactose, and disaccharides, e.g. sucrose, maltose and lactose. Lactose is present in milk only. Other sugars are present in fruits, vegetables, honey, etc. Sucrose or cane sugar is commonly used as a sweetening agent. Jaggery is also used as a sweetening agent. Besides sucrose, it provides iron also.

Roughage

Cellulose is present in most vegetable foods in varying proportions. It can not be digested by human beings, and constitutes roughage or **fibre** in the diet. Some other polysaccharides, e.g. hemicellulose, pectin, lignin, inulin, etc also contribute to roughage. Presence of roughage in diet is also essential as it stimulates peristalsis and prevents constipation. A high fibre intake has been reported to decrease the incidence of colorectal cancer, hypertension, diabetes mellitus, etc.

No quantitative requirement can be laid down for carbohydrates. After calculating the total energy requirement of an individual and deducting the contribution of proteins and lipids, the remainder of energy requirement should be met from carbohydrates. The carbohydrate content of some common foods is given in Table 26.10.

Carbohydrates also have a **protein sparing effect**. An adequate intake of carbohydrates spares the proteins for tissue formation rather than being used as a source of energy.

BALANCED DIET

The daily food intake (diet) should be such that the daily requirements of all the essential nutrients are met. There should be neither a deficiency nor an excess of any nutrient in the diet. These objectives can be achieved from a balanced diet.

A balanced diet is defined as a diet which contains a variety of foods in such quantities and proportions that the requirements for energy, proteins, lipids, carbohydrates,

Table 26.8: Fatty acid content (%)of common oils and fats

Oil or fat	Saturated fatty acids	Monoun-saturated fatty acids	Polyun-saturated fatty acids
Coconut oil	92	6	2
Palm oil	46	44	10
Groundnut oil	20	50	30
Cottonseed oil	25	25	50
Soya bean oil	15	25	60
Corn oil	8	27	65
Sunflower oil	8	27	65
Safflower oil	10	15	75
Butter	60	37	3

Table 26.10: Carbohydrate content (%) of some common foods

Food	Carbohydrate	Food	Carbohydrate
Wheat	72	Sweet potato	34
Rice	78	Carrot	9
Maize	66	Radish	4
Sorghum (Jowar)	73	Peas	18
Pearl millet (Bajra)	67	Apple	11
Bengal gram	60	Banana	23
Black gram	60	Grape	15
Green gram	60	Guava	11
Red gram	56	Mango	18
Groundnut	22	Orange	11
Soya bean	21	Milk, cow's	4.8
Onion	10	Milk, buffalo's	4.8
Potato	20	Cane sugar	100

vitamins, essential minerals and other nutrients are adequately met, and a small provision is also made for extra nutrients to tide over short durations of lean intake.

The major **food groups** in a usual diet are cereals, pulses, vegetables and fruits, milk, fats and oils, and sugar. In addition to these, a non-vegetarian diet contains egg, meat and fish. Each of these food groups has a specific **nutritional profile**. Some of these are rich in carbohydrates, some are rich in lipids, some are rich in proteins and some are rich in vitamins and minerals. The daily diet should contain each of these food groups in such a combination that our daily requirements of energy and all the essential nutrients are met. Before planning a diet, we should know the nutritional profile of each of these food groups.

Cereals

Cereals are the largest component of an average diet. The major cereals are rice, wheat and maize. Millets, which are smaller grains, are also included in this group. The important millets are sorghum and pearl millet. The cereals are a major source of **energy**. Their energy content is about 350 kcal/100 gm. The major nutrient in cereals is carbohydrate which is present in the form of **starch**. It makes up 70 to 80 percent of the weight of cereals.

The protein content of rice is about 7 percent while other cereals contain 10 to 12 percent protein. The proteins present in cereals are deficient in lysine. Some are deficient in threonine also. Maize is, in addition, deficient in tryptophan. The fat content of cereals is low. It is less than 2 percent in rice, wheat and sorghum, and less than 5 percent in maize and pearl millet.

The cereals contain significant amounts of minerals but absorption of calcium, phosphorus and iron, present in cereals, is not very efficient. Several members of **B-complex** group of vitamins are present in cereals, mainly in the outer layer of the grain. The removal of outer layer leads to a significant loss of vitamins, and some loss of proteins as well.

Pulses

Energy content of pulses is about 350 kcal/100 gm. Carbohydrate content is 60 to 65 percent, fat content less than 5 percent and protein content 22 to 24 percent. Pulses are a major source of **proteins** for vegetarians. The proteins present in pulses are deficient in methionine, but pulses and cereals supplement the limiting amino acids of each other. Minerals and some members of **B-complex** group of vitamins, e.g. thiamin, riboflavin, niacin, etc. are also present in pulses. **Germinating pulses** contain vitamin C also, and contain higher concentrations of B-complex vitamins.

Vegetables and Fruits

Vegetables and fruits are known as protective foods as they are rich in **vitamins** and **minerals**. They also provide **roughage**. Some vegetables and fruits contain significant amounts of carbohydrates also. The vegetables are generally divided into three groups:

1. Roots and Tubers

This group includes potato, sweet potato, colocasia, onion, carrot, radish, etc. Potato and sweet potato are fair sources of carbohydrates. Carrot is rich in carotenes. Potato contains some vitamin C also.

2. Green Leafy Vegetables

These include spinach, coriander leaves, fenugreek (methi) leaves, mint, cabbage, etc. They are good sources of carotenes, vitamins of B-complex group, vitamin C, calcium, iron and other trace elements. They also add roughage to the diet.

3. Other Vegetables

Vegetables other than green leafy vegetables, and roots and tubers are included in this group, e.g. cauliflower, brinjal, tomato, lady's finger, cucumber, pumpkin, bitter gourd, etc. These are rich in vitamins and minerals. They also add roughage to diet.

Fruits should also be considered alongwith vegetables as they are excellent sources of vitamins and minerals. An added advantage of fruits is that they are generally eaten raw and, therefore, the heat-labile vitamins present in them are not destroyed. Some fruits and/or raw vegetables (salads), e.g. tomato, cucumber, carrot, radish, etc. must be included in the daily diet.

Milk

Milk can form a nearly balanced diet by itself. It contains all the essential nutrients **except** iron and vitamin C. **Proteins** of milk contain all the essential amino acids. Lactose, the carbohydrate present in milk, is particularly useful for infants and children as it provides **galactose** for the formation of nervous tissue. Infants should be fed **mother's milk** as long as possible as it provides **antibodies** against many infectious diseases. Milk fat is rich in saturated fatty acids.

Fats and Oils

These are pure lipids. A certain amount of fats and oils has to be used during cooking to improve the taste of food but excess should be avoided. Vegetable oils should be preferred as they provide essential fatty acids.

Sugar

Cane sugar is used as sweetening agent. It is pure sucrose, and provides nothing except energy. Jaggery provides some iron also.

Egg

Egg is an excellent food as it contains all the essential nutrients **except** carbohydrates and vitamin C. Egg **proteins** are considered to be the best out of all the dietary proteins. Raw egg contains **avidin** which forms a complex with **biotin** and prevents its intestinal absorption. Avidin is heat-labile, and is inactivated during cooking. Cooking also coagulates albumin and globulin, and makes them easily digestible. Egg **yolk** is rich in **cholesterol** and saturated fatty acids, and should avoided by those who are at a high risk of developing coronary artery disease.

Meat

Meat is another good source of high-quality **proteins**. The protein content of meat is about 20 percent. It is also a good source of easily available **iron**. Iron of meat is much better absorbed than iron present in vegetable foods. Many other **minerals** and **vitamins** are present in meat. Liver is rich in many nutrients. Fat content of meat is variable, and contains mostly saturated fatty acids. Organ meats are rich in nucleic acids and purines, and should be avoided by those prone to gout.

Fish

Fish is also a good source of **proteins** of high biological value. Protein content of fish is about 22 percent. Fish is also a good source of **vitamins A** and **D**. Fat present in fish contains α-linolenic acid and some other **omega-3 unsaturated fatty acids**. Sea fish are good sources of iodine.

The inclusion of these food groups in appropriate proportions in the daily diet can provide all the essential nutrients. Within a group, one food can be replaced by another. For instance, rice can be replaced by wheat and vice versa. One pulse can be replaced by another. Attention should also be paid to the cost of a food item. A costly food item is not necessarily superior. Balanced diets for males and females of different age groups and different occupations are given in Tables 26.11 to 26.14.

Adjustment in Pregnancy

Additional allowances of 35 gm of cereals, 15 gm of pulses, 100 ml of milk and 10 gm of sugar and jaggery are required in pregnancy.

Adjustments during Lactation

Additional allowances of 60 gm of cereals, 30 gm of pulses, 100 ml of milk, 10 gm of oil and fat, and 10 gm of sugar and jaggery are to be made during lactation.

Adjustments for Non-vegetarians

Egg, meat and fish can replace some of the requirement for pulses. Half of the requirement for pulses can be

Table 26.11: Balanced diet for adult men (vegetarian)		
	Sedentary work	Moderate work	Heavy work
Cereals (gm/day)	460	520	670
Pulses (gm/day)	40	50	60
Roots and tubers (gm/day)	50	60	80
Leafy vegetables (gm/day)	40	40	40
Other vegetables (gm/day)	60	70	80
Milk (ml/day)	150	200	250
Oil and fat (gm/day)	40	45	65
Sugar and jaggery (gm/day)	30	35	55

Table 26.12: Balanced diet for adult women (vegetarian)

	Sedentary work	Moderate work	Heavy work
Cereals (gm/day)	410	440	575
Pulses (gm/day)	40	45	50
Roots and tubers (gm/day)	50	50	60
Leafy vegetables (gm/day)	100	100	100
Other vegetables (gm/day)	40	40	50
Milk (ml/day)	100	150	200
Oil and fat (gm/day)	20	25	40
Sugar and jaggery (gm/day)	20	20	40

Table 26.13: Balanced diet for children (vegetarian)

	Children (1–3 years)	Children (4–6 years)	Children (7–9 years)
Cereals (gm/day)	175	270	325
Pulses (gm/day)	35	35	40
Roots and tubers (gm/day)	20	30	30
Leafy vegetables (gm/day)	35	35	40
Other vegetables (gm/day)	40	50	50
Milk (ml/day)	300	250	250
Oil and fat (gm/day)	15	25	35
Sugar and jaggery (gm/day)	30	40	40

Table 26.14: Balanced diet for adolescents (vegetarian)

	Boys (10–12 years)	Girls (10–12 years)
Cereals (gm/day)	420	380
Pulses (gm/day)	45	45
Roots and tubers (gm/day)	30	30
Leafy vegetables (gm/day)	50	50
Other vegetables (gm/day)	50	50
Milk (ml/day)	250	250
Oil and fat (gm/day)	40	35
Sugar and jaggery (gm/day)	45	45

replaced by one egg (or 30 gm of meat or fish) and 5 gm of oil and fat. The entire requirement for pulses can be replaced by two eggs (or 50 gm of meat or fish) and 10 gm of oil and fat.

NUTRITIONAL DISORDERS

Diseases resulting from inadequate or excessive intake of nutrients are known as nutritional disorders. Disorders resulting from deficient or excessive intake of vitamins and minerals have been discussed earlier. Disorders arising from inadequate or excessive intake of proximate principles are described below:

Kwashiorkor

Kwashiorkor occurs when the diet is severely deficient in **proteins** but adequate in calories. This usually occurs when infants are weaned from breast milk and top feeding is started. If the diet is poor in proteins, it fails to meet the protein requirements of the growing child.

Growth is retarded in kwashiorkor. There is muscle wasting. Skin is hyperpigmented in some areas and hypopigmented in others. Hair is brittle and discoloured. Lack of apolipoprotein synthesis leads to fatty liver. Anaemia develops due to a decrease in globin synthesis. There is a marked decrease in serum albumin concentration which leads to generalised oedema. Oedema masks muscle wasting, and gives a **rounded appearance**. Diarrhoea is common and leads to losses of nutrients including vitamins. Concentrations of amino acids and urea in serum are decreased.

Kwashiorkor can be prevented by correct feeding practices in the post-weaning period. A small amount of animal foods (milk, skimmed milk, egg, meat, fish, etc.) or a mixture of cereals and pulses should be included in the post-weaning diet. Once kwashiorkor has occurred, it can be treated by increasing the protein intake to a level that proteins supply 20 percent of the total energy. The protein intake may be raised by addition of skimmed milk powder to the diet. Or a mixture containing three parts of groundnut flour and one part of Bengal gram flour or three parts of wheat flour and one part of cottonseed flour may be added to the diet.

Marasmus

Marasmus results from a **generalised decrease** in food intake. There is deficiency of calories as well as proteins in the diet. The available proteins are used as a source of energy rather than for tissue formation. Growth is retarded. There is muscle wasting. Subcutaneous fat disappears. The child gives a **shrunken appearance**. Diarrhoea is frequently present and aggravates the problem by increasing the loss of nutrients in stools. Multiple vitamin deficiencies and infections are commonly present.

Marasmus can be treated by increasing the energy and protein intake, by supplementing vitamins and minerals, by correcting dehydration and by controlling the infections.

Recently, a term **'Protein-Energy Malnutrition (PEM)'** has been coined which includes both kwashiorkor and marasmus. It has been proposed that deficiencies of proteins and energy always co-exist. When proteins are relatively more deficient, a kwashiorkor-like syndrome develops. When energy intake is relatively more deficient a marasmus-like picture develops. In between these two extremes, a picture having features of kwashiorkor as well as marasmus (marasmic kwashiorkor) develops.

Starvation

Starvation can occur due to scarcity of food in famine-affected areas. It can also occur in ship-wrecked sailors and in travellers stranded in desert. Sometimes, it may be due to a psychiatric condition, anorexia nervosa. Or it may result from voluntary fasting.

When food intake stops, the body begins to use stored carbohydrates, lipids and proteins. The energy reserves of an average well-fed adult are, 125 gm (or 500 kcal) of glycogen, 9,000 gm (or 81,000 kcal) of triglycerides and 5,000 gm (or 20,000 kcal) of proteins (mainly muscle proteins). Even if the starving person is lying in bed, his basal energy expenditure would be about 1,600 kcal/day. Thus, the carbohydrate reserves are not sufficient for even one day. The lipid reserves can last 50 to 60 days. The protein reserves can last 10 to 15 days.

After glycogen depletion, lipids become the major energy source but some proteins are also utilised for gluconeogenesis to provide glucose to brain, and to form citric acid cycle intermediates to metabolise the fatty acids. Major metabolic readjustments would occur to prevent unnecessary wastage of proteins. Unnecessary enzymes are not synthesised. These include the digestive enzymes, glucokinase, enzymes of urea cycle, enzymes required for fatty acid synthesis, etc. Synthesis of gluconeogenic enzymes is increased.

When fatty acid oxidation increases and availability of glucose is poor, the rate of formation of **ketone bodies** is increased. Ketone bodies begin to appear in urine 3 to 4 days after complete starvation. The brain tissue may adapt itself to use ketone bodies as a source of energy. But when gluconeogenesis fails to keep pace with the requirements due to decreasing protein reserves, severe ketosis develops, and disturbs the **acid-base balance** and **electrolyte** balance. Death usually occurs from acidosis and electrolyte imbalance.

The treatment consists of resumption of feeding. Since the synthesis of digestive enzymes is decreased and intestinal mucosa may be atrophied, re-feeding should begin with glucose-water, fruit juices and skimmed milk.

Later on, bread, biscuits, potatoes and eggs may be added to the diet. Normal diet may be given after a few days.

Severely starved persons may require intravenous fluids and correction of acid-base and electrolyte imbalance.

Obesity

Obesity may be defined as accumulation of **excess fat** in the body. In some subjects, it may be due to hereditary factors or hormonal disorders. But in majority of subjects, it is due to excessive calorie intake. When energy intake exceeds the energy expenditure, the extra calories are converted into fat, and are deposited in fat depots.

Obesity predisposes the individual to many diseases, e.g. dyspnoea on exertion, hypertension, diabetes mellitus, coronary artery disease, cerebral thrombosis, gall bladder stones, arthritis of weight-bearing joints, etc. Surgical operations and labour are more risky in obese subjects.

Before starting the treatment of obesity, we should ascertain whether one is obese and, if yes, what is the degree of obesity. One way to assess obesity is by measuring **skin-fold thickness** with calipers. Skin-fold thickness is increased in obesity. Another method is based on **standard height and weight** charts. Height and weight charts of Life Insurance Corporation of India are considered as standard for Indian subjects. If the weight of a subject exceeds the ideal body weight by 10 percent or more, he is considered to be obese. A simpler alternative is the calculation of **body mass index (BMI)**.

$$BMI = \frac{Weight\ in\ kg}{(Height\ in\ metres)^2}$$

The normal BMI is 20 to 25 in males and 19 to 24 in females. A BMI above the upper limit of normal signifies obesity.

The basic principle of treatment is to decrease energy intake and to increase energy expenditure. Energy expenditure is increased by increasing physical activity. Walking at moderate speed increases the energy expenditure to 300 kcal/hour. The energy expenditure during brisk walking, running, swimming and heavy exercise is 500 to 600 kcal/hour.

The energy intake should be reduced to 1,000 kcal/day until the ideal body weight or BMI is achieved. Protein intake should be maintained at 1 gm/kg of body weight. Fats should provide about 10 percent energy, and should be in the form of vegetable oils rich in essential fatty acids. The remaining calories should be provided by carbohydrates. Intake of sugar and jaggery should be restricted to 15 gm/day or less. Potatoes and sweet potatoes should be excluded from the diet. Other vegetables, raw, boiled or steamed, may be taken as desired. 200 to 250 gm of fruits and 400 ml of skimmed milk should be included in the daily diet. Vitamin supplements may be given in the form of one multivitamin tablet daily.

DIET PRESCRIPTION

Special dietary advice is required in some non-nutritional disorders also, e.g. diabetes mellitus, coronary artery disease, liver diseases, kidney diseases, etc. While giving dietary advice to a patient, the following points should be kept in mind:

1. One need not be mathematically precise in prescribing a diet. There is considerable variation in the composition of a given food item. Efficiency of digestion, absorption and metabolism also vary from person to person. Therefore, absolute accuracy is impossible to achieve.

2. Quantities of food items should be prescribed in terms of usual serving measures, e.g. teaspoon, tablespoon, cup, glass, etc. and not in terms of gm or ml as a patient is unlikely to weigh or measure food items.

3. The cost of food items and purchasing power of the patient should always be kept in mind. It is always possible to substitute a costly fruit with a cheaper one or a costly vegetable with a cheaper one without compromising the nutritional value.

4. One should also enquire whether a patient is allergic to some food.

Diabetes Mellitus

Diet control is one of the cornerstones in the treatment of diabetes mellitus. Many mild to moderate diabetics can be controlled by diet alone. One of the important considerations while recommending diet is the weight of the diabetic patient. The weight should be brought to, and maintained, as near the ideal body weight as possible. An underweight diabetic should gain weight and an over-weight diabetic should lose weight until the ideal body weight is attained.

Total energy intake is more important than the proportions of proteins, carbohydrates and fats. Intake of saturated fatty acids and cholesterol should be restricted as diabetics are relatively more prone to atherosclerosis. Intake of mono- and di-saccharides should also be restricted as these lead to sharper elevations of blood glucose than polysaccharides. In drug-dependent diabetics, timing and carbohydrate content of meals are important. Missing or delaying a meal or taking insufficient carbohydrate after taking an antidiabetic drug can cause hypoglycaemia which may sometimes be fatal.

Diet for an Underweight Diabetic

The total energy intake should be 2,400 kcal/day which should come from 90 gm of proteins, 350 gm of carbohydrates and 70 gm of fats. Visible fat intake should be about three tablespoons a day, preferably in the form of vegetable oils. Sugar and jaggery should not exceed four teaspoons a day. The daily milk intake should be five cups of skimmed milk or three cups of whole milk.

Diet for Normal Weight Diabetic

The total energy intake should be 1,700 kcal/day which should come from 250 gm of carbohydrates, 65 gm of proteins and 50 gm of fat. The intake of visible fat is reduced to two tablespoons a day and that of sugar and jaggery to three teaspoons a day. The milk ration is four cups of skimmed milk a day.

Diet for An Overweight Diabetic

The total energy intake is 1,400 kcal/day which come from 225 gm of carbohydrates, 65 gm of proteins and 30 gm of fat. The daily ration of visible fat is one tablespoon. Sugar and jaggery is excluded. The milk ration is three cups of skimmed milk a day. To produce a feeling of fullness, intake of vegetables, salads and low-carbohydrate fruits may be increased.

Liver Diseases

Liver is a major site for metabolism of carbohydrates, lipids and proteins. Therefore, the diet has to be modified in a number of liver disorders. Major hepatic disorders which require diet readjustments are cirrhosis of liver, hepatic or obstructive jaundice and hepatic precoma or coma.

Cirrhosis of Liver

A high-calorie, high-protein diet is required for regeneration of liver but the patient is unable to take large meals because of poor appetite and sub-normal hepatic function. A diet providing 2,000 kcal/day can usually be tolerated by the patient. These should come from 110 gm of proteins, 290 gm of carbohydrates and 45 gm of fat. Vitamin supplements are usually required. If the patient has oedema, salt should not be added to food.

Jaundice

In moderate to severe hepatic or obstructive jaundice (serum bilirubin exceeding 15 mg/dl), protein intake is restricted to decrease the production of ammonia, and fat intake is restricted as the patient is unable to digest, absorb and metabolise it. The total energy intake should be about 1,700 kcal/day which should come from 40 gm of proteins, 25 gm of fat and 325 gm of carbohydrates. The total ration of visible fat is one tablespoon a day. Total ration of milk is two cups of skimmed milk/day. Egg, meat, chicken, fish, pulses and nuts are totally excluded.

Hepatic Pre-coma and Coma

Severe viral hepatitis and cirrhosis can lead to hepatic pre-coma which may culminate into coma. The patient is unable to eat. Hence, the feeding has to be parenteral or through a nasogastric tube.

Nasogastric tube feeding is preferable as it is easier and cheaper. Protein and fat are completely withheld. The following solution may be given by nasogastric tube every six hours.

Glucose or cane sugar	:	75 gm
Vegetable soup	:	100 ml
Fruit juice	:	100 ml
Sodium chloride	:	½ teaspoon
Potassium chloride	:	½ teaspoon
Liquid multivitamin syrup	:	1 teaspoon
Water, to make	:	500 ml

Kidney Diseases

Dietary modifications are required in renal failure and nephrotic syndrome. In renal failure, protein intake is restricted as the kidneys are unable to excrete urea. In nephrotic syndrome, extra proteins are required as there is excessive loss of proteins in urine.

Renal Failure

The total energy intake should be 1,700 kcal/day which should come from 30 gm of proteins, 60 gm of fat and 260 gm of carbohydrates. The intake of visible fat should be two tablespoons a day, and milk, three cups a day. Egg, meat, fish, pulses, nuts and beans are totally excluded. If there is oedema or hypertension, no salt should be added during cooking.

Nephrotic Syndrome

A diet providing 2,100 kcal/day is recommended. These calories should be provided by 110 gm of proteins, 70 gm of fat and 260 gm of carbohydrates. Intake of visible fat should be two tablespoons a day. No salt should be added to the food.

Coronary Artery Disease

A patient with coronary artery disease is likely to be obese and with elevated serum cholesterol. Therefore, the weight should be reduced until ideal body weight is reached by giving the diet advised for obesity. To reduce serum cholesterol, butter, cream, egg yolk and organ meats should be excluded from the diet. Fish is preferable over meat and chicken. When body weight becomes normal, carbohydrate intake should be gradually raised to a level that doesn't increase body weight.

Hypertension

A hypertensive patient is also generally obese, and is prone to coronary artery disease. Therefore, the dietary guidelines for coronary artery disease apply to hypertension also. In addition, salt restriction is also required in hypertension.

Peptic Ulcer

Peptic ulcers can occur in stomach or duodenum. Hypersecretion of gastric hydrochloric acid was believed to be a major factor in causation and aggravation of peptic ulcers. For decades, peptic ulcer patients were advised to take a bland diet consisting mainly of milk and cream with the assumption that it would not stimulate gastric acid secretion and would help in the healing of ulcers.

Later evidence showed that most of the peptic ulcers are caused by *H. pylori* infection which can be treated by antibiotics. The only dietary advice given nowadays is avoidance of coffee and alcohol, and any food that aggravates the symptoms.

EXERCISE

1. Describe the metabolic readjustments in starvation.

2. Write short notes on:
   a. Basal metabolic rate
   b. Specific dynamic action
   c. Dietary fibre
   d. Balanced diet
   e. Kwashiorkor
   f. Marasmus

3. Write 'true' or 'false':
   a. Calorific value of protein in living persons is less than that in a bomb calorimeter.
   b. Calorific value of alcohol is more than that of fats.
   c. Specific dynamic action of carbohydrates is more than that of proteins.
   d. Limiting amino acid is pulses is methionine.
   e. Kwashiorkor occurs due to deficient intake of calories.

4. Fill in the blanks:
   a. Calorific value of .... is about 9 kcal/gm.
   b. One kcal is roughly equal to .... kilojoules.

c. BMR is .... in hyperthyroidism.

d. .... occurs from a severe dietary deficiency of proteins.

e. Cholesterol is present only in .... foods.

ANSWERS TO SHORT QUESTIONS

3. a. True
   c. False
   e. False

   b. False
   d. True

4. a. Fats
   c. Increased
   e. Animal

   b. 4.2
   d. Kwashiorkor

Metabolism of Xenobiotics

Xenobiotics are foreign compounds (strangers) entering our body. They may be divided into: (a) Pharmacological xenobiotics and (b) Environmental xenobiotics. Pharmacological xenobiotics include the drugs that we take intentionally. Environmental xenobiotics include food additives, food adulterants and various pollutants present in food, water and air. Environmental xenobiotics may enter our body with or without our knowledge. Human beings may be exposed to more than 100,000 foreign chemicals. The long list of manufactured chemicals is increasing every year. Foreign compounds, which are antigenic, are dealt with by our immune system. Non-antigenic foreign chemicals are metabolised to convert less soluble chemicals into more soluble ones, and to convert toxic chemicals into non-toxic or less toxic compounds. The relatively soluble metabolites are excreted, mainly in urine or bile.

Liver is the major site for metabolism of xenobiotics though metabolism can occur in some other tissues as well. The metabolic reactions can be divided into two phases:

Phase 1 Reactions

These are non-synthetic reactions, and include hydroxylation, oxidation, reduction, hydrolysis, etc. Some xenobiotics are excreted directly after phase 1 reactions. Others undergo phase 2 reactions before excretion.

Phase 2 Reactions

These are synthetic reactions, and include conjugation and methylation. The conjugated or methylated metabolites are highly soluble, and can be easily excreted.

PHASE 1 REACTIONS

A. Hydroxylation

Hydroxylation is the major reaction in phase 1, and is catalysed by the microsomal hydroxylase system. Microsomal hydroxylase system is associated with microsomal (endoplasmic reticulum) membrane, and consists of cytochrome P-450 (abbreviated as CYP), NADPH-CYP reductase (mono-oxygenase), FAD, FMN

and, sometimes, cytochrome b_5. The substrate and an oxygen molecule are attached to CYP. One of the oxygen atoms of the oxygen molecule is introduced into the substrate, and the other oxygen atom combines with two hydrogen atoms to form water. The hydrogen atoms are provided by NADPH, and pass via FAD and FMN before reacting with oxygen (Fig. 27.1).

The overall reaction catalysed by the microsomal hydroxylase system may be summed up as:

$$XH + O_2 + NADPH + H^+ \longrightarrow X\text{-}OH + H_2O + NADP^+$$

A variety of substrates can undergo hydroxylation reactions such as:

i. Codeine is converted into morphine by hydroxylation:

$$R - O - CH_3 \longrightarrow R - OH + HCHO$$

ii. Phenytoin and amphetamine are partly metabolized by hydroxylation of their benzene ring:

iii. Amphetamine is partly metabolized by hydroxylation of its amino group:

$$R - NH_2 \longrightarrow R - NH - OH$$

iv. Some unsaturated aliphatic compounds are first converted into epoxides and are, then, hydroxylated:

Cytochrome P-450 is not a single protein. More than 200 isoforms of CYP, encoded by different genes, have been identified. Important **families** of CYP in human

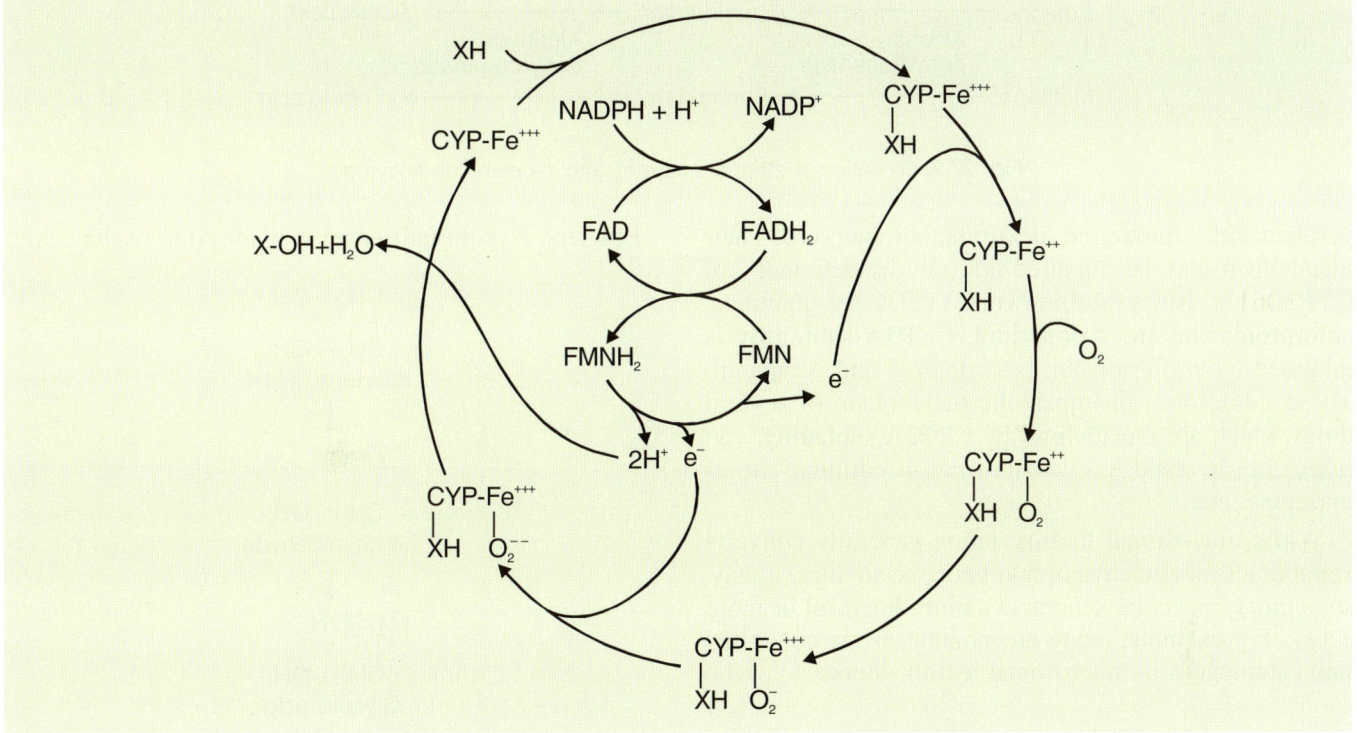

Fig. 27.1: Microsomal hydroxylation of a xenobiotic (XH)

beings include CYP1, CYP2, CYP3, CYP4, CYP11, CYP17 CYP19 and CYP21. Members of a particular family show at least 40 percent homology in amino acid sequence. Many families have **subfamilies**. For example, CYP2 has five subfamilies (CYP2A, CYP2B, CYP2C, CYP2D and CYP2E). Members of a particular subfamily have at least 55 percent homology in amino acid sequence. Subfamilies comprise individual members, e.g. CYP1A1 and CYP1A2 are members of CYP1A subfamily.

CYP1, CYP2 and CYP3 are the major families of CYP involved in the metabolism of drugs. Other families of CYP hydroxylate endogenous substrates. The largest number of drugs are metabolised by CYP3A subfamily followed by CYP2D6 and CYP2C subfamily. Different isoforms of CYP have different substrate specificities but there are exceptions. Some drugs may be metabolised by more than one isoform of CYP. Conversely, one isoform of CYP may metabolise more than one drug. Some isoforms may be induced by one drug but may metabolise some other drugs also. Some isoforms or even subfamilies may be inhibited by some drugs which can alter the metabolism of other drugs. Some isoforms may be genetically deficient in some persons or races. These differences require alertness on the part of the physician while prescribing a drug or a combination of drugs.

Many CYPs are **inducible**. CYP2C9 is induced by phenobarbital, CYP2E1 by ethanol and CYP3A4 by rifampicin. Since a single CYP may metabolise more than one substrates, CYP induction can result in altered

metabolism of some drugs. For example, CYP2C9 metabolises phenobarbital as well as warfarin. In a patient taking both these drugs, the CYP induction by phenobarbital results in rapid metabolism of warfarin leading to decreased anti-coagulant effect of warfarin. Therefore, the dose of warfarin has to be increased. Subsequently, if phenobarbital is withdrawn, the CYP2C9 concentration decreases, necessitating a decrease in the dose of warfarin. Similarly, CYP3A4 metabolises rifampicin as well as oral contraceptives. If a woman taking oral contraceptives is put on rifampicin, an anti-tubercular drug, there will be induction of CYP3A4 by rifampicin leading to rapid metabolism of the oral contraceptive which may result in failure of contraception. Sildenafil is also metabolised by CYP3A4.

Mutations in CYP genes can lead to **deficiency** of certain isoforms of CYP resulting in poor metabolism of some drugs. For example, nearly 20% of Asian people are genetically deficient in CYP2C19 which metabolises mephenytoin, diazepam and omeprazole. Genetic deficiency of CYP2D6 can lead to poor metabolism of several drugs. Debrisoquin and codeine are metabolised exclusively by CYP2D6. Debrisoquin is used as a test substrate to detect CYP2D6 deficiency. Codeine is converted into its active metabolite, morphine by hydroxylation. Therefore, codeine is less effective in persons deficient in CYP2D6.

Several other drugs are metabolised, but not exclusively, by CYP2D6. These include timolol, nortryptiline,

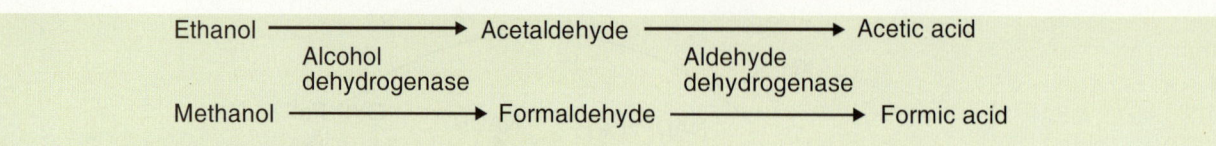

Fig. 27.2: Oxidation of ethanol and methanol by common enzymes

perphenazine, fluoxetine, dextromethorphan, etc. Their metabolism may be impaired not only by deficiency of CYP2D6 but also by **inhibitors** of CYP2D6, e.g. quinidine, chlorpromazine and haloperidol. CYP3A subfamily is inhibited by erythromycin, ketoconazole and verapamil. These inhibitors can impair the metabolism of several drugs which are metabolised by CYP3A subfamily, e.g. lidocaine, lovastatin, cyclosporine, nifedipine, carbamazepine, etc.

While microsomal hydroxylation generally converts xenobiotics into inactive or non-toxic metabolites, it may, sometimes, make the xenobiotics **more harmful** or more active. For example, many procarcinogens are converted into carcinogens by microsomal hydroxylation.

B. Oxidation

Ethanol and methanol are first oxidised to acetaldehyde and formaldehyde respectively by alcohol dehydrogenase. Acetaldehyde and formaldehyde are oxidised to acetic acid and formic acid respectively by aldehyde dehydrogenase (Fig. 27.2).

By oxidation, methanol is converted into more toxic metabolites, formaldehyde and formic acid, which cause atrophy of optic nerves. Ethanol is used to treat methanol poisoning as the common enzymes which metabolise these two have a far greater affinity for ethanol than for methanol.

Benzaldehyde is oxidised to benzoic acid:

CHO → COOH
Benzaldehyde   Benzoic acid

Chloral (trichloroacetaldehyde) is oxidised to trichloroacetic acid:

$$Cl-\underset{\underset{Cl}{|}}{\overset{\overset{Cl}{|}}{C}}-CHO \longrightarrow Cl-\underset{\underset{Cl}{|}}{\overset{\overset{Cl}{|}}{C}}-COOH$$

Chloral   Trichloroacetic acid

Ethylene glycol (antifreeze) is oxidised to oxalic acid:

$$\underset{CH_2-OH}{\overset{CH_2-OH}{|}}$$
Ethylene glycol

↓

$$\underset{CH_2-OH}{\overset{CHO}{|}}$$
Glycol aldehyde

↓

$$\underset{CH_2-OH}{\overset{COOH}{|}}$$
Glycolic acid

↓

$$\underset{CHO}{\overset{COOH}{|}}$$
Glycoxylic acid

↓

$$\underset{COOH}{\overset{COOH}{|}}$$
Oxalic acid

C. Reduction

Nitrobenzene is reduced to aminobenzene:

NO₂ → NH₂
Nitrobenzene   Aminobenzene

Chloral is partly reduced to trichloroethanol:

$$Cl-\underset{\underset{Cl}{|}}{\overset{\overset{Cl}{|}}{C}}-CHO \longrightarrow Cl-\underset{\underset{Cl}{|}}{\overset{\overset{Cl}{|}}{C}}-CH_2-OH$$

Chloral   Trichloroethanol

p-Nitrophenol is reduced to p-aminobenzene:

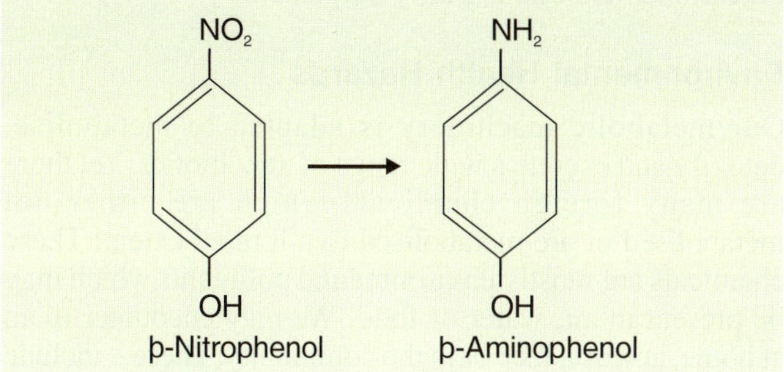

þ-Nitrophenol → þ-Aminophenol

Chloramphenicol and metyrapone are partly metabolised by reduction. Picric acid is metabolised by reduction to picramic acid.

D. Hydrolysis

Aspirin (acetylsalicylic acid), clofibrate, indomethacin, procainamide and procaine are hydrolysed.

Procaine is hydrolysed into p-aminobenzoic acid and diethylethanolamine:

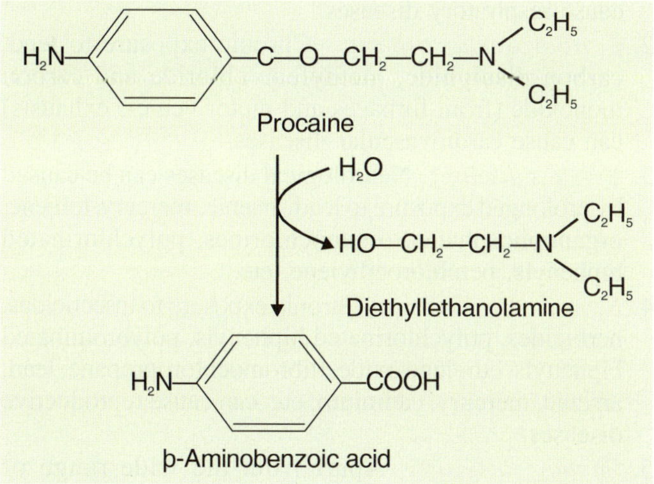

Procaine

Diethyllethanolamine

þ-Aminobenzoic acid

Acetaminophen (paracetamol) is metabolised partly by hydrolysis:

Acetaminophen

þ-Aminophenol

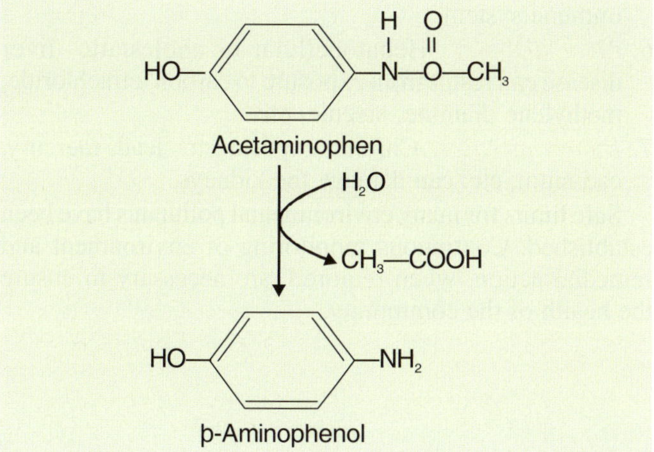

Aspirin is hydrolysed into acetic acid and salicylic acid:

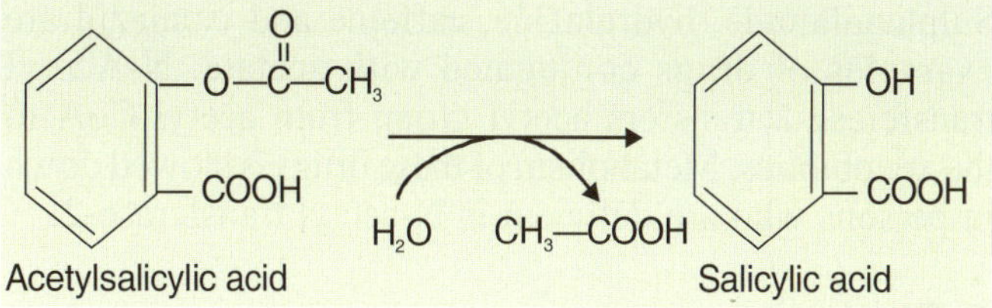

Acetylsalicylic acid → Salicylic acid

Cardiac glycosides (e.g. digoxin) are inactivated by hydrolysis of their glycosidic bond, releasing the carbohydrate moiety and the aglycone. Clofibrate and indomethacin are metabolised partly by hydrolysis.

Drugs like azathioprine (immunosuppressant) and 6-mercaptopurine (anticancer) are oxidised to 6-thiouric acid. Azathioprine is first converted into 6-mercaptopurine which is then oxidised to 6-thiouric acid by xanthine oxidase. Inhibitors of xanthine oxidase, e.g. allopurinol, can decrease the metabolism of azathioprine and 6-mercaptopurine.

PHASE 2 REACTIONS

The major reaction in phase 2 is **conjugation**. The conjugated products are highly soluble, and are easily excreted. Conjugation may occur with:

1. Glucuronic Acid

Glucuronyl moiety of UDP-glucuronic acid is conjugated with the xenobiotic by UDP-glucuronyl transferase, the same enzyme which conjugates bilirubin with glucuronic acid. Acetylaminofluorene, acetaminophen, diazepam, meprobamate, morphine, phenytoin, chloramphenicol, aniline, salicylic acid and benzoic acid are examples of xenobiotics conjugated with glucuronic acid.

2. Sulphate

Some alcohols and phenols are conjugated with sulphate. Sulphotransferases transfer sulphate from phosphoadenosine phosphosulphate (PAPS) to the xenobiotics, for example, acetaminophen is partly metabolised by sulphation:

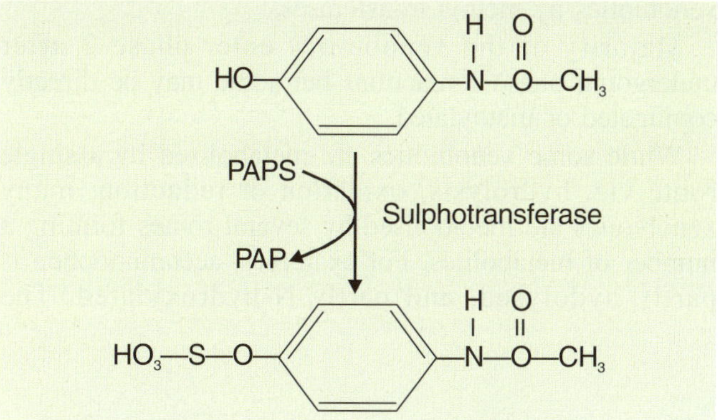

Steroids, methyldopa, phenol and indole are also sulphated.

3. Acetate

Sulphanilamide, hydralazine, caffeine and isoniazid are examples of drugs conjugated with acetate. N-Acetyl transferase-2 transfers acetyl group from acetyl CoA to the xenobiotics. Metabolism of these drugs is slowed down in persons who are deficient in N-acetyl transferase-2.

4. Glycine

Benzoic acid, after conversion into benzoyl CoA, is conjugated with glycine to form hippuric acid. Salicylic acid is partly conjugated with glycine to form salicyluric acid:

Salicylic acid

H_2N—CH_2—COOH
Glycine

H_2O

Salicyluric acid

5. Glutathione

Acetaminophen and some carcinogens are conjugated with glutathione. Glutathione is γ-glutamyl-cysteinylglycine. Conjugation occurs with the sulphydryl group of the cysteine residue. The glutamate and glycine residues are split off, and the cysteine residue is acetylated to form the mercapturic acid derivative of the xenobiotic, which is excreted.

The second phase 2 reaction is **methylation.** Some xenobiotics, e.g. thiouracil are methylated. The methyl group is transferred from S-adenosyl methionine to the xenobiotics by methyl transferases.

Majority of the xenobiotics enter phase 2 after undergoing phase 1 reactions but some may be directly conjugated or methylated.

While some xenobiotics are metabolised by a single route viz. hydrolysis, oxidation or reduction, many xenobiotics are metabolised by several routes forming a number of metabolites. For examples, acetaminophen is partly hydolysed, and partly N-hydroxylated. The hydroxylated metabolite is partly conjugated with glucuronic acid and is partly sulphated.

Environmental Health Hazards

Our metabolic machinery is adapted to metabolise, detoxify and excrete a wide range of xenobiotics. Yet there are many foreign chemicals which are either not metabolised or are metabolised to a limited extent. These chemicals are mostly environmental pollutants which may be present in air, water or food. We may encounter them at home, at workplace or in the community. These include industrial chemicals, insecticides, pesticides, lead, mercury, cadmium, arsenic, asbestos, silica, oxides of nitrogen and sulphur, carbon monoxide, solid particulate matter (spm), etc. Exposure to these pollutants beyond certain limits can cause disease. Such diseases may affect respiratory system, cardiovascular system, nervous system, reproductive system, immune system, liver, kidneys, etc. The following examples are illustrative of diseases caused by environmental pollutants:

1. *Respiratory diseases:* Exposure to smoke (amongst firemen), welding fumes, epoxy resins and asbestos can cause respiratory diseases.
2. *Cardiovascular diseases:* Chronic exposure to lead, carbon disulphide, methylene chloride and carbon monoxide (from furnaces and motor vehicle exhausts) can cause cardiovascular diseases.
3. *Nervous diseases:* Neurological diseases can be caused by prolonged exposure to lead, arsenic, mercury, toluene, organophosphates, organochlorines, polychlorinated biphenyls, perchloroethylene, etc.
4. *Reproductive diseases:* Chronic exposure to insecticides, herbicides, polychlorinated biphenyls, polybrominated biphenyls, ethylene oxide, dibromochloropropane, lead, arsenic, mercury, cadmium, etc. can cause reproductive diseases.
5. *Immune diseases:* Apart from the wide range of allergens that evoke an allergic response, exposure to polybrominated biphenyls, methylcholanthrene, dieldrin, mercury, etc can disturb the functioning of immune system.
6. *Liver diseases:* Hepatocellular or cholestatic liver disease can result from exposure to carbon tetrachloride, methylene diamine, arsenic, etc.
7. *Kidney diseases:* Chronic exposure to lead, mercury, cadmium, etc. can damage the kidneys.

Safe limits for many environmental pollutants have been established. Continuous monitoring of environment and remedial action, when required, are necessary to ensure the health of the community.

EXERCISE

1. Describe the detoxification and excretion of xenobiotics.

2. Write 'true' or 'false':
    a. Liver is the major site for metabolism of xenobiotics.
    b. All xenobiotics undergo microsomal hydroxylation before further reactions and excretion
    c. Cytochrome P-450 participates in hydroxylation of endogenous substrates as well as xenobiotics.
    d. There are several isoforms of cytochrome P-450.
    e. Cytochrome b_5 hydroxylates only xenobiotics.

3. Fill in the blanks:
    a. Members of one family of cytochrome P-450 share at least .... % homology in amino acid sequence.
    b. Members of one sub-family of cytochrome P-450 share at least .... % homology in amino acid sequence.
    c. Procarcinogens are converted into carcinogens generally by ....
    d. Acetylsalicylic acid is metabolised by ....
    e. Ethanol and .... are metabolised by common enzymes.

ANSWERS TO SHORT QUESTIONS

2. a. True   b. False   c. True
   d. True   e. False

3. a. 40   b. 55   c. Microsomal hydroxylation
   d. Hydrolysis   e. Methanol

Tests for Liver, Kidney, Pancreatic and Thyroid Functions

Liver, kidneys, pancreas and thyroid gland perform a variety of functions which are deranged in diseases involving these organs. Laboratory investigations are often required to make a diagnosis of these diseases and to assess the functional status of the organs concerned. A group of tests is often required to evaluate the functional efficiency and to confirm the diagnosis. These tests are known as function tests or organ profiles.

LIVER FUNCTION TESTS

Liver function tests are performed usually:

a. To detect hepatocellular damage,

b. To evaluate the functional status of liver, and

c. To distinguish between different types of jaundice.

As liver performs a multitude of functions, a number of tests are required to assess hepatic function. All the tests need not be performed in every case. The tests should be selected according to the clinical symptoms and signs. Several tests used earlier, e.g. icterus index, Van den Bergh test, thymol turbidity, zinc sulphate turbidity, cholesterol-cephalin flocculation, serum cholesterol: cholesteroyl ester ratio, etc. have now become obsolete due to lack of specificity and/or sensitivity. The following are the commonly used liver function tests:

Serum Bilirubin

Total serum bilirubin ranges from 0.2 to 1.0 mg/dl in healthy subjects, the unconjugated fraction being 0.1 to 0.6 mg/dl and the conjugated fraction 0.1 to 0.4 mg/dl. A rise in total serum bilirubin above 2 mg/dl leads to yellow staining of tissues known as jaundice. Jaundice may be haemolytic (prehepatic), hepatocellular (hepatic) or obstructive (posthepatic). Measurement of total, unconjugated and conjugated bilirubin in serum can help in the detection of jaundice and in distinguishing between different types of jaundice. In haemolytic jaundice, total and unconjugated bilirubin is raised. In hepatocellular jaundice, total, unconjugated and conjugated bilirubin is raised. In obstructive jaundice, total and conjugated bilirubin is raised (*see* Chapter 20 also).

Bile Pigments in Urine

Bilirubin is the major bile pigment in human beings. Normally, it is not present in urine. Only conjugated bilirubin is soluble in water, and can be excreted in urine. Therefore, a rise in conjugated bilirubin in serum, which occurs in hepatocellular and obstructive jaundice, leads to the appearance of bilirubin in urine.

Urobilinogen in Urine

Urobilinogen is formed from bilirubin in the intestine, is absorbed into portal circulation, and is mostly re-excreted by the liver in bile. Some urobilinogen escapes from liver into systemic circulation, and is excreted in urine. Normal urine contains a very small amount of urobilinogen. Urinary urobilinogen is increased in haemolytic jaundice due to increased formation of bilirubin and, hence, increased formation of urobilinogen. In obstructive jaundice, no bilirubin reaches the intestine, no urobilinogen is formed in the intestine, and no urobilinogen is present in urine. In hepatocellular jaundice, urinary urobilinogen is normal or decreased.

Bile Salts in Urine

Bile salts are formed in liver, and are excreted in bile. In obstructive jaundice, bile salts can not be excreted in bile due to biliary obstruction, and are regurgitated into systemic circulation. Being water-soluble, they are excreted in urine. In hepatocellular jaundice also, bile salts appear in urine due to intrahepatic obstruction of biliary canaliculi. In normal subjects and in haemolytic jaundice, bile salts are not present in urine as there is no obstruction to the flow of bile (Table 28.1).

Serum Proteins and Albumin: Globulin Ratio

Albumin is synthesised only in liver. Albumin synthesis is decreased in liver desease and, hence, serum albumin is decreased. Globulin synthesis may be increased, specially in infective diseases. Therefore, the ratio of albumin: globulin in serum is decreased or even reversed in liver

Table 28.1: Serum bilirubin and urinary bile pigments, urobilinogen and bile salts in haemolytic, hepatocellular and obstructive jaundice

	Haemolytic jaundice	*Hepatocellular jaundice*	*Obstructive jaundice*
Serum bilirubin (total)	↑	↑	↑
Serum bilirubin (unconjugated)	↑	↑	Normal
Serum bilirubin (conjugated)	Normal	↑	↑
Bile pigments in urine	Absent	Present	Present
Urobilinogen in urine	↑	Normal or ↓	Absent
Bile salts in urine	Absent	Present	Present

disease. However, this may happen in some non-hepatic diseases as well.

Serum Enzymes

Several enzymes of hepatic origin are released in blood in diseases involving acute necrosis of liver cells, e.g. viral hepatitis. This leads to an increase in serum lactate dehydrogenase (LDH), glutamate oxaloacetate transaminase (GOT) and glutamate pyruvate transaminase (GPT). The rise in serum GPT is generally greater than that in GOT in liver disease. Determination of isoenzymes of LDH may be more informative than that of total LDH.

Serum γ-glutamyl transpeptidase (GGT) is increased in many liver diseases, especially alcoholic hepatitis. Alkaline phosphatase (ALP) is synthesised in liver, bones, intestine and placenta. In liver, ALP is synthesised by parenchymal cells as well as epithelial cells of biliary canaliculi. Serum ALP is mildly elevated in viral hepatitis due to necrosis of parenchymal cells. A marked elevation in serum ALP occurs in obstructive jaundice due to irritation of epithelial cells of biliary canaliculi resulting in increased synthesis of ALP (*see* Chapter 7).

Prothrombin Time

Prothrombin time is prolonged when the concentration of prothrombin in plasma is decreased. Prothrombin is synthesised in liver, and its synthesis is decreased in hepatocellular disease leading to a prolongation of prothrombin time. Prothrombin time is also prolonged in vitamin K deficiency as vitamin K is required for post-translational modification of newly synthesised prothrombin (pre-prothrombin). Parenteral administration of vitamin K restores the prothrombin time in vitamin K deficiency but not in hepatocellular disease.

Galactose Tolerance Test

Dietary galactose is converted into glucose in liver. In hepatocellular disease, capacity of the liver to convert galactose into glucose is decreased, and blood galactose remains elevated for a long time after ingestion of galactose. In the oral galactose tolerance test, 40 gm of galactose, dissolved in a glass of water, is given by mouth to the subject after an overnight fast. Blood galactose is measured after 60 minutes. A blood galactose level above 60 mg/dl indicates impairment of hepatic function.

Hippuric Acid Test

Benzoic acid, given orally or intravenously, is conjugated in liver with glycine to form hippuric acid which is excreted in urine. If liver function is impaired, formation and excretion of hippuric acid is decreased. The oral test is done after an overnight fast or 2 to 3 hours after a light breakfast. The subject is asked to void, and is given 6 gm of sodium benzoate dissolved in a glass of water by mouth. The urine passed over the next four hours is collected, and the total amount of hippuric acid present in urine is measured. Excretion of less than 4 gm of hippuric acid indicates impairment of hepatic function.

In the intravenous test, the subject is asked to void and 1.77 gm of sodium benzoate dissolved in 2 ml of water is injected intravenously. The urine passed over the next one hour is collected, and hippuric acid present in it is measured. Excretion of less than 0.8 gm of hippuric acid indicates impairment of hepatic function.

Bromsulphthalein Test

Bromsulphthalein (BSP) is a dye which is conjugated in liver, and is excreted in bile. Rate of disappearance of BSP from circulation after an intravenous injection is a sensitive indicator of hepatobiliary function. After an overnight fast, a 5% solution of BSP is injected intravenously in the dose of 5 mg/kg of body weight. A blood sample is collected after three minutes, and again after 15 minutes. BSP concentration is measured in each sample. If the concentration at 45 minutes is more than 6% of the initial concentration, it indicates impairment of hepatobiliary function.

KIDNEY FUNCTION TESTS

Kidney function tests are done:

a. To detect the presence of an active lesion in the excretory system, and

b. To assess the functional efficiency of the kidneys.

During early stages of renal disease, functional efficiency may be normal despite the presence of an active lesion. Conversely, functional efficiency may be impaired even though the active lesion has healed but has left behind permanent tissue damage.

Kidney function tests may be broadly divided into:
a. Tests of glomerular function, and
b. Tests of tubular function.

Some of these tests may be affected by extra-renal factors and, therefore, the results should be interpreted in the light of clinical features. The following tests are commonly employed to assess kidney function:

Urine Examination

A routine qualitative examination of urine should be undertaken before quantitative analysis of blood and urine. A careful physical examination and qualitative tests for abnormal constituents of urine, e.g. proteins and blood, may provide useful information, especially about the presence of an active lesion in the urinary tract.

Serum Urea

Urea is the end product of protein catabolism. It is synthesised in liver, and is excreted by kidneys. Normal range of serum urea is 20 to 45 mg/dl. Impairment of glomerular function leads to decreased glomerular filtration of urea and its retention in blood. However, it is not a sensitive test of glomerular function as serum urea begins to rise only when the glomerular filtration rate decreases below 50% of the normal. Still, it is a widely used test of renal function, and **uraemia** (a rise in serum urea) has practically become a synonym of renal failure. Serum urea may be altered in some extra-renal diseases also. Therefore, the results should be interpreted in conjunction with the clinical findings and the results of other investigations. In some laboratories, the concentration of urea in blood is expressed as blood urea nitrogen (BUN) which represents the nitrogen content of urea present in blood. Molecular weight of urea is 60 in which the contribution of nitrogen atoms is 28. Therefore, BUN equals blood urea multiplied by 28/60, i.e. nearly 0.47. The normal range of BUN is 9–21 mg/dl. A rise in nitrogen content of blood is called azotaemia.

Serum Creatinine

Creatinine is formed from creatine in muscles, and is excreted by kidneys in urine. Normal range of serum creatinine is 0.6 to 1.5 mg/dl. Serum creatinine is raised in renal failure due to decreased glomerular filtration and, consequently, increased retention of creatinine in blood. Serum creatinine is a more sensitive indicator of glomerular function than serum urea.

Urea Clearance

Since a simple measurement of serum urea is not a sensitive test, Moller, MacIntosh and Van Slyke devised the concept of urea clearance in which the rate of urinary excretion of urea is compared with the concentration of urea in serum. Urea clearance is the hypothetical volume of blood from which urea is completely removed by kidneys in one minute. If the substance chosen for clearance is completely filtered by glomeruli in a single circulation of blood through the kidneys and is neither secreted nor reabsorbed by tubules, its clearance will be equal to the glomerular filtration rate (GFR). Urea is completely filtered by glomeruli but is partially reabsorbed by tubules. Therefore, urea clearance is less than the GFR.

Urea clearance is generally measured over two consecutive periods of 60 minutes each, and their mean is calculated. The patient takes two glasses of water and empties his bladder completely. The time is noted. Exactly 60 minutes later, he micturates again, and the entire urine specimen is collected. A specimen of blood is also collected at the same time. The patient is asked to micturate again after another 60 minutes, and the entire urine specimen is collected. Volume of each urine specimen is measured accurately. Concentration of urea is measured in serum and each urine specimen. Urea clearance is calculated from U (concentration of urea in urine in mg/dl), V (volume of urine in ml/minute) and S (concentration of urea in serum in mg/dl). If the output of urine is more than 2 ml/minute, "maximum urea clearance" is calculated from the formula:

$$\text{Maximum urea clearance (ml/minute)} = \frac{UV}{S}$$

If the urine output is less than 2 ml/minute, "standard urea clearance" is calculated from the formula:

$$\text{Standard urea clrearance (ml/minute)} = \frac{U\sqrt{V}}{S}$$

Maximum urea clearance is 75 ml/minute and standard urea clearance 54 ml/minute in a normal person having a body surface area of 1.73 square metres. For body surface area other than this, the calculated clearance has to be corrected by multiplying it by 1.73/body surface area of the subject. Urea clearance below 60% of the normal indicates impaired glomerular function.

Creatinine Clearance

Creatinine clearance is closer to GFR than is urea clearance as there is little tubular reabsorption of creatinine. It is usually measured over a 24-hour period. The urine passed in the 24-hour period is collected carefully. A blood sample is also collected during this period. Volume of the urine is measured accurately, and concentration of creatinine in urine and serum is measured. Creatinine clearance is calculated using the formula UV/S. The normal range of creatinine clearance is 100 to 120 ml/minute in males and 95 to 105 ml/minute in females. Values below normal indicate impairment of glomerular function.

Inulin Clearance

True GFR may be measured by inulin clearance. Inulin is a polysaccharide of relatively low molecular weight made up of fructose. It is non-toxic, is not metabolised in human beings, is completely filtered by glomeruli, and is neither secreted nor reabsorbed by tubules. Therefore, its clearance is equal to GFR.

Inulin is given by slow intravenous infusion to maintain a constant level in blood during the test period. Initially, 30 ml of 10 percent inulin solution diluted with 250 ml of isotonic saline is infused at the rate of 20 ml/minute to achieve the desired concentration of inulin in blood. Then, 70 ml of 10 percent inulin solution diluted with 500 ml of isotonic saline is infused at the rate of 4 ml/minute to maintain the inulin concentration in blood. The subject is asked to micturate 20 minutes after starting the second infusion. The urine is discarded and the time is noted. Exactly 60 minutes later, the subject micturates again, and the urine is collected. A blood sample is also collected during the test period. Urine volume is measured, and the concentration of inulin in urine and serum is measured. Inulin clearance is calculated using the formula UV/S. Normal inulin clearance is 120 to 130 ml/minute for a body surface are of 1.73 square metres. Decreased clearance indicates impairment of glomerular function.

Phenolsulphonephthalein (PSP) Excretion Test

This is a test of tubular function. PSP, injected intravenously, is not filtered by the glomeruli but is secreted by the tubules. PSP excretion in urine indicates the efficiency of tubular function. The test is done after an overnight fast which is preferable but not essential. The subject is asked to drink two glasses of water to ensure an adequate output of urine. One ml of 0.6 percent solution of PSP (a total dose of 6 mg of PSP) is injected intravenously. Urine is collected 15 minutes and 70 minutes after the injection. The total amount of PSP present in each urine sample is measured. Normal subjects excrete 20 to 25 percent of the injected dose within 15 minutes and 55 to 70 percent within 70 minutes. Decreased excretion indicates impairment of tubular function.

Concentration Test

This is a test of tubular function. When the water content of the body decreases, tubular reabsorption of water is increased to conserve water, and the urine becomes concentrated. To perform the test, the subject is not allowed to take any food or drink after the evening meal. The first three urine specimens passed in the morning are collected, and their specific gravity is measured. In normal subjects, at least one of the urine specimens should have a specific gravity of 1.025 or more. If it remains below 1.025 in all the specimens, it shows impairment of tubular function.

Dilution Test

This is also a test of tubular function. When an excess of water enters the body, tubular reabsorption of water decreases, and a dilute urine is excreted. The test is done in the morning after an overnight fast. The subject is asked to drink 1,200 ml of water within 30 minutes. Urine specimens are collected every hour for four hours, and their specific gravity is measured. In normal subjects, at least one of the specimens should have a specific gravity of 1.003 or less. Specific gravity above 1.003 in all the specimens shows impairment of tubular function.

Para-amino Hippurate Clearance

Para-amino hippurate (PAH) is an exogenous compound which is filtered by glomeruli and is also secreted by tubules. At low plasma PAH levels, the entire PAH present in blood is removed by the kidneys in a single circulation of blood through the kidneys. Therefore, PAH clearance is a measure of renal plasma flow (RPF) at low plasma PAH levels. The procedure is similar to that of inulin clearance. First, a loading dose of PAH is given by intravenous injection to achieve the desired concentration of PAH in plasma and, then, a slow intravenous infusion is given to maintain the plasma PAH level during the test period. The loading dose is 3 ml of 20 percent PAH solution diluted with 250 ml of isotonic saline infused at the rate of 20 ml/minute. This is followed by an infusion of 14 ml of 20 percent PAH diluted with 500 ml of isotonic saline at the rate of 4 ml/minute. Urine and blood samples are collected as in inulin clearance. Urine output and PAH concentrations in urine and serum are measured. PAH clearance is calculated by the formula UV/S. This equals the RPF.

Normal RPF is about 600 ml/minute for a body surface area of 1.73 square metres. Normal filtration fraction (GFR/RPF) is about 0.2. Filtration fraction decreases in glomerulonephritis.

PANCREATIC FUNCTION TESTS

These tests are performed to diagnose diseases of the exocrine portion of the pancreas. The tests include the following:

Serum Amylase

Amylase is a digestive enzyme synthesised in the pancreas and salivary glands. Most of the amylase present in circulation is of pancreatic origin. Serum amylase is greatly increased in acute pancreatitis due to leakage of the enzyme

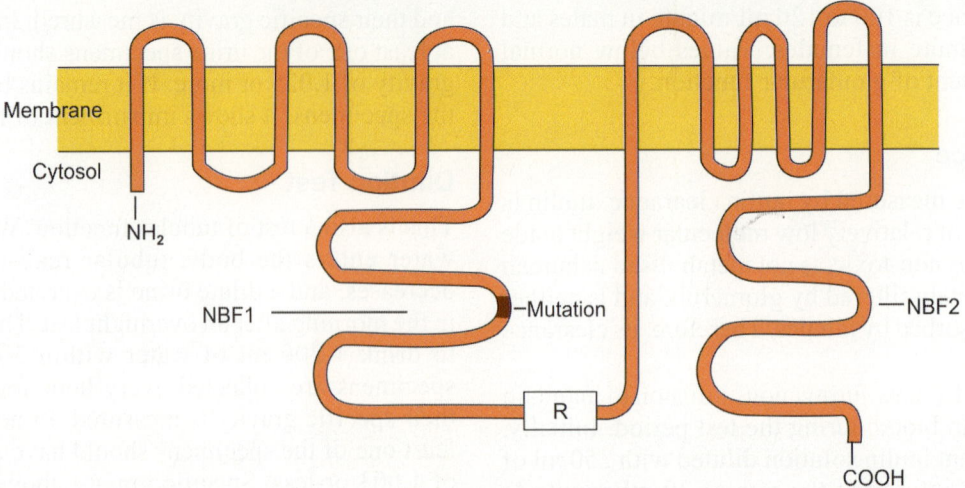

Fig. 28.1: Cystic fibrosis transmembrane conductance regulator (NBF1, nucleotide-binding fold 1; NBF 2, nucleotide-binding fold 2; R, regulatory domain)

from the pancreatic cells. A smaller increase occurs in acute parotitis.

Serum Lipase

Lipase is another digestive enzyme synthesised in the pancreas. Serum lipase is increased in acute pancreatitis.

Sweat Chloride

This test is very useful in the diagnosis of **cystic fibrosis** (fibrocystic disease of the pancreas or mucoviscidosis). Cystic fibrosis is a recessively inherited autosomal disease affecting a number of exocrine glands including the pancreas. Very viscous mucus is secreted by exocrine glands in this disease clogging pancreatic ducts and bronchioles. In addition, the chloride content of sweat is increased.

The gene which undergoes mutation in cystic fibrosis has been recently identified and sequenced. It is located on chromosome 7, and encodes a transmembrane protein, **CFTR (cystic fibrosis transmembrane conductance regulator)**. This protein has two membrane-spanning regions, two nucleotide-binding folds in the cytosol and a regulatory domain in the cytosol. Nucleotide-binding folds are the sites for binding of ATP. Regulatory domain can be phosphorylated by protein kinase A and protein kinase C. CFTR protein acts as a chloride channel (Fig. 28.1).

The gene encoding CFTR protein is known as CFTR gene. In 70 percent of the patients with cystic fibrosis, a three base-pair deletion in the gene leads to deletion of a phenylalanine residue from nucleotide-binding fold 1. This impairs chloride transport across the membrane. In the remaining patients, other mutations have been detected.

Diagnosis of cystic fibrosis can be made by measuring the chloride concentration in sweat. A concentration above 60 mEq/L is diagnostic of cystic fibrosis.

THYROID FUNCTION TESTS

Thyroid function tests are commonly performed for the diagnosis of hyper- and hypo-thyroidism. Most of the patients with these disorders have only a few isolated signs and symptoms, and a clinical diagnosis is usually difficult. Therefore, laboratory investigations are often required to confirm the diagnosis.

Production of Thyroid Hormones

Dietary iodide is absorbed by the alimentary tract, and released into circulation. Some of it is excreted in urine. Some is taken up by the thyroid gland, and is converted into iodine. Iodine reacts with the tyrosine residues of thyroglobulin to form mono-iodo-tyrosine (MIT) and di-iodotyrosine (DIT). Two DIT residues react with each other to form tetra-iodo-thyronine (thyroxine or T_4). One residue each of MIT and DIT react with each other to form tri-iodo-thyronine (T_3).

T_3 and T_4 are stored in thyroid acini attached to thyroglobulin. The hormones are released into circulation as needed. In circulation, they are transported by thyroxine-binding globulin (TBG). Small amounts are transported by thyroxine-binding pre-albumin and albumin. The TBG-bound hormones are inactive. Small amounts of T_3 and T_4 are released from TBG and exist as free T_3 and T_4 in circulation.

Free T_3 and T_4 are the biologically active forms of the hormones. T_4 is more abundant but T_3 is more powerful. Synthesis of T_3 and T_4 in thyroid gland and their release in circulation are increased by thyroid-stimulating hormone (TSH) of anterior pituitary. TSH secretion is increased by thyrotropin-releasing hormone (TRH) of hypothalamus. High levels of T_3 and T_4 in circulation decrease the secretion of TSH and TRH by feedback inhibition (Fig. 28.2).

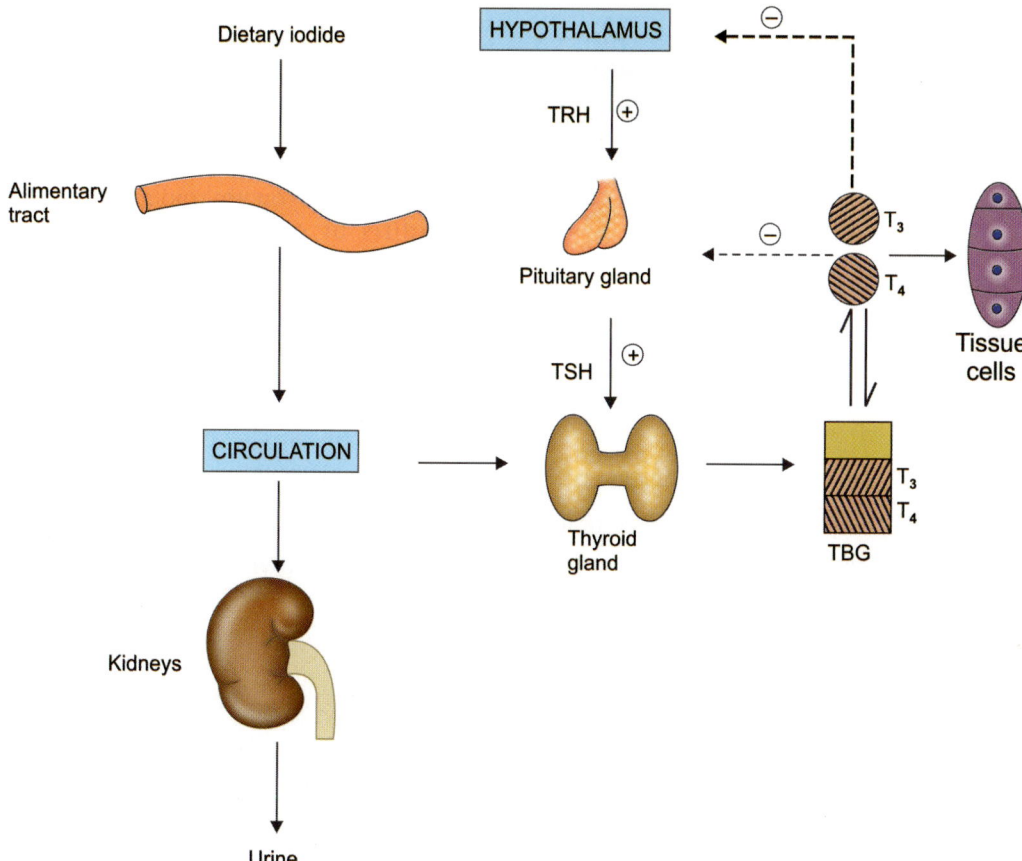

Fig. 28.2: An outline of production and secretion of thyroid hormones (TRH, Thyrotropin- releasing hormone; TSH, Thyroid-stimulating hormone; TBG, Thyroxine-binding globulin; T_3, Tri-iodo-thyronine; T_4, Thyroxine)

Before the advent of radio-immuno-assay for hormones, the tests for assessing thyroid function were indirect and and lacked specificificity and sensitivity. The following are some of the older tests:

Basal Metabolic Rate

Thyroid hormones stimulate all metabolic activities and raise the basal metabolic rate (BMR). Therefore, BMR is increased in hyperthyroidism and decreased in hypo-thyroidism. However, this test lacks specificity as BMR is affected in a number of physiological and pathological conditions.

Serum Cholesterol

Serum cholesterol is decreased in hyperthyroidism and increased in hypothyroidism, but again, serum cholesterol is affected in a number of other diseases.

Serum Protein-bound Iodine

In this test, the iodine bound to serum proteins is measured. Most of the protein-bound iodine (PBI) is present in T_3 and T_4. Therefore, serum PBI is increased in hyper-thyroidism and decreased in hypothyroidism. However, the accuracy of the measurement is poor.

Radioactive Iodine Uptake

This test measures the uptake of circulating iodide by the thyroid gland. A small dose of radioactive isotope of iodine (5 μc of $Na^{131}I$) is given to the subject orally in a fasting condition. The radioactivity over the thyroid gland is measured by a Geiger Muller counter after 2, 24 and 48 hours. This is a measure of the radioactive iodine present in the thyroid gland. The normal uptake is 1.5 to 15 percent of the ingested dose at two hours, 25 to 50 percent of the ingested dose at 24 hours and 15 to 40 percent of the ingested dose at 48 hours. The uptake is increased in hyperthyroidism and decreased in hypothyroidism.

All these tests have now become obsolete as sensitive and specific assays of hormones by radio-immuno-assay or enzyme immuno-assay are now available. The tests commonly done now are the following:

1. Serum T_4

The normal range of total T_4 in serum is 5-12 μg/dl. Serum total T_4 is increased in hyperthyroidism and is decreased in hypothyroidism.

2. Serum T_3

The normal range of total T_3 in serum is 0.1–0.2 µg/dl. It is increased in hyperthyroidism and is decreased in hypothyroidism. An increase in serum T_3 with normal T_4 is seen in T_3 toxicosis.

3. Serum Free T_4 (FT_4)

Sometimes, serum total T_4 may be normal inspite of the presence of a thyroid disorder. In such cases, measurement of serum FT_4 can clinch the diagnosis. The normal range of serum FT_4 is 0.8–2 ng/dl. It is increased in hyperthyroidism and is decreased in hypothyroidism.

4. Serum Free T_3 (FT_3)

Like serum FT_4, serum FT_4 may be of greater value in the diagnosis of subtle disorders of thyroid. The normal range of serum FT_3 is 0.3–0.6 ng/dl.

5. Serum TSH

Serum TSH assay is useful in differentiating between hyperthyroidism and hypothyroidism of thyroid origin and those secondary to pituitary or hypothalamic disease. In primary hyperthyroidism, serum TSH is decreased due to feedback inhibition. In hyperthyroidism secondary to pituitary or hypothalamic disease, serum TSH is raised.

In primary hypothyroidism, serum TSH is increased due to lack of feedback inhibition. In hypothyroidism secondary to pituitary or hypothalamic disease, serum TSH is decreased. The normal range of serum TSH is 0.5 to 5 µU/ml.

6. Thyroperoxidase Antibodies (TPO Ab)

Many cases of hyopothyroidism are due to Hashimoto's thyroiditis or post-partum thyroiditis in which an autoimmune response against thyroperoxidase results in hypothyroidism. These cases can be diagnosed by detection of thyroperoxidase antibodies in serum.

7. TRH Stimulation Test

Stimulation of anterior pituitary by TRH administration followed by measurement of serum T_3, T_4 and TSH can help distinguish between thyroid disorders of hypothalamic and pituitary origin. TRH stimulation test is rarely required in hyperthyroidism. In hypothyroidism with low TSH, low T_4 and low T_3, a response to TRH stimulation points to the hypothalamic origin of the disorder.

Subclinical Hypothyroidism

Subclinical hypothyroidism usually results from auto-immune thyroiditis. The patients present with vague signs and symptoms, have a normal serum T_4 and a high serum TSH. These patients can progress to frank hypothyroidism later on. It is recommended that these patients should be screened for TPO Ab. If TPO Ab is present, treatment is indicated. If TPO Ab is absent, annual follow up is recommended.

EXERCISE

1. Describe liver function tests.
2. Describe kidney function tests.
3. Write short notes on:
   a. Tests for exocrine function of pancreas
   b. Thyroid function tests
4. Write 'true' or 'false':
   a. Bile pigments are absent from urine in haemolytic jaundice.
   b. Urobilinogen is increased in urine in obstructive jaundice.
   c. Bile salts are synthesised in liver.
   d. Serum albumin is decreased in liver diseases.
   e. Urea clearance is a very sensitive test of glomerular function.
   f. GFR can be measured by inulin clearance.
   g. PSP excretion test is a test of tubular function.
   h. Serum amylase and lipase are increased in acute pancreatitis.
   i. Sweat chloride is increased in pancreatitis.
   j. Serum TSH is increased in primary hyperthyroidism.
5. Fill in the blanks:
   a. .... bilirubin is soluble in water.
   b. Urobilinogen is absent from urine in .... jaundice.

c. Albumin is synthesised in ....only.

d. Prothrombin time is prolonged in .... diseases and .... deficiency.

e. Creatinine clearance is a more sensitive test of glomerular function than .... clearance.

f. Concentration test is a test of .... function.

g. Renal plasma flow can be measured by .... clearance.

h. Sweat chloride is .... in cystic fibrosis.

i. .... gene is abnormal in cystic fibrosis.

j. Radioactive iodine uptake by the thyroid gland is .... in hyperthyroidism.

ANSWERS TO SHORT QUESTIONS

4. a. True
   b. False
   c. True
   d. True
   e. False
   f. True
   g. True
   h. True
   i. False
   j. False

5. a. Conjugated
   b. Obstructive
   c. Liver
   d. Liver, vitamin K
   e. Urea
   f. Tubular
   g. Para-amino hippurate
   h. Increased
   i. CFTR
   j. Increased

Normal Range of Some Common Laboratory Investigations

Acid phosphatase (ACP)	1–5 King-Armstrong Units (KAU)/dl
Alanine aminotransferase (ALT)	0–35 U/L
Albumin	3.5–5.5 gm/dl
Alkaline phosphatase (ALP)	4–17 King-Armstrong Units (KAU)/dl
Ammonia	10–80 µg/dl
Amylase	80–180 Somogyi Units (SU)/dl
Ascorbic acid	0.5–1.5 mg/dl
Aspartate aminotransferase (AST)	0–35 U/L
Bicarbonate	24–30 mEq/L
Bilirubin	
Total	0.2–1.0 mg/dl
Conjugated	0.1–0.4 mg/dl
Unconjugated	0.1–0.6 mg/dl
Calcium	
Total	9–11 mg/dl
Ionised	4.5–5.5 mg/dl
Ceruloplasmin	25–45 mg/dl
Chloride	96–106 mEq/L
Cholesterol (fasting)	
Total	150–220 mg/dl
HDL (desirable)	Above 40 mg/dl
LDL (desirable)	Below 180 mg/dl
VLDL (desirable)	Below 40 mg/dl
Copper	100–200 µg/dl

Creatine kinase (CK)	
Total	10–50 IU/L
BB	0% of the total
MB	0–3% of the total
MM	97–100% of the total
Creatinine	0.6–1.5 mg/dl
Ferritin	1–40 µg/dl
Gamma-glutamyl transpeptidase (GGT)	Below 30 U/L
Globulins	1.8–3.6 gm/dl
Glucose (fasting)	65–110 mg/dl
Iron	50–175 µg/dl
Iron-binding capacity	250–400 mg/dl
Lactate dehydrogenase (LDH)	60–200 IU/L
Magnesium	2–3 mg/dl
pH (arterial blood)	7.35–7.45
Phosphorus, inorganic (adults)	2.5–4.5 mg/dl
Phosphorus, inorganic (children)	4.0–7.0 mg/dl
Potassium	3.5–5 mEq/L
Proteins (total)	6–8 gm/dl
Sodium	136–145 mEq/L
Thyroxine (T_4), total	5–12 µg/dl
Transferrin	200–400 mg/dl
Triglycerides (fasting)	Below 160 mg/dl
Tri-iodothyronine (T_3)	0.1–0.2 µg/dl
Urea	20–45 mg/dl
Uric acid	2–6.5 mg/dl
Zinc	50–150 µg/dl

Common Abbreviations used in Biochemistry

A	Adenosine	CDK	Cyclin-dependent kinase
ABP	Androgen-binding protein	CDP	Cytidine diphosphate
ACE	Angiotensin-converting enzyme	CEA	Carcinoembryonic antigen
ACP	Acid phosphatase	cGMP	Cyclic guanosine monophosphate
ACP	Acyl carrier protein	CK	Creatine kinase
ACTH	Adrenocorticotropic hormone	CLIP	Corticotropin-like intermediate lobe peptide
ADA	Adenosine deaminase	CM	Chylomicron
ADH	Antidiuretic hormone	CMP	Cytidine monophosphate
ADP	Adenosine diphosphate	Co A	Coenzyme A, free or bound
AFP	α-Fetoprotein	Co A-SH	Coenzyme A, free
AIDS	Acquired immunodeficiency syndrome	Co Q	Coenzyme Q (oxidised)
Ala	Alanine	COMT	Catechol O-methyl transferase
ALA	Aminolevulinic acid	CPK	Creatine phosphokinase (also called creatine kinase or CK)
ALP	Alkaline phosphatase		
ALT	Alanine aminotransferase	CRBP	Cellular retinol-binding protein
AMP	Adenosine monophosphate	CRH	Corticotropin-releasing hormone
ANP	Atrial natriuretic peptide	CRP	C-reactive protein
Arg	Arginine	CTP	Cytidine triphosphate
Asn	Asparagine	Cys	Cysteine
Asp	Aspartate	1,25-DHCC	1,25-Dihydroxycholecalciferol
AST	Aspartate aminotransferase	dA	Deoxyadenosine
ATP	Adenosine triphosphate	DAG	Diacylglycerol
AVP	Arginine-vasopressin	dATP	Deoxyadenosine triphosphate
BMI	Body mass index	dC	Deoxycytidine
BMR	Basal metabolic rate	dG	Deoxyguanosine
bp	Base pairs	DHT	Dihydrotestosterone
BPG	Biphosphoglycerate	DIT	Di-iodo-tyrosine
BV	Biological value	DNA	Deoxyribonucleic acid
C	Cytidine	DOPA	Dihydroxyphenylalanine
cAMP	Cyclic adenosine monophosphate	dT	Deoxythymidine
CBG	Corticosteroid-binding globulin	dTMP	Deoxythymidine monophosphate
CCK-PZ	Cholecystokinin-pancreozymin	dUMP	Deoxyuridine monophosphate
CD	Cluster of differentiation	EC	Enzyme commission number

ECF	Extracellular fluid	IDP	Inosine diphosphate
EF	Elongation factor	IF	Intrinsic factor
EGF	Epidermal growth factor	IFN	Interferon
FAD	Flavin adenine dinucleotide (oxidised)	IGF	Insulin-like growth factor
$FADH_2$	Flavin adenine dinucleotide (reduced)	IL	Interleukin
FFA	Free fatty acids	Ile	Isoleucine
FGF	Fibroblast growth factor	IMP	Inosine monophosphate
Figlu	Formiminoglutamate	IP_3	Inositol triphosphate
FMN	Flavin mononucleotide (oxidised)	ITP	Inosine triphosphate
$FMNH_2$	Flavin mononucleotide (reduced)	IU	International unit(s)
Fp	Flavoprotein	IUB	International Union of Biochemistry
FSH	Follicle-stimulating hormone	kb	Kilobases
G	Guanosine	kcal	Kilocalories
GAG	Glycosaminoglycan	kJ	Kilojoules
GAP	GnRH-associated peptide	K_m	Michaelis constant
GAP	GTPase-activating protein	LCAT	Lecithin cholesterol acyl transferase
GDP	Guanosine diphosphate	LDH	Lactate dehydrogenase
GFR	Glomerular filtration rate	LDL	Low density lipoprotein
GH	Growth hormone	Leu	Leucine
GHRH	Growth hormone-releasing hormone	LH	Luteinising hormone
GHRIH	Growth hormone release-inhibiting hormone	LTH	Luteotropic hormone
GIP	Gastric inhibitory polypeptide	Lys	Lysine
Gln	Glutamine	MAO	Mono-amine oxidase
Glu	Glutamate	MDH	Malate dehydrogenase
Gly	Glycine	Met	Methionine
GMP	Guanosine monophosphate	MHC	Major histocompatibility complex
GnRH	Gonadotropin-releasing hormone	MIT	Mono-iodo-tyrosine
GTP	Guanosine triphosphate	mRNA	Messenger RNA
Hb	Haemoglobin	MSH	Melanocyte-stimulating hormone
hCG	Human chorionic gonadotropin	MUFA	Monounsaturated fatty acid(s)
HDL	High density lipoprotein	MW	Molecular weight
H_2-Folate	Dihydrofolate	NAD^+	Nicotinamide adenine dinucleotide (oxidised)
H_4-Folate	Tetrahydrofolate	NADH	Nicotinamide adenine dinucleotide (reduced)
hGH	Human growth hormone		
His	Histidine	$NADP^+$	Nicotinamide adenine dinucleotide phosphate (oxidised)
HIV	Human immunodeficiency virus		
HMG CoA	β-Hydroxy-β-methyl glutaryl CoA	NADPH	Nicotinamide adenine dinucleotide phosphate (reduced)
hnRNA	Heterogeneous nuclear RNA		
HPL	Human placental lactogen	NGF	Nerve growth factor
HPLC	High performance liquid chromatography	NPU	Net protein utilisation
Hyl	Hydroxylysine	PAF	Platelet-activating factor
Hyp	Hydroxyproline	Pi	Inorganic phosphate
ICD	Isocitrate dehydrogenase	PCR	Polymerase chain reaction
IDL	Intermediate density liproprotein	PDGF	Platelet-derived growth factor

PEP	Phosphoenol pyruvate		SHBG	Sex hormone-binding globulin
PER	Protein efficiency ratio		snRNA	Small nuclear RNA
PFK	Phosphofructokinase		snRNP	Small nuclear ribonucleoprotein particle
PG	Prostaglandin		T_3	Tri-iodothyronine
Phe	Phenylalanine		T_4	Tetra-iodothyronine
PL	Placental lactogen		TBG	Thyroxine-binding globulin
PLP	Pyridoxal phosphate		TBPA	Thyroxine-binding pre-albumin
PNMT	Phenylethanolamine N-methyl transferase		TEBG	Testosterone-estrogen-binding globulin
POMC	Pro-opiomelanocortin		TF	Transcription factor
PPi	Inorganic pyrophosphate		TG	Triglyceride (or triacylglycerol)
PRH	Prolactin-releasing hormone		TGF	Transforming growth factor
PRIH	Prolactin release-inhibiting hormone		Thr	Threonine
Pro	Proline		TLC	Thin layer chromatography
PRPP	5-Phosphoribosyl-1-pyrophosphate		Tm_G	Tubular maximum for glucose
PTH	Parathormone		TMP	Thymidine monophosphate
PUFA	Polyunsaturated fatty acid(s)		TNF	Tumour necrosis factor
RBC	Red blood cell		TRH	Thyrotropin-releasing hormone
RBP	Retinol-binding protein		tRNA	Transfer RNA
RE	Retinol equivalent		Trp	Tryptophan
RF	Releasing factor		TSH	Thyroid-stimulating hormone
RFLP	Restriction fragment length polymorphism		TTP	Thymidine triphosphate
RNA	Ribonucleic acid		Tyr	Tyrosine
RQ	Respiratory quotient		UDP	Uridine diphosphate
rRNA	Ribosomal RNA		UMP	Uridine monophosphate
RT	Reverse transcriptase		UTP	Uridine triphosphate
S	Sedimentation constant		Val	Valine
SCID	Severe combined immunodeficiency disease		V_{max}	Maximum velocity
SDA	Specific dynamic action		VIP	Vasoactive intestinal polypeptide
Ser	Serine		VLDL	Very low density lipoprotein
Sf	Svedberg floatation unit		VMA	Vanillylmandelic acid
SFA	Saturated fatty acid(s)		VNTR	Variable number of tandem repeats
SGOT	Serum glutamate oxaloacetate transaminase (same as AST)		WBC	White blood cell
SGPT	Serum glutamate pyruvate transaminase (same as ALT)			

3

Atomic Weights of Some Common Elements

Element	Symbol	Atomic number	Atomic weight
Aluminium	Al	13	26.981
Antimony	Sb	51	121.75
Arsenic	As	33	74.922
Barium	Ba	56	137.34
Beryllium	Be	4	9.012
Bismuth	Bi	83	208.980
Boron	B	5	10.81
Bromine	Br	35	79.904
Cadmium	Cd	48	112.40
Calcium	Ca	20	40.08
Carbon	C	6	12.011
Cerium	Ce	58	140.12
Cesium	Cs	55	132.905
Chloride	Cl	17	35.453
Chromium	Cr	24	51.996
Cobalt	Co	27	58.933
Copper	Cu	29	63.546
Fluoride	F	9	18.998
Gold	Au	79	196.966
Helium	He	2	4.002
Hydrogen	H	1	1.008
Iodine	I	53	126.904
Iron	Fe	26	55.847
Lead	Pb	82	207.20
Lithium	Li	3	6.941
Magnesium	Mg	12	24.305
Manganese	Mn	25	54.938
Mercury	Hg	80	200.59
Molybdenum	Mo	42	95.94
Nickel	Ni	28	58.70
Nitrogen	N	7	14.007
Osmium	Os	76	190.2
Oxygen	O	8	15.999

Contd...

Contd...

Element	Symbol	Atomic number	Atomic weight
Phosphorus	P	15	30.974
Platinum	Pt	78	195.09
Potassium	K	19	39.098
Rubidium	Rb	37	85.468
Selenium	Se	34	78.96
Silicon	Si	14	28.086
Silver	Ag	47	107.868
Sodium	Na	11	22.990
Strontium	Sr	38	87.62
Sulphur	S	16	32.06
Tin	Sn	50	118.69
Tungsten	W	74	183.85
Uranium	U	92	239.029
Vanadium	V	23	50.941
Zinc	Zn	30	65.38

Based on IUPAC (1973)

Index

Multiple Choice Questions

Chapter 3: Chemistry of Carbohydrates

1. α-1,4-Glycosidic bond is present in:
   (a) Maltose (b) Lactose (c) Sucrose (d) Cellulose
2. Fructose is present in hydrolysate of:
   (a) Lactose (b) Sucrose (c) Maltose (d) Starch
3. Sucrose can be hydrolysed by:
   (a) Lactase (b) Maltase (c) Invertase (d) α-1,6-Glycosidase
4. Deoxyribose is a:
   (a) Triose (b) Tetrose (c) Pentose (d) Hexose
5. A disaccharide made up of one glucose and one fructose unit is:
   (a) Trehalose (b) Lactose (c) Maltose (d) Sucrose
6. Inulin is a:
   (a) Homopolysaccharide (b) Heteropolysaccharide
   (c) Oligosaccharide (d) Disaccharide
7. Furanose ring can be present in:
   (a) Glyceraldehyde (b) Dihydroxyacetone (c) Erythrose
   (d) Ribose
8. α-1,6-Glycosidic bonds are present in:
   (a) Glycogen (h) Hyaluronic acid (c) Chondroitin
   sulphate (d) Heparin
9. Sedoheptulose is a:
   (a) Ketose (b) Pentose (c) Disaccharide (d) Constituent of
   heparin
10. A lubricant present in joints is:
    (a) Heparin (b) Heparan sulphate (c) Chondroitin
    sulphate (d) Hyaluronic acid

Chapter 4: Chemistry of Lipids

1. Polyunsaturated fatty acids have:
   (a) One carbon-carbon double bond (b) One carbon-oxygen
   double bond (c) More than one carbon-carbon double bonds
   (d) More than one carbon-oxygen double bonds
2. Omega carbon in fatty acids is:
   (a) The carboxyl carbon (b) The methyl carbon (c) The side
   chain carbon (d) None of these
3. α-Linolenic acid is an:
   (a) Omega-3 fatty acid (b) Omega-6 fatty acid (c) Omega-
   9 fatty acid (d) Omega-12 fatty acid
4. Triglycerides are:
   (a) Polar (b) Heavier than water (c) Made up of glycerol
   and fatty acids (d) All of these
5. All of the following are polyunsaturated fatty acid
   except:
   (a) Oleic acid (b) Linoleic acid (c) Linolenic acid
   (d) Arachidonic acid
6. Sphingosine is:
   (a) An aliphatic alcohol (b) An amino alcohol (c) A
   branched-chain fatty acid (d) A cerebroside

7. Ceramide is made up of:
   (a) Serine and palmitic acid (b) Serine and glycerol
   (c) Glycerol and fatty acid (d) Sphingosine and fatty acid
8. Protein content of chylomicrons is about:
   (a) 1% (b) 7% (c) 21% (d) 33%
9. Lecithin is made up of:
   (a) Glycerol and fatty acids (b) Glycerol, fatty acids and
   phosphoric acid (c) Glycerol, fatty acids, phosphoric acid
   and choline (d) Glycerol, fatty acids, phosphoric acid and
   serine
10. High-density lipoproteins transport:
    (a) Triglycerides from liver to extrahepatic tissues
    (b) Triglycerides from extrahepatic tissues to liver
    (c) Cholesterol from liver to extrahepatic tissues
    (d) Cholesterol from extrahepatic tissues to liver

Chapter 5: Chemistry of Amino Acids and Proteins

1. All the following amino acids have an asymmetric
   carbon atom *except*:
   (a) Glycine (b) Alanine (c) Serine (d) Cysteine
2. All the following are essential amino acids *except*:
   (a) Leucine (b) Lysine (c) Serine (d) Valine
3. All the following are sulphur-containing amino acids
   except:
   (a) Cysteine (b) Cystine (c) Threonine (d) Methionine
4. All the following are aromatic amino acids *except*:
   (a) Phenylalanine (b) Tyrosine (c) Tryptophan (d) Histidine
5. Two amino groups and one carboxyl group are present
   in:
   (a) Lysine (b) Leucine (c) Isoleucine (d) Glutamate
6. A disulphide bond is present in:
   (a) Cysteine (b) Cystine (c) Methionine (d) None of these
7. Selenocysteine is formed from:
   (a) Cysteine (b) Cystine (c) Methionine (d) Serine
8. Ionizable side chain is present in:
   (a) Alanine (b) Aspartate (c) Valine (d) Leucine
9. An amino acid that disrupts α-helix is:
   (a) Glycine (b) Glutamate (c) Proline (d) Phenylalanine
10. A chromoprotein among the following is:
    (a) Albumin (b) Globulin (c) Ferritin (d) Myoglobin
11. A phosphoprotein among the following is:
    (a) Albumin (b) Casein (c) Gelatin (d) Peptone
12. Quaternary structure is present in all of the following
    except:
    (a) Insulin (b) Haemoglobin (c) Creatine kinase
    (d) Lactate dehydrogenase
13. All the following are lost during denaturation *except*:
    (a) Primary structure (b) Secondary structure (c) Tertiary
    structure (d) Quaternary structure

14. The most abundant plasma protein is:
(a) Albumin (b) β-Globulin (c) γ-Globulin (d) Fibrinogen

15. All the following statements about ceruloplasmin are true *except*:
(a) It is a copper-containing protein (b) It is an acute phase protein (c) It is present in plasma (d) It is a β-globulin

Chapter 6: Chemistry of Nucleotides and Nucleic Acids

1. A methyl group is present as a substituent in:
(a) Thymine (b) Cytosine (c) Adenine (d) Guanine

2. An amino group is present as a substituent at position 6 in:
(a) Thymine (b) Cytosine (c) Adenine (d) Guanine

3. All the following are present in DNA *except*:
(a) Adenine (b) Guanine (c) Uracil (d) Cytosine

4. All the following are present in RNA *except*:
(a) Adenine (b) Guanine (c) Uracil (d) Thymine

5. A phosphate group is attached to carbon atoms 3 and 5 of ribose in:
(a) Cyclic AMP (b) AMP (c) ADP (d) ATP

6. Hypoxanthine is present in:
(a) XMP (b) IMP (c) AMP (d) GMP

7. Complementary base of cytosine is:
(a) Uracil (b) Thymine (c) Adenine (d) Guanine

8. Complementary base of thymine is:
(a) Guanine (b) Adenine (c) Cytosine (d) Uracil

9. Diameter of double helix of B-DNA is:
(a) 3.4 nm (b) 34 nm (c) 2 nm (d) 20 nm

10. Number of base pairs in each turn of helix of B-DNA is:
(a) 10 (b) 11 (c) 12 (d) 14

11. In eukaryotes, the precursor of mRNA is:
(a) snRNA (b) hnRNA (c) 7S RNA (d) None of these

12. In prokaryotes, the precursor of mRNA is:
(a) snRNA (b) hnRNA (c) 7S RNA (d) None of these

13. 7-Methyl GTP cap is present in:
(a) hnRNA (b) mRNA (c) tRNA (d) rRNA

14. Poly-A tail is present in:
(a) mRNA (b) tRNA (c) rRNA (d) snRNA

15. In eukaryotes, some DNA is present in:
(a) Ribosomes (b) Lysosomes (c) Endoplasmic reticulum (d) Mitochondria

Chapter 7: Enzymes

1. A group specific enzyme among the following is:
(a) Amylase (b) Glucokinase (c) Fructokinase (d) Galactokinase

2. A substrate specific enzyme among the following is:
(a) Amylase (b) Hexokinase (c) Fructokinase (d) Aminopeptidase

3. Chymotypsin hydrolyses peptide bonds in which carboxyl group is contributed by:
(a) An aliphatic amino acid (b) A sulphur-containing amino acid (c) An aromatic amino acid (d) A dicarboxylic amino acid

4. A coenzyme that participates in hydrogen transfer reactions is:
(a) Tetrahydrofolate (b) Pyridoxal phosphate (c) Coenzyme A (d) FAD

5. A coenzyme that helps transfer a group other than hydrogen is:
(a) Thiamin pyrophosphate (b) Coenzyme Q (c) FMN (d) FAD

6. Transamination reactions require:
(a) Tetrahydrofolate (b) Pyridoxal phosphate (c) Coenzyme A (d) FAD

7. Tetrahydrofolate is required for transfer of:
(a) Hydrogen (b) Phosphate (c) Amino groups (d) Single-carbon moieties

8. Pantothenic acid is present in:
(a) Coenzyme Q (b) Coenzyme A (c) Cobamides (d) FAD

9. The following enzyme is a transferase:
(a) Acetyl CoA carboxylase (b) Trypsin (c) Hexokinase (d) Fumarase

10. The following enzyme is a hydrolase:
(a) Amylase (b) Aldolase (c) Enolase (d) Fumarase

11. The following enzyme is a lyase:
(a) Pepsin (b) Fumarase (c) Hexokinase (d) Ornithine carbamoyl transferase

12. Lipase is:
(a) An oxidoreductase (b) A transferase (c) A lyase (d) None of these

13. Aldolase is:
(a) An oxidoreductase (b) A lyase (c) A transferase (d) None of these

14. Acetyl CoA carboxylase is:
(a) A ligase (b) A lyase (c) A transferase (d) An oxidoreductase

15. Alanine racemase is:
(a) A ligase (b) A lyase (c) A transferase (d) An isomerase

16. Allosteric enzymes:
(a) Possess at least two binding sites (b) Are catalytically inactive (c) Are regulated by covalent modification (d) None of these

17. Allosteric enzymes:
(a) Generally catalyze an early reaction in a long pathway (b) Are affected by an allosteric modifier (c) Can be regulated positively or negatively (d) All of these

18. Km of an enzyme can be determined by:
(a) Sanger's method (b) Lineweaver-Burk plot (c) Koshland's method (d) Fischer's method

19. Lineweaver-Burk plot is a plot between:
(a) Substrate concentration on x-axis and velocity on y-axis (b) Substrate concentration on y-axis and velocity on x-axis (c) Reciprocal of substrate concentration on x-axis and reciprocal of velocity on y-axis (d) Reciprocal of substrate concentration on y-axis and reciprocal of velocity on x-axis

20. A competitive inhibitor:
(a) Is a substrate analogue (b) Binds to the enzyme reversibly (c) Can displace the substrate from the substrate site (d) All of these

21. **Allopurinol is a:**
(a) Competitive inhibitor of acetylcholinesterase (b) Non-competitive inhibitor of acetylcholinesterase (c) Competitive inhibitor of xanthine oxidase (d) Non-competitive inhibitor of xanthine oxidase

22. **An early indicator of myocardial infarction is:**
(a) Serum LDH (b) Serum CK (c) Serum GOT (d) Serum GPT

23. **A serum enzyme elevated in acute pancreatitis is:**
(a) Creatine kinase (b) Amylase (c) Lactate dehydrogenase (d) Acid phosphatase

24. **Serum alkaline phosphatase is elevated in:**
(a) Acute pancreatitis (b) Cancer of prostate (c) Obstructive jaundice (d) Myocardial infarction

25. **Ceruloplasmin is:**
(a) A copper-containing protein (b) A ferroxidase (c) Absent or greatly decreased in Wilson's disease (d) All of these

Chapter 8: Bio-energetics and Oxidative Phosphorylation

1. **A high-energy phosphate among the following is:**
(a) 1,3-Biphosphoglycerate (b) Carbamoyl phosphate (c) Creatine phosphate (d) All of these

2. **ADP can receive a phosphate group from:**
(a) GTP (b) Phosphoenolpyruvate (c) Creatine kinase (d) All of these

3. **The correct order of the following in respiratory chain is:**
(a) Cyt a, Cyt b, Cyt c, Cyt c_1 (b) Cyt b, Cyt c, Cyt c_1, Cyt a (c) Cyt b, Cyt c_1, Cyt a, Cyt c (d) Cyt b, Cyt a, Cyt c, Cyt c_1

4. **Cytochrome P-450 is present in:**
(a) Outer mitochondrial membrane (b) Cytosol (c) Membrane of endoplasmic reticulum (d) Peroxisomes

5. **Cytochrome a_3 transfers reducing equivalents to:**
(a) Coenzyme Q (b) Oxygen (c) Cytochrome a (d) Cytochrome b

6. **When reducing equivalents are accepted in the respiratory chain by FAD, P:O ratio is:**
(a) 1:1 (b) 2:1 (c) 3:1 (d) 4:1

7. **F_o component of vectorial ATP synthetase is:**
(a) Present in inner mitochondrial membrane (b) A channel for passage of hydrogen ions (c) Made up of a, b and c subunits (d) All of these

8. **Oligomycin inhibits:**
(a) Cytochrome c (b) Cytochrome a_3 (c) F_o component of vectorial ATP synthetase (d) F_1 component of vectorial ATP synthetase

9. **Dinitrophenol:**
(a) Uncouples oxidation and phosphorylation (b) Inhibits oxidative phosphorylation (c) Inhibits F_o component of vectorial ATP synthetase (d) Inhibits F_1 component of vectorial ATP synthetase

10. **An endogenous uncoupler of oxidative phosphorylation is:**
(a) Thermogenin (b) Rotenone (c) Piericidin A (d) None of these

Chapter 9: Citric Acid Cycle

1. **Oxidative decarboxylation of pyruvate converts it into:**
(a) Oxaloacetate (b) Alanine (c) Acetyl CoA (d) Propionyl CoA

2. **A tricarboxylic acid among the following is:**
(a) Oxaloacetate (b) cis-Aconitate (c) Succinate (d) Malate

3. **Citric acid cycle is located in:**
(a) Mitochondria (b) Cytosol (c) Endoplasmic reticulum (d) Peroxisomes

4. **Correct order of the following in citric acid cycle is:**
(a) Oxaloactate, Malate, Fumarate, Succinate (b) Malate, Oxaloactate, Fumarate, Succinate (c) Fumarate, Oxaloactate, Malate, Succinate (d) Succinate, Fumarate, Malate, Oxaloactate

5. **In three reactions of citric acid cycle:**
(a) NAD is reduced (b) FAD is reduced (c) GDP is phosphorylated (d) None of these

6. **In the reaction catalyzed by succinate dehydrogenase:**
(a) NAD is reduced (b) FAD is reduced (c) GDP is phosphorylated (d) None of these

7. **Acetyl CoA is an allosteric inhibitor of:**
(a) Succinate dehydrogenase (b) Malate dehydrogenase (c) Pyruvate dehydrogenase (d) Isocitrate dehydrogenase

8. **α-Ketoglutrate dehydrogenase is inhibited by:**
(a) Succinyl CoA (b) NADH (c) Arsenite (d) All of these

9. **Succinate dehydrogenase is inhibited by:**
(a) Arsenite (b) Fluoroacetate (c) Malonate (d) ATP

10. **Energy captured in one complete revolution of citric acid cycle is:**
(a) Fifteen ATP equivalents (b) Twelve ATP equivalents (c) Eight ATP equivalents (d) Two ATP equivalents

Chapter 10: Metabolism of Carbohydrates

1. **Lactate is the end product of:**
(a) Aerobic glycolysis (b) Anaerobic glycolysis (c) Gluconeogenesis (d) Metabolism of lactose

2. **Glucokinase acts mainly in:**
(a) Fed condition (b) Fasting condition (c) Muscles (d) Brain

3. **Enolase is inhibited by:**
(a) ATP (b) Pyruvate (c) Fluoride (d) Arsenate

4. **The reaction catalyzed by the following is functionally irreversible:**
(a) Phosphohexose isomerase (b) Phosphoglucomutase (c) Enolase (d) Pyruvate kinase

5. **A coenzyme required in glycolysis is:**
(a) NAD (b) NADP (c) FMN (d) FAD

6. **An allosteric enzyme among the following is:**
(a) Phosphohexose isomerase (b) Phosphofructokinase (c) Aldolase (d) Enolase

7. **Allosteric inhibitor of hexokinase is:**
(a) ATP (b) Citrate (c) Glucose-6-phosphate (d) Fructose-6-phosphate

8. **2,3-Biphosphoglycerate is a by-product of glycolysis in:**
(a) Liver (b) Myocardium (c) Brain (d) Erythrocytes

9. Inorganic phosphate is required in the reaction catalyzed by:
(a) Hexokinase (b) Phosphofructokinase (c) Glyceraldehyde-3-phosphate dehydrogenase (d) Pyruvate kinase

10. A coenzyme required in HMP shunt is:
(a) FMN (b) FAD (c) NAD (d) NADPH

11. Transketolase is required in:
(a) Glycolysis (b) HMP shunt (c) Glycogenesis (d) Gluconeogenesis

12. Free glucose is liberated from glycogen by:
(a) Phosphorylase (b) Amylo-1,6-glucosidase (c) UDPG pyrophosphorylase (d) None of these

13. GTP is required in the reaction catalyzed by:
(a) Pyruvate carboxylase (b) Phosphoenolpyruvate carboxykinase (c) Fructose-1,6-biphosphatase (d) Glucose-6-phosphatase

14. Cori cycle transports:
(a) Lactate from muscles to liver (b) Lactate from liver to muscles (c) Pyruvate from muscles to liver (d) Pyruvate from liver to muscles

15. Glucose-alanine cycle transports:
(a) Lactate from muscles to liver (b) Lactate from liver to muscles (c) Pyruvate from muscles to liver (d) Pyruvate from liver to muscles

16. Cori's disease results from absence of:
(a) Debranching enzyme (b) Branching enzyme (c) Glucose-6-phosphatase (d) Phosphorylase

17. Phosphorylase is deficient in muscles in:
(a) von Gierke's disease (b) Cori's disease (c) Her's disease (d) McArdle's disease

18. Aldolase B deficiency impairs the metabolism of:
(a) Glucose (b) Fructose (c) Galactose (d) None of these

19. Congenital absence of galactose-1-phosphate uridyl transferase can cause:
(a) Hepatomegaly (b) Premature cataract (c) Mental retardation (d) All of these

20. Amylo-1,6-glucosidase is absent in:
(a) Tarui's disease (b) Andersen's disease (c) Pompe's disease (d) Cori's disease

21. A hypoglycaemic hormone among the following is:
(a) Epinephrine (b) Growth hormone (c) Insulin (d) Glucagon

22. An insulin-dependent glucose transporter is:
(a) SGLT 1 (b) GLUT 1 (c) GLUT 4 (d) GLUT 5

23. Renal threshold for glucose is:
(a) 180 mg/minute (b) 180 mg/dl (c) 350 mg/minute (d) 350 mg/dl

24. Long-term control of diabetes mellitus can be monitored by measuring:
(a) Fasting blood glucose (b) Post-prandial blood glucose (c) Glycosylated haemoglobin (d) Plasma insulin

25. HbA$_{1c}$ is:
(a) Formed non-enzymatically (b) Normally 4–6% of total haemoglobin (c) A measure of the average blood glucose level over the preceding 6–8 weeks (d) All of these

Chapter 11: Metabolism of Lipids

1. Beta-oxidation of fatty acids occurs in:
(a) Cytosol (b) Mitochondria (c) Partly in cytosol and partly in mitochondria (d) Partly in cytosol and partly in endoplasmic reticulum

2. Carnitine is required to:
(a) Transport short-chain fatty acids into mitochondria (b) Transport long-chain fatty acids into mitochondria (c) Transport short-chain fatty acids out of mitochondria (d) Transport long-chain fatty acids out of mitochondria

3. Propionyl CoA is formed during β-oxidation of:
(a) Monounsaturated fatty acids (b) Polyunsaturated fatty acids (c) Fatty acids having an odd number of carbon atoms (d) Fatty acids having an even number of carbon atoms

4. Activation of fatty acids requires:
(a) No energy (b) One ATP equivalent (c) Two ATP equivalents (d) Four ATP equivalents

5. Unsaturated fatty acids are oxidized by:
(a) α-Oxidation (b) β-Oxidation (c) γ-Oxidation (d) ω-Oxidation

6. A defect in the α-oxidation of fatty acids can cause:
(a) Refsum's disease (b) Wilson's disease (c) Niemann-Pick disease (d) Hartnup disease

7. De novo synthesis of fatty acids is regulated by:
(a) Acyltransferase (b) Acetyl CoA carboxylase (c) Malonyl transferase (d) Thio esterase

8. De novo synthesis of fatty acids is increased by:
(a) Glucagon (b) Insulin (c) Glucocorticoids (d) Epinephrine

9. Acetyl CoA carboxylase is inhibited by:
(a) Acetyl CoA (b) Acetoacetyl CoA (c) Malonyl CoA (d) Palmitoyl CoA

10. A coenzyme required for de novo synthesis of fatty acids is:
(a) NADPH (b) NAD (c) FMN (d) FAD

11. Cerebrosides are synthesized from:
(a) Sphingosine and UDP-galactose (b) Ceramide and UDP-galactose (c) Sphingosine and UDP-glucose (d) Ceramide and UDP-glucose

12. Cerebrosides contain:
(a) Short-chain fatty acids (b) Medium-chain fatty acids (c) Long-chain fatty acids (d) Very long-chain fatty acids

13. N-Acetyl neuraminic acid is required for the synthesis of:
(a) Cerebrosides (b) Sulphatides (c) Gangliosides (d) Plasmalogens

14. Gaucher's disease results from deficiency of:
(a) Hexosaminidase A (b) β-Glucosidase (c) β-Galactosidase (d) None of these

15. Deficiency of arylsulphatase A causes:
(a) Metachromatic leukodystrophy (b) Gaucher's disease (c) Krabbe's disease (d) None of these

16. Tay-Sachs disease results from deficiency of:
(a) Arylsulphatase A (b) Hexosaminidase A (c) β-Galactosidase (d) β-Glucosidase

17. Sphingomyelinase is deficient in:
(a) Krabbe's disease (b) Gaucher's disease (c) Tay-Sachs disease (d) Niemann-Pick disease

18. Very long-chain fatty acids are oxidized in:
(a) Lysosomes (b) Peroxisomes (c) Cytosol (d) Mitochondria

19. All the following are ketone bodies *except*:
(a) Acetone (b) Acetoacetate (c) β-Hydroxybutyrate (d) β-Hydroxy-β-methyl glutarate

20. Cholesterol synthesis is regulated by:
(a) HMG CoA synthetase (b) HMG CoA hydrolase (c) HMG CoA reductase (d) HMG CoA oxidase

21. Very low density lipoproteins are synthesized in:
(a) Small intestine (b) Liver (c) Adipose tissue (d) Muscles

22. Lecithin cholesterol acyl transferase converts:
(a) Nascent chylomicrons into mature chylomicrons (b) Nascent VLDL into mature VLDL (c) Nascent LDL into mature LDL (d) Nascent HDL into mature HDL

23. In Tangier disease:
(a) Synthesis of apoprotein A is decreased (b) Synthesis of apoprotein A is increased (c) Synthesis of apoprotein B is decreased (d) Synthesis of apoprotein B is increased

24. HMG CoA reductase is inhibited by:
(a) Statins (b) Gemfibrozil (c) Nicotinic acid (d) Cholestyramine

25. Aspirin causes:
(a) Irreversible inhibition of cyclo-oxygenase (b) Reversible inhibition of cyclo-oxygenase (c) Irreversible inhibition of phospholipase A_2 (d) Reversible inhibition of phospholipase A_2

Chapter 12: Metabolism of Amino Acids

1. The main acceptor of amino groups of amino acids for urea synthesis is:
(a) Aspartate (b) γ-Aminobutyrate (c) α-Ketoglutarate (d) Glutamate

2. Ubiquitin is required for:
(a) Lysosomal degradation of proteins (b) Cytosolic degradation of proteins (c) Synthesis of urea (d) Synthesis of ubiquinone

3. In adult human beings, daily protein turnover is:
(a) 1–2% (b) 2–5% (c) 5–10% (d) 10–20%

4. Half-life of a protein depends upon its:
(a) Secondary structure (b) Tertiary structure (c) C-Terminal amino acid (d) N-Terminal amino acid

5. Normal concentration of ammonia in blood is:
(a) 10–80 µg/dl (b) 100–200 µg/dl (c) 0.6–1.5 mg/dl (d) 20–40 mg/dl

6. N-Acetylglutamate:
(a) Activates carbamoyl phosphate synthetase I (b) Inhibits carbamoyl phosphate synthetase I (c) Activates carbamoyl phosphate synthetase II (d) Inhibits carbamoyl phosphate synthetase II

7. Glucose can be synthesized from all of the following *except*:
(a) Valine (b) Leucine (c) Serine (d) Proine

8. All the following are required for synthesizing creatine *except*:
(a) Glycine (b) Arginine (c) ATP (d) S-Adenosyl methionine

9. All the following can be synthesized from tyrosine *except*:
(a) Epinephrine (b) Norepinephrine (c) Thyroxine (d) Melatonin

10. All the following can be synthesized from tryptophan *except*:
(a) Nicotinic acid (b) Serotonin (c) Melatonin (d) Melanin

11. Nitric oxide is synthesized from:
(a) Ornithine (b) Citrulline (c) Arginine (d) None of these

12. Maple syrup urine disease is a disorder of:
(a) Sulphur-containing amino acids (b) Branched-chain amino acids (c) Aromatic amino acids (d) Dicarboxylic amino acids

13. A low-phenylalanine diet is given for the treatment of:
(a) Alkaptonuria (b) Phenylketonuria (c) Tyrosinaemia (d) Albinism

14. Homogentisate oxidase is absent in:
(a) Alkaptonuria (b) Phenylketonuria (c) Tyrosinaemia (d) Albinism

15. A pellagra-like picture can appear in:
(a) Primary hyperoxaluria (b) Albinism (c) Histidinaemia (d) Hartnup disease

Chapter 13: Metabolism of Nucleotides

1. During de novo synthesis, the following carbon atom of purine nucleus is contributed by carbon dioxide:
(a) 2 (b) 4 (c) 6 (d) 8

2. De novo synthesis of purine nucleotides begins with the formation of:
(a) 5-Phosphoribosyl-1-pyrophosphate (b) Glycinamide ribosyl-5-phosphate (c) Inosine monophosphate (d) Xanthosine monophosphate

3. The first reaction unique to de novo synthesis of purine nucleotides is catalyzed by:
(a) PRPP synthetase (b) PRPP glutamyl amidotransferase (c) Phosphoribosyl glycinamide synthetase (d) Formyl transferase

4. The following purine base can be salvaged:
(a) Adenine (b) Guanine (c) Hypoxanthine (d) All of these

5. In human beings, uric acid is the end product of:
(a) Purine catabolism (b) Pyrimidine catabolism (c) Protein catabolism (d) All of these

6. Conversion of ribonucleotides into deoxyribonucleotides requires:
(a) NADPH (b) Thioredoxin (c) Thioredoxin reductase (d) All of these

7. Hyperuricaemia occurs in:
(a) Gout (b) Adenosine deaminase deficiency (c) Purine nucleoside phosphorylase deficiency (d) All of these

8. Uric acid begins to precipitate when its plasma level *exceeds*:
(a) 2 mg/dl (b) 5 mg/dl (c) 7 mg/dl (d) 10 mg/dl

9. A drug that decreases the synthesis of uric acid is:
   (a) Colchicine (b) Allopurinol (c) Probenecid (d) Alcohol

10. A non-competitive inhibitor of xanthine oxidase is:
    (a) Allopurinol (b) Febuxostat (c) Probenecid (d) Colchicine

11. Immunodeficiency occurs in inherited deficiency of:
    (a) HGPRT (b) Adenosine deaminase (c) PRPP synthetase (d) Xanthine oxidase

12. Inherited absence of HGPRT causes:
    (a) Primary gout (b) Immunodeficiency (c) Retardation of growth (d) Neurological abnormalities

13. Lesch-Nyhan syndrome results from inherited absence of:
    (a) PRPP synthetase (b) Adenine phosphoribosyl transferase (c) Hypoxanthine-guanine phosphoribosyl transferase (d) Adenosine deaminase

14. Immunodeficiency can occur in deficiency of:
    (a) Adenosine deaminase (b) Purine nucleoside phosphorylase (c) Orotate phosphoribosyl transferase (d) All of these

15. Megaloblastic anaemia occurs in:
    (a) Primary gout (b) Adenosine deaminase deficiency (c) Orotic aciduria (d) None of these

Chapter 14: Metabolism of Nucleic Acids

1. Replication means:
   (a) Synthesis of RNA (b) Synthesis of proteins (c) Synthesis of DNA (d) Supercoiling of DNA

2. Synthesis of DNA is:
   (a) Discontinuous (b) Semi-discontinuous (c) Conservative (d) Non-conservative

3. DNA polymerase can:
   (a) Add a mononucleotide to another mononucleotide (b) Add a mononucleotide to an oligonucleotide (c) Add an oligonucleotide to another oligonuleotide (d) Do all of these

4. RNA primer is required to initiate:
   (a) Replication (b) Transcription (c) Translation (d) None of these

5. Primase is required for synthesis of:
   (a) DNA (b) hnRNA (c) tRNA (d) rRNA

6. Telomerase is a:
   (a) DNA polymerase (b) RNA polymerase (c) Reverse transcriptase (d) None of these

7. DNA polymerase γ is present in:
   (a) Eukaryotes (b) Bacteria (c) Viruses (d) All of these

8. DNA polymerase γ is present in:
   (a) Nucleus (b) Nucleolus (c) Mitochondria (d) Cytosol

9. A drug that inhibits the synthesis of DNA in prokaryotes is:
   (a) Rifampicin (b) Oligomycin (c) Ciprofloxacin (d) α-Amanitin

10. Sigma factor is required to recognize:
    (a) Initiation site for transcription (b) Termination site for transcription (c) Initiation site for replication (d) Termination site for replication

11. In eukaryotes, the precursor of mRNA is:
    (a) snRNA (b) hnRNA (c) 7S RNA (d) siRNA

12. Introns are present in:
    (a) rRNA (b) tRNA (c) mRNA (d) hnRNA

13. Primers are:
    (a) Polypeptides (b) Polyribonucleotides (c) Polydeoxyribonucleotides (d) None of these

14. Intragenic promoters are present in:
    (a) mRNA genes (b) tRNA genes (c) rRNA genes (d) None of these

15. 7-MethylGTP cap is present in:
    (a) tRNA (b) rRNA (c) mRNA (d) hnRNA

Chapter 15: Genetic Code and Protein Synthesis

1. Nonsense codons are responsible for:
   (a) Degeneracy of genetic code (b) Unambiguity of genetic code (c) Chain termination (d) Wobble in base pairing

2. Nonsense codons:
   (a) Do not encode amino acids (b) Have no complementary anticodons (c) Are different in nuclear and mitochondrial DNA (d) All of these

3. Introns:
   (a) Are non-coding sequences (b) Are present in between exons (c) Are not present in prokaryotes (d) All of these

4. ATPase activity is present in:
   (a) Eukaryotic Initiation Factor 4A (b) Eukaryotic Initiation Factor 4B (c) Eukaryotic Initiation Factor 4F (d) Eukaryotic Initiation Factor 5

5. Streptomycin inhibits binding of:
   (a) Formylmethionyl tRNA to 30S ribosomal subunit (b) Formylmethionyl tRNA to 50S ribosomal subunit (c) Methionyl tRNA to 40S ribosomal subunit (d) Methionyl tRNA to 60S ribosomal subunit

6. Binding of all amino acyl tRNAs to 30S ribosomal subunits is inhibited by:
   (a) Streptomycin (b) Chloramphenicol (c) Erythromycin (d) Tetracyclins

7. Peptidyl transferase activity in 50S ribosomal subunit is inhibited by:
   (a) Streptomycin (b) Chloramphenicol (c) Erythromycin (d) Tetracyclins

8. Elongation Factor G is inhibited by:
   (a) Streptomycin (b) Chloramphenicol (c) Erythromycin (d) Tetracyclins

9. In eukaryotes, peptidyl transferase activity is present in:
   (a) 5S rRNA (b) 5.8S rRNA (c) 18S rRNA (d) 28S rRNA

10. Shine-Dalgarno sequence is present in:
    (a) Prokaryotic mRNA (b) Prokaryotic tRNA (c) Prokaryotic rRNA (d) Eukaryotic hnRNA

11. Cistron is the coding unit for one:
    (a) Amino acid (b) Polypeptide (c) Protein (d) None of these

12. Signal sequence is present in proteins destined for:
    (a) Export from the cell (b) Nucleus (c) Mitochondria (d) Peroxisomes

13. An example of acceptable mis-sense mutation is:
(a) Haemoglobin S (b) Haemoglobin M (c) Haemoglobin Sydney (d) None of these

14. Mannose-6-phosphate prosthetic group of proteins targets them to:
(a) Peroxisomes (b) Lysosomes (c) Nucleus (d) Mitochondria

15. Thymine dimers can be formed on exposure of DNA to:
(a) Nitrosamine (b) Nitrous oxide (c) Ultraviolet light (d) All of these

Chapter 16: Recombinant DNA Technology

1. Restriction endonucleases act on:
(a) Double-stranded DNA (b) 4–8 Base pair sequences (c) Palindromic sequences (d) All of these

2. All of the following are cloning vectors *except*:
(a) Baculovirus (b) Plasmid (c) Cosmid (d) Bacteriophage

3. Southern blotting is used to recognize a particular:
(a) Protein (b) DNA (c) RNA (d) All of these

4. Northern blotting is used to recognize a particular:
(a) Protein (b) DNA (c) RNA (d) All of these

5. Western blotting is used to recognize a particular:
(a) Protein (b) DNA (c) RNA (d) All of these

6. A radio active cDNA probe is commonly used in:
(a) Western blotting (b) Southern blotting (c) Sanger's method of DNA sequencing (d) Maxam-Gilbert method of DNA sequencing

7. A radio active antibody probe is commonly used in:
(a) Southern blotting (b) Northern blotting (c) Eastern blotting (d) Western blotting

8. Taq polymerase is commonly used in polymerase chain reaction because:
(a) It does not require a primer (b) It acts more rapidly than any other DNA polymerase (c) It is not denatured at 95°C (d) It is not destroyed by antibiotics

9. Polymerase chain reaction requires all of the following *except*:
(a) Template DNA (b) Deoxyribonucleoside triphosphates (c) Primase (d) Taq polymerase

10. A DNA up to 45 kb in size can be amplified using:
(a) Polymerase chain reaction (b) Cosmids (c) Plasmids (d) Bacteriophages

11. Taq polymerase acts optimally at:
(a) 95°C (b) 72°C (c) 56°C (d) 37°C

12. In polymerase chain reaction, the primer binds to target DNA at:
(a) 95°C (b) 72°C (c) 56°C (d) 37°C

13. All the following can be used as expression vectors *except*:
(a) Cosmid (b) Plasmid (c) Baculovirus (d) Vaccinia virus

14. VNTR pattern is used commonly in:
(a) DNA sequencing (b) DNA finger-printing (c) Diagnosis of genetic diseases (d) Production of recombinant proteins

15. Severe combined immunodeficiency disease:
(a) Causes severe impairment of humoral and cell-mediated immunity (b) Is caused by adenosine deaminase deficiency (c) Is being treated successfully by gene therapy (d) All of these

Chapter 17: Hormones

1. All the following are hydrophilic hormones *except*:
(a) Catecholamines (b) Thyroid hormones (c) Peptide hormones (d) Protein hormones

2. All of the following have intracellular receptors *except*:
(a) Insulin (b) Calcitriol (c) Thyroid hormones (d) Steroid hormones

3. Tyrosine kinase/phosphatase is involved in the action of:
(a) Oxytocin (b) Growth hormone (c) Nitric oxide (d) Glucagon

4. All the following have membrane-bound receptors *except*:
(a) Epinephrine (b) Insulin (c) Thyroxine (d) Glucagon

5. A hormone-response element is involved in the action of:
(a) Glucocorticoids (b) Glucagon (c) Growth hormone (d) All of these

6. Hormone-response elements are located in:
(a) Nucleus (b) Mitochondria (c) Cell membrane (d) Cytosol

7. cAMP mediates the action of:
(a) Glucagon (b) Insulin (c) Oxytocin (d) Atrial natriuretic peptide

8. cGMP mediates the action of:
(a) Glucagon (b) Insulin (c) Oxytocin (d) Atrial natriuretic peptide

9. Ca^{++} and/or phosphoinositides mediate the action of:
(a) Glucagon (b) Insulin (c) Oxytocin (d) Atrial natriuretic peptide

10. Tyrosine kinase/phosphatase is involved in the action of all the following *except*:
(a) Growth hormone (b) Nerve growth factor (c) Epidermal growth factor (d) Insulin

11. The second messenger for insulin is:
(a) cAMP (b) cGMP (c) Tyrosine kinase (d) Diacyl glycerol

12. All the following are second messengers for hormones *except*:
(a) cAMP (b) cGMP (c) Nitric oxide (d) Diacyl glycerol

13. G-proteins:
(a) Are trimers (b) Have a GDP/GTP binding site (c) Act as signal transducers (d) All of these

14. Signal transducers are:
(a) Located in the cell membrane (b) G-proteins (c) Required by all the hormones (d) All of these

15. Signal transducers:
(a) Are proteins (b) Are made up of α-, β- and γ-subunits (c) Carry the signal from receptor to effector (d) All of these

16. Insulin receptor is:
(a) A tetramer (b) Made up of α, β, γ and δ subunits (c) Located in the cytosol (d) All of these

17. Phospholipase C:
(a) Is located in the cell membrane (b) Acts on phosphatidyl inositol-4,5-biphosphate (c) Produces inositol triphosphate and diacylglycerol (d) All of these

18. Diacylglycerol activates:
    (a) Protein kinase A (b) Protein kinase C (c) Protein kinase G (d) Calmodulin kinase

19. The only correct statement about insulin receptor is:
    (a) It is made up of two α and two β subunits (b) Its β subunits are extracellular (c) Its α subunits are trans-membrane (d) Its α subunits possess tyrosine kinase domain

20. All the following are required for radioimmunoassay of hormones *except*:
    (a) Radio-labeled hormone (b) Unlabeled hormone (c) Receptor for hormone (d) Antibody against hormone

21. A hormone synthesized from tryptophan is:
    (a) Melatonin (b) Melanin (c) Melanocyte-stimulating hormone (d) None of these

22. Glucagon is secreted by the following cells of islets of Langerhans:
    (a) α cells (b) β cells (c) δ cells (d) F cells

23. Lispro insulin:
    (a) Is a genetically engineered insulin (b) Does not polymerize (c) Acts very rapidly (d) All of these

24. Diabetes mellitus, type 1 is caused by:
    (a) Destruction of β cells of islets of Langerhans (b) Decreased number of insulin receptors (c) Antibodies against insulin receptors (d) Any of these

25. Long-term control of diabetes mellitus can be monitored by periodical measurement of:
    (a) Fasting blood glucose (b) Post-prandial blood glucose (c) Hb A_{1c} (d) Any of these

Chapter 18: Cancer: Proto-oncogenes, Oncogenes and Anti-oncogenes

1. Cancer can be caused by all of the following *except*:
   (a) Oncogenic bacteria (b) Oncoviruses (c) Mutagenic chemicals (d) Ionizing radiation

2. Oncogenes are present in:
   (a) Oncoviruses (b) Oncogenic bacteria (c) Healthy human cells (d) Healthy animals

3. Proto-oncogenes are present in:
   (a) Oncoviruses (b) Oncogenic bacteria (c) Healthy human cells (d) All of these

4. Proto-oncogenes may encode all of the following *except*:
   (a) Growth factors (b) Receptors for growth factors (c) Signal transducers (d) Carcinogenic proteins

5. All the following statements about proto-oncogenes are correct *except*:
   (a) They encode some essential proteins (b) They are dominant genes (c) They protect us against cancer (d) They can undergo mutations

6. All the following are proto-oncogenes *except*:
   (a) sis gene (b) p 16 gene (c) ras gene (d) fos gene

7. All the following are anti-oncogenes *except*:
   (a) p 53 gene (b) p 16 gene (c) myc gene (d) NF-1 gene

8. Platelet-derived growth factor is encoded by:
   (a) An oncogene (b) A proto-oncogene (c) An anti-oncogene (d) A tumour suppressor gene

9. Malignant transformation may be caused by:
   (a) Point mutation in a proto-oncogene (b) Deletion of a part of a proto-oncogene (c) Chromosomal translocation involving a proto-oncogene (d) All of these

10. If DNA is found to be damaged, p 53 arrests the cell cycle in:
    (a) M phase (b) G_1 phase (c) S phase (d) G_2 phase

11. Li-Fraumeni syndrome is caused by an inherited mutation in:
    (a) p 16 gene (b) p 53 gene (c) NF-1 gene (d) BRCA-1 gene

12. Xeroderma pigmentosum results from a:
    (a) Defect in nucleotide excision repair system (b) Mutation in NF-1 gene (c) Mutation in DCC gene (d) None of these

13. A tumour marker useful in the diagnosis of chorio-carcinoma is:
    (a) CA 125 (b) AFP (c) CEA (d) hCG

14. Ames' assay is a rapid method for detecting:
    (a) Malignant transformation (b) Oncoviruses (c) Mutant oncogenes (d) Mutagenicity of chemicals

15. The tester strain of *Salmonella typhimurium* used in Ames' assay cannot grow in the absence of:
    (a) Tryptophan (b) Tyrosine (c) Histidine (d) Methionine

Chapter 19: Immunochemistry

1. Antigenic determinant is present in:
   (a) Antigen (b) Light chain of antibody (c) Heavy chain of antibody (d) Complement C_1

2. An antibody recognizes the following part of the antigen:
   (a) Hapten (b) Epitope (c) Paratope (d) Variable region

3. Paratope is present in:
   (a) Hapten (b) Antigen (c) Antibody (d) None of these

4. An antibody molecule possesses at least:
   (a) Two polypeptide chains (b) Four polypeptide chains (c) Eight polypeptide chains (d) Ten polypeptide chains

5. The light chains of antibodies:
   (a) Are of two types (b) Have a molecular weight of about 23,000 (c) Have a constant region and a variable region (d) All of these

6. The heavy chains of antibodies are of following types:
   (a) α, β, γ, κ and λ (b) α, β, γ, δ and λ (c) α, γ, δ, ε and μ (d) α, β, γ, κ and μ

7. Antibodies are classified on the basis of their:
   (a) Size (b) Heavy chains (c) Light chains (d) Idiotypes

8. The antibody present in the highest concentration in plasma is:
   (a) Immunoglobulin A (b) Immunoglobulin D (c) Immunoglobulin E (d) Immunoglobulin G

9. The antibody present in lowest concentration in plasma is:
   (a) Immunoglobulin A (b) Immunoglobulin D (c) Immunoglobulin E (d) Immunoglobulin G

10. The variable regions of light chains and heavy chains have:
    (a) One hypervariable region (b) Two hypervariable

regions (c) Three hypervariable regions (d) Four hypervariable regions

11. **The antibody having the largest size is:**
(a) Immunoglobulin M (b) Immunoglobulin G (c) Immunoglobulin D (d) Immunoglobulin A

12. **The following can cross the placental barrier:**
(a) Immunoglobulin M (b) Immunoglobulin G (c) Immunoglobulin D (d) Immunoglobulin A

13. **The following can act against parasites:**
(a) Immunoglobulin M (b) Immunoglobulin G (c) Immunoglobulin E (d) Immunoglobulin A

14. **Four light chains and four heavy chains are present in:**
(a) Secretory IgA (b) IgG (c) IgE (d) IgM

15. **The antigen receptor on B lymphocytes is made up of:**
(a) IgA (b) IgG (c) IgE (d) IgM

16. **An effector function of antibodies is:**
(a) Neutralization (b) Opsonization (c) Complement activation (d) All of these

17. **The following can activate the complement system:**
(a) Immunoglobulin E (b) Immunoglobulin M (c) Immunoglobulin D (d) Immunoglobulin A

18. **We can synthesize a huge variety of antibodies from a small number of immunoglobulin genes because of:**
(a) Gene re-arrangement (b) Gene amplification (c) Alternate splicing of hnRNA (d) mRNA editing

19. **Secretory component of secretory IgA is formed from:**
(a) Immunoglobulin light chains (b) Immunoglobulin heavy chains (c) J chains (d) Immunoglobulin receptor

20. **A light chain gene is made up of:**
(a) Variable, joining and constant segments (b) Variable and joining segments (c) Joining and constant segments (d) Variable and constant segments

21. **A heavy chain gene is made up of:**
(a) Variable, joining and constant segments (b) Variable, joining, diversity and constant segments (c) Diversity, joining and constant segments (d) Variable and constant segments

22. **Antibody diversity arises from:**
(a) Gene re-arrangement (b) Junctional diversity (c) Somatic hypermutation (d) All of these

23. **The first antibody to be formed upon first entry of any antigen is:**
(a) Immunoglobulin G (b) Immunoglobulin A (c) Immunoglobulin M (d) Immunoglobulin E

24. **Hybridoma cells are formed by fusion of:**
(a) B lymphocytes and T lymphocytes (b) B lymphocytes and myeloma cells (c) T lymphocytes and myeloma cells (d) B lymphocytes and macrophages

25. **Hybridoma cells are cultured in a medium containing:**
(a) Hypoxanthine, aspartate and thymidine (b) Hypoxanthine, aminopterin and thymidine (c) Hypoxanthine, asparagine and thymidine (d) Hypoxanthine, aminopterin and thymine

26. **The following enzyme is not present in hybridoma cells:**
(a) Thymidine kinase (b) Thymine phosphoribosyl transferase (c) Adenine phosphoribosyl transferase (d) Hypoxanthine guanine phosphoribosyl transferase

27. **Hybridoma cells:**
(a) Are formed by fusion of B cells and myeloma cells (b) Are immortal cells (c) Secrete a particular monoclonal antibody (d) All of these

28. **The classic complement cascade can be activated by:**
(a) IgG and IgM (b) IgA and IgG (c) IgM and IgA (d) IgE and IgG

29. **The alternate complement pathway can be activated by:**
(a) IgG and IgM (b) IgA and IgG (c) IgM and IgA (d) None of these

30. **The correct sequence of events in the classic complement cascade is:**
(a) Recognition phase, activation phase and membrane attack phase (b) Recognition phase and membrane attack phase (c) Activation phase and membrane attack phase (d) Recognition phase and activation phase

31. **T lymphocytes are responsible for:**
(a) Complement activation (b) Humoral immunity (c) Cell-mediated immunity (d) Innate immunity

32. **Diversity of T cell receptors arises from:**
(a) Differential processing in thymus (b) Altered splicing of hnRNA (c) Gene re-arrangement (d) None of these

33. **MHC proteins:**
(a) Are present on the surface of all the cells (b) Are unique to each individual (c) Have antigen-binding site (d) All of these

34. **Antigen-binding site on T cell receptor is formed of:**
(a) Variable regions of light and heavy chains (b) Variable regions of α and β chains (c) Variable region of MHC I proteins (d) Variable region of MHC II proteins

35. **Cytotoxic T cells recognize:**
(a) Antigen fragments attached to MHC I proteins (b) Antigen fragments attached to MHC II proteins (c) Antigen fragments attached to MHC III proteins (d) Antigens bound to antibodies

36. **Antigen-presenting cells are:**
(a) Follicular dendritic cells (b) B lymphocytes (c) Macrophages (d) All of these

37. **Antigen fragments bound to antigen-presenting cells are recognized by:**
(a) Plasma cells (b) Cytotoxic T cells (c) Helper T cells (d) Suppressor T cells

38. **CD4 is a transmembrane protein present in:**
(a) Plasma cells (b) Cytotoxic T cells (c) Helper T cells (d) Suppressor T cells

39. **CD8 is a transmembrane protein present in:**
(a) Plasma cells (b) Cytotoxic T cells (c) Helper T cells (d) Suppressor T cells

40. **Perforin, granzymes and granulysin are released by:**
(a) Plasma cells (b) Cytotoxic T cells (c) Helper T cells (d) Suppressor T cells

41. **Interleukins, tumour necrosis factor and interferon-γ are released by:**
(a) Plasma cells (b) Cytotoxic T cells (c) Helper T cells (d) Suppressor T cells

42. **Acquired immunodeficiency can occur due to:**
(a) Severe undernutrition (b) Irradiation (c) HIV infection (d) All of these

43. HIV binds avidly to:
    (a) B cells (b) Cytotoxic T cells (c) Helper T cells (d) Suppressor T cells

44. Allergens bind to:
    (a) IgA (b) IgG (c) IgD (d) IgE

45. IgE is bound to the surface of:
    (a) Plasma cells (b) Mast cells (c) Macrophages (d) T cells

Chapter 20: Porphyrins, Haemoglobin and Bilirubin

1. All the following contain porphyrin *except*:
   (a) Trytophan pyrrolase (b) Tryptophan hydroxylase (c) Catalase (d) Peroxidase

2. All the following substituents are present in haem *except*:
   (a) Acetate (b) Propionate (c) Methyl group (d) Vinyl group

3. Porphyrin present in haem is of the type:
   (a) Coproporphyrin (b) Uroporphyrin (c) Protoporphyrin (d) None of these

4. An amino acid required for porphyrin synthesis is:
   (a) Proline (b) Phenylalanine (c) Valine (d) Glycine

5. The most abundant porphyrin is:
   (a) Protoporphyrin I (b) Protoporphyrin III (c) Uroporphyrin I (d) Uroporphyrin III

6. The enzyme that regulates porphyrin synthesis is:
   (a) δ-Aminolevulinic acid synthetase (b) δ-Aminolevulinic acid dehydrase (c) Ferrochelatase (d) Haem synthetase

7. δ-Aminolevulinic acid synthetase is regulated by:
   (a) Induction (b) Repression (c) Covalent modification (d) Allosteric mechanism

8. The polypeptide chains in haemoglobin are of following types:
   (a) α and β (b) α, β and γ (c) α, β, γ and δ (d) α, β, γ, δ and ε

9. Embryonic haemoglobin contains:
   (a) Two α and two β chains (b) Two α and two γ chains (c) Two α and two δ chains (d) Two α and two ε chains

10 Foetal haemoglobin contains:
   (a) Two α and two β chains (b) Two α and two γ chains (c) Two α and two δ chains (d) Two α and two ε chains

11. Hb A contains:
   (a) Two α and two β chains (b) Two α and two γ chains (c) Two α and two δ chains (d) Two α and two ε chains

12. Hb A_2 contains:
   (a) Two α and two β chains (b) Two α and two γ chains (c) Two α and two δ chains (d) Two α and two ε chains

13. One molecule of haemoglobin can bind:
   (a) One oxygen molecule (b) Two oxygen molecules (c) Three oxygen molecules (d) Four oxygen molecules

14. Oxygenated myoglobin releases oxygen when pO_2 falls to about:
   (a) 80 mm Hg (b) 60 mm Hg (c) 40 mm Hg (d) 20 mm Hg

15. In Hb S, an amino acid substitution occurs in:
   (a) α chain (b) β chain (c) γ chain (d) δ chain

16. In Hb S, the amino acid substitution is:
   (a) Replacement of glutamate by valine (b) Replacement of valine by glutamate (c) Replacement of glutamate by leucine (d) Replacement of leucine by glutamate

17. Uroporphyrin I synthetase is deficient in:
   (a) Acute intermittent porphyria (b) Porphyria cutanea tarda (c) Hereditary coproporphyria (d) Protoporphyria

18. Uroporphyrinogen decarboxylase is deficient in:
   (a) Acute intermittent porphyria (b) Porphyria cutanea tarda (c) Hereditary coproporphyria (d) Protoporphyria

19. Coproporphyrinogen oxidase is deficient in:
   (a) Acute intermittent porphyria (b) Porphyria cutanea tarda (c) Hereditary coproporphyria (d) Protoporphyria

20. Ferrochelatase is deficient in:
   (a) Acute intermittent porphyria (b) Porphyria cutanea tarda (c) Hereditary coproporphyria (d) Protoporphyria

Chapter 21: Water-soluble Vitamins

1. Transketolase require the following as a coenzyme:
   (a) Thiamin diphosphate (b) Flavin mononucleotide (c) Flavin adenine dinucleotide (d) Nicotinamide adenine dinucleotide

2. Thiamin diphosphate is required in all the following *except*:
   (a) Citric acid cycle (b) Glycolysis (c) Hexose monophosphate shunt (d) Oxidative decarboxylation of pyruvate

3. Requirement for thiamin is greater than normal in:
   (a) Hypothyroidism (b) Anaemia (c) Alcoholics (d) None of these

4. Blood level of the following is raised in beriberi:
   (a) Thiamin (b) Thiamin diphosphate (c) Lactic acid (d) Pyruvic acid

5. The daily requirement for riboflavin is:
   (a) 0.1 mg/1,000 kcal (b) 0.6 mg/1,000 kcal (c) 5 mg/day (d) 20 mg/day

6. Angular stomatitis, cheilosis and glossitis occur in deficiency of:
   (a) Thiamin (b) Riboflavin (c) Niacin (d) Pantothenic acid

7. Pellagra-preventing factor is:
   (a) Thiamin (b) Riboflavin (c) Niacin (d) Pantothenic acid

8. Human beings can synthesize niacin from:
   (a) NAD (b) Leucine (c) Tryptophan (d) Proline

9. Excess of leucine inhibits the synthesis of:
   (a) Niacin (b) NAD (c) NADP (d) None of these

10. One mg of niacin can be synthesized from:
   (a) 30 mg of leucine (b) 60 mg of leucine (c) 30 mg of tryptophan (d) 60 mg of tryptophan

11. Diarrhoea, dermatitis and dementia occur in deficiency of:
   (a) Niacin (b) Pantothenic acid (c) Pyridoxine (d) None of these

12. Coenzyme A is formed from the vitamin:
   (a) Riboflavin (b) Niacin (c) Pantothenic acid (d) Pyridoxine

13. Vitamin B_6 activity is present in:
    (a) Pyridoxal (b) Pyridoxine (c) Pyridoxamine (d) All of these

14. Pyridoxal phosphate acts as a coenzyme in:
    (a) Oxidation-reduction (b) Oxidative decarboxylation (c) Oxidative deamination (d) Transamination

15. Pyridoxal phosphate is required for the catabolism of:
    (a) Haem (b) Tryptophan (c) Ketone bodies (d) Cholesterol

16. Urinary excretion of xanthurenic acid is increased in deficiency of:
    (a) Riboflavin (b) Niacin (c) Pantothenic acid (d) Pyridoxine

17. Synthesis of pyridoxal phosphate can be inhibited by:
    (a) Thiacetazone (b) Isoniazid (c) Rifampicin (d) None of these

18. Avidin prevents the intestinal absorption of:
    (a) Biotin (b) Niacin (c) Pantothenic acid (d) Pyridoxine

19. A vitamin that acts as a co-caboxylase is:
    (a) Lipoic acid (b) Biotin (c) Pantothenic acid (d) Pyridoxine

20. All the following are required in oxidative decarboxylation of α-keto acids *except*:
    (a) Coenzyme A (b) Pyridoxal phosphate (c) Thiamin diphosphate (d) Lipoic acid

21. A coenzyme that transfers one-carbon units is:
    (a) Biotin (b) Lipoic acid (c) Tetrahydrofolate (d) CoA

22. Tetrahydrofolate can receive one-carbon units from:
    (a) Formiminoglutamic acid (b) Methionine (c) Serine (d) All of these

23. Tetrahydrofolate can transfer its one-carbon units to:
    (a) Homocysteine (b) Deoxyuridine monophosphate (c) Serine (d) All of these

24. Daily requirement of folic acid in adults is:
    (a) 1 μg/day (b) 10 μg/day (c) 100 μg/day (d) 1,000 μg/day

25. Folic acid deficiency causes:
    (a) Megaloblastic anaemia (b) Normocytic anaemia (c) Microcytic anaemia (d) Polycythaemia

26. Urinary FIGLU is increased:
    (a) In histidine deficiency (b) In folic acid deficiency (c) After excessive intake of histidine (d) After excessive intake of folic acid

27. Intrinsic factor is required for:
    (a) Absorption of vitamin B_{12} (b) Absorption of folic acid (c) Activation of vitamin B_{12} (d) Activation of folic acid

28. Intrinsic factor is a:
    (a) Vitamin (b) Coenzyme (c) Glycoprotein (d) Carbohydrate

29. Synthesis of methionine from homocysteine requires:
    (a) Hydroxycobalamin (b) Methylcobalamin (c) Nitrocobalamin (d) None of these

30. Methylmalonic aciduria occurs in deficiency of:
    (a) Vitamin B_{12} (b) Folic acid (c) Lipoic acid (d) Pyridoxine

31. Pernicious anaemia results from:
    (a) Combined dietary deficiency of folic acid and vitamin B_{12} (b) Combined dietary deficiency of iron and folic acid
    (c) Combined dietary deficiency of iron and vitamin B_{12}
    (d) Absence of intrinsic factor

32. Subacute combined degeneration of spinal cord occurs in:
    (a) Pernicious anaemia (b) Nutritional deficiency of vitamin B_{12} (c) Folic acid deficiency (d) Thiamin deficiency

33. Folate trap occurs due to:
    (a) Folic acid deficiency (b) Vitamin B_{12} deficiency (c) Folic acid antagonists (d) Methionine deficiency

34. L-Gulonolactone oxidase is required to synthesize:
    (a) Gulonic acid (b) Ascorbic acid (c) Dehydroascorbic acid (d) Folic acid

35. A vitamin required for formation of intercellular cement substance is:
    (a) Vitamin C (b) Vitamin A (c) Folic acid (d) Vitamin B_{12}

36. An anti-oxidant among the following is:
    (a) Niacin (b) Vitamin B_{12} (c) Vitamin C (d) Pantothenic acid

37. Scurvy is caused by deficiency of:
    (a) Ascorbic acid (b) Vitamin B_{12} (c) Pyridoxine (d) Pantothenic acid

38. The vitamin having the lowest daily requirement is:
    (a) Niacin (b) Vitamin B_{12} (c) Vitamin C (d) Pantothenic acid

39. The vitamin having the highest daily requirement is:
    (a) Niacin (b) Vitamin B_{12} (c) Vitamin C (d) Pantothenic acid

40. Anaemia can occur in deficiency of:
    (a) Pyridoxine (b) Folic acid (c) Vitamin B_{12} (d) All of these

Chapter 22: Fat-soluble Vitamins

1. Retinal is:
   (a) Vitamin A (b) Vitamin D (c) Vitamin E (d) Vitamin K

2. A β-ionone ring attached to a polyene chain is present in:
   (a) Vitamin A (b) Vitamin D (c) Vitamin E (d) Vitamin K

3. Carotenes are:
   (a) Provitamin A (b) Provitamin D (c) Provitamin E (d) Provitamin K

4. A precursor of vitamin A is:
   (a) α-Carotene (b) β-Carotene (c) γ-Carotene (d) All of these

5. Two β-ionone rings are present in:
   (a) α-Carotene (b) β-Carotene (c) γ-Carotene (d) All of these

6. Albumin transports:
   (a) Carotenes (b) Retinol (c) Retinoic acid (d) All of these

7. Chylomicrons transport:
   (a) Retinal (b) Retinol (c) Retinoic acid (d) Carotenes

8. The prosthetic group in rhodopsin is:
   (a) All-cis-retinal (b) All-trans-retinal (c) 11-cis-retinal (d) 11-trans-retinal

9. When light falls on rod cells, 11-cis-retinal is converted into:
   (a) 11-trans-retinal (b) All-trans-retinal (c) 11-cis-retinol (d) All-trans-retinol

10. **Dark adaptation time depends upon:**
    (a) Vitamin A stores in retina (b) Retinene reductase activity in retina (c) Vitamin A stores in liver (d) Retinol isomerase activity in liver

11. **Transducin is:**
    (a) Present in rod cells (b) A G-protein (c) A trimer (d) All of these

12. **Transducin is a:**
    (a) Photoreceptor (b) Second messenger (c) GDP/GTP binding protein (d) None of these

13. **When light falls on rod cells, the following enzyme is activated:**
    (a) Guanylate cyclase (b) cGMP phosphodiesterase (c) Retinene reductase (d) Adenylate cyclase

14. **When light falls on rod cells, the concentration of:**
    (a) cGMP increases (b) cGMP decreases (c) cAMP increases (d) cAMP decreases

15. **Decreased concentration of cGMP in rod cells causes:**
    (a) Closure of cation-specific channels (b) Opening of cation-specific channels (c) Closure of anion-specific channels (d) Opening of anion-specific channels

16. **One retinol equivalent is the vitamin A activity present in:**
    (a) 1 μg of retinol (b) 6 μg of β-carotene (c) 12 μg of α-carotene (d) All of these

17. **The earliest clinical abnormality in vitamin A deficiency is:**
    (a) Night blindness (b) Prolonged dark adaptation time (c) Bitot's spots (d) Xerophthalmia

18. **The anti-rachitic factor is:**
    (a) Vitamin A (b) Vitamin D (c) Vitamin E (d) Vitamin K

19. **The precursor of vitamin D_3 is:**
    (a) 7-Dehydrocholesterol (b) Cholecalciferol (c) Ergosterol (d) Ergocalciferol

20. **A fat-soluble vitamin that can be synthesized in human beings is:**
    (a) Vitamin A (b) Vitamin D (c) Vitamin E (d) Vitamin K

21. **Active form of vitamin D is:**
    (a) 1-Hydroxycholecalciferol (b) 25-Hydroxychole-calciferol (c) 1,25-Dihydroxycholecalciferol (d) None of these

22. **1,25-Dihydroxycholecalciferol induces the synthesis of:**
    (a) Calcium-binding protein (b) Ca^{++}-dependent ATPase (c) Alkaline phosphatase (d) All of these

23. **One international unit of vitamin D is the activity present in:**
    (a) 0.025 μg of cholecalciferol (b) 0.25 μg of cholecalciferol (c) 1 μg of cholecalciferol (d) 2.5 μg of cholecalciferol

24. **The requirement of vitamin D in children is:**
    (a) 100 IU/day (b) 200 IU/day (c) 300 IU/day (d) 400 IU/day

25. **Hypercalcaemia occurs in:**
    (a) Hypervitaminosis D (b) Rickets (c) Osteomalacia (d) None of these

26. **Vitamin E activity is present in:**
    (a) Carotenes (b) Tocopherols (c) Ergosterol (d) None of these

27. **The highest vitamin A activity is present in:**
    (a) α-Tocopherol (b) β-Tocopherol (c) γ-Tocopherol (d) δ-Tocopherol

28. **Anti-oxidant activity present in:**
    (a) Vitamin D (b) Vitamin E (c) Vitamin K (d) None of these

29. **The requirement of vitamin E in adult men is:**
    (a) 5 IU/day (b) 15 IU/day (c) 30 IU/day (d) 100 IU/day

30. **The main function of Vitamin E in human beings is to:**
    (a) Act as an anti-oxidant (b) Prevent sterility (c) Prevent muscular dystrophy (d) Prevent hepatic necrosis

31. **A water-soluble form of vitamin K activity is:**
    (a) Phylloquinone (b) Menaquinone (c) Menadione (d) None of these

32. **Vitamin K is required for:**
    (a) Bone growth (b) Maintenance of epithelial tissues (c) Coagulation of blood (d) Prevention of oxidative damage

33. **Vitamin K is required for carboxylation of:**
    (a) Glutamate residues of pre-prothrombin (b) Glutamine residues of pre-prothrombin (c) Aspartate residues of pre-prothrombin (d) Asparagine residues of pre-prothrombin

34. **Deficiency of vitamin K causes:**
    (a) Prolongation of dark adaptation time (b) Prolongation of prothrombin time (c) Delayed wound healing (d) Oxidative damage

35. **A fat-soluble vitamin that can be synthesized by intestinal bacteria is:**
    (a) Vitamin A (b) Vitamin D (c) Vitamin E (d) Vitamin K

Chapter 23: Minerals

1. **The most abundant mineral in our body is:**
   (a) Sodium (b) Calcium (c) Chloride (d) Potassium

2. **All the following are micronutrients *except*:**
   (a) Iron (b) Magnesium (c) Iodine (d) Manganese

3. **Total calcium concentration in plasma is:**
   (a) 9–11 mg/dl (b) 6–8 mg/dl (c) 4.5–5.5 mg/dl (d) 2–4 mg/dl

4. **Concentration of ionized calcium in plasma is:**
   (a) 9–11 mg/dl (b) 6–8 mg/dl (c) 4.5–5.5 mg/dl (d) 2–4 mg/dl

5. **The following is required for coagulation of blood:**
   (a) Sodium (b) Potassium (c) Magnesium (d) Calcium

6. **When plasma calcium rises above normal, it inhibits:**
   (a) Calcitriol secretion (b) Calcitonin secretion (c) Parathormone secretion (d) None of these

7. **A sudden decrease in plasma calcium can cause:**
   (a) Muscular paralysis (b) Tetany (c) Excessive bleeding (d) Osteoporosis

8. **Daily calcium requirement in adults is:**
   (a) 800 mg (b) 800 mg (c) 4–6 mg (d) 4–6 gm

9. **Normal range of serum inorganic phosphorus in adults is:**
   (a) 60–100 mg/dl (b) 20–45 mg/dl (c) 9–11 mg/dl (d) 2–4.5 mg/dl

10. **Daily phosphorus requirement in adults is:**
    (a) 800 mg (b) 800 mg (c) 4–6 mg (d) 4–6 gm

11. The correct statement about renal rickets is:
(a) It is an inherited disease (b) Its inheritance is X-linked dominant (c) Renal tubular reabsorption of phosphate is decreased in it (d) All of these

12. A high aldosterone level decreases renal tubular absorption of:
(a) Sodium (b) Calcium (c) Phosphate (d) Magnesium

13. Major cation in extracellular fluids is:
(a) Sodium (b) Potassium (c) Calcium (d) Magnesium

14. Major cation in intracellular fluids is:
(a) Sodium (b) Potassium (c) Calcium (d) Magnesium

15. Major anion in extracellular fluids is:
(a) Sulphate (b) Phosphate (c) Chloride (d) Bicarbonate

16. In tropical countries, daily requirement of elemental sodium is:
(a) 10–15 gm (b) 6–9 gm (c) 4–6 gm (d) 2–3 gm

17. Normal range of serum sodium is:
(a) 96–106 mEq/L (b) 136–145 mEq/L (c) 96–106 mg/dl (d) 136–145 mg/dl

18. Normal range of serum potassium is:
(a) 5–10 mEq/L (b) 3.5–5 mEq/L (c) 5–10 mg/dl (d) 3.5–5 mg/dl

19. Normal range of serum chloride is:
(a) 100–106 mEq/L (b) 136–145 mEq/L (c) 100–106 mg/dl (d) 136–145 mg/dl

20. The most abundant trace metal in an adult is:
(a) Iodine (b) Iron (c) Zinc (d) Copper

21. Total amount of iron in an adult is:
(a) 3.5–4.5 mg (b) 3.5–4.5 gm (c) 5–10 mg (d) 5–10 gm

22. About 70% of total body iron is present in:
(a) Haemoglobin (b) Myoglobin (c) Haemosiderin (d) Ferritin

23. Iron is transported in plasma by:
(a) Ferritin (b) Haemosiderin (c) Transferrin (d) Albumin

24. Major storage form of iron is:
(a) Cytochromes (b) Haemosiderin (c) Ferritin (d) Myoglobin

25. Four iron atoms are present in each molecule of:
(a) Transferrin (b) Haemosiderin (c) Haemoglobin (d) Myoglobin

26. One iron atom is present in each molecule of:
(a) Transferrin (b) Haemosiderin (c) Haemoglobin (d) Myoglobin

27. About 5,000 iron atoms are present in each molecule of:
(a) Transferrin (b) Ferritin (c) Haemoglobin (d) Myoglobin

28. A transferrin molecule can bind:
(a) One ferric ion (b) Two ferric ions (c) Four ferric ions (d) Eight ferric ions

29. Total iron binding capacity of plasma is:
(a) 250–400 mg/dl (b) 250–400 mg/dl (c) 50–175 mg/dl (d) 50–175 mg/dl

30. Normal iron concentration in plasma is:
(a) 250–400 µg/dl (b) 250–400 µg/dl (c) 50–175 µg/dl (d) 50–175 µg/dl

31. Daily iron loss in an adult man is about:
(a) 1 mg (b) 2–4 mg (c) 5–8 mg (d) 9–10 mg

32. Daily iron requirement of an adult man is about:
(a) 1 mg (b) 2.5 mg (c) 5 mg (d) 10 mg

33. From a mixed diet, iron absorption is about:
(a) 1–2% (b) 3–4% (c) 5–10% (d) 10–20%

34. Bronzed diabetes:
(a) Is a complication of diabetes mellitus (b) Is a disorder of intestinal absorption of iron (c) Causes microcytic anaemia (d) Leads to iron deposition in reticulo-endo-thelial cells

35. Consumption of iodized salt is recommended to:
(a) Treat hypothyroidism (b) Treat hyperthyroidism (c) Prevent endemic goitre (d) Prevent hypertension

36. Anaemia can occur in deficiency of:
(a) Copper (b) Chromium (c) Manganese (d) Selenium

37. Wilson's disease and Menkes disease have all the following similarities except:
(a) Plasma copper is decreased in both (b) Copper is deposited around cornea in both (c) Both are inherited diseases (d) Copper-binding P-type ATPase is deficient in both

38. Hypogonadism can occur in:
(a) Copper deficiency (b) Zinc deficiency (c) Manganese deficiency (d) Selenium deficiency

39. Acrodermatitis enteropathica can cause:
(a) Chromium deficiency (b) Chromium overload (c) Zinc deficiency (d) Zinc overload

40. The following possesses anti-oxidant activity:
(a) Manganese (b) Molybdenum (c) Chromium (d) Selenium

Chapter 24: Water Balance

1. Out of total body water, the extracellular compartment contains about:
(a) 20% (b) 30% (c) 40% (d) 50%

2. Normal osmolality of plasma is:
(a) 200–225 mOsm/kg (b) 235–250 mOsm/kg (c) 255–270 mOsm/kg (d) 275–290 mOsm/kg

3. Normal oncotic pressure of plasma is:
(a) 25 mg/dl (b) 25 mg Hg (c) 50 mg/dl (d) 50 mg Hg

4. Oncotic pressure of plasma is the pressure exerted by:
(a) Sodium (b) Sodium and chloride (c) Colloids (d) All of these

5. Osmoreceptors are present in:
(a) Capillaries (b) Aortic arch (c) Carotid sinus (d) Hypothalamus

6. V_2 receptors for ADH are present in:
(a) Proximal convoluted tubules (b) Loop of Henle (c) Distal convoluted tubules (d) None of these

7. Diabetes insipidus results from deficient secretion/action of:
(a) Antidiuretic hormone (b) Aldosterone (c) Insulin (d) Glucagon

8. All the following are true about antidiuretic hormone except:
(a) It is secreted by posterior pituitary (b) Its secretion increases when osmolality of plasma rises (c) It increases

obligatory reabsorption of water (d) Its deficiency causes diabetes insipidus

9. **Acetazolamide:**

(a) Is a competitive inhibitor of carbonic anhydrase (b) Acts on distal convoluted tubules (c) Decreases facultative reabsorption of water (d) Can cause alkalosis if used in excess

10. **Spironolactone:**

(a) Is a structural analogue of antidiuretic hormone (b) Binds to V_2 receptors (c) Translocates aquaporins from cytosol to cell membrane (d) Acts as a diuretic

Chapter 25: Acid–base Balance

1. **If hydrogen ion concentration in a fluid is 40 nanomol/litre, its pH would be:**
   (a) 7.2 (b) 7.4 (c) 7.6 (d) 7.8

2. **If the pH of a fluid containing bicarbonate-carbonic acid buffer is 7.4, the ratio of bicarbonate to carbonic acid would be:**
   (a) 20:1 (b) 1:20 (c) 4:1 (d) 1:4

3. **If the pH of a fluid containing phosphate buffer is 7.4, the ratio of monohydrogen phosphate to dihydrogen phosphate would be:**
   (a) 20:1 (b) 1:20 (c) 4:1 (d) 1:4

4. **Of the total buffering capacity of blood, haemoglobin is responsible for:**
   (a) 60% (b) 40% (c) 20% (d) 0%

5. **Respiratory alkalosis results from:**
   (a) Accumulation of carbon dioxide (b) Accumulation of bicarbonate (c) Excessive elimination of carbon dioxide (d) Excessive loss of bicarbonate

6. **Respiratory acidosis results from:**
   (a) Accumulation of carbon dioxide (b) Accumulation of bicarbonate (c) Excessive elimination of carbon dioxide (d) Excessive loss of bicarbonate

7. **Anion gap in plasma is the difference between the concentrations of:**
   (a) [Total cations] – [Total anions] (b) [Sodium] – [Chloride] (c) [Sodium + Potassium] – [Chloride + Bicarbonate] (d) [Chloride] – [Bicarbonate]

8. **Normal anion gap in plasma is about:**
   (a) 15 mEq/L (b) 10 mEq/L (c) 5 mEq/L (d) 0 mEq/L

9. **Anion gap in plasma represents the concentration of:**
   (a) Unmeasured anions (b) Unmeasured cations (c) Anionic proteins (d) None of these

10. **Metabolic alkalosis can occur due to:**
    (a) Severe diarrhoea (b) Severe vomiting (c) Uncontrolled diabetes mellitus (d) Prolonged starvation

Chapter 26: Nutrition and Diet

1. **If a protein is combusted completely outside the body, each gram will give:**
   (a) 4 kcal (b) 5.4 kcal (c) 7 kcal (d) 9 kcal

2. **Calorific value of fats is:**
   (a) 4 kcal (b) 5.4 kcal (c) 7 kcal (d) 9 kcal

3. **Calorific value of carbohydrates is:**
   (a) 4 kcal (b) 5.4 kcal (c) 7 kcal (d) 9 kcal

4. **Calorific value of proteins in living persons is:**
   (a) 4 kcal (b) 5.4 kcal (c) 7 kcal (d) 9 kcal

5. **Respiratory quotient depends upon:**
   (a) Atmospheric pO_2 (b) Rate and depth of respiration (c) Type of fuel being consumed (d) All of these

6. **If carbohydrate is the sole source of energy, respiratory quotient would be:**
   (a) 0.7 (b) 0.8 (c) 0.85 (d) 1.0

7. **If a person is taking a mixed diet containing carbohydrates, fats and proteins, respiratory quotient would be:**
   (a) 0.7 (b) 0.8 (c) 0.85 (d) 1.0

8. **Basal metabolic rate of adult males is about:**
   (a) 30 kcal/hour/square metres (b) 40 kcal/hour/square metres (c) 50 kcal/hour/square metres (d) 60 kcal/hour/square metres

9. **Basal metabolic rate is higher in:**
   (a) Women than in men (b) Adults than in children (c) Vegetarians than in non-vegetarians (d) Pregnant women than in non-pregnant women

10. **Correct increasing order of specific dynamic action of following nutrients is:**
    (a) Proteins, fats, carbohydrates (b) Proteins, carbohydrates, fats (c) Carbohydrates, fats, proteins (d) Fats, proteins, carbohydrates

11. **If 25 gm of protein is consumed by a person, the net gain of energy would be:**
    (a) 70 kcal (b) 100 kcal (c) 130 kcal (d) 225 kcal

12. **If a mixed diet having a calculated energy value of 3,000 kcal is consumed in a day, the net energy gain would be:**
    (a) 3,000 kcal (b) 3,300 kcal (c) 2,700 kcal (d) 2,500 kcal

13. **Lysine is the limiting amino acid in:**
    (a) Milk (b) Cereals (c) Pulses (d) Soya bean

14. **Soya bean has higher protein content than:**
    (a) Wheat (b) Pulses (c) Meat (d) All of these

15. **Protein requirement per kg of body weight is higher in:**
    (a) Children than in adults (b) Adults than in children (c) Adult men than in adult women (d) Adult women than in adult men

16. **Dietary lipids should provide:**
    (a) 10% of total calories (b) 20% of total calories (c) 30% of total calories (d) 40% of total calories

17. **Cholesterol is not present in:**
    (a) Pulses (b) Skimmed milk (c) Cheese (d) Fish

18. **Amino acids present in wheat can supplement the limiting amino acid of:**
    (a) Milk (b) Fish (c) Pulses (d) None of these

19. **Biotin deficiency can occur following consumption of:**
    (a) Raw milk (b) Raw eggs (c) Raw vegetables (d) All of these

20. **Fats have a higher calorific value than:**
    (a) Carbohydrates (b) Proteins (c) Ethanol (d) All of these

Chapter 27: Metabolism of Xenobiotics

1. **Cytochrome P-450 is present in the membrane of:**
   (a) Mitochondria (b) Endoplasmic reticulum (c) Both of these (d) Neither of these

2. **Microsomal hydroxylase system contains all of the following *except*:**
   (a) Cytochrome P-450 (b) FMN (c) FAD (d) NAD

3. **In mitochondria, cytochrome P-450 is a component of:**
   (a) Mitochondrial hydroxylase system (b) Respiratory chain (c) Both of these (d) Neither of these

4. **Some isoforms of cytochrome P-450 may be:**
   (a) Induced (b) Genetically deficient (c) Inhibited by some drugs (d) All of these

5. **All the following families of cytochrome P-450 are involved in metabolism of drugs *except*:**
   (a) CYP 1 (b) CYP 2 (c) CYP 3 (d) CYP 11

6. **Phase 1 reactions for the metabolism of xenobiotics include all of the following *except*:**
   (a) Hydroxylation (b) Oxidation (c) Methylation (d) Hydrolysis

7. **Ethanol is used to treat:**
   (a) Methanol poisoning (b) Ethylene glycol poisoning (c) Salicylic acid poisoning (d) All of these

8. **Ethanol is used to treat methanol poisoning because:**
   (a) A common enzyme system metabolizes these two (b) This enzyme system has greater affinity for ethanol than for methanol (c) Metabolites of methanol are toxic while those of ethanol are not (d) All of these

9. **Xenobiotics may be conjugated with all of the following *except*:**
   (a) Cysteine (b) Glycine (c) Glutathione (d) Glucuronic acid

10. **All the following are true about cytochrome P-450 *except*:**
    (a) It is a haemoprotein (b) There are more than 200 isoforms of cytochrome P-450 (c) It is a component of microsomal and mitochondrial hydroxylase systems (d) It hydroxylates only exogenous compounds

Chapter 28: Tests for Liver, Kidney, Pancreatic and Thyroid Functions

1. **In obstructive jaundice, urine contains:**
   (a) Urobilinogen but not bile pigments (b) Bile pigments but not urobilinogen (c) Urobilinogen and bile pigments (d) Neither bile pigments nor urobilinogen

2. **In haemolytic jaundice, urine contains:**
   (a) Urobilinogen but not bile pigments (b) Bile pigments but not urobilinogen (c) Urobilinogen and bile pigments (d) Neither bile pigments nor urobilinogen

3. **In hepatic jaundice, urine contains:**
   (a) Urobilinogen but not bile pigments (b) Bile pigments but not urobilinogen (c) Urobilinogen and bile pigments (d) Neither bile pigments nor urobilinogen

4. **The following is increased in acute necrosis of liver cells:**
   (a) Serum LDH (b) Serum GPT (c) Serum GOT (d) All of these

5. **Serum alkaline phosphatase is markedly increased in:**
   (a) Haemolytic jaundice (b) Hepatocellular jaundice (c) Obstructive jaundice (d) None of these

6. **All the following occur in obstructive jaundice *except*:**
   (a) Rise in unconjugated bilirubin in serum (b) Presence of bile pigments in urine (c) Presence of bile salts in urine (d) Absence of urobilinogen from urine

7. **All the following occur in haemolytic jaundice *except*:**
   (a) Rise in total bilirubin in serum (b) Rise in unconjugated bilirubin in serum (c) Presence of bile salts in urine (d) Increase in urobilinogen in urine

8. **All the following occur in obstructive jaundice *except*:**
   (a) Rise in conjugated bilirubin in serum (b) Presence of bile pigments in urine (c) Presence of bile salts in urine (d) Increase in urobilinogen in urine

9. **Normal range of serum BUN is:**
   (a) 9–21 mg/dl (b) 9–21 mmol/litre (c) 20–45 mg/dl (d) 20–45 mmol/litre

10. **Creatinine is:**
    (a) A metabolite of creatine (b) Formed in muscles (c) Excreted in urine (d) All of these

11. **Glomerular filtration rate is equal to:**
    (a) Inulin clearance (b) Creatinine clearance (c) Urea clearance (d) p-Amino hippurate clearance

12. **A test of renal tubular function is:**
    (a) Inulin clearance (b) Urea clearance (c) Phenolsulfonphthalein excretion test (d) p-Amino hippurate clearance

13. **Tubular function of kidneys can be evaluated by:**
    (a) Concentration test (b) Dilution test (c) Phenolsulfonphthalein excretion test (d) All of these

14. **Renal plasma flow can be measured by:**
    (a) Inulin clearance (b) Creatinine clearance (c) Urea clearance (d) p-Amino hippurate clearance

15. **Serum amylase is greatly increased in:**
    (a) Acute parotitis (b) Acute pancreatitis (c) Chronic pancreatitis (d) Pancreatic cancer

16. **All the following about cystic fibrosis are true *except*:**
    (a) It is a recessively inherited autosomal disease (b) It affects a number of exocrine glands (c) Sweat chloride is decreased in it (d) It results from mutated CFTR gene

17. **Serum T_3, T_4 and TSH increased in:**
    (a) Hypothyroidism of pituitary origin (b) Hyperthyroidism of pituitary origin (c) Primary hypothyroidism (d) Primary hyperthyroidism

18. **Serum T_3, T_4 and TSH decreased in:**
    (a) Hypothyroidism of pituitary origin (b) Hyperthyroidism of pituitary origin (c) Primary hypothyroidism (d) Primary hyperthyroidism

19. **Serum T_3 and T_4 are decreased and serum TSH increased in:**
    (a) Hypothyroidism of pituitary origin (b) Hyperthyroidism of pituitary origin (c) Primary hypothyroidism (d) Primary hyperthyroidism

20. **Serum T_3 and T_4 are raised and serum TSH decreased in:**
    (a) Hypothyroidism of pituitary origin (b) Hyperthyroidism of pituitary origin (c) Primary hypothyroidism (d) Primary hyperthyroidism

Answers

Chapter 3
| 1 a | 2 b | 3 c | 4 c | 5 d | 6 c | 7 d | 8 a | 9 a | 10 d |

Chapter 4
| 1 c | 2 b | 3 a | 4 c | 5 a | 6 b | 7 d | 8 a | 9 c | 10 d |

Chapter 5
| 1 a | 2 c | 3 c | 4 d | 5 a | 6 b | 7 d | 8 a | 9 c | 10 d |
| 11 b | 12 a | 13 a | 14 a | 15 d | | | | | |

Chapter 6
| 1 a | 2 c | 3 c | 4 d | 5 a | 6 b | 7 d | 8 b | 9 c | 10 a |
| 11 b | 12 d | 13 b | 14 a | 15 d | | | | | |

Chapter 7
1 a	2 c	3 c	4 d	5 a	6 b	7 d	8 b	9 c	10 a
11 b	12 d	13 b	14 a	15 d	16 a	17 d	18 b	19 c	20 d
21 c	22 b	23 b	24 c	25 d					

Chapter 8
| 1 d | 2 d | 3 c | 4 c | 5 b | 6 b | 7 d | 8 c | 9 a | 10 a |

Chapter 9
| 1 c | 2 b | 3 a | 4 d | 5 a | 6 b | 7 c | 8 d | 9 c | 10 b |

Chapter 10
1 b	2 a	3 c	4 d	5 a	6 b	7 c	8 d	9 c	10 d
11 b	12 b	13 b	14 a	15 b	16 a	17 d	18 b	19 d	20 d
21 c	22 c	23 b	24 c	25 d					

Chapter 11
1 b	2 b	3 c	4 c	5 b	6 a	7 c	8 b	9 d	10 a
11 b	12 d	13 c	14 b	15 a	16 b	17 d	18 b	19 d	20 c
21 b	22 d	23 a	24 a	25 a					

Chapter 12
| 1 c | 2 b | 3 a | 4 d | 5 a | 6 a | 7 b | 8 c | 9 d | 10 d |
| 11 c | 12 b | 13 b | 14 a | 15 d | | | | | |

Chapter 13
| 1 c | 2 a | 3 b | 4 d | 5 a | 6 d | 7 a | 8 c | 9 b | 10 b |
| 11 b | 12 d | 13 c | 14 d | 15 c | | | | | |

Chapter 14
| 1 c | 2 b | 3 b | 4 a | 5 a | 6 c | 7 a | 8 c | 9 c | 10 a |
| 11 b | 12 d | 13 b | 14 b | 15 c | | | | | |

Chapter 15
| 1 c | 2 d | 3 d | 4 a | 5 a | 6 d | 7 a | 8 c | 9 d | 10 a |
| 11 b | 12 a | 13 a | 14 b | 15 c | | | | | |

Chapter 16
| 1 d | 2 a | 3 b | 4 c | 5 a | 6 b | 7 d | 8 c | 9 c | 10 b |
| 11 b | 12 c | 13 a | 14 b | 15 d | | | | | |

Chapter 17
1 b	2 a	3 b	4 c	5 a	6 a	7 a	8 d	9 c	10 a
11 c	12 c	13 d	14 b	15 d	16 a	17 d	18 b	19 a	20 c
21 a	22 a	23 d	24 a	25 c					

Chapter 18
| 1 a | 2 a | 3 c | 4 d | 5 c | 6 b | 7 c | 8 b | 9 d | 10 b |
| 11 b | 12 a | 13 d | 14 d | 15 c | | | | | |

Chapter 19
1 a	2 b	3 c	4 b	5 d	6 c	7 b	8 d	9 c	10 c
11 a	12 b	13 c	14 a	15 d	16 d	17 b	18 a	19 d	20 a
21 b	22 d	23 c	24 b	25 b	26 d	27 d	28 a	29 d	30 a
31 c	32 c	33 d	34 b	35 a	36 d	37 c	38 b	39 c	40 b
41 c	42 d	43 c	44 d	45 b					

Chapter 20
| 1 b | 2 a | 3 c | 4 d | 5 b | 6 a | 7 b | 8 d | 9 d | 10 b |
| 11 a | 12 c | 13 d | 14 d | 15 b | 16 a | 17 a | 18 b | 19 c | 20 d |

Chapter 21
1 a	2 b	3 c	4 d	5 b	6 b	7 c	8 c	9 a	10 d
11 a	12 c	13 d	14 d	15 b	16 d	17 b	18 a	19 b	20 B
21 c	22 d	23 d	24 c	25 a	26 b	27 a	28 c	29 b	30 a
31 d	32 a	33 b	34 b	35 a	36 c	37 a	38 b	39 c	40 d

Chapter 22
1 a	2 a	3 a	4 d	5 b	6 c	7 d	8 c	9 b	10 c
11 d	12 c	13 b	14 b	15 a	16 d	17 b	18 b	19 a	20 b
21 c	22 d	23 a	24 d	25 a	26 b	27 a	28 b	29 b	30 a
31 c	32 c	33 a	34 a	35 d					

Chapter 23
1 b	2 b	3 a	4 c	5 d	6 c	7 b	8 a	9 d	10 a
11 d	12 c	13 a	14 b	15 c	16 c	17 b	18 b	19 a	20 b
21 b	22 a	23 c	24 c	25 c	26 d	27 b	28 b	29 a	30 a
31 a	32 d	33 c	34 b	35 c	36 a	37 b	38 b	39 c	40 a

Chapter 24
| 1 b | 2 d | 3 b | 4 c | 5 d | 6 c | 7 a | 8 a | 9 a | 10 d |

Chapter 25
| 1 b | 2 a | 3 c | 4 a | 5 c | 6 a | 7 c | 8 a | 9 a | 10 b |

Chapter 26
| 1 b | 2 d | 3 a | 4 a | 5 c | 6 d | 7 c | 8 b | 9 d | 10 c |
| 11 a | 12 c | 13 b | 14 d | 15 a | 16 b | 17 a | 18 c | 19 b | 20 d |

Chapter 27
| 1 c | 2 d | 3 a | 4 d | 5 d | 6 c | 7 a | 8 d | 9 a | 10 d |

Chapter 28
| 1 b | 2 a | 3 c | 4 d | 5 c | 6 a | 7 c | 8 d | 9 a | 10 d |
| 11 a | 12 c | 13 d | 14 d | 15 b | 16 c | 17 b | 18 a | 19 c | 20 d |